UNDERSTANDING THE ORIGIN AND GLOBAL SPREAD OF COVID-19

UNDERSTANDING THE ORIGIN AND GLOBAL SPREAD OF COVID-19

Editors

Chandra Wickramasinghe
University of Buckingham, UK

Reginald M Gorczynski
University of Toronto, Canada

Edward J Steele
Melville Analytics Pty Ltd, Melbourne, Australia

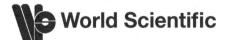

World Scientific

NEW JERSEY · LONDON · SINGAPORE · BEIJING · SHANGHAI · HONG KONG · TAIPEI · CHENNAI · TOKYO

Published by

World Scientific Publishing Co. Pte. Ltd.

5 Toh Tuck Link, Singapore 596224

USA office: 27 Warren Street, Suite 401-402, Hackensack, NJ 07601

UK office: 57 Shelton Street, Covent Garden, London WC2H 9HE

British Library Cataloguing-in-Publication Data

A catalogue record for this book is available from the British Library.

UNDERSTANDING THE ORIGIN AND GLOBAL SPREAD OF COVID-19

ISBN 978-981-125-907-4 (hardcover)
ISBN 978-981-125-908-1 (ebook for institutions)
ISBN 978-981-125-909-8 (ebook for individuals)

For any available supplementary material, please visit
https://www.worldscientific.com/worldscibooks/10.1142/12911#t=suppl

Printed in Singapore

On The Fragility of Empires and Paradigms

N Chandra Wickramasinghe[1,2,3,4*], Edward J Steele[2,9], Reginald M Gorczynski[6], Robert Temple[7], Gensuke Tokoro[4], Daryl H. Wallis[4] and Brig Klyce[8]

[1]Buckingham Centre for Astrobiology, University of Buckingham, MK18 1EG, England, UK

[2]Centre for Astrobiology, University of Ruhuna, Matara, Sri Lanka

[3]National Institute of Fundamental Studies, Kandy, Sri Lanka

[4]Institute for the Study of Panspermia and Astroeconomics, Gifu, Japan

[5]C Y O'Connor, ERADE Village, Foundation, Piara Waters,Perth 6112 WA, Australia

[6]University Toronto Health Network, Toronto General Hospital, University of Toronto, Canada

[7]History of Chinese Science and Culture Foundation, Conway Hall, London, UK

[8]Astrobiology Research Trust, Memphis, TN, USA

Letter to the Editor

In the perspective of deep time we can see that empires do not last indefinitely; nor indeed do scientific paradigms. The rise and fall of empires have punctuated human history throughout the ages. The collapse of an empire often comes suddenly and follows on the heels of major catastrophes such as wars and pestilences. Scientific paradigms are similarly fragile and can be overturned by a few transformative discoveries, as for instance happened in the case of the geocentric world view with the observations of Galileo Galilei. The two historical processes can be seen to be related in a fundamental way.

The way in which scientific paradigms are successively overturned has been meticulously described in the famous book by Thomas S. Kuhn [1]. All historians of science today are familiar with this seminal work by Kuhn, which provided insights which have guided our thoughts on this subject since the sixties. As for the decay and collapse of empires, ever since Edward Gibbon (The History of the Decline and Fall of the Roman Empire, London, 1832), those processes, apparently all following the same series of steps, have haunted the minds of all serious historians and are ever present in the anxieties of forecasters. Fortunately, these processes, although often ignored or put out of mind, have been absolutely clear to all thinking people for some time. Most of us alive today witnessed the sudden fall of the Soviet Empire, which we all thought, were so strong, and we saw it collapse like a house of cards in a short time. The most impressive empires and the most passionately held scientific theories (remember that until the 1950s 'outer space' was firmly believed by all to be 'empty'?) can vanish in moments when reality meets them head on.

We believe that a horrific global catastrophe in relation to the COVID-19 pandemic looms large if urgent action is not taken so as to honestly understand its true cause. Pronouncements given from the highest pulpits are worth nothing if they are not based on facts. Based on unpublished work by EJS it has recently been argued that the premise [2]. If that assumption is threatened all that rests upon it is open to question

If we remain content to adhere to obsolete paradigms and thereby arrive at wrong conclusions we face the risk of replacing one human tragedy with another on a more horrific scale – an economic disaster that could threaten to destroy the cohesion of modern society and wreak untold misery on hundreds of millions of people worldwide. We have discussed some of these issues in a series of recent articles [2-4]. It is of the utmost importance and urgency to lay aside false ideologies and to look at the body of emerging evidence dispassionately and without prejudice. It is only then that we would gain even a glimmer of hope to understand the facts and thus forge a way that may eventually lead to a lasting solution.

The societal reluctance to come to grips with the present disaster is, in our view, due to a deep-rooted reluctance to accept a body of evidence that points inexorably to a connection between terrestrial life and a wider cosmic biosphere. If we look at all the evidence dispassionately, the proposition that COVID-19 could have a cosmic connection is no longer seen as bizarre. This would be the first step towards constructively coping with COVID-19 whilst also helping to plan for the avoidance of similar disasters in the future. Such plans could take the form of regularly monitoring the stratosphere for incoming microorganisms that we have suggested earlier [5]. We noted that collections of stratospheric material have consistently revealed the presence of bacteria, including new bacterial species, at

*Corresponding author: Dr N Chandra Wickramasinghe, Buckingham Centre for Astrobiology, University of Buckingham MK18 1EG, England, UK, Tel: +44 (0)2920752146/+44 (0)7778389243; E-mail: ncwick@gmail.com

Received: March 18, 2020; Accepted: April 08, 2020; Published: April 15, 2020

DOI: 10.37421/vcrh.2020.4.112

Wickramasinghe NC, et al.

Virol Curr Res, Volume 4: 1, 2020

the height of 41 km [5-7]; and the presence of bacteria on the exterior of the International Space Station at 400 km has also been reported [8]. Because the descent through the atmosphere of viral and bacterial-sized particles from heights above 40 km could take several months, the desirability of monitoring the stratosphere is amply clear. Aircraft, balloons and rockets could be deployed for this purpose along with next generation gene sampling technologies to give us advanced warning of future pandemic-causing pathogens before they fall to Earth [9].

References

1. Thomas, S Kuhn. "The Structure of Scientific Revolutions, University of Chicago Press reprinted many times." since then (1962).

2. Lindley, RA and Steele EJ. "ADAR and APOBEC editing signatures in viral RNA during acute- phase Innate Immune responses of the host-parasite relationship to Flaviviruses." Research Reports 2 (2018):e1- e22.

3. Wickramasinghe, NC, Steele EJ, Gorczynski RM and Temple R. "Comments on the Origin and Spread of the 2019 Coronavirus." VirolCurr Res 4 (2020):1.

4. Wickramasinghe, NC, Steele EJ, Gorczynski RM and Temple R. "Growing Evidence against Global Infection-Driven by Person-to-Person Transfer of COVID-19." VirolCurr Res (2020) Vol.4 (2020):1.

5. Wickramasinghe, NC, Steele EJ, Gorczynski RM and Temple R, et al. "Predicting the Future Trajectory of COVID-19." VirolCurr Res (2020) 4:1.

6. Harris, MJ, Wickramasinghe NC and Loyd DL. "Detection of living cells in stratospheric samples." Proceedings of SPIE (2002) 4495:192-198.

7. Shivaji, S, Chaturvedi P and Suresh K. "Bacillus aerius sp. nov., Bacillus aerophilus sp. nov., Bacillus stratosphericus sp. nov. and Bacillus altitudinis sp. nov., isolated from cryogenic tubes used for collecting air samples from high altitudes." Int J Syst Evol Microbiol (2006) 56(2006):7.

8. Shivaji, S, Chaturvedi P and Begum Z. "Janibacter hoylei sp. nov., Bacillus isronensis sp. nov. and Bacillus aryabhattai sp. nov., isolated from cryotubes used for collecting air from the upper atmosphere." Int J Syst Evol Microbiol 59(2009): 12.

9. Grebennikova, TV, Syroeshkin AV and Shubralova EV. "The DNA of Bacteria of the World Ocean and the Earth in Cosmic Dust at the International Space Station." Scientific World Journal (2018) 7360147.

How to cite this article: N Chandra Wickramasinghe, Gensuke Tokoro, Robert Temple and Daryl H Wallis et al. "On The Fragility of Empires and Paradigm". *Virol Curr Res* 4 (2020) doi:10.37421/Virol Curr Res.2020.4.112

Correction Note to Published Version

Author Affiliation: Edward J Steele[2,9] should read as Edward J Steele[2,5]

Text Error: Incorrect text at the end of the third paragraph, so it should read as follows: "Based on unpublished work by EJS it has recently been argued that the premise that the virus came from animals rests on the shakiest imaginable ground, a questionable premise and circular logic based on that premise [2]. If that assumption is threatened all that rests upon it is open to question. Also now read Chapter 12 this volume."

Citation Errors: Incorrect citation numbers in the fifth sentence of the last paragraph. The correct reference numbers are "the height of 41 km [5–8]; and the presence of bacteria on the exterior of the International Space Station at 400 km has also been reported [9]."

Contents

SECTION 1

Introduction

This book is for sober reflection when the SARS-CoV-2 (COVID-19) pandemic has finally passed into history. The book is a compendium — a curation — of our published scientific papers just prior (2018, 2019) to the sudden origin and emergence of COVID-19 and its further global spread (2019–2022).

All of us have spent the best part of two years continuously monitoring and providing plausible explanations, albeit often contested, of unfolding events of the pandemic from its putative meteorite origins in the stratosphere over Jilin NE China on the night of October 11, 2019, to the last twists and turns of the Omicron variant in early 2022. The explanations we provide are diametrically at odds with all other mainstream views that have been published in both the scientific media and the popular press over the past two years. Our explanations range from the first region-wide set of large numbers (in the millions?) of sudden "mystery" infections throughout China from late November through early December 2019 to January 2020; to the haplotype switching adaptive-genetics of the virus as it navigated different human hosts first in China, then to Europe, the USA and the rest of the world including Australia (Jan 2020–Aug 2020); to the innate and adaptive immune mechanisms arising from the host-parasite interaction; to the putative protective efficiency and adverse events of the vaccine roll out from Dec 2020; to COVID-19's global spread and transport within putative dust-associated viral clouds by prevailing wind systems; to the downstream role of tropospheric plumes of human passaged (and often attenuated) viral-laden clouds.

Towards the end of the pandemic (from mid Dec 2021) we noted a clear association of the increased vulnerability of the Earth to tropospheric in-falls of COVID-19 (Omicron/Delta mix?) and, we predict, likely other pathogen-clouds with the minima of the Solar Sun Spot Cycle (through which we are now passing between solar cycles 24 and 25). The role of this putative "Space Weather" association external to the Earth is not understood in detail but is discussed in Chapter 19.

Since 2018, we have published a series of papers of data analysis and overviews in both the peer-reviewed journals (released as Open Access) and in accelerated Open Access non-peer review journals. The central theme depends on the arrival of living systems from space, a process known as Panspermia; cryopreserved viruses, micro-organisms and their spores, and even on rare occasions perhaps more complex cellular organisms, their seeds and fertilized eggs. This corpus of work (Chapters 2 and 3) summarises the prior astrobiology data published in a long series of books and papers over the past decades (1970s–2001) by Professors Sir Fred Hoyle and N. Chandra Wickramasinghe, and then continued by Professor N. Chandra Wickramasinghe and his associates to the present day, as manifest in this compendium.

This book is then for scientific posterity and provides lessons on how suddenly emergent pandemics in the future should be understood and best handled by scientific, medical, epidemiological and government authorities.

When the COVID-19 pandemic emerged overtly and suddenly throughout China, not just in Wuhan and regions, in late December 2019 and through January 2020 we were therefore in a unique position. This allowed us to analyse the emerging observations and data in the public domain and to explain the various phases of the unfolding pandemic.

So this book collects together, in one place, all of our recent key papers both just prior to COVID-19 (Prelude, Chapters 2 and 3) as well as our regular analytical reports through to January–February 2022. Our understanding is based on the *unfolding data and observations sequentially over time*. The data patterns we interpret are consistent with a unique strike from space in the stratosphere of a life-bearing cometary bolide over Jilin NE China on the 40° N latitude line on the night of October 11, 2019 (Chapters 4–6). The evidence we marshal to support this claim is multifactorial: geophysical location and timing and viral genomics (Chapters 4–6, 11 and 12); immuno-logic (type of immunity levels in SARS-CoV-2 victims) including vaccine appraisal (Chapters 11, 13 and 18); epidemiologic analysis of mystery cases first in China (e.g. Chapters 6 and 18) then particularly in Australia (Chapter 15); the sudden epidemic strikes on ships at sea, on islands and remote regions (Chapters 9, 10 and 12); how new variants become dominant and plumed in dust clouds into the troposphere (Chapters 13–15) and the transport therefrom to distant global regions by application of familiar knowledge of known global prevailing wind systems, both in the lower troposphere and higher stratosphere (Chapters 14 and 15). Many key issues include countering several popular myths on the origins of the virus either as sudden jumps from animal reservoirs or human-engineered coronavirus variants ("Wuhan Lab leak" explanations) are comprehensively dealt with in Chapters 12 and 18. The lack of evidence for the "jab in the arm" vaccine roll out bringing the pandemic to an end is discussed in Chapter 16 and the evidence discussed for the poor protective efficacy of the vaccines analysed in Chapters 13, 17–19 and 21.

We do not claim to know or understand *every piece* of evidence — that many other groups are no doubt collecting — but we do believe we have focused on the *key relevant* data and observations necessary to understand the discrete cometary origin of COVID-19 and its subsequent global spread via prevailing wind systems. All our papers address these central issues. In the later phases of the pandemic (late 2020 into 2021), the evidence points to a clear contribution of aerosol rising plumes of human passaged virions from localized regions such as the Indian, UK, Brazil, South African epidemics, rather than the cometary meteorite dust form of the virus that appeared to dominate in the first six months (first over China and other European and North American countries on the 40° N latitude band, then to the Southern Hemisphere to South America and South Africa via Atlantic prevailing winds, Chapters 14 and 15.

The analyses of full-length genomic data on COVID-19 isolated in the first six months of 2020 contributes to the genetic understanding of the viral adaptation process in different human populations (China, Spain, USA, New York in particular) and especially also in Victoria, Australia (in both 2020 and 2021 epidemics) — Chapters 11–13. The high incidence of genuine mystery cases in Australia is best understood as viral laden dust clouds contaminating the environment in defined regions thereby igniting community transmissions without a known patient X. In these regions it has caused COVID-19 infections in hapless victims who cannot understand how they have been infected (who they got it from) if person-to-person spread was the main and only mode of viral transmission (Chapters 13 and 16). All the evidence we outline for explosive epidemics fits the infection model just outlined: the virus is airborne in its primary mode of global spread whether as raw virus associated with meteorite dust particles, or plumed human-passaged variants distributed as clusters in similar dust particles. Person-to-person spreads certainly do occur but these have been of secondary importance in understanding the epidemiology of sudden explosive outbreaks in different regions (e.g. see Chapters 18 and 19 in particular).

Just prior to COVID-19 in 2018 then late in 2019, we published two very large critical reviews of the state of play of all the evidence consistent with Panspermia, gathered largely by Sir Fred Hoyle and Professor N. Chandra Wickramasinghe and their many colleagues over the previous 45 years (H–W). We first dealt with the perennial evolutionary conundrum — from a strict and conventional neo-Darwinian perspective — of *what exactly caused* the Cambrian explosion of emergent complex animal and plant life on Earth about 550 million years ago? This was then followed by adding a distinct biomedical focus to the emerging H-W astrobiology paradigm — namely by the addition of Lamarckian evolutionary concepts, an imperative in our view to the understanding of the putative rapid spread of living systems across the cosmos (Chapter 3):

> *"For example, a viable, or cryo-preserved, living system travelling through space in a protective matrix will need of necessity to **rapidly adapt and proliferate** on landing in a new cosmic niche. Lamarckian mechanisms thus come to the fore and supersede the slow (blind and random) genetic processes expected under a traditional neo-Darwinian evolutionary paradigm."*

A cosmos which is clearly teeming with life becomes acutely apparent during Pandemics such as COVID-19.

SECTION 2

Prelude to COVID-19

Contents lists available at ScienceDirect

Progress in Biophysics and Molecular Biology

journal homepage: www.elsevier.com/locate/pbiomolbio

Cause of Cambrian Explosion - Terrestrial or Cosmic?

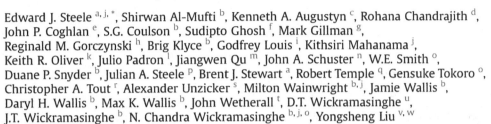

Edward J. Steele [a, j, *], Shirwan Al-Mufti [b], Kenneth A. Augustyn [c], Rohana Chandrajith [d], John P. Coghlan [e], S.G. Coulson [b], Sudipto Ghosh [f], Mark Gillman [g], Reginald M. Gorczynski [h], Brig Klyce [b], Godfrey Louis [i], Kithsiri Mahanama [j], Keith R. Oliver [k], Julio Padron [l], Jiangwen Qu [m], John A. Schuster [n], W.E. Smith [o], Duane P. Snyder [b], Julian A. Steele [p], Brent J. Stewart [a], Robert Temple [q], Gensuke Tokoro [o], Christopher A. Tout [r], Alexander Unzicker [s], Milton Wainwright [b, j], Jamie Wallis [b], Daryl H. Wallis [b], Max K. Wallis [b], John Wetherall [t], D.T. Wickramasinghe [u], J.T. Wickramasinghe [b], N. Chandra Wickramasinghe [b, j, o], Yongsheng Liu [v, w]

[a] CY O'Connor ERADE Village Foundation, Piara Waters, WA, Australia
[b] Buckingham Centre for Astrobiology, University of Buckingham, UK
[c] Center for the Physics of Living Organisms, Department of Physics, Michigan Technological University, Michigan, United States
[d] Department of Geology, University of Peradeniya, Peradeniya, Sri Lanka
[e] University of Melbourne, Office of the Dean, Faculty Medicine, Dentistry and Health Sciences, 3rd Level, Alan Gilbert Building, Australia
[f] Metallurgical & Materials Engineering IIT, Kanpur, India
[g] South African Brain Research Institute, 6 Campbell Street, Waverly, Johannesburg, South Africa
[h] University Toronto Health Network, Toronto General Hospital, University of Toronto, Canada
[i] Department of Physics, Cochin University of Science and Technology Cochin, India
[j] Centre for Astrobiology, University of Ruhuna, Matara, Sri Lanka
[k] School of Veterinary and Life Sciences Murdoch University, Perth, WA, Australia
[l] Studio Eutropi, Clinical Pathology and Nutrition, Via Pompei 46, Ardea, 00040, Rome, Italy
[m] Department of Infectious Disease Control, Tianjin Center for Disease Control and Prevention, China
[n] School of History and Philosophy of Science, Faculty of Science, University of Sydney, Sydney, Australia
[o] Institute for the Study of Panspermia and Astrobiology, Gifu, Japan
[p] Centre for Surface Chemistry and Catalysis, KU Leuven, Celestijnenlaan 200F, 3001, Leuven, Belgium
[q] The History of Chinese Culture Foundation, Conway Hall, London, UK
[r] Institute of Astronomy, The Observatories, Madingley Road, Cambridge, CB3 0HA, UK
[s] Pestalozzi- Gymnasium, 11, D-81247, München, Germany
[t] School of Biomedical Sciences, Perth, Curtin University, WA, Australia
[u] College of Physical and Mathematical Sciences, Australian National University, Canberra, Australia
[v] Henan Collaborative Innovation Center of Modern Biological Breeding, Henan Institute of Science and Technology, Xinxiang, 453003, China
[w] Department of Biochemistry, University of Alberta, Edmonton, AB T6G 2H7, Canada

ARTICLE INFO

Article history:
Available online 13 March 2018

Keywords:
Cosmic biology
Cambrian Explosion
Retroviruses
Panspermia
Hypermutation & evolution
Origin epidemics & pandemics

ABSTRACT

We review the salient evidence consistent with or predicted by the Hoyle-Wickramasinghe (H-W) thesis of Cometary (Cosmic) Biology. Much of this physical and biological evidence is multifactorial. One particular focus are the recent studies which date the emergence of the complex retroviruses of vertebrate lines at or just before the Cambrian Explosion of ~500 Ma. Such viruses are known to be plausibly associated with major evolutionary genomic processes. We believe this coincidence is not fortuitous but is consistent with a key prediction of H-W theory whereby major extinction-diversification evolutionary boundaries coincide with virus-bearing cometary-bolide bombardment events. A second focus is the remarkable evolution of intelligent complexity (Cephalopods) culminating in the emergence of the Octopus. A third focus concerns the micro-organism fossil evidence contained within meteorites as well as the detection in the upper atmosphere of apparent incoming life-bearing particles from space. In our view the totality of the multifactorial data and critical analyses assembled by Fred Hoyle, Chandra Wickramasinghe and their many colleagues since the 1960s leads to a very plausible conclusion — life

* Corresponding author. CY O'Connor ERADE Village Foundation, Piara Waters, WA, Australia.
E-mail address: ejsteele@cyo.edu.au (E.J. Steele).

https://doi.org/10.1016/j.pbiomolbio.2018.03.004

4   *E.J. Steele et al. / Progress in Biophysics and Molecular Biology 136 (2018) 3—23*

may have been seeded here on Earth by life-bearing comets as soon as conditions on Earth allowed it to flourish (about or just before 4.1 Billion years ago); and living organisms such as space-resistant and space-hardy bacteria, viruses, more complex eukaryotic cells, fertilised ova and seeds have been continuously delivered ever since to Earth so being one important driver of further terrestrial evolution which has resulted in considerable genetic diversity and which has led to the emergence of mankind.

Contents

" **The historian of science may be tempted to claim that when paradigms change, the world itself changes with them.**" *The Structure of Scientific Revolutions* (Thomas S Kuhn, 1962, 2nd ed. 1970)

When presented with the uncanny survival attributes of Tardigrades, a friend exclaimed: " **How on earth did they evolve?**" (*Anon.* 2017)

" The idea that in the whole universe life is unique to the Earth is essentially pre-Copernican. Experience has now repeatedly taught us that this type of thinking is very likely wrong. Why should our own infinitesimal niche in the universe be unique? Just as no one country has been the centre of the Earth, so the Earth is not the centre of the universe." *Life Cloud* (Fred Hoyle and N Chandra Wickramasinghe, 1978 J.M. Dent & Sons, London, p.132).

1. Purpose of article

This review article is intended to represent, in the main, the collective knowledge and wisdom of over 30 scientists and scholars across many disciplines of the Physical and Biological sciences. We review much of the key experimental and observational data gathered over the past 60 years consistent with or predicted by the Hoyle-Wickramasinghe (H-W) thesis of Cometary (Cosmic) Biology.

We are acutely aware that mainstream thinking on the origin and further evolution of life on Earth is anchored firmly in the "Terrestrial" paradigm. Our aim here is to facilitate further discussion in the biophysical, biomedical and evolutionary science communities to the quite different H-W "Cosmic" origins viewpoint which better handles, in our opinion, a wider range of physical, astrophysical, biological and biophysical facts often quite inexplicable, if not contradictory, under the dominant Terrestrial neo-Darwinian paradigm. Further, if some readers are hoping to read a disquisition based on Population Genetics-type analyses, as one reviewer has put it, " … analyses of evolutionary rates, examples of appearance of new genes with no homology to old ones, etc" they will mostly be disappointed; although some genetic features from recent data in the Octopus and other Cephalopods provide challenging examples to conventional evolutionary thinking. But that is not the main thrust of this review.

The general, and admittedly unusual, scientific writing style is to ensure clear plain-English communications across many scientific disciplines. However of iconic specific interest, we discuss the recent phylogenetic data which date the emergence of the complex retroviruses of vertebrate lines at or just before the Cambrian Explosion of ~500 Ma (the widely agreed epochal event in the evolutionary history of multicellular life on Earth). These types of reverse transcribing and genome integrating viruses are speculated to be plausibly associated with major evolutionary genomic processes. We believe this coincidence with the Cambrian Explosion

E.J. Steele et al. / Progress in Biophysics and Molecular Biology 136 (2018) 3–23   5

may not be fortuitous but consistent with a key prediction of H-W theory whereby major extinction-diversification evolutionary boundaries coincide with cometary-bolide bombardment events delivering hypothesized viruses, microorganism, and more complex eukaryotic systems to Earth during the past 4.5 Billion years of Earth history. Not all of such incoming living systems would necessarily take hold, and substantial terrestrial based evolutionary processes (whatever the actual molecular genetic mechanisms) are also expected to be on going.

In our considered view the totality of the multifactorial data and critical analyses assembled by Fred Hoyle, Chandra Wickramasinghe and their many colleagues leads to the bare minimum yet plausible scientific conclusion — that life was seeded here on Earth by life-bearing comets as soon as conditions on Earth allowed it to flourish (at or just before 4.1 Billion years ago); and living organisms such as space-resistant and space-hardy bacteria, viruses, more complex eukaryotic cells and organisms (e.g. Tardigrades), perhaps even fertilised ova and plant seeds, may have been continuously delivered ever since to Earth helping to drive further the progress of terrestrial biological evolution. This process, since the time of Lord Kelvin (1871) and Svante Arrhenius (1908) has the scientific name "Panspermia".

Perhaps the most important astronomical data relevant to the theory of cosmic life to emerge in the past decade are the detections of habitable exoplanets — planets outside of our solar system. The total estimated tally of such Earth-like planets in our Milky Way galaxy alone now stands at 100 billion, and with 100 billion or so galaxies in the observable universe the grand total stands at 10^{22}. Because exchanges of possibly fecund material between neighbouring habitats is more than likely, panspermia and the theory of cosmic life could be argued to become inevitable facts.

The paradigm shift to this critical viewpoint, whilst underway, is by no means complete - yet we believe the historical moment has now arrived for a comprehensive and considered cross-disciplinary review of much of the relevant evidence, which this paper endeavours to represent. There are many and far reaching consequences of this new scientific awareness which we believe would be the privilege of future generations to explore.

2. Introductory remarks

The Aristotlean paradigm of the spontaneous generation of life — the idea that the simplest life-forms emerged spontaneously on Earth (fireflies from mixtures of warm earth and morning dew) - has survived in one form or other for over 2000 years. It has withstood contradictory evidence on several occasions during this time. Pasteur's 1862 experiments on the fermentation of wine and the souring of milk led him to enunciate the dictum "*Omne vivum ex vivo*" or "All life comes from life". The implication of the Pasteur experiment was that every generation of every microbe, plant or animal was preceded by a generation of the same organism. This view was endorsed enthusiastically by others particularly by physicists, prominent amongst whom John Tyndall, who on 21 January 1870 lectured at the Royal Institution in London on the implications for panspermia. It is interesting and noteworthy that the newly established magazine *Nature* objected to this lecture in its Editorial columns with some passion. Behind the objection was the realisation that were Pasteur's dictum to be strictly true then the origin of life would need to be external to the Earth. The continuing antagonism to the panspermic implications of Pasteur's dictum led the way to the emergence of the dominant biological paradigm - abiogenesis in a primordial soup. The latter idea was developed at a time when the earliest living cells were considered to be exceedingly simple structures that could subsequently evolve in a Darwinian way. These ideas should of course have been

critically examined and rejected after the discovery of the exceedingly complex molecular structures involved in proteins and in DNA. But this did not happen. Modern ideas of abiogenesis in hydrothermal vents or elsewhere on the primitive Earth have developed into sophisticated conjectures with little or no evidential support.

Even if we concede that the dominant neo-Darwinian paradigm of natural selection can explain aspects of the evolutionary history of life once life gets started, independent abiogenesis on the cosmologically diminutive scale of oceans, lakes or hydrothermal vents remains a hypothesis with no empirical support and is moreover unnecessary and redundant. With astronomical data now pointing to the existence of hundreds of billions of habitable planets in our galaxy alone (Abe et al., 2013; Kopparapu, 2013) such an hypothesis seeking an independent origin of life on any single planet seems to be no longer hardly necessary.

The recent report indicating evidence of microbial life in Canadian rocks that formed 4.1—4.23 billion years ago (Dodd et al., 2017), if accepted, makes it more difficult in our view to envisage the option of abiogenesis taking place anywhere on the Earth. The claim that these rocks may have been associated with hydrothermal vents still raises the question of how life could have originated *in situ* during the early Hadean epoch that was riddled with frequent and violent collisions by asteroids and comets. Rather we think it more reasonable to suggest that the particular evidence of microbial life in the Canadian rocks was delivered by cometary bolides, only to be instantly destroyed or carbonised on impact.

The conditions that would most likely have prevailed near the impact-riddled Earth's surface 4.1—4.23 billion years ago were too hot even for simple organic molecules to survive let alone evolve into living complexity. This leaves panspermia as the most plausible valid option for the origin of terrestrial life; the first microbes were most likely delivered to the planet along with impacting comets and meteorites. This study, together with that of Bell and associates (2015) dating zircons in the Jack Hills of Western Australia to a similar time point, constitute the most recent discoveries that lead naturally into the data-based ideas that we discuss at length in this review.

From the turn of the 20th century the resistance to panspermia had become ever more deeply entrenched in our scientific culture. Attempts by Hoyle and Wickramasinghe (Hoyle and Wickramasinghe, 1979, 1981, 1986, 1993; Wickramasinghe, 2015a,b) to re-examine and re-instate panspermia in the light of new evidence from astronomy and biology were often met with hostility (Hoyle and Wickramasinghe, 1986; Wickramasinghe, 2015a).

A similar fate often befell attempts to re-instate certain crucial aspects of Lamarckism - the pre-Darwinian notion that the genes in our genome can be enriched in a 'directional' fashion through the inheritance of adaptive, environmentally-driven, acquired characteristics (Steele, 1979; Steele et al., 1998; Jablonka and Lamb, 1995, 2005; Lindley, 2010). This latter inheritance mechanism can be more precisely described as soma-to-germline feedback penetration of a semi-permeable (not absolute) *Weisman's Barrier*, a concept fashioned in the 19th Century at about the time of Darwin's death. There is now considerable evidence (Steele et al., 1998; Lindley, 2010; Steele and Lloyd, 2015; Steele, 2016a) consistent with the original 'somatic selection hypothesis' (proposed by one of us (EJS) in the late 1970s) which is hypothesized to operate via the agency of endogenous retroviral gene vectors and reverse transcriptase (Steele, 1979). Indeed there is much contemporary discussion, observations and critical analysis consistent with this position led by Corrado Spadafora, Yongsheng Liu, Denis Noble, John Mattick and others, that developments such as Lamarckian Inheritance processes (both direct DNA modifications and indirect,

6   *E.J. Steele et al. / Progress in Biophysics and Molecular Biology 136 (2018) 3–23*

viz. epigenetic, transmissions) in evolutionary biology and adjacent fields now necessitate a complete revision of the standard neo-Darwinian theory of evolution or "New Synthesis " that emerged from the 1930s and 1940s (https://royalsociety.org/science-events-and-lectures/2016/11/evolutionary-biology/, Spadafora, 2008; Liu, 2007; Noble, 2011,2013; Noble et al., 2016; https://royalsociety.org/science-events-and-lectures/2016/11/evolutionary-biology/; Mattick, 2012; Liu and Li, 2016a,2016b). This call was indeed also made by two of the present co-authors (EJS, NCW) many years ago based on the then available data and the plethora of inherent contradictions in the extant data (Hoyle and Wickramasinghe, 1979,1981, 1982; Steele, 1979).

We certainly do not want this paper to read, as one reviewer has put it ...

" somewhat like a last-ditch and exasperated attempt to convince the main stream of the scientific community that in following neo-Darwinism they have gone seriously astray, because life has been carried to this planet from elsewhere in the universe on comets/meteorites and does not result from abiogenesis on Earth." We actually consider that certain mechanistic aspects of neo-Darwinian and Population Genetic thinking is invaluable in biomedical research and clinical medicine (development of the "big data" algorithms that allow "personalised" navigation around the genetic features of thousands of human genomes by, for example, the Broad Institute in Boston and the Welcome Trust Sanger Institute in Cambridge). However these basic Darwinian based-concepts need to be circumscribed, in our opinion, and be placed in a Cosmic rather than a solely Terrestrial setting. In our view then both Panspermia and Lamarckian issues therefore contribute to our wider understanding as they go to the very heart of how life originated on Earth and how it subsequently evolved and diversified to the higher levels of sophisticated complexity that we witness today. In our view "Natural Selection" in its essence (survival of fittest) still plays a crucial role in a changing environment but it is now in a Cosmic, rather than a pure Terrestrial, setting; and it occurs in concert with both non-Darwinian and non-Mendelian inheritance mechanisms. Yet we recognize that the whole topic of 'evolutionary mechanisms' is, like political beliefs, both fraught and is a heated area of social and cultural discourse - certainly in all those areas lying outside of normal scientific investigation. Yet the simple fact that cannot be denied is that the terrestrial biosphere is an infinitesimal part of the far, far bigger system which is the astronomer's cosmos and the two systems are inextricably connected.

This then is a trigger warning: Accurate scientific terminology can be unsettling because of their history, yet sometimes unavoidable - the terms *Panspermia* and *Lamarckian Inheritance* despite their emotive implications and prejudicial overtones will be used where deemed appropriate in this paper.

Our additional epistemological argument for reviving these admittedly controversial issues here is this: Wrong theories are simply *not fecund*. Correct theories however *always lead* in logical ways to successive confirmatory instances and predict the discovery of novel phenomena in the real world - that is, they do not self-refute themselves by severe experimental and observational tests beyond their immediate explanatory domain. It is therefore in this spirit that we also discuss in the present paper, the exciting new virological evidence recently published in *Nature Communications* by Aiewsakun and Katzourakis (2017) which confirms an important prediction of the Hoyle-Wickramasinghe (H-W) theory of Cosmic Biology for the causes of the greatest epochal evolutionary event on Earth - the Cambrian Explosion of multicellular life a half billion years ago.

However, before we move into that detail, we set the scene for a better understanding of the Aiewsakun-Katzourakis discovery by discussing the salient experimental and observational data behind

the H-W concept of an all pervasive Cosmic Biology impacting continuously on Earth and other general evolutionary issues and about virus particles and their general properties.

3. Cosmic theory of life

In the mid-1970's the idea of prebiotic molecules existing in interstellar space or in comets was initially not part of mainstream of scientific opinion. The original proposal by one of us (NCW) for organic polymers in interstellar space in 1974 (Wickramasinghe, 1974) was followed by a long series of articles in collaboration with Fred Hoyle confronting head-on the reigning scientific paradigm of an origin of life on the Earth — the so-called Haldane-Oparin primordial soup theory (Hoyle and Wickramasinghe, 1976, 1977a, 1977b, 1978a, 1978b). After discussing a variety of possible interstellar and circumstellar settings for the beginnings of biochemistry (prebiotic evolution), Hoyle and Wickramasinghe (1978b) turned to the ensemble of the estimated 10^{11} comets in our solar system alone as the favoured setting for the origin of life on Earth (Hoyle and Wickramasinghe, 1985, 1986). The anticipated radioactively heated interiors of these icy bodies containing liquid water domains (see below) replete with interstellar organics were argued to be enormously more favorable for an origin of life than anything that can be accomplished on the Earth.

4. Condition of liquid water

The existence of liquid water is a prerequisite not only for the origin of life but for active microbiology as well. This requirement has come to the fore and been much publicised with the recent conclusion of NASA's Cassini mission. When Fred Hoyle and one of us (NCW) first proposed and developed the theory of cometary panspermia (Hoyle and Wickramasinghe, 1979, 1981,1985) there was no direct evidence for liquid water anywhere outside the Earth. The inference of the presence of liquid water in comets and giant icy bodies of the solar system came from theoretical studies alone. Hoyle and Wickramasinghe (1985) argued that a largely icy body comprised of a normal solar system fraction of uranium and thorium would, through radioactive heating, maintain warm interior oceans of liquid water thus providing microbial habitats for billions of years. Hoyle and Wickramasinghe (1985) wrote: "There would evidently be no difficulty for a body of lunar size R > 1000km, maintaining a liquid condition in its interior, and some comets may have been able to do so over at least the first 500 million years history of the Solar System. Excess energy output would simply lead to a thinner surface shell, while a reduction of output would thicken the shell, in effect with the shell thickness adjusting itself to the reactor output. This solves the problem for the existence of chemoautotrophic biological systems under anaerobic conditions." More detailed studies of the same processes were carried out later by Wickramasinghe et al. (1996) and J.T. Wickramasinghe et al. (2009).

It was long afterwards that direct evidence of liquid water in comets as well as other icy solar system bodies came to be firmly established through space exploration. The Jovian moon Europa, the Saturnian moon Enceladus and the dwarf planet Ceres all have evidence of liquid water, maintained either through tidal energy dissipation or radioactive heating.

5. Earliest terrestrial life

Three decades ago the earliest evidence for microbial life in the geological record was thought to be in the form of cyanobacteria-like fossils dating back to 3.5 Billion Years (Ga) ago. From the time of formation of a stable crust on the Earth at 4.3 Ga following

E.J. Steele et al. / Progress in Biophysics and Molecular Biology 136 (2018) 3–23   7

an episode of violent impacts with comets (the Hadean Epoch to which we have already referred) there seemed to be available a 800 million years timespan during which the canonical Haldane-Oparin primordial soup may have developed. Very recent discoveries, however, have shown that this time interval has been effectively closed (Dodd et al., 2017). Further, detrital zircons ≥4.1 Ga, discovered in rocks belonging to a geological outcrop in the Jack Hills region of Western Australia, have been found to contain micron-sized graphite spheres with an isotopic signature of biogenic carbon (Bell et al., 2015). The ^{12}C-enrichment found within these inclusions may thus be taken as plausible unequivocal evidence for the existence of microbial life on Earth before 4.1 Ga, during the epoch of comet and asteroid impacts. These data are consistent with the dating of first life on Earth for the just discussed data for early signs of cell-based life (>4.1Ga) in Canada's oldest hydrothermal vent precipitates (Dodd et al., 2017). The requirement now, on the basis of orthodox abiogenic thinking, is that an essentially instantaneous transformation of non-living organic matter to bacterial life occurs, an assumption we consider strains credibility of Earth-bound abiogenesis beyond the limit. A far more plausible possibility is that fully-developed microorganisms and maybe other eukaryotic organisms arrived at the Earth via impacting comets, and these later became carbonized and trapped within condensing mineral grain conglomerates. It is now becoming amply clear that Earth-like planets and other life-friendly planetary bodies exist in their hundreds of billions and exchanges of material between them (meteorites, cometary bolides) must routinely occur (Wickramasinghe et al., 2012; Kopparapu, 2013; Appendix A). One is thus forced in our view to conclude that the entire galaxy (and perhaps our local group of galaxies) constitutes a single connected biosphere.

6. Origin of life

A facile criticism that is often leveled against the cosmic life theory is that it does not solve the problem of life's origin, but merely transfers it elsewhere (Appendix A). Whilst this may be true in the strictest sense, the importance of knowing whether or not life originated, or could have done so *de novo*, in the most minuscule of cosmic environments (here on Earth) as against the cosmos as a whole is a scientific question of paramount importance and one that needs to be addressed. The cosmic theory of life that extends the interactive biosphere of all life to encompass a cosmological volume connecting all habitable niches in the Universe has profound ramifications within evolutionary biology itself. Some of these ramifications will emerge in other sections of this article, and see the further extended discussion of view-points on the origin of life *per se* in the Universe in the supplementary information, Appendix A.

The transformation of an ensemble of appropriately chosen biological monomers (e.g. amino acids, nucleotides) into a primitive living cell capable of further evolution appears to require overcoming an information hurdle of superastronomical proportions (Appendix A), an event that could not have happened within the time frame of the Earth except, we believe, as a miracle (Hoyle and Wickramasinghe, 1981, 1982, 2000). All laboratory experiments attempting to simulate such an event have so far led to dismal failure (Deamer, 2011; Walker and Wickramasinghe, 2015). It would thus seem reasonable to go to the biggest available "venue" in relation to space and time. A cosmological origin of life thus appears plausible and overwhelmingly likely to us, and various ideas that have a bearing on this question have been explored in great depth by Hoyle and Wickramasinghe (1979, 1981,1982, 2000) and Gibson et al. (2011).

7. Organic molecules and biological dust in space and in comets

Detections of interstellar organic molecules of ever-increasing complexity have continued with the deployment of newer and better instruments and telescopes. Infrared, microwave, and radio observations are used to detect the presence of such molecules, and the current list of positive detections is likely to be circumscribed only by limitations of available techniques. Historically, the first mid-infrared spectrum of the Galactic Centre infrared source GC-IRS7 was shown to be very similar to the spectrum that was predicted earlier for a partially degraded (freeze dried) bacterium (Fig. 1) and this striking exact correlation between laboratory data and astrophysical observation was reasonably interpreted by Hoyle and Wickramasinghe as tenable evidence for life being a cosmic phenomenon (Hoyle et al., 1982, 1984). Evidence accumulated in the subsequent 3 decades has only served to strengthen this claim; a mixture of semi-bituminous coals and desiccated *E-coli* bacteria gave a similar match to the IR spectral features of GC-IRS7 over 3.2–3.8 µm as in Fig. 2 (Coulson and Wickramasinghe, 2000), suggesting that the process of bacterial degradation leads to the formation of interstellar coal. The standard rebuttal of this biological interpretation of spectroscopic data was to assert that an appropriately weighted ensemble of organic functional groups (produced abiotically) could be conceived in the biochemistry/biophysical laboratory that exactly matched such a biological spectrum. But the conditions needed to produce such a finely tuned mixture infallibly and ubiquitously were never actually explored or published by those motivated by such a viewpoint. (While a skeptical scientific attitude in such matters is essential we nevertheless re-emphasize that deducing chemical and physical properties of extraterrestrial objects and entities in the wider Solar System and Universe from correlative spectroscopic data in Earth-

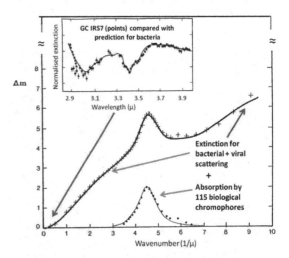

Fig. 1. A composite of absorption and scattering properties of interstellar dust from the infrared to the far ultraviolet. Lowest curve is the predicted behaviour around 2175A of an ensemble of biological aromatic molecules compared with average properties of interstellar dust; the middle curve is the total extinction (absorption + scattering) behaviour of an ensemble of bacterial and viral dust compared with astronomical data points for interstellar dust; the upper curve is the measured extinction of desiccated bacteria. The points are astronomical observations of D.T. Wickramasinghe and D.A. Allen for the Galactic Centre source GC-IRS7 (1986). Drawn from published data by NCW. For more details see refs. (Wickramasinghe, 2015a, 2015b; Hoyle et al., 1982, 1984).

8   *E.J. Steele et al. / Progress in Biophysics and Molecular Biology 136 (2018) 3–23*

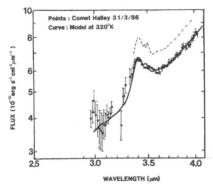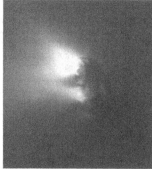

Fig. 2. **Emission by dust coma of Comet Halley on March 31, 1986 (points) compared with normalized fluxes for desiccated *E-coli* at an emission temperature of 320K.** The solid curve is for unirradiated bacteria; the dashed curve is for X-ray irradiated bacteria (Allen and Wickramasinghe, 1981; Wickramasinghe and Allen, 1986). Left hand graph drawn from published data by NCW. Right hand image Giotto image of the cometary nucleus is on the right frame (Courtesy of the European Space Agency).

based laboratories and telescopes, has been the bread and butter of Astrophysical deductive science at least since Galileo and the Renaissance, e.g. as illustrated in the extant data in Figs. 1–3).

The evidence based arguments in favour of complex organics in comets were first put forward by Vanýsek and Wickramasinghe (1975). In 1986 the presence of organic dust in comets was confirmed by D.T. Wickramasinghe and Allen (1986), Fig. 2. Hoyle and N.C. Wickramasinghe thereafter (1986) pointed out that the infrared spectrum of Comet Halley suggestively indicated bacteria-like material in comets (Fig. 1), and also that comets appear to have a tar-like surface layer resulting from the degradation of biological material near its closest orbital point near the Sun, or perihelion.

These data posed a serious challenge to Whipple's 'dirty snowball' comet model that was the reigning paradigm at the time. Space probes to Halley's comet in 1986 established its dust as high in carbonaceous compounds and its surface as very dark, quite unlike ice or snow. Later exploration of several comets, using a variety of space technologies, has strengthened the case for microbial life in comets (and in carbonaceous chondrite residues) but this is not readily admitted in conservative astronomical and meteoritic circles. Solar system short-period comets as well as long period comets whose source is the Oort Cloud and adjacent star systems are hypothesized to be the carriers and amplifiers of microbial life on a galactic or even cosmological scale (Hoyle and Wickramasinghe, 1981, 1993). On this model it follows that interstellar dust should include a fraction of material that represents the detritus of biology.

Since 1980 the existence in interstellar clouds of complex organic molecules such as polycyclic aromatic hydrocarbons, is beyond dispute (Hoyle and Wickramasinghe, 1991, 2000). In addition to infrared data the ubiquitous 2175A absorption band in interstellar dust, although still "unidentified", appears fully consistent with either biochemical chromophores (break-up of microbiology) or radiation-processed microbial entities. Another astronomical dataset pointing to ubiquitous microbiology are the diffuse interstellar absorption bands in the visual spectra of stars that have defied identification for over 8 decades, but which match the properties of porphyrins (Hoyle and Wickramasinghe, 1991). It should also be noted that during the past 15 years the correspondences shown in Fig. 1 have been greatly extended to include the most distant galaxies (Wickramasinghe, 2015a). This would mean that a fortuitous match of biochemical spectra with astronomy must (according to critics and skeptics) stretch out to the very edge of the observable universe (redshift z = 4).

The Rosetta Mission's Philae lander has recently provided us novel information about the comet 67P/C-G (Capaccionne et al., 2015; Wallis and Wickramasinghe, 2015; Wickramasinghe et al., 2015). Jets of H_2O vapour and organics issuing from cracks and holes in the black crust (Fig. 3) are plausibly consistent with biological activity occurring within sub-surface pools (Wickramasinghe et al., 1996, 2009). The most recent report of O_2 along with evidence for the occurrence of water and organics provides, in our view, a further compelling argument for ongoing biological activity (Bieler et al., 2015). Such a mixture of gases cannot be produced under thermodynamic conditions, since organics are readily destroyed in an oxidizing environment. The freezing of an initial mixture of compounds, including O_2, not in thermochemical equilibrium, has been proposed, but there is no evidence to support such a claim. On the other hand the $O_2/H_2O/$

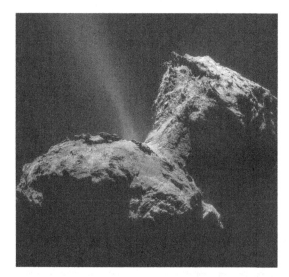

Fig. 3. **Jets of organic molecules, and molecular oxygen were found emerging from comet 67P/C-G** (Courtesy of the European Space Agency). P/C ratio of gas analysed by the Rosetta orbiter revealed values of 1% that are consistent with degradation of bacteria (Capaccionne et al., 2015; Bieler et al., 2015; Altwegg et al., 2016).

E.J. Steele et al. / Progress in Biophysics and Molecular Biology 136 (2018) 3–23   9

organics outflow from the comet can be elegantly explained on the basis of subsurface microbiology. Photosynthetic microorganisms operating at the low light levels near the surface at perihelion could produce O_2 along with organics. Many species of fermenting bacteria can also produce ethanol from sugars, so the recent discovery that Comet Lovejoy emits ethyl alcohol amounting to 500 bottles of wine per second may well be an indication that such a microbial process is operating (Biver et al., 2015).

8. Evidence for extant life on mars

The scientific history of the issue of life on Mars is a story in itself, yet very significant in the cosmic biology context (Hoyle and Wickramasinghe, 1997; Wickramasinghe, 2015a). The early positive results of Gilbert Levin and Patricia Straat (1976) on extant microbial life detected on the surface of Mars by the 1976 Viking Labelled Release (LR) experiment have never been properly refuted (Levin and Straat, 2016), and Levin and colleagues have fully considered and dealt with all the various comments and criticisms (Levin, 2007, 2013, 2015; Bianciardi et al., 2012). Indeed the prospects for a better quality of scientific search for life missions on Mars with Gilbert Levin's involvement have improved considerably (University of Buckingham Press Release, July 23, 2016). The pioneering 1976 studies are supported by the new results of Ruff and Farmer (2016) from the Mars Spirit rover which show silica deposits on Mars containing features resembling hot spring biosignatures at El Taion in Chile. Ruff and Farmer conclude that "Although only abiotic processes are not ruled out for the Martian silica structures, they satisfy an *a priori* definition of potential biosignatures." It is therefore appropriate that the extensive dataset relating to the possibility of extant Martian life is fully appraised, and Levin and Straat's discoveries of 4 decades ago placed in context and they be accorded full credit for their discoveries.

9. Microbial material in the stratosphere and meteorites

Data from cometary studies continue to be backed up by recoveries of microbial material in the stratosphere (under conditions where upwelling terrestrial contamination can be plausibly ruled out). Biological entities ranging from viable but non-culturable microbes to unexplained aggregates of microscopic biological entities continue to be recovered from heights in the range 30—41 km in the stratosphere (Wainwright et al., 2014, 2015a, 2015b). The entities are composed of carbon and nitrogen and exhibit bilateral symmetry and organism-like morphologies. The evidence has been interpreted to show it is consistent with the plausible conclusion that these micro-organism-like entities are incoming to Earth from space, possibly transported by small comets (Frank and Sigwarth, 2001). The likely survival of biological materials descending through the Earth's atmosphere has been demonstrated in micron-sized meteoroids (Coulson and Wickramasinghe, 2003) and in icy comet meteors with radii of ~1 m (Coulson et al., 2014). Early evidence of fossilized micro-organisms internal to carbonaceous meteorites has become well-established, with skepticism over terrestrial contamination now firmly countered (Pflug and Heinz, 1997; Hoover, 2005, 2011; Miyake et al., 2010; Wickramasinghe, 2015a). The most recent discovery of microbial fossils in meteorites that fell in Sri Lanka in 2012, and the unequivocal determination (based on Oxygen isotope data) that the rocks are not of Earth origin provides further strong evidence of panspermia (Wallis et al., 2013). Another related phenomenon concerns the red rain events recorded throughout history (McCafferty, 2008) but most recently in Kerala, India (Louis and Kumar 2006) and Sri Lanka in 2012. All the available evidence point to red pigmented organisms that are unlikely to have a terrestrial origin.

In spite of rigorous precautions and controls that have been undertaken for the investigations we have discussed in this section, the general trend has been to dismiss such discoveries that contradict the reigning paradigm as contaminants.

10. Principles of virology - viruses as dense information-rich control systems

Before embarking on a discussion of the new evidence on retroviral evolution (Aiewsakun and Katzourakis, 2017) it is important we recap the basic processes of the biology of viruses and their *modus operandi* as genetic vectors within and between cells.

All DNA and RNA viruses infecting bacterial or eukaryotic cells are tightly ordered and dense information systems. All known cellular systems carry integrated virus genetic information, or fragments thereof, or are potentially targets of virus attack and infection. These axioms do not contradict any principle in any modern textbook. Indeed, since Felix d'Herrelle and Frederick Twort in 1915-17 discovered the "filterable" agents that could infect and kill bacterial cells, we now have an almost complete understanding of the essential principles of virology.

To continue a short list summary we know that:

- The experience over decades from experimental transformation and transfection systems leads to the conclusion that any given virus particle or nucleic acid agent (viroid) can in principle potentially enter any cell.
- Replication within the cell is another matter, as the incoming information-rich molecular system must both gel, mesh and integrate with the host cell's complex biochemical and genetic circuits (Fig. 4).
- But florid replication can lead to explosive production of virions and death of the host cell (cf. cytopathic viruses). Such events occur because both the cell's immediate Innate Immunity mechanism and then later the organism's more delayed Adaptive Immune Response fail to stop the virus infection. The explosive production of virions is rarer than a more measured replication and extracellular virion export, accommodating both viral and host cell growth (or even integration of the viral DNA/RNA into the host cell genome, as latent virus). These then are the essential three main outcomes of the first stage of the host-parasite relationship (Fig. 4).
- Usually the explosive cytopathic growth type of infection (leading to the rapid death of the host) is rare because most terrestrially circulating (and evolving) viruses have established 'host-parasite' rules of engagement (in both their Innate and Adaptive defence arms).
- So the explosive cytopathic infections, typical of unexpected fast emerging epidemics and pandemics are likely, on a first pass, to have causes unrelated to the normal constraints of the host-parasite relationship (below).
- Thus, the host-range of all plant, animal and bacterial viruses is defined not by entry of the virion into the cellular microenvironment, but by whether it can productively replicate or integrate and then express itself (such as a retrovirus). In practice this is usually manifest as an observable viral disease with characteristic non-life threatening first symptoms.
- Viruses then are dense information-rich polynucleotide macromolecules of $\geq$ 3000 bp (SanJuan, 2010, 2012; Sanjuan and Domingo-Calap, 2016). They are in a sense, in susceptible host cells, condensed regulatory blueprints in tune with the essential transcriptional regulator genes and nodal biochemical pathways critical to the growth and viability of the cell.

• We should then plausibly view viruses as among the most information-rich natural systems in the known Universe (Fig. 4). Their size dictates they are very small targets minimizing the probability of destruction by flash heating or ionizing radiation, Hoyle and Wickramasinghe (1979) e.g. Chapter 1. Their nanometer dimensions plausibly allow easy transport and dispersal by micrometer sized dust grains and other protective physical matrices of similar size. They are then nanoparticle-sized genetic vectors which contain all the essential information to take over and drive the physiology of any given target cell within which they mesh. Their replicative growth means they are produced, and exist, in huge numbers on cosmic scales; so that they (and to a lesser quantitative extent their cellular reservoirs) can suffer huge losses by inactivation while still leaving a residue of millions of surviving particles potentially still infective. A virus then is a type of compressed module in touch with the whole of the cell's very ability to grow and divide to produce progeny cells and thus to evolve.

This check list is underpinned by the important experiments on RNA viruses by Sanjuan and his associates (Sanjuan, 2010, 2012; SanJuan et al., 2004, 2010; Combe et al., 2015). It will be expected that finely tuned information-dense viral genomes are susceptible to random mutations which cripple their speed of replication and infectivity. Using site-directed mutagenesis to produce randomized mutations in viral genomes (SanJuan et al., 2004; Sanjuan, 2010) up to 40% of such mutated nucleotides result in clear lethals. This is only an estimate as substitutions leading to amino acid replacements (non-synonymous mutations) is not the only mutation hazard a virus can encounter. Silent substitutional changes in the 3rd position 'Wobble Site' in a codon can have functional consequence affecting replication and infective efficacy caused by co-translational pausing/delays as the polypeptide exits the Ribosome. These effects lead to anomalies in folding kinetics due to variations in the composition of the nucleotide triphosphate precursor pool (Buhr et al., 2016). Well-conserved RNA structures in the HCV RNA genome when manipulated at 3rd position synonymous sites can alter the ability of the virus to replicate, and hence infect (Pirakitikulr et al., 2016).

The sophistication of viral infectivity and their *modus operandi* of cell-cell spreading does not end here. To ensure maximal gene complementation defective viral genomes carrying stop codons (Aaskov et al., 2006) can be propagated almost indefinitely (Combe et al., 2015) as "virion clusters" of mixtures of infective and crippled genomes with significant numbers of newly minted virus particles enwrapped in protective membrane vesicles - a type of multiunit nanoparticle. This then constitutes the actual infective dose rather than just a single exported virion entering a nearby target cell to cause a productive infection as is commonly believed (Combe et al., 2015; Chen et al., 2015).

However it needs pointing out again that most terrestrial viruses have already evolved established molecular-interactive host-parasite relationships. Many, by themselves are benign and non-cytolytic, such that many initial infections are usually silent and asymptomatic. Physicians and Clinicians now understand that the main health problem is often the unintended tissue damage caused by inflammatory responses by the host's adaptive immune response launched prior to the establishment of chronic infection states e.g. HCV induced hepatitis (in those patients who fail to naturally and quickly clear the initial infection).

There seems no end to the inventive strategies that viruses employ to infect and take over their target cells, whether they are bacterial (normal prokaryotes, extremophile archaebacteria) or eukaryotic metazoan cells. If we just consider a recent RNA virome sample for invertebrate hosts, the complex magnitude of which,

with the swapping and sharing of viral gene sequences, is staggering in its scope (Shi et al., 2016). In the more extensively studied vertebrates, where similar sharing and gene swapping has occurred, the evasion of both the innate and adaptive immune responses are key facets of the viral life cycle. Recently it has been pointed out that one possible reason why the HIV retrovirus cannot be controlled by conventional immunological vaccines (producing neutralizing antibodies in advance of the infection by a HIV-1 variant) is because the main cellular focus of proviral integration may not be the T lymphocyte or the macrophage/dendritic cell as commonly supposed, but more likely the B lymphocyte (Steele and Dawkins, 2016), the cellular home of the somatic hypermutation mechanism (Franklin et al., 2004; Steele, 2016b; Steele and Lindley, 2017). Thus it was reasonably postulated that HIV by co-opting the adaptive somatic hypermutation mechanism of the antibody system will always be a mutational step ahead of the patient's own adaptive immune response (Steele and Dawkins, 2016). This proposal has not been publicly challenged by mainstream critics in immunology and virology since it was circulated and remains a conceptual option in better understanding the *modus operandi* of HIV and retroviruses related to it.

11. Criticism of host specificity and survival under space conditions

A criticism that has been levelled against the concept of viruses causing disease and contributing to the evolution of life is encapsulated in a single rhetorical question: how can a virus from space know ahead of its coming here the range of organisms that are available with which it can interact? In the previous section we have elaborated on the correct answer to this question: viruses originating in a cosmic context and evolution on the Earth are inextricably intertwined. The host specificity of viruses is maintained only over fairly narrow ranges of species that are defined by their evolutionary history. Thus the influenza A virus can be cultured in hen's eggs so attesting to host specificity to within 50 million years of evolutionary history (and is known to infect many vertebrate and mammalian species). Again the Ebola virus affects the class of primates.

The criticism that bacteria and/or viruses are incapable of surviving under the harsh conditions of space is certainly not borne out by all the data that has accumulated over the past 3 decades. Bacteria and viruses embedded in grains of rock, carbonaceous material or ice, are protected effectively from radiation damage and can remain fully viable for millions of years under space conditions. Microorganisms including virions deep frozen within cometary bodies could remain viable indefinitely, and certainly for cosmological timescales. Recent space experiments including those conducted aboard the International Space Station have shown remarkable survival properties of bacteria and viruses.

Thus Hiel et al. (2014) have recently conducted an experiment in which plasmid DNA was placed on the outer surface of a TEXUS-49 sounding rocket that was blasted through the atmosphere into space and which subsequently re-entered the atmosphere. The conditions endured by the DNA would closely mimic what actually happens in the high-speed entry of viruses attached to meteor/comet dust. The data of Hiel et al. (2014) show that a significant fraction of DNA remained viable and infective - a clear indication that extraterrestrial viruses can indeed arrive at the Earth in viable form.

The microorganism (*D. audaxviator*) discovered at a depth of 2.8km in a South African gold mine has been found to derive its energy from radiolysis induced by particles emitted from the decay of U, Th and K (Chivian et al., 2008). A bacterium such as *D. audaxviator* would survive not only in interstellar transits but

E.J. Steele et al. / Progress in Biophysics and Molecular Biology 136 (2018) 3–23   11

they would thrive on the energy derived from galactic cosmic rays that reach the interstellar or interplanetary frozen bodies.

12. Retroviral induction model

We now also have a far better understanding of clear non-Darwinian and non-Mendelian evolutionary inheritance mechanisms shaping both the immune and central nervous systems in particular (e.g. retroviral and RNA/RT-based Lamarckian Inheritance (Steele, 1979; Gorczynski and Steele, 1980, 1981; Steele et al., 1984; Steele et al., 1998; Steele, 2016a) as well as retroviral/retro-element drivers of segmental duplications and genomic block structure of Ancestral Haplotypes and related non-Darwinian inheritance phenomena of medical significance (Dawkins et al., 1999; Dawkins, 2015; Steele, 2014, 2015; Steele and Lloyd, 2015). The plethora of adaptive Lamarckian-like inheritance mechanisms in general are discussed elsewhere (Campbell and Perkins, 1988; Jablonka and Lamb, 1995; Lindley, 2010; Liu, 2007; Noble, 2013; Mattick, 2012; Liu and Li, 2016a, 2016b) some involving mobile lymphocytes delivering endogenous retroviruses and somatic genes to the germline (Rothenfluh, 1995) or other types of soma-to-germline transfer mechanisms involving vesicles or exosomes have been considered (Spadafora, 2008; Cossetti et al., 2014; Devanapally et al., 2015; Sharma et al., 2015). A clear causal chain of new viruses arriving from space potentially driving evolution on Earth can thus be discerned and rationally understood (Wickramasinghe and Steele, 2016). Indeed LINE retro-element transposition (and Alu repeat element co-mobility, Appendix B) is a normal part of genomic rearrangement during specific neuron commitment, much like the V-> DJ rearrangement in specific B and T lymphocyte commitment in the Immune System (Erwin et al., 2016).

With respect to HIV and retroviral evolution in general viz. the genomic duplicative processes generating the polymorphic block (Ancestral) haplotype structure of the human genome, the key concepts can be traced to what is now known as the *"Retroviral-Induction Model "* (Dawkins et al., 1999; Steele, 2014) and Steele (2015, p.95). Thus when a retrovirus infects a human cell all measure of mutagenic processes are unleashed, including: AID/APOBEC-deaminase induced C-to-U events leading to C-to-T mutations, Abasic sites, and ssDNA nicks, as well as ADAR-deaminase induced A-to-I RNA editing events. Both of these DNA and RNA deaminations are now identified as strand-biased and codon-context Targeted Somatic Mutations (TSM) in the human cancer genome (Lindley, 2013; Lindley and Steele, 2013; Lindley et al., 2016; Steele and Lindley, 2017). As well as these we have LINE/Alu–retro-element mutagenic mobility (Harris and Liddament, 2004; Chiu et al., 2006; Muotri et al., 2007; Doria et al., 2009; Refsland and Harris, 2013; Jones et al., 2013). So as discussed already LINE/Alu retro-mobility now appears as a normal part of specific synaptic neuronal Brain development (Erwin et al., 2016). RNA editing (A-to-I) targeting neural Alu inverted elements (in the introns, creating alternative spliced isoforms) is an established synaptic neural diversification process in the Brain (Paz-Yaacov et al., 2010). Thus retroviruses and other viruses hypothezed to be liberated in cometary debris trails both can potentially add new DNA sequences to terrestrial genomes and drive further mutagenic change within somatic and germline genomes (Appendix B). Indeed Frank Ryan has termed virus-driven terrestrial evolution with the appropriate catch-phrase, 'virolution' and this concept has been supported and expanded by Oliver and Greene (2012) in the Transposable-Element Thrust Hypothesis (Appendix B).

Yohn et al. (2005) have stated that their data are consistent with a retroviral infection that bombarded the genomes of chimpanzees and gorillas independently and concurrently, 3–4 million years ago, with no horizontal transmission being implied. Recently Diehl et al.

(2016) have shown that a specific endogenous retrovirus group (ERV-Fc) has somehow come to be spread globally across many mammalian species about 33-15 million years ago. There have also been suggestions that the later evolutionary development of hominids, including enhanced cognitive capacity, may also have viral origins (Villareal, 2004). A plausible externally driven viral involvement appears to have been identified in the development of mammalian placenta in ancestors of all mammals including humans about 150 million years ago (Katzourakis (2013)).

13. Evolution of intelligent complexity

Evidence of the role of extraterrestrial viruses in affecting terrestrial evolution has recently been plausibly implied in the gene and transcriptome sequencing of Cephalopods. The genome of the Octopus shows a staggering level of complexity with 33,000 protein-coding genes more than is present in *Homo sapiens* (Albertin et al., 2015). Octopus belongs to the coleoid sub-class of molluscs (Cephalopods) that have an evolutionary history that stretches back over 500 million years, although Cephalopod phylogenetics is highly inconsistent and confusing (see Carlini et al., 2000; Strugnell et al., 2005, 2006, 2007; Bergmann et al., 2006). Cephalopods are also very diverse, with the behaviourally complex coleoids, (Squid, Cuttlefish and Octopus) presumably arising under a pure terrestrial evolutionary model from the more primitive nautiloids. However the genetic divergence of Octopus from its ancestral coleoid sub-class is very great, akin to the extreme features seen across many genera and species noted in Eldridge-Gould punctuated equilibria patterns (below). Its large brain and sophisticated nervous system, camera-like eyes, flexible bodies, instantaneous camouflage via the ability to switch colour and shape are just a few of the striking features that appear suddenly on the evolutionary scene. The transformative genes leading from the consensus ancestral Nautilus (e.g. *Nautilus pompilius*) to the common Cuttlefish (*Sepia officinalis*) to Squid (*Loligo vulgaris*) to the common Octopus (*Octopus vulgaris*, Fig. 5) are not easily to be found in any pre-existing life form — it is plausible then to suggest they seem to be borrowed from a far distant "future" in terms of terrestrial evolution, or more realistically from the cosmos at large. Such an extraterrestrial origin as an explanation of emergence of course runs counter to the prevailing dominant paradigm.

However consistent with this conclusion are the recent RNA editing transcriptome-wide data on the somatic RNA diversification mechanisms in the behaviourally sophisticated Cephalopods such as Octopus. These data demonstrate extensive evolutionary conserved adenosine to inosine (A-to-I) mRNA editing sites in almost every single protein-coding gene in the behaviorally complex coleoid Cephalopods (Octopus in particular), *but not in nautilus* (Liscovitch-Brauer et al., 2017). This enormous qualitative difference in Cephalopod protein recoding A-to-I mRNA editing compared to nautilus and other invertebrate and vertebrate animals is striking. Thus in transcriptome-wide screens only 1–3% of *Drosophila* and human protein coding mRNAs harbour an A-to-I recoding site; and there only about 25 human mRNA messages which contain a conserved A-to-I recoding site across mammals. In *Drosophila* lineages there are about 65 conserved A-sites in protein coding genes and only a few identified in *C. elegans* which support the hypothesis that A-to-I RNA editing recoding is mostly either neutral, detrimental, or rarely adaptive (reviewed in Liscovitch-Brauer et al., 2017). Yet in Squid and particularly Octopus it is the norm, with almost every protein coding gene having an evolutionary conserved A-to-I mRNA editing site isoform, resulting in a nonsynonymous amino acid change (Liscovitch-Brauer et al., 2017). This is a virtual qualitative jump in molecular genetic strategy in a supposed smooth and incremental evolutionary lineage - a type of

12   *E.J. Steele et al. / Progress in Biophysics and Molecular Biology 136 (2018) 3—23*

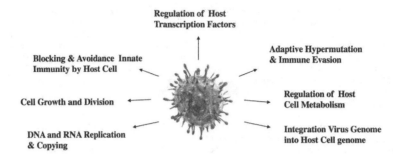

Fig. 4. Typical main functions of viruses. They are in tune with all the essential growth aspects of their own production and the wider cellular machinery. Virus image from: https://www.dreamstime.com/royalty-free-stock-photo-h1n1-viruses-image11898035.

sudden "great leap forward". Unless all the new genes expressed in the squid/octopus lineages arose from simple mutations of existing genes in either the squid or in other organisms sharing the same habitat, there is surely no way by which this large qualitative transition in A-to-I mRNA editing can be explained by conventional neo-Darwinian processes, even if horizontal gene transfer is allowed. One plausible explanation, in our view, is that the new genes are likely new extraterrestrial imports to Earth - most plausibly as an already coherent group of functioning genes within (say) cryopreserved and matrix protected fertilized Octopus eggs.

Thus the possibility that cryopreserved Squid and/or Octopus eggs, arrived in icy bolides several hundred million years ago should not be discounted (below) as that would be a parsimonious cosmic explanation for the Octopus' sudden emergence on Earth ca. 270 million years ago. Indeed this principle applies to the sudden appearance in the fossil record of pretty well all major life forms, covered in the prescient concept of "punctuated equilibrium" by Eldridge and Gould advanced in the early 1970s (1972, 1977); and see the conceptual cartoon of Fig. 6. Therefore, similar living features like this "as if the genes were derived from some type of pre-existence" (Hoyle and Wickramasinghe, 1981) apply to many other biological ensembles when closely examined. One little known yet cogent example is the response and resistance of the eye structures of the *Drosophila* fruit fly to normally lethally damaging UV radiation at 2537 Å, given that this wavelength does not penetrate the ozone layer and is thus not evident as a Darwinian selective factor

at the surface of the Earth (Lutz and Grisewood, 1934) and see Hoyle and Wickramasinghe (1981, p.12—13). Many of these "unearthly" properties of organisms can be plausibly explained if we admit the enlarged cosmic biosphere that is indicated by modern astronomical research — discoveries of exoplanets already discussed. The average distance between habitable planets in our galaxy now to be reckoned in light years — typically 5 light years (Wickramasinghe et al., 2012). Virion/gene exchanges thus appear to be inevitable over such short cosmic distances. The many features of biology that are not optimised to local conditions on the Earth may be readily understood in this wider perspective.

Given that the complex sets of new genes in the Octopus may have not come solely from horizontal gene transfers or simple random mutations of existing genes or by simple duplicative expansions, it is then logical to surmise, given our current knowledge of the biology of comets and their debris, the new genes and their viral drivers most likely came from space. However, it is also clear that to accept such a proposition also requires that we diminish the role for highly localised Darwinian evolution on Earth which is likely to be strongly resisted by traditional biologists. That should not, of course, be of concern as the focus of our attention, for general evolutionary molecular processes, now shifts to the Cosmos and beyond our immediate solar system. This evidence provides for, and allows the study of, *Cosmic Gene Pools* — and these are capable of driving, and, dare we say, controlling and thus steering biological evolution here on Earth (via Darwinian and non-

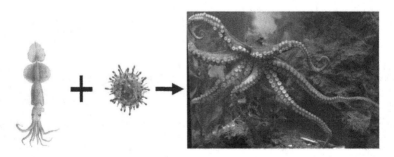

Fig. 5. The evolution from squid to octopus is compatible with a suite of genes inserted by extraterrestrial viruses. An alternative extraterrestrial scenario discuused is that a population of cryopreserved octopus embryos soft-landed *en mass* from space 275 million years ago.
Squid image - Grimalditeuthis bonplandi. jpg.From Wikimedia Commons -Author: Jeanne Le Roux & L. Joubin URL (http://www.archive.org/stream/rsultatsdescam17albe#page/n165/mode/2up)
Octopus Image - File:Octopus at Kelly Tarlton's.jpg From Wikimedia Commons Author: Pseudopanax at English Wikipedia
https://upload.wikimedia.org/wikipedia/commons/f/ff/Octopus_at_Kelly_Tarlton%27s.jpg
Virus image from: https://www.dreamstime.com/royalty-free-stock-photo-h1n1-viruses-image11898035.

E.J. Steele et al. / Progress in Biophysics and Molecular Biology 136 (2018) 3–23   13

Consequences of the Paradigm Shift for Phylogenetic Sequence Relationships

Separate In-fall Cosmic-Derived Lines with Some Branch Terrestrial Evolution

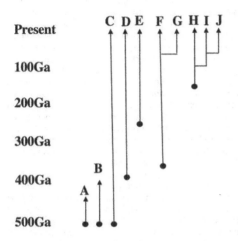

A Phylogenetic Tree is Forced by Assuming Evolutionary Precursor Relationships

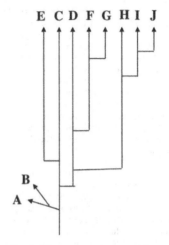

Fig. 6. Conceptual Cartoon - Cosmic Evolution after an in-fall versus Terrestrial Evolutionary Relationships. Evolutionary patterns for an essential conserved protein such as, for example, Haemoglobin (O_2 transfer) or Cytochrome C (electron transfer). The 10 different variant proteins are A through to J. This cartoon illustrates the conceptual differences for evolutionary schemes caused by the in-fall of a species of organism from space followed by subsequent terrestrial evolution (on the left) versus the evolutionary relationships between the same groups of conserved proteins after a phylogenetic tree is forced on the data by quantitative assessment of the homology relationships based on, for example, Kimura's Neutral Theory (of third position synonymous variation). On the left independent lines are initiated at different times on in-fall from space (from the •). On the right a "Tree" is formed by the algorithm which assumes direct precursor evolutionary relationships for all the homologous variants of the conserved protein. The branched groups F, G and HIJ are genuine terrestrial evolutionary diversifications. A, and B go extinct shortly after in-fall. Adapted from the concepts outlined in Hoyle and Wickramasinghe (1981). Fig. 6.3 and 6.4 pages 83–85. The essential concept on the left fits the punctuated equilibria scheme of Eldredge and Gould (1972), Gould and Eldredge (1977). Conventional phylogenetics of any type thus operates on the tacit assumption that all homologies are related by arising *only on Earth* ignoring the contribution of a Cosmic evolutionary dimension to the data.

Darwinian adaptation mechanisms). The main effect of terrestrial Darwinian evolution is to act on these new cosmic-derived genes and fine-tune them by further somatic and germline Lamarckian gene feedback and haplotype-block shuffling mechanisms to fit the environment and also the recipient organism (Wickramasinghe and Steele, 2016). Indeed it has been shown that viral footprints are evident in human brain tissue which seem to mark important steps that led up to the present human condition (Villarreal, 2004; Ryan, 2009).

14. Evolutionary origin of vertebrate retroviruses

This now leads us to the crux and an important take home lesson of this review. While all viruses, when looked at closely, are exceedingly clever, the Retroviruses (family *Retroviridiae*) are up there with the most sophisticated and compact of all known viruses. These viruses and their elements (reverse transcriptase enzymes, associated with induced mobile retro-elements) now appear to be important viral-drivers of major evolutionary genetic change on Earth over the past few hundred million years (Wickramasinghe, 2012), and see (Hoyle and Wickramasinghe, 1979, 1981). Cell-derived reverse transcriptase (RT) activity is also a principal molecular player in adaptive somatic hypermutation of antibody genes (Franklin et al., 2004; Steele, 2016b; Steele and

Lindley, 2017). As just discussed endogenous retroviral vectors as well as RT activities are likely to be involved in soma-to-germline Lamarckian transmissions in the immune system (Steele, 1979; Steele et al., 1984; Steele et al., 1998; Steele and Lloyd, 2015; Steele, 2016a) including the shaping, duplicative expansions and the adaptive shuffling of the block-ancestral haplotype structures of the human and higher mammalian genome (Dawkins et al., 1999; McLure et al., 2013; Steele, 2014, 2015; Dawkins, 2015).

The main genetic and evolutionary feature of an RNA retrovirus is that on productive infection the virus ensures that a double stranded (ds) DNA copy of the viral single stranded (ss) RNA genome is made and that this is integrated as a provirus into the host cell genome (Temin, 1974). When active this potentially latent provirus is transcribed and produces viral progeny in the infected cell for export to other cells. If the host cell is a germline cell then the integrated provirus can be transmitted vertically to progeny organisms.

Retroviruses can infect a wide range of animal cells and the integrated proviruses produced can leave their trace as "genomic fossils" termed endogenous retroviruses (ERVs). These DNA sequences are therefore relics of past, and probably, virulent HIV-like epidemics whereby the survivors, and now partially immune to the immediate HIV-like variant, have genomic integrations in their germ-line cells (leading, as discussed, to the duplicative expansion and diversification of functional ancestral haplotype blocks

(Dawkins et al., 1999; Dawkins, 2015).

These fields of retroviral research are now blossoming with much data in public databases. Many ancient ERVs have now been discovered, allowing the examination of the early evolutionary history of retroviruses by bioinformatic techniques. Until just recently the oldest age estimates from analyses of mammalian retroviruses and ERVs were directly inferred to be dated back about 100 million years, to the beginning of the mammalian radiation. It is now clear in a comprehensive co-evolutionary phylogenetic analysis (Aiewsakun and Katzourakis, 2017) that bony fish endogenous retroviruses display a *co-speciation pattern* with their hosts (yet not so clear for amphibian endogenous retroviruses). However the *overall co-speciation pattern* of an ERV with the known times of emergence of their vertebrate host species is very convincing. Other possible ancient viral cross-species and class transmissions have taken place at a low rate (involving lobe-finned fish, shark and frog) yet the analyses reveal two major lineages of ray-finned fish ERVs: one line of which gained two novel accessory genes within their much larger genomes (~20 Kb, or twice the size of extant mammalian retroviruses). This major retroviral lineage (and retroviruses as a whole) appears therefore to have an ancient marine origin which " ... originated together with, if not before, their jawed vertebrate hosts >450 million years ago in the Ordovician period, early Palaeozoic Era " (Aiewsakun and Katzourakis, 2017). This is a very important result, and the authors conclude " ....our analyses provide evidence, both phylogenetically and temporally, that retroviruses emerged together with their vertebrate hosts in the ocean. ~460 - 550Ma, in the early Palaeozoic Era, if not earlier".

This of course dates these sophisticated viral gene vectors - and their associated gene-manipulative evolutionary driver effects - to just at or before the Cambrian Explosion. Certainly they are emerging before the later evolutionary appearance of the far more complex animal and plant species now extant on Earth. In other words, we can now make the plausible scientific argument that a key feature of information-dense genetic systems to make more complex organisms was already here on Earth before the actual emergence of subsequent greater terrestrial complexity. This is a contradiction if we consider our just discussed viewpoint that all viruses, and particularly the retroviruses, are a "reflection in microcosm of the host's genetic regulatory make-

15. Cambrian Explosion

It is well known that a mass extinction event, or events, occurred at the end of the Ediacaran period about 542 million years ago. This was the immediate forerunner of the Cambrian explosion and the mass extinction scale suggests the passage of our Solar System through a Giant Molecular Cloud dislodging multiple long period Oort Cloud comets into the inner Solar System setting up impacts with the Earth (Hoyle and Wickramasinghe, 1981, 1993). It takes little imagination to consider that the pre-Cambrian mass extinction event(s) was correlated with the impact of a giant life-bearing comet (or comets), and the subsequent seeding of Earth with new cosmic-derived cellular organisms and viral genes (Hoyle and Wickramasinghe, 1979, 1981). There may indeed have been a complex comet debris stream implying multiple impacts over the estimated 25 million years at the start of the Cambrian explosion.

The pre-Cambrian impact event is not unique. There is other evidence for the coincidence of cosmic bolide impacts at mass extinction event-diversification boundaries (e.g. K-T Boundary 65 Million years ago extinction of the Dinosaurs and rise of small mammals) and the now well established 26 Million yr periodicity (Galactic Tide-Holmes cycle) with cometary impacts coinciding with mass extinction events (Clube et al., 1996) and evolutionary diversifications (Napier et al., 2007). The exotic amino acids in the K-T boundary rocks and the rise of microfungi are also indicative of novel genetic material arriving in the impact (Wallis, 2007).

In this regard the work of Martin Brasier showing a 20–30 million year periodicity in foraminifera-alga coevolution could be interpreted from a Cosmic perspective rather than the Terrestrial perspective favoured by Brasier (2012, p156 -157) viz. that the 20–30 million year periodicity is an uproven systems property of large organisms to be vulnerable to small changes. Although H-W theory and analyses predicts such a large Cosmic-driven environmental change, our conclusion is consistent with Noble's recent view that "Causality is multiple in biology" (Noble, 2011). It should also be stressed in this context that Eldridge-Gould "punctuated equilibrium" (Fig. 6) is often presented as an explanation of the observed facts of evolution, but it is not. It is the use of words to describe a striking phenomenon which itself lacks a plausible explanation within the framework of Earth-centred biology.

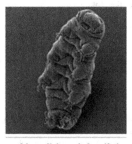

Hypsibius dujardini

" Tardigrades (0.5 mm long fully grown) form the phylum Tardigrada, part of the superphylum Ecdysozo.. an ancient group, with fossils dating from 530 million years ago, in the Cambrian period. About 1,150 species of tardigrades have been described .. [and they] can be found throughout the world, from the Himalayas (above 6,000 m (20,000 ft)), to the deep sea (below 4,000 m (13,000 ft)) and from the polar regions to the equator. [They] are water-dwelling, eight-legged, segmented micro-animals. and have been found everywhere from mountaintops to the deep sea, from tropical rain forests to the Antarctic....the most resilient animal known.(able to). survive extreme conditions that would be rapidly fatal to nearly all other known life forms, withstand[ing] temperature ranges from 1 K (~458 °F; ~272 °C) (close to absolute zero) to about 420 K (300 °F; 150 °C)..pressures about six times greater than those found in the deepest ocean trenches, ionizing radiation at doses hundreds of times higher than the lethal dose for a human, and the vacuum of outer space.. They can go without food or water for more than 30 years, drying out to the point where they are 3% or less water, only to rehydrate, forage, and reproduce." *Wikipedia*

up". That is, " a type of compressed module of genetic information in touch with the whole of the cell's very ability to grow and divide to produce progeny cells and to evolve."(Fig. 4).

It goes without saying that Tardigrades, micro-segmented tiny eukaryotic animals, which emerged in the Cambrian period pose a serious challenge to traditional neo-Darwinian thinking (see

E.J. Steele et al. / Progress in Biophysics and Molecular Biology 136 (2018) 3–23   15

Wikipedia summary Box above and the further detailed references at the Wikipedia site https://en.wikipedia.org/wiki/Tardigrade, and the data discussed in Jönsson et al., 2008). The catalogue of 'living' space-hardy properties is entirely consistent with 'evolutionary natural selective events' acting on Tardigrades evolving in extra-terrestrial space environments. These properties are incompatible with known purely terrestrial 'natural selection' conditions, either now or 500 million years ago. A plausible evidentiary case for proof of Cosmic Panspermia could rest entirely on this one example. However as has been discussed at some length there are many other living examples like this (space-hardy bacterial species and their spores), the Tardigrades being an extreme case which appears to prove the rule (Hoyle and Wickramasinghe, 1981, 1993).

The results reported recently (Leya et al., 2017) of an experiment conducted by Dr. Thomas Leya at the Fraunhofer Institute for Cell Therapy and Immunology IZI in Potsdam, Germany, in cooperation with German and international partners are consistent with this picture.

The group reports evidence that two algae species survived 16 months on the exterior of the International Space Station (ISS) despite extreme temperature fluctuations and the vacuum of space — as well as considerable UV and cosmic radiation (http://www.algaeindustrymagazine.com/algae-survive-outside-space-station/). The logical implications of these data for a Cosmic Biology are obvious - indeed we argue such findings make far better sense under the cosmic evolutionary paradigm of H-W Cosmic Biology-Panspermia (Appendix A).

16. Implications of Cambrian Explosion and retroviral data

Before the extensive sequencing of DNA became available it would have been reasonable to speculate that random copying errors in a gene sequence could, over time, lead to the emergence of new traits, body plans and new physiologies that could explain the whole of evolution. However the data we have reviewed here challenge this point of view. It suggests that the Cambrian Explosion of multicellular life that occurred 0.54 billion years ago led to a sudden emergence of essentially all the genes that subsequently came to be rearranged into an exceedingly wide range of multi-celled life forms - Tardigrades, the Squid, Octopus, fruit flies, humans — to name but a few.

The expression of an entire new suite of retroviral genes (of presumed external origin) appears to have taken place mainly via genomic rearrangements that followed ERV integrations. This was precisely the logic of evolution proposed by the late Sir Fred Hoyle and one of us (NCW) as far back as 1981. It was argued that copying errors of existing genes could not, on the average, produce new genes with functional utility. By analogy with computer programming, it was pointed out that errors generated in copying a computer code would not lead to enhanced or new capabilities but over-whelmingly to degradation of the original program. It was argued therefore that new genes for evolution must logically be supplied by the ingress of extraterrestrial virions and other micro-organisms.

17. Cosmic biology and the rise of mankind

Hoyle and Wickramasinghe (1979, 1981,1986) thus argued and predicted on the basis of the then available evidence (Figs. 1 and 2) - as well as the species mass extinction record and astronomical infra-red spectra on interstellar and cometary bodies and, more recently on the known periodic cratering and comet impact records (Clube et al., 1996) - that microorganisms and virus populations in the comets and related cosmic bolides appear to have regularly delivered living systems (organisms, viruses and seeds) to the Earth

since its formation, and continue to do so. Of course the Earth needed to be a 'hospitable' place and thus receptive to these comet-derived living systems. This then provides one plausible explanation as to why Cambrian-like explosions did not occur in the previous 3500 million years prior to 500 Ma despite the likely passage of our Solar System through many other Galactic Molecular Clouds in that time interval, given our Sun's approximately 240 Million Year galactic periodicity in its orbit around the Galactic Centre (Hoyle and Wickramasinghe, 1993; JT Wickramasinghe et al., 2010). The alternative is that a large dump stream of cosmically-derived complex eukaryotic organisms (plants, animals, fungi) arrived during the 25 million years at the start of the Cambrian, a rare and large cosmic seeding-event that happened ca. 500-550Ma but not in the previous 2000–3000 million years. The discussion here therefore, is by necessity, on Cosmic space-time scales.

So the evidence consistent with the H-W Cosmic Biology viewpoint has grown both in quantity and strength over the past decade (Napier et al., 2007; Rauf and Wickramasinghe, 2010; Wickramasinghe, 2010, 2011, 2012, 2015a, 2015b; Smith, 2013; Wickramasinghe and Smith, 2014). We are of the conviction that an extensive Cosmic Biology is the most plausible driver of the evolutionary complexity on Earth, and the recent report by Aiewsakun and Katzourakis (2017) provides a major jig-saw piece of evidence fitting in and consistent with this picture.

Darwinian evolution and its various non-Darwinian terrestrial drivers (Wickramasinghe and Steele, 2016) are therefore most likely caused by the continuing supply of new virions and micro-organisms from space with their genetic impact events written all over our genomes (Wickramasinghe, 2012). Indeed a strong case can be made for hominid evolution involving a long sequence of viral pandemics, each one of which was a close call to total extinction of an evolving line. The most crucial genes relevant to evolution of hominids, as indeed all species of plants and animals, seems likely in many instances to be of external origin, being transferred across the galaxy largely as information rich virions. In some cases it is possible to imagine — fanciful as it might seem - multicellular life-forms that were established on an icy cometary or planetary body to be transferred as frozen eggs, embryos or seeds (Tepfer and Leach, 2017) in large icy bolides that have been trans-ported to the Earth in soft landings (Frank and Sigwarth, 2001; Snyder, 2015); certainly the terrestrial evidence for Earth's own pervasive Icy Biosphere is compelling and consistent with such a picture (Priscu and Christner, 2004; Fox, 2014; Christner et al., 2014). It is plausible that in the warmed and liquid subsurface in-teriors of the comets, or planetary moons such as Jupiter's Europa and Saturn's Enceladus (Hoover, 2011; Snyder, 2015) cellular res-ervoirs for viral replication would, by necessity, need to exist.

18. The causes of epidemics and pandemics: a new virology principle

That many disease epidemics and pandemics have afflicted mankind is beyond dispute. HIV/AIDS is one of the biggest and most recent. A sexually transmitted retroviral disease apparently tar-geting the immune system and causing its eventual collapse came out of the blue - and it was not science fiction! Major monitoring centres such CDC in Atlanta, and Pirbright in the UK were caught completely unawares and unprepared. However the 1918 Spanish Flu Pandemic was probably just as devastating and equally unex-pected. The highly unusual epidemiology of the 1918 Spanish Flu Influenza virus pandemic - in the pre-air travel era - has been analysed in great detail, as have the epidemiological minutiae of more recent Influenza epidemics (Hoyle and Wickramasinghe, 1979). These analyses completely refute the popular and tradi-tional biomedical view that the Influenza virus spreads in such

16   *E.J. Steele et al. / Progress in Biophysics and Molecular Biology 136 (2018) 3–23*

epidemics largely by person-to-person transmission. This extremely strong evidence is analyzed and documented in detail in Hoyle and Wickramasnghe (1979). The many colleagues of co-author NCW in this review article would argue that this cogent evidence should be confronted in its totality by all biologists and biomedical scientists wanting to understand the most likely drivers of many apparently unexpected (and fully unexplained) infectious epidemics that occur all the time, many with annual periodicities or periodicities that coincide with the 11 year sun-spot cycle (Wickramasinghe et al., 2017). In the case of Influenza the sudden appearance of multiple yet patchy location strikes (many, as indicated, before the advent of air travel) cannot be explained by simple infectious person-to-person disease models. However they are more completely understandable by multiple strikes or in-falls from space at widely disparate global locations dependent on vagaries like weather, topography and geography, and in particular the periodicity of the significant correlation with the 11 year Sun Spot flare cycle (Hope-Simpson, 1978; Hoyle and Wickramasinghe, 1979; reviewed in Qu, 2016; Wickramasinghe et al., 2017). With respect to the latter correlation "..the peaks of solar activity will be expected to assist in the descent of charged molecular aggregates (including viruses) from the stratosphere to ground level..along magnetic field lines that connect the Sun and the Earth" (Wickramasinghe, 2015a, p.81; Wickramasinghe et al., 2017).

It could be argued that both H-W theory and person-to-person (P-P) contact are responsible for epidemics, some epidemics being more of the H-W kind and some more of the P-P kind. In apparent support of this we all will have had experiences of catching a cold from someone else, and can remember exactly who and when we encountered the person who gave it to us. This experience of course gives us all a bias in thinking that "this is the only way to catch a virus, directly or indirectly from someone else." Yet it is precisely this widely held belief which is directly refuted in the detailed analyses of suddenly appearing Influenza epidemics (Hoyle and Wickramasinghe, 1979, see in particular Chapter 6 " Anatomy of an epidemic" and Chapter 5, the critical analysis of the 1968 Influenza pandemic): where such potential intimate P-P physical transfers cannot explain the patterns in Influenza spread (i.e. spread by body fluid vehicles such as saliva, blood, semen or in your face explosive P-P aerosols). In other cases such as *Vibrio cholerae*, a water borne bacterium, contaminated water can be identified as the direct physical vector causing Cholera diarrohea - consumed straight into the mouth and digestive tracts of susceptible victims. Salmonella food poisoning outbreaks are another familiar example of this type. So while there is clearly a mix of H-W and P-P transmission modes it does depend on the disease being studied. But if it is unexpected and explosive and on a large epidemic or pandemic scale then "in-fall from space" should be one possible default first cause to fall under suspicion. This is all discussed in detail elsewhere (Hoyle and Wickramasinghe, 1979). And it is still the case now, despite many years of flu vaccine research and improved understanding of avian flu viral reservoirs that seasonal Influenza and epidemics/pandemics are poorly understood. This ignorance is both with respect to the emergence of new antigenically unpredictable strains as well as the *actual mode* of transmission of the disease during outbreaks and epidemics (Paules et al., 2017).

An all pervasive Cosmic Biology means that many novel emergent disease-causing micro-organisms and viruses will show phylogenetic relationships with existing viral species and genera, as we are now considering a "Cosmic Gene Pool" under this viewpoint (Fig. 6). We should then assume, as one first reactive response, they have come from space - even if there are also plausible alternative terrestrial explanations of first cause i.e. the cosmic cause should be part of the possible mix of causative explanations to be ruled either in or out.

But what to do about the Cosmic possibility? At this juncture our response can only be a long-term surveillance strategy building up knowledge of the warning signs of impending pathogenic cometary debris strikes. This means organised deployment of spacecraft monitoring and recording stations, as well as more wide-spread and systematic higher atmosphere balloon-lifted sampling techniques (Wainwright et al., 2014, 2015a, 2015b) and a sophisticated monitoring system for which a prototype known as the "Hoyle Shield" has been proposed and is in very early design (Smith, 2013).

19. Paradigm shift

In our considered view Mankind is now entering a historic paradigm shifting moment in both our understanding of the evolution of life on Earth and the origins of the many pandemics that have exacted huge tolls on mankind in the recent past. Indeed all of us have contributed directly as co-authors of this paper because, in our considered opinion in confronting the wide range of scientific data, all the scientific and societal evidence seemingly points in one direction, an all-pervasive Cosmic Biology, mediated mainly by cometary transfers, being a driver for life on Earth. We believe the signs of this change are now so apparent that one of the biggest back-flips in the history of science is now on our door step (Appendix C).

If you think that our position here is farfetched, or even alarmist, we quote the late great Cornell Professor, Thomas Gold, a farsighted and creative astronomer and geophysicist (Gold, 1992, 1999) who observed closely many scientific back-flips in his long career, the most notable being in the Geosciences in the mid to late 1960s with the gigantic about-face over Alfred Wegner's 1912 theory of Continental Drift. In 1989 Tom Gold wrote:

" What does the refereeing procedure really look like? How does it really go on? If, for example, an application was made in the early 60's or late 50's suggesting that the person wanted to investigate the possibility that continents are moving around a little, it would have been ruled out absolutely instantly without questions. That was crack-pot stuff, and had long been thought dead. Wegener, of course, was an absolute crack-pot, and everybody knew that and you wouldn't have any chance.

Six years later you could not get a paper published that doubted continental drift. The herd had swung around - but it was still a firm and arrogant herd." Check it out at http://amasci.com/freenrg/newidea1.html.

A related example was the wide-spread institutional denial of the reality of meteorites during Lavoisier's time (1768) who "rejected eye-witness accounts of the fall of meteorites for the sound common sense reason that 'stones cannot fall from the sky as there are no stones in the sky' (Haynes, 1980)."

The Hoyle-Wickramasinghe thesis on the influence of an all pervasive Cosmic Biology delivered to Earth mainly via Comets is wholly in keeping with the experimental and observational evidence that has been accumulated over the past 40–50 years since first proposal. While the acceptance of these multifactorial and specific data will be long overdue this will still be a great scientific advance and we hope and trust that the new devotees will be kind, considerate and respectful to those who pioneered the field and acknowledge the priority of their scientific discoveries.

So with an avalanche of data from diverse fields all pointing to an all pervasive Cosmic Biology implying an origin of life external to Earth, the continuing reluctance of the scientific community to recognise this fact might seem strange. Yet as Tom Gold clearly shows - and we are all aware of this force in our daily lives - "Group Think" and the safety of "Running with the Herd" are powerful driving motivating forces both in science and society (Gold, 1989). These forces are quite irrational (scientifically speaking) yet very

E.J. Steele et al. / Progress in Biophysics and Molecular Biology 136 (2018) 3—23   17

powerful socially and culturally. However, the long-overdue scientific paradigm shift from Earth-centred biology to Cosmic Life will have profound implications that would extend well outside the bounds of Science (Wickramasinghe and Tokoro, 2014a, 2014b). Certainly just within biomedical sciences the straightforward implication for phylogenetic analyses based on DNA or amino acid sequence data will require a fundamental reappraisal (compare Left and Right evolutionary conceptual trajectories in Fig. 6). However the resulting upheaval in the realms of politics, religion and human self-understanding is likely to be even more dramatic and more profound than any that has happened in the past 500 years.

In a final reckoning it would have to be admitted that ultimately all of evolution has been controlled and continues to be controlled by space-borne organisms, microbes and viruses. It is important that we not allow Science to be stifled by a reign of dogmatic authority that strives to restrict its progress along narrow conservative lines. The current situation is strikingly reminiscent of the Middle Ages in Europe — Ptolemaic epicycles that delayed the acceptance of a Sun-centred planetary system for over a century (Appendix C). The current evidence suggests we came from space, we are made of viral genes, and eventually our evolutionary legacy would in full measure return to space. This will then complete the second and final phase of the Copernican revolution that was started over half a millennium ago.

Conflicts of interest

The authors declare no conflict of interest.

Author contributions

Conceptualization: Edward J Steele, N. Chandra Wickramasinghe, John P Coghlan, Kenneth A. Augustyn, Brig Klyce, Gensuke Tokoro, John A Schuster.

Contributing Data Assembly and Publications 1970s to 2017: Edward J. Steele, Shirwan Al-Mufti, S.G. Coulson, Reginald M. Gorczynski, Brig Klyce, Godfrey Louis, Keith R. Oliver, Jiangwen Qu, W.E. Smith, Duane P Snyder, Brent J. Stewart, Christopher A. Tout, Milton Wainwright, Daryl H. Wallis, Jamie Wallis, Max K. Wallis, D.T. Wickramasinghe, J.T. Wickramasinghe, N. Chandra Wickramasinghe, Yongsheng Liu.

Formal Analysis and Interpretations of Different Aspects of the Data: Edward J. Steele, Shirwan Al-Mufti, S.G. Coulson, Reginald M. Gorczynski, Brig Klyce, Godfrey Louis, Keith R. Oliver, Jiangwen Qu, W.E. Smith, Duane P Snyder, Gensuke Tokoro, Christopher A. Tout, Milton Wainwright, Daryl H. Wallis, Jamie Wallis, Max K. Wallis, D.T. Wickramasinghe, J.T. Wickramasinghe, N. Chandra Wickramasinghe, Yongsheng Liu.

Writing — Original Draft: Edward J. Steele, Gensuke Tokoro, N. Chandra Wickramasinghe.

Writing — Review & Editing: Edward J. Steele, Shirwan Al-Mufti, Kenneth A. Augustyn, Rohana Chandrajith, John P Coghlan, S.G. Coulson, Sudipto Ghosh, Mark Gillman, Reginald M. Gorczynski, Brig Klyce, Godfrey Louis, Kithsiri Mahanama, Keith R. Oliver, Julio Padron, Jiangwen Qu, John A. Schuster, W.E. Smith, Duane P Snyder, Julian A. Steele, Brent J. Stewart, Robert Temple, Gensuke Tokoro, Christopher A. Tout, Alexander Unzicker, Milton Wainwright, Jamie Wallis, Max K. Wallis, Max K. Wallis, John Wetherall, D.T. Wickramasinghe, J.T. Wickramasinghe, N. Chandra Wickramasinghe, Yongsheng Liu.

Note added in proof

A crucial prediction of the Hoyle-Wickramasinghe cosmic theory of life is that new genetic material (DNA/RNA) in the form of

bacteria and viruses arrives at the Earth from space both continuously as well as in sporadic bursts. Such a process is envisioned to extend the processes of biological evolution to involve horizontal gene transfer over galactic or cosmic dimensions. The search for such incoming bacteria and viruses using balloon-borne equipment lofted to the stratosphere has been carried out for nearly two decades (Harris et al, 2002; Wainwright et al, 2003; Shivaji et al, 2009). Stratospheric air samples recovered from heights ranging from 28 to 41 km have indeed yielded evidence of microorganisms, but these have been widely regarded as most likely to have been lofted from the Earth's surface. The situation has changed dramatically in recent months, however. T.V. Grebennikova et al (2018) have now confirmed the discovery of several microbial species associated with cosmic dust on the exterior windows of the International Space Station (ISS), and contamination at source and in the laboratory has been ruled out. The results of PCR amplification followed by DNA sequencing and phylogenetic analysis have established the presence of bacteria of the genus *Mycobacteria* and the extremophile genus *Delftia*, amongst others, associated with deposits of cosmic dust, which are now from a height of some 400km above the Earth's surface. A terrestrial origin seems most unlikely. Studies by Wickramasinghe and Rycroft (2018) have shown that all possible mechanisms for lofting these organisms against gravity to heights of 400km in the ionosphere fall short by many orders of magnitude.

Appendix A. Origins of life and scientific alternatives to the H-W cosmic panspermia?

> " "Let us seek to fathom those things that are fathomable and reserve those things that are unfathomable for reverence in solitude.." Johann Wolfgang von Goethe"

At this stage of our scientific understanding we need to place on hold the issue of life's actual biochemical origins - where, when and how may be too difficult to solve on the current evidence. The current paper is focused on the evidence for an all pervasive Cosmic Biology and its effects on the emergence of life on Earth and its further evolution. Certainly all attempts at abiogenesis in the laboratory on Earth have been unsuccessful. It is many orders of magnitude more likely that it emerged in one of the trillions of comet-like incubators or water-bearing planets (cosmic-wide versions of Darwin's 'warm little ponds') at a very early time in the growth of this Universe, perhaps 12 Billion years ago (Wickramasinghe, 2015a) which then went on to infect via knock-on effects other life-favourable sites (planets, moons, comets) throughout that Galaxy and then in an interconnected and interactive way throughout the Cosmos as the Universe expanded. The spherical Oort Cloud, the source of long period Comets around our solar system provides a causal connection and explanation. Possibly the majority of these billions of comets *did not* originate from our Solar System accretion plane — they have most likely arisen by capture of Comets by our Sun's gravity from other passing Solar Systems (Levison et al., 2010).

One of us (BK) thinks " that the complexity and sophistication of life cannot *originate* (from non-biological) matter under any scenario, over any expanse of space and time, however vast. If this were to be so, then, supernatural intervention or intelligence would be required, following the standard big bang (see also Walker and Wickramasinghe, 2015). A strictly scientific way around this dilemma would be to amend or tweak the big bang theory to allow for life from the eternal past. After all, the big bang theory is relatively new and still occasionally amended. Therefore it seems unready to forever overrule the unviolated principle and consistent evidence that life comes from life."

18   *E.J. Steele et al. / Progress in Biophysics and Molecular Biology 136 (2018) 3–23*

Another of us (EJS) might state this same scenario a little differently, based on the positions published in Hoyle and Wickramasinghe (1978b, 1979, 1981): "Is the Universe an Infinite Steady-State (a rolling series of big bangs and contractions) - as advanced in 1948 by Fred Hoyle, Tom Gold and Herman Bondi - or just the conventional "Big Bang"? The latter is what most Mathematical Physicists and Astronomers adhere to at the present time, but it cannot by any means be regarded as set in stone (Tegmark, 2014). Both alternatives make the rational scientific mind boggle. But if we are to choose, then on the basis of the existence of Cosmic-wide, mutually interactive Biology, a Steady-State Universe (or a Quasi-Steady State Universe, Hoyle et al., 2000) with infinite time provides all the time needed for abiogenesis by trial-and-error elimination in trillions of warm-little ponds throughout the Cosmos (to put together the incredible phenomenon of the living cell with its thousands of interacting genes driving the processes of cellular life on a cosmic scale). Thus Hoyle and Wickramasinghe (1981) concluded that the improbabilities for the non-random assemblage of living proteins and nucleic acids are so huge (1 part in $10^{40,000}$) that maybe an 'Infinite Universe' or super intelligent God would be required to produce a living miracle, which then spread and evolved on a Cosmic scale." It is the confrontation with these profound empirical-based issues that may well explain the honest and very public back-flip of the late noted humanist philosopher, Antony Flew (2007).

However with respect to the immediate origin of life on Earth we think, based on the evidence, there is no serious alternative scientific theory to the Hoyle-Wickramasinghe model of Cosmic (Cometary) Panspermia as the major driver of life on Earth. About 1960 Tom Gold when asked in public, and then after surveying the evidence before him, apparently stated in half jest: " A space-ship landed on the Earth in the early days, scattering living cells, which have evolved and persisted ever since." Hoyle and Wickramasinghe, 1981, p.30]. And this was given some considerable gravitas in 1973 by Francis Crick and Leslie Orgel who published their own theory of "Directed Panspermia" ie. a super intelligent civilization seeded life by sending space ships three to four billions of years ago. Their scientific reason for advancing such a theory was to explain the extraordinary facts of the exquisite complexity yet 'generality' of the Genetic Code: which indeed allows us to clone and express human genes in bacteria and vice versa - and underpins all modern biotechnology, biomedical therapeutics and biomedical research. The H-W explanation is far more reasonable and scientific in our view (a parsimonious model).

It has been suggested by a critical co-author (KAA) that both H-W theory and life emerging from non-life on Earth are both possibly true. Thus for KAA " Life could have emerged from non-life in many different ways and places, *including* here on Earth." Thus Panspermia is perfectly consistent with life *also* having emerged here on Earth. In a recent book *The Vital Question* Nick Lane (2015) provides a possible theory of life emerging from non-life on Earth and suggests that life could have emerged in a similar fashion independently at many locations in the Universe. Hoyle and Wickramasinghe have already considered this possibility for terrestrial origins in depth. To Hoyle and Wickramasinghe it is a sophisticated variant of the spontaneous generation view refuted by Louis Pasteur in the 19th Century. Moreover, it merely compounds indefinitely the gross difficulties envisaged with an origin of life at one site only. It also takes no account of the recognised modern fact that hundreds of billions of habitable planets exist in the galaxy alone, with average separations of the order of a few light years. Exchanges of biotic material between adjacent planets and therefore a single connected biosphere appears inevitable. We suggest an extraterrestrial emergence of life in the early Cosmos as the most likely based on all the current evidence (again H-W is the

more parsimonious model).

However what is very strange about the book *The Vital Question* by Nick Lane (2015) is that he dismisses panspermia as irrelevant: " Panspermia fails utterly to address those principles (the steps he outlines as important in life's abiogenic origin), and so is irrelevant." (p.94n). This completely misses the point of an extant all pervasive extraterrestrial Biology, throughout the Solar System, and almost certainly from the interstellar infra red extinction data, throughout the wider Cosmos. Of this Nick Lane seems oblivious. Yet in a striking contradiction in the same book (p.55–56) Lane discusses the Tardigrades (Wiki Box) and accurately describes in detail their space-hardy characteristics! The key issue then is the extensive evidence, briefly reviewed here in our paper, for an all pervasive Cosmic Biology that mankind now needs to confront. This knowledge will allow us to better understand the ongoing evolutionary process and also the emergence of new explosive disease epidemics in our domestic animals and plants, as well as in human beings.

Writers of popular science books such as Nick Lane of University College London, have considered it fashionable to dismiss the Hoyle-Wickramasinghe thesis in one-line disproofs. This is disappointing because his book displays much innovative and imaginative thinking on likely scenarios for the emergence of life, not only on Earth but also throughout the Cosmos. There is no need to be dismissive of the manifest data all around us for Cosmic Biology. While abiogenesis causation may be unlikely for Earth, his vivid and knowledgeable scenarios for porous alkaline hydrothermal (temperate) deep sea vents as sites of early likely bioenergenesis (early mitochondrial-like proton-gradient driven membrane bounded energy systems) are being tested in the laboratory. Indeed the plethora of experiments that Nick Lane's thinking inspires (with his collaborators such as Bill Martins and his PhD students) needs to be encouraged and funded. Sooner or later, after much Popperian trial and error elimination of the numerous steps to self-replicating energetic living systems, we have no doubt that mankind led by people like Nick Lane will eventually execute a successful abiogenesis experiment. This will be informed by the integrated insight of past failures to pull off an "origins of life" demonstration from simple cosmic-wide starting materials (H_2, CO_2, CO, silicates, phosphates, iron-sulphur aggregates, H_2O, etc) in the test tube. That would truly be an epoch-changing experiment for mankind. But at the moment we have the mountain of parsimonious data of extraterrestrial life all around us to integrate and understand the full consequences.

Another co-author and theoretical physicist (AZ) takes the Tom Gold scenario further and considers the probabilities of a Cosmic origin thus: " Since the idea of a cosmic origin of life is not yet accepted in the field of evolutionary biology, it has not entered the mainstream of general scientists either - however, that might change. In his 2014 book "Superintelligence", Oxford philosopher Nick Bostrom argues that humanity sooner or later will develop forms intelligence that vastly exceed the human level. Whether this will occur on a short timescale (via artificial intelligence generated by new algorithms in existing hardware) or in the more distant future when nanotechnology will allow building copies of the human brain, is irrelevant for our discussion here - on astronomical timescales, it will be a blink of an eye in both cases. Such a superintelligence will easily be able (and likely willing) to build spacecraft (or smaller units) that can efficiently distribute primitive forms of life in other regions of the Milky Way far from the solar system - thus panspermia. The timescale for this would be thousands rather than millions of years, that is, negligible. So it is certainly a reasonable hypothesis that such a superintelligent planet could have 10–100 descending civilizations. That would imply however we have an *a priori* likelihood of 90–99 percent of

E.J. Steele et al. / Progress in Biophysics and Molecular Biology 136 (2018) 3–23   19

being of cosmic origin - that's what a simple Bayesian analysis suggests after just one 'generation'.

AZ goes further: " It is remarkable that Bostrom's thesis has passed unchallenged so far - it appears that no serious counterarguments exist (see, e.g. Wikipedia - Superintellligence). Yet it has profound consequences for our discussion here. Science is sometimes schizophrenic - a hypothesis can be interesting and convincing in one field (here: Neurobiology) whereas in another field it is considered not worth debating (Evolutionary Biology)."

But there is clearly one very fundamental process discovered and developed by Irena Cosic and her colleagues, the molecular resonance recognition between receptor-ligand macromolecules (proteins, nucleic acids), that needs to be integrated *into all thinking* of how life may have emerged in the first place and continues to evolve. This is electromagnetic-mediated intermolecular recognition and functional activation *prior to* actual binding which is essential in all living systems and should be factored into all models and experiments on abiogenesis (Cosic, 1994; Cosic et al., 2015, 2016; Cosic and Cosic, 2016).

With the rapidly increasing number of exoplanets that have been discovered in the habitable zones of long-lived red dwarf stars (Gillon et al., 2016), the prospects for genetic exchanges between life-bearing Earth-like planets cannot be ignored. In our view the idea of life emerging *de novo* in multiple locations through a process of *in situ* abiogenesis appears far-fetched and merely compounds the difficulty of a single origination on the Earth. The internal evidence from terrestrial biology that we have discussed in this paper suggests that the entire ensemble of habitable planets in the galaxy constitutes a single interconnected biosphere. Lifeforms elsewhere, on this viewpoint, will be expected to exhibit a converging pattern of genotypes and phenotypes, subject to natural selection (Darwinian and Lamarckian) within individual planetary habitats. The recent announcement of 7 "habitable" planets around the star Trappist 1 located 40 light years away is therefore timely (Gillon et al., 2016) and relevant to the thesis discussed in the present paper. Future investigations are planned to search for spectral signatures of molecular oxygen and methane in the planetary atmospheres as indicators of life; although such molecules (and much more) have indeed been detected in dwarf planets and comets within the solar system with no reference being made to biology.

Finally, the idea of 'Necropanspermia should be addressed (Wesson, 2011) - the idea that organisms are continually arriving on Earth but are so degraded by ionizing radiation and the desiccation rigours of space, they are dead on arrival. Yet they will add to the terrestrial gene pool (DNA/RNA) albeit dead. We had considered this in an earlier draft but decided not to include it in the main section. We thought then (Wickramasinghe, 2011), and still think, Wesson's ideas are contradictory and thus non-viable scientifically in the broad sweep of all the evidences for the continued arrival of living organisms to Earth (with their space—hardy and space-resistant properties over the past 4 Billion years).

Appendix B. Retroviruses, Alu and LINE retroelements - structure, function, genome mobility and significance

The interspersed short (SINE) and long (LINE) repetitive retro-elements elements (RLEs) in the human and mammalian genome are major features of genome structure and drivers of genomic evolutionary diversity (see reviews by Kapitonov and Jurka, 1996; Arcot et al., 1996; Cordaux and Batzer, 2009) and germline retro-transpositions of this type discussed much earlier as general evolutionary mechanisms in Steele et al. (1984). They exist in multiple copies dispersed by reverse transcriptase-mediated retrotransposition across the genome. The LINE RLEs are long

interspersed nuclear elements (about $\geq 500,000$ copies in the human genome) and different families of elements have been continuously active (in their genomic mobility) for the past 150 Mya, and the current activity of the main L1 elements are in the Brian, where each neurone has a unique mobilized L1 element indicative of a normal physiological role in the healthy human Brain and CNS development in specific neurone commitment (Erwin et al., 2016). They are about 6Kb and encode their own reverse transcriptase (RT) and supply this RT activity to co-mobilise the smaller Alu elements (approx. 300 bp, about 1.1 million copies in the human genome). LINE and Alu RLEs are located in the tran-scriptionally active gene rich regions of the genome, usually in in-trons (as their insertion in coding regions, while it happens, usually leads to such dramatic gene disruptions, that strong purifying se-lection purges the organism of such lethal mutations, only toler-ating harmless and 'neutral' LINE and Alu insertions which usually lie outside protein-coding portions). However, LINE and Alu ret-roelements are of functional importance (Steele, 2015; Erwin et al., 2016) with Alu repeats located in the intronic regions of Brain and CNS neurones of major significance (Paz-Yaacov et al., 2010). The Alu elements have a dimeric structure originally derived from the RNA of the 7SL RNA of gene-signal recognition particle and in their central portions they are adenosine (A)-rich and thus ideal targets in dsRNA structures for Adenosine-to-Inosine (A-to-I) pre-mRNA editing mediated by ADAR deaminases, again a prominent activity of great significance in the human and higher primate Brain and CNS (Paz-Yaacov et al., 2010). Indeed "Alu-exonization", or new gene creation via RNA editing leading to new pre-mRNA splice sites (thus exon skipping during pre-mRNA splicing) both generates and destroys existing exons and thus make new gene isoforms (on which physiological somatic selection may act to enhance the synaptic functions of the Brain and CNS). Such somatic neuronal gene re-arrangements can of course, also lead to pathology and diseases such as Alzheimer's Diseases, Parkinson Disease, Autism Spectrum Disorder. Recognised Alu families are very good evolu-tionary markers. Based on consensus sequences they can be divided into at least three families (and their subfamilies). The oldest Alu J, expanded by transcription/reverse transcription 81 mya; the pri-mate specific Alu S, subfamilies Sx, Sq, Sp, Sc all platyrrhine specific, expanded across the genome 35–44 mya; and Sg about 31 mya. The Primate specific Alu Y subfamily spread 19 mya to as recently as several hundred thousand years ago. Such markers linked to other emerging new genes allow molecular "dating" of emergence of new germline gene families in the Primate lines leading to Homo Sapi-ens. Along with the similar endogenous retroviruses (ERVs, about 10 Kb and >200,000 copies per haploid human genome) the mul-tiple copies of the LINE and Alu retroelements elements are drivers of duplicative genomic expansions as their similar sequences, separated yet physically in tandem nearby, can drive large segmental duplications by unequal crossing over during meiosis thus increasing both genome size and functional diversity (Dawkins et al., 1999; McLure et al., 2013; Steele, 2014, 2015).

A feature of retroviruses is their ability to incorporate non-randomly host cell enzymes and small RNAs of various types into virions. As well as reverse transcriptase (RTs) proteins (>50 per virion) and host-derived APOBEC3G enzymes which are DNA mutators (C-to-U deamination of ssDNA) and host specific pre-tRNAs that prime reverse transcription, selective packaging of multiple host cell noncoding RNAs also includes signal recognition particle 7SL RNA, (the 300 nt RNA precursors of Alu RNA retro-elements) as well as host Alu RNAs themselves, specific regulato-ry microRNAs and spliceosomal U6 small nuclear RNA (snRNA), normally thought of as residing only in mammalian nuclei, sug-gesting new mechanisms involving these RNAs in retroviral as-sembly and infectivity. Thus whilst the two 10 kb viral genomes are

20   *E.J. Steele et al. / Progress in Biophysics and Molecular Biology 136 (2018) 3–23*

the main occupants of mature retroviral virions it is now recognised that the infecting virus delivers many more additional specific proteins and nucleic acid species to the intended target cell than previously thought (Tian et al., 2007; Bach, 2008; Hu et al., 2012; Lin et al., 2012; Eckwahl et al., 2016; Telesnitsky et al., 2016) - no doubt assisting the very mutagenic cellular environment triggered by the infection of HIV and other viruses.

In the text the "The Transposable -Element (TE) -Thrust Hypothesis " of Oliver and Greene was mentioned (2012). This is envisaged as an intrinsic force, intermittently thrusting adaptation, speciation, and the evolution of novelties forward, often, but not always, in a punctuated equilibrium manner. When most of the TEs become deactivated by accumulated mutations, and if they are not replaced by horizontal transposon transfer, or by endogenised retroviruses, etc. lineages can become "Living Fossils", and further, if this lack of TE-Thrust continues then lineages can become extinct, as a part of the background extinction, which appears to accounts for the overwhelming majority of the extinctions on Earth.

Appendix C. Visualizing the causes and drivers of the history of life on earth implied by this paper

(By co-author John A Schuster, Historian and Philosopher of Science, an authority on Descartes and the Copernican Revolution who did his PhD under Thomas S Kuhn). "The foregoing paper implies a radical challenge to the present scientific consensus about the causes that are taken to explain the history of life on Earth. The presently accepted Darwinian mechanisms, related to best practice geological history of the Earth, are not questioned. They are, however, placed in a new set of relations to a wider theoretical nexus, grounded, on the one hand, in developments in astrophysics, then astrobiology since the original and ongoing contributions of Fred Hoyle and N. Chandra Wickramasinghe and their colleagues, and on the other hand, in the developments in virology and molecular biology, including, most importantly, the ongoing improvements in neo-Lamarckian models in molecular immunology developed by Edward J. Steele and various colleagues over the past forty years.

One may initially envision the nature and scope of the new synthesis on analogy to how differential equations describing known laws interact with the boundary conditions that need to be fed into them to produce concrete solutions. We may say that the normally agreed Darwinian processes, along with Steele's neo-Lamarckian ones, always operate on Earth. They are analogous to the routine equations or algorithms employed to describe a system. As to the boundary conditions applied to the equations in order to produce concrete solutions, we now have a radical new vision. There are shifting, unpredictable and, in geological terms, sudden astrobiological inputs. It is as though someone were insisting on changing the boundary conditions randomly from time to time. The history of life on Earth becomes the temporal record of the outputs of the underlying Darwinian/neo Lamarckian mechanisms or equations as they have worked over time upon a concatenation of randomly timed, quickly and radically altered boundary conditions. At the time of a new astrobiological input, the state of life on Earth will have been the product of all previous workings of the fundamental mechanisms upon and through the sequence of previous astrobiological inputs. With a new input, the system will further evolve, based on the input, the mechanisms and the previously achieved state.

As the paper argues, the causal elements taken to be involved in biological evolution need to radically modified beyond the neo-Darwinian consensus. This is achieved by grasping and conceptually articulating to each other findings and models in previously widely disparate domains such as astrobiology and molecular immunology. The new synthesis suggests that the concrete history

of life on Earth will necessarily reveal facts about, and mappings amongst, biological groupings significantly different from those imposed by reading the evidence solely in the light of Neo-Darwinism. Just as the promise of Nicholas Copernicus' first proposal in 1543 was only fully realized several generations later on the basis of Kepler's adducing of laws and possible causal mechanisms for planetary motion and Galileo's discovery of dramatic confirmatory empirical evidence, so the Hoyle-Wickramasinghe panspermia model can now be fleshed out and articulated by means of two generations of findings in astrobiology and molecular biology. In each case the initial claims were potentially revolutionary and quite brilliantly executed in themselves. But in each case it was necessary for wider and deeper empirical and theoretical foundations to be laid under the original claim—foundations making use of factual and theoretical materials not necessarily available at the time of the founders' inaugural claims.

Finally, let us take an even wider view and speculate about the kinds of challenges the new synthesis poses to a range of political, cultural and religious beliefs. Revolutionary theories almost always have such a penumbra of wider consequences. The paper hints at this, without of course being able to enter into any detail. For example, amongst the wider scientifically literate public, the dominant popular versions of neo-Darwinism are threatened, along with the many cultural, philosophical and public policy claims that have been leveraged from it. For religious believers of all stripes, the new synthesis, even more than orthodox Darwinism, demystifies the history of life on Earth and embeds it in a history of cosmic events, that is, the history of the Universe at large. Finally, as intellectual historians and historians of science have long recognized, there is a central question that has energized both biological and socio-political theorizing since the early 19th century; that is, even before Darwin. That question concerns 'Man's place in nature'- where 'nature' meant 'the immediate terrestrial environment'. The new synthesis re-invents and extends that question: We will now be inquiring about humankind's place in, and relations to, the entire cosmos, and, in particular, we will be viewing humankind's situation as the result of a concatenation of cosmic processes and events that have impacted the Earth in a decidedly ruptural and randomly causative manner. " (*Note*: The Evolutionary Physiologist Denis Noble of Oxford has also used the argument from boundary and initial conditions (Chapter 6 of *Dance to the Tune of Life* (2017) and was first used first used in Noble (2011).

References

Aaskov, J., et al., 2006. Long- term transmission of defective RNA viruses in humans and Aedes mosquitoes. Science 311, 236–238.

Abe, F., et al., 2013. Extending the planetary mass function to Earth mass by microlensing at moderately high magnification. Mon. Not. Roy. Astron. Soc. 431 (4), 2975–2985.

Aiewsakun, P., Katzourakis, A., 2017. Marine origin of retroviruses in the early Palaeozoic Era. Nat. Commun. 8, 13954. https://doi.org/10.1038/ncomms13954.

Albertin, C.B., et al., 2015. The octopus genome and the evolution of cephalopod neural and morphological novelties. Nature 524, 220–224.

Allen, D.A., Wickramasinghe, D.T., 1981. Diffuse interstellar absorption bands between 2.9 and 4.0 μm. Nature 294, 239–240.

Altwegg, K., et al., 2016. Prebiotic chemical – amino acid and phosphorus in the coma of comet 67P/Churyumov-Gerasimenko. Sci. Adv 2, e1600285, 27 May.

Arcot, S.S., et al., 1996. Alu fossil relics - distribution and insertion polymorphism. Genome Res. 6, 1084–1092.

Bach, D., 2008. Characterization of APOBEC3G binding to 7SL RNA. Retrovirology 5, 54. https://doi.org/10.1186/1742-4690-5-54.

Bell, E.A., et al., 2015. Potentially biogenic carbon preserved in a 4.1 billion-year-old zircon. Proc. Natl. Acad. Sci. U.S.A. 112, 14518–14521.

Bergmann, S., et al., 2006. The hemocyanin from a living fossil, the cephalopod Nautilus pompilius: protein structure, gene organization, and evolution. J. Mol. Evol. 62, 362–374.

Bianciardi, G., et al., 2012. Complexity analysis of the viking labelled Release experiments. Intl J. Aeronautical & Space Sci. 13, 14–26. https://doi.org/10.5139/IJASS.2012.13.1.14.

Bieler, K., et al., 2015. Abundant molecular oxygen in the coma of comet 67P/

E.J. Steele et al. / Progress in Biophysics and Molecular Biology 136 (2018) 3–23   21

Churyumov—Gerasimenko. Nature 526, 678—681. https://doi.org/10.1038/nature15707.

Biver, N., et al., 2015. Ethyl alcohol and sugar in comet C/2014 Q2 (Lovejoy). Sci. Adv. 1, e1500863, 23 October 2015.

Bostrom, N., 2014. Superintelligence: Paths, Dangers, Strategies. Oxford University Press, Oxford, UK.

Brasier, M., 2012. Secret Chambers. Oxford University Press. ISBN 9780199644001.

Buhr, F., et al., 2016. Synonymous codons direct co-translational folding towards different protein conformations. Mol. Cell 61, 342—351.

Campbell, J.H., Perkins, P., 1988. Transgenerational effects of drug and hormonal treatments in mammals: a review of observations and ideas. In: Boer, G.J., Feenstra, M.G.P., Mirmiran, M., Swaab, D.F., van Haaren, F. (Eds.), Progress in Brain Research, vol. 73, pp. 535—553.

Capaccione, F., et al., 2015. The organic-rich surface of comet 67P/Churyumov-Gerasimenko as seen by VIRTIS/Rosetta. Science 347 (6220).

Carlini, D.B., et al., 2000. Actin gene family evolution and the phylogeny of coleoid cephalopods (Mollusca: cephalopoda). Mol. Biol. Evol. 17, 1353—1370.

Chen, Y.-H., et al., 2015. Phosphatidylserine vesicles enable efficient en bloc transmission of enteroviruses. Cell 160, 619—630. https://doi.org/10.1016/j.cell.2015.01.032.

Chiu, Y.-L., Greene, W.C., 2006. APOBEC3 Cytidine Deaminases: distinct antiviral actions along the retroviral life cycle. J. Biol. Chem. 281, 8309—8312. https://doi.org/10.1074/jbc.R500021200.

Chivian, D, et al., 2008. Environmental genomics reveals a single-species ecosystem deep within the Earth. Science 322, 275—278.

Christener, B.C., et al., 2014. A microbial ecosystem beneath the West Antarctic ice sheet. Nature 512, 310—313. https://doi.org/10.1038/nature13667.

Clube, S.V.M., et al., 1996. Giant comets, evolution and civilization. Astrophys. Space Sci. 245, 43—60.

Combe, M., et al., 2015. Single-cell analysis of RNA virus infection identifies multiple genetically diverse viral genomes within single infectious units. Cell Host Microbe 18, 424—432. https://doi.org/10.1016/j.chom.2015.09.009.

Cordaux, R., Batzer, M.A., 2009. The impact of retrotranspositions on human genome evolution. Nat. Rev. Genet. 10, 691—703.

Cosic, I., 1994. Macromolecular bioactivity: is it resonant interaction between macromolecules? - Theory and applications. IEEE Trans. Biomed. Eng. 41, 1101—1114.

Cosic, I., Cosic, D., 2016. The treatment of crigler-najjar syndrome by blue light as explained by resonant recognition model. EPJ Nonlinear Biomedical Physics 4, 9. https://doi.org/10.1140/epjnbp/s40366-016-0016-x.

Cosic, I., et al., 2015. Is it possible to predict electromagnetic resonances in proteins, DNA and RNA? EPJ Nonlinear Biomedical Physics 3, 5. https://doi.org/10.1140/s40366-015-0020-6.

Cosic, I., et al., 2016. Environmental light and its relationship with electromagnetic resonances of biomolecular interactions, as predicted by the Resonant Recognition Model. Int. J. Environ. Res. Publ. Health 13 (7), 647,. https://doi.org/10.3390/ijerph13070647.

Cossetti, C., et al., 2014. Soma-to- germline transmission of RNA in mice xenografted with human tumour cells: possible transport by exosomes. PLoS One 9, e101629.

Coulson, S.G., Wickramasinghe, N.C., 2000. IR spectrometry of coals. In: Celnikier, L.M., Tran Thanh Van, J. (Eds.), Frontiers of Life, Proceedings of the XIIth Recontres de Blois, pp. 233—236.

Coulson, S.G., Wickramasinghe, N.C., 2003. Frictional and radiation heating of micron-sized meteoroids in the Earth's upper atmosphere. Mon. Not. Roy. Astron. Soc. 343, 1123—1130.

Coulson, S.G., et al., 2014. On the dynamics of volatile meteorites. Mon. Not. Roy. Astron. Soc. 445, 3669—3673.

Crick, F.H.C., Orgel, L.E., 1973. Directed panspermia. Icarus 19, 341—346.

Dawkins, R.L., 2015. Adapting Genetics: Quantal Evolution after Natural Selection — Surviving the Changes to Come. Nearurban Publishing, Dallas, TX. ISBN 978-0-9864115-1-9.

Dawkins, R.L., et al., 1999. Genomics of the major histocompatibility complex: haplotypes, duplication, retroviruses and disease. Immunol. Rev. 167, 275—304.

Deamer, D., 2011. First Life: Discovering the Connections between Stars, Cells, and How Life Began. University of California Press, Berkeley, USA.

Devanapally, S., et al., 2015. Double-stranded RNA made in C. elegans neurons can enter the germline and cause transgenerational gene silencing. Proc. Natl. Acad. Sci. U.S.A. 112, 2133—2138. https://doi.org/10.1073/pnas.1423333112.

Diehl, W.E., et al., 2016. Tracking interspecies transmission and long-term evolution of an ancient retrovirus using the genomes of modern mammals. eLife 5, e12704.

Dodd, M.C., et al., 2017. Evidence for early life in Earth's oldest hydrothermal vent precipitates. Nature 543, 60—65.

Doria, M., et al., 2009. Editing of HIV-1 RNA by the double-stranded RNA deaminase ADAR1 stimulates viral infection. Nucleic Acids Res. 37, 5848—5858.

Eckwahl, M.J., et al., 2016. Host RNA packaging by retroviruses: a newly synthesized story. mBio 7 (1). https://doi.org/10.1128/mBio.02025-15 e02025—15.

Eldredge, N., Gould, S.J., 1972. Punctuated equilibria : an alternative to phyletic gradualism. In: Schopf, T.J.M. (Ed.), Models in Paleobiology. Freeman Cooper, San Francisco, pp. 82—115.

Erwin, J.A., et al., 2016. L1-associated genomic regions are deleted in somatic cells of the healthy human brain. Nat. Neurosci. 19, 1583—1591. https://doi.org/10.1038/nn.4388.

Flew, A., 2007. There Is a God : How the World's Most Notorious Atheist Changed

His Mind. Harper Collins, New York.

Fox, D., 2014. Antartica's secret garden. Nature 512, 244—246.

Frank, L.A., Sigwarth, J.B., 2001. Detection of small comets with a ground-based telescope. J. Geophys. Res. 106, 3665—3683.

Franklin, A., et al., 2004. Human DNA polymerase-η, an A-T mutator in somatic hypermutation of rearranged immunoglobulin genes, is a reverse transcriptase. Immunol. Cell Biol. 82, 219—225. https://doi.org/10.1046/j.0818-9641.2004.01221.x.

Gibson, C., et al., 2011. The origin of life from primordial planets. Int. J. Astrobiol. 10, 83—98. https://doi.org/10.1017/S1473550410000352. https://arxiv.org/abs/1004.0504.

Gillon, et al., 2016. Temperate earth size planets transiting a nearby ultracool dwarf star. Nature 533, 221—224.

Gold, T., 1989. New ideas in science. J. Sci. Explor. 3 (2), 103—112. http://amasci.com/freenrg/newidea1.html.

Gold, T., 1992. The deep hot biosphere. Proc. Natl. Acad. Sci. U.S.A. 89, 6045—6049.

Gold, T., 1999. The Deep Hot Biosphere: the Myth of Fossil Fuels. Copernicus. Springer Verlag, New York.

Gorczynski, R.M., Steele, E.J., 1980. Inheritance of acquired immunologic tolerance to foreign histocompatibility antigens in mice. Proc. Natl. Acad. Sci. U.S.A. 77, 2871—2875.

Gorczynski, R.M., Steele, E.J., 1981. Simultaneous yet independent inheritance of somatically acquired tolerance to two distinct H-2 antigenic haplotype determinants in mice. Nature 289, 678—681. https://doi.org/10.1038/289678a0.

Gould, S.J., Eldredge, N., 1977. Punctuated equilibria: the tempo and mode of evolution reconsidered. Paleobiology 3, 115—151.

Grebennikova, T.V., Syroeshkin, A.V., Shubralova, E.V., et al., 2018. The DNA of bacteria of the World Ocean and the Earth in cosmic dust at the International Space Station. Sci. World J. In press.

Harris, M.J., et al., 2002. The detection of living cells in the stratosphere. Proc.SPIE Conf. 4495, 192—198.

Harris, R.S., Liddament, M.T., 2004. Retroviral restriction by APOBEC proteins. Nat. Rev. Immunol. 4, 868—877.

Haynes, R., 1980. The boggle threshold. Encounter 92—96. Aug 1980.

Hiel, C.S., et al., 2014. Functional activity of plasmid DNA after entry into the atmosphere of Earth investigated by a new biomarker stability assay for Ballistic Spaceflight Experiments. e112979 PLoS One 9.

Hoover, R.B., 2005. Microfossils, biominerals, and chemical biomarkers in meteorites. In: Hoover, R.B., Rozanov, A.Y., Paepe (Eds.), Perspectives in Astrobiology. RR IOS Press, Amsterdam, pp. 43—65.

Hoover, R.B., 2011. Fossils of cyanobacteria in CI1 carbonaceous meteorites: implications for life on comets, Europa and Enceladus. J. Cosmology 16, 7070—7111.

Hope-Simpson, R.E., 1978. Sunspots and flu: a correlation. Nature 275, 86.

Hoyle, F., Wickramasinghe, N.C., 1976. Primitive grain clumps and organic compounds in carbonaceous chondrites. Nature 264, 45.

Hoyle, F., Wickramasinghe, N.C., 1977a. Polysaccharides and the infrared spectra of galactic sources. Nature 268, 610—612.

Hoyle, F., Wickramasinghe, N.C., 1977b. Identification of the 2200A interstellar absorption feature. Nature 270, 323.

Hoyle, F., Wickramasinghe, N.C., 1978a. Calculations of infrared fluxes from galactic sources for a polysaccharide grain model. Astrophys. Space Sci. 53, 489—505.

Hoyle, F., Wickramasinghe, N.C., 1978b. Life Cloud. J.M. Dent Ltd, London.

Hoyle, F., Wickramasinghe, N.C., 1979. Diseases from Space. J.M. Dent Ltd, London.

Hoyle, F., Wickramasinghe, N.C., 1981. Evolution from Space. J.M. Dent Ltd, London.

Hoyle, F., Wickramasinghe, C., 1982. Why Neo-Darwinism Does Not Work. University College Cardiff Press. ISBN 0 906449 50 2.

Hoyle, F., Wickramasinghe, N.C., 1985. Living Comets. Univ. College, Cardiff Press, Cardiff.

Hoyle, F., Wickramasinghe, N.C., 1986. The case for life as a cosmic phenomenon. Nature 322, 509—511.

Hoyle, F., Wickramasinghe, N.C., 1991. The Theory of Cosmic Grains. Kluwer, Dordrecht.

Hoyle, F., Wickramasinghe, N.C., 1993. Our Place in the Cosmos : the Unfinished Revolution. J.M. Dent Ltd, London.

Hoyle, F., Wickramasinghe, N.C., 1997. Life on Mars? : the Case for a Cosmic Heritage. Clinical Press Ltd, Bristol.

Hoyle, F., Wickramasinghe, N.C., 2000. Astronomical Origins of Life: Steps towards Panspermia. Kluwer, Dordrecht.

Hoyle, F., et al., 1982. Infrared spectroscopy over the 2.9-3.9μm waveband in biochemistry and astronomy. Astrophys. Space Sci. 83, 405—409.

Hoyle, F., et al., 1984. The spectroscopic identification of interstellar grains. Astrophys. Space Sci. 98, 343—352.

Hu, W.-S., et al., 2012. HIV-1 reverse transcription. Cold Spring Harb Perspect Med 2 a006882, 22 pages.

Jablonka, E., Lamb, M.J., 1995. Epigenetic Inheritance and Evolution:The Lamarckian Dimension. Oxford University Press, Oxford.

Jablonka, E., Lamb, M.J., 2005. Evolution in Four Dimensions: Genetic, Epigenetic, Behavioral, and Symbolic Variation in the History of Life. MIT Press, Boston. ISBN 0-262-10107-6.

Jones, R.B., et al., 2013. LINE-1 retrotransposable element DNA accumulates in HIV-1- infected cells. J. Virol. 87, 13307—13320.

Jönsson, K.I., et al., 2008. Tardigrades survive exposure to space in low Earth orbit. Curr. Biol. 18, R729—R731.

Kapitonov, V., Jurka, J., 1996. The age of Alu subfamilies. J. Mol. Evol. 42, 59—65.

Katzourakis, A., 2013. Paleovirology: inferring viral evolution from host genome

22 *E.J. Steele et al. / Progress in Biophysics and Molecular Biology 136 (2018) 3–23*

sequence data. Phil. Trans. Roy. Soc. Lond. 368, 20120493.

Kopparapu, R.K., 2013. A revised estimate of the occurrence rate of terrestrial planets in habitable zones around Kepler M-Dwarf. Astrophys. J. 767, L8.

Kuhn, T.S., 1970. The Structure of Scientific Revolutions, second ed. Univ. Chicago Press, Chicago.

Lane, N., 2015. The Vital Question: Energy, Evolution, and the Origins of Complex Life. W.W. Norton & Company, London.

Levin, G.V., 2007. Modern myths of Mars. Int. J. Astrobiol. 6, 95–108.

Levin, G.V., 2013. Implications of Curiosity's findings for the viking labelled Release experiment and life on Mars. Instruments, methods, and missions for astrobiology XVI. In: SPIE Proc., 8865, 8865–8862.

Levin, G.V., 2015. The curiousness of Curiosity. Astrobiology 15, 101–103. https://doi.org/10.1089/ast.2014.1406.

Levin, G.V., Straat, P.A., 1976. Viking Labeled Release biology experiment: interim results. Science 194, 1322–1329.

Levin, G.V., Straat, P.A., 2016. The case for extant life on Mars and its possible detection by the Viking Labelled Release Experiment. Astrobiology 16, 798–810.

Levison, H.F., et al., 2010. Capture of the Sun's Oort cloud from stars in its birth cluster. Science 329, 187–190. https://doi.org/10.1126/science.1187535.

Leya, T., et al., 2017. Algae Survive outside Space Station. AlgaeIndustryMagazine.Com, 7th February, 2017. http://www.algaeindustrymagazine.com/algae-survive-outside-space-station/.

Liscovitch-Brauer, et al., 2017. Trade-off between transcriptome plasticity and genome evolution in cephalopods. Cell 169, 191–202.

Lin, X., 2012. MicroRNAs and unusual small RNAs discovered in Kaposi's Sarcoma-Associated Herpesvirus virions. J. Virol. 86, 12717–12730. https://doi.org/10.1128/JVI.01473-12.

Lindley, R., 2010. The Soma: How Our Genes Really Work and How that Changes Everything! CYO Foundation. ISBN1451525648, POD book Amazon.com.

Lindley, R., 2013. The importance of codon context for understanding the Ig-like somatic hypermutation strand-biased patterns in TP53 mutations in breast cancer. Cancer Genet. 206, 222–226.

Lindley, R.A., Steele, E.J., 2013. Critical analysis of strand-biased somatic mutation signatures in TP53 versus Ig genes. In: Genome -wide Data and the Etiology of Cancer ISRN Genomics, vol. 2013. Article ID 921418, 18 pages.

Lindley, R.A., et al., 2016. Association between targeted somatic mutation (TSM) signatures and HGS-OvCa progression. Cancer Med 5, 2629–2640.

Liu, Y., 2007. Like father like son. EMBO Rep. 8, 798–803.

Liu, Y., Li, X., 2016a. Darwin's Pangenesis as a molecular theory of inherited diseases. Gene 582, 19–22. https://doi.org/10.1016/j.gene.2016.01.051.

Liu, Y., Li, X., 2016b. Darwin and Mendel today: a comment on "Limits of imagination: the 150th Anniversary of Mendel's Laws, and why Mendel failed to see the importance of his discovery for Darwin's theory of evolution". Genome 59, 75–77. https://doi.org/10.1139/gen-2015-0155.

Louis, G., Kumar, A.S., 2006. The red rain phenomenon in Kerala and its possible extraterrestrial origin. Astrophys. Sp.Sci. 302, 175–187.

Lutz, F.E., Grisewood, E.N., 1934. Reactions of Drosophila to 2537A radiation. Am. Mus. Novit. 706. March 1934.

Mattick, J.S., 2012. Rocking the foundations of molecular genetics. Proc. Natl. Acad. Sci. U. S. A. 109, 16400–16401.

McCafferty, P., 2008. Bloody red rain again! Red rain in meteors and myth. Int. J. Astrobiol. 7, 9–15.

McLure, C.A., et al., 2013. Genomic evolution and polymorphism: segmental duplications and haplotypes at 108 regions on 21 chromosomes. Genomics 102, 15–26.

Miyake, N., et al., 2010. Identification of micro-biofossils in space dust. J. Cosmology 7, 1743–1749.

Muotri, A.R., et al., 2007. The necessary junk: new functions for transposable elements. Hum. Mol. Genet. 16 (2), R159–R167. https://doi.org/10.1093/hmg/ddm196.

Napier, W.M., et al., 2007. The origin of life in comets. Int. J. Astrobiol. 6, 321–323.

Noble, D., 2011. A Theory of Biological Relativity: No Privileged Level of Causation Interface Focus Royal Society Publishing. https://doi.org/10.1098/rsfs.2011.0067. Published 9 November 2011.

Noble, D., 2013. Physiology is rocking the foundations of evolutionary biology. Exp. Physiol. 98 (8), 1235–1243.

Noble, D., 2017. Dance to the Tune of Life. Cambridge University Press. ISBN 1-107-17624-9.

Noble, D., et al., 2016. New Trends in Evolutionary Biology: Biological, Philosophical and Social Science Perspectives. The Royal Society, London, 6–9 Carlton House Terrace, London, SW1Y 5AG Nov 7 -9, 2016. Editors-Organisors. https://royalsociety.org/science-events-and-lectures/2016/11/evolutionary-biology/.

Oliver, K.R., Greene, W.K., 2012. Transposable elements and viruses as factors in adaptation and evolution: an expansion and strengthening of the TE-Thrust hypothesis. Ecol. Evol. 2 (11), 2912–2933. https://doi.org/10.1002/ece3.400.

Paules, C.I., et al., 2017. The pathway to a universal influenza vaccine. Immunity 47, 599–603.

Paz-Yaacov, N., et al., 2010. Adenosine-to-inosine RNA editing shapes transcriptome diversity in primates. Proc. Natl. Acad. Sci. U.S.A. 107, 12174–12179.

Pflug, H.D., Heinz, B., 1997. Analysis of fossil organic nanostructures: terrestrial and extraterrestrial. SPIE Proc. Instrum. Methods Missions Investigation Extraterr. Microorg.. 86, 3111. https://doi.org/10.1117/12.278814. July 11, 1997.

Pirakitikulr, N., et al., 2016. The coding region of the HCV genome contains a network of regulatory RNA structures. Mol. Cell 61, 1–10.

Priscu, J.C., Christner, B.C., 2004. Earth's icy biosphere. In: Bull, A. (Ed.), Microbial Diversity and Bioprospecting. ASM Press, Washington, D.C., pp. 130–145. Chap 13.

Qu, J., 2016. Is sunspot activity a factor in influenza pandemics? Rev. Med. Virol. 26, 309–313. https://doi.org/10.1002/rmv.1887.

Rauf, K., Wickramasinghe, C., 2010. Evidence for biodegradation products in the interstellar medium. Int. J. Astrobiol. 9, 29–34.

Refsland, E.W., Harris, R.S., 2013. The APOBEC3 family of retroelement restriction factors. Curr. Top. Microbiol. Immunol. 371, 1–27. https://doi.org/10.1007/978-3-642-37765-5_1.

Rothenfluh, H.S., 1995. Hypothesis: a memory lymphocyte specific soma-to-germline genetic feedback loop. Immunol. Cell Biol. 73, 174–180.

Ruff, S.W., Farmer, J.D., 2016. Silica deposits on Mars with features resembling hot spring biosignatures at El Tatio in Chile
Nat. Commun. Now. 7, 13554. https://doi.org/10.1038/ncomms13554.

Ryan, F., 2009. Virolution. Collins, London.

Sanjuan, R., 2010. Mutational fitness effects in RNA and single-stranded DNA viruses: common patterns revealed by site-directed mutagenesis studies. Phil Trans R Soc B 365, 1975–1982. https://doi.org/10.1098/rstb.2010.0063.

Sanjuan, R., 2012. From molecular genetics to phylodynamics: evolutionary relevance of mutation rates across viruses. PLoS Pathog. 8 (5), e1002685. https://doi.org/10.1371/journal.ppat.1002685.

Sanjuan, R., Domingo-Calap, P., 2016. Mechanisms of viral mutation. Cell. Mol. Life Sci. 3, 4433–4448. https://doi.org/10.1007/s00018-016-2299-6.

Sanjuan, R., et al., 2004. The distribution of fitness effects caused by single-nucleotide substitutions in an RNA virus. Proc. Natl. Acad. Sci. U.S.A. 101, 8396–8401. https://doi.org/10.1073/pnas.0400146101.

Sanjuan, R., et al., 2010. Viral mutation rates. Virology 84, 9733–9748. https://doi.org/10.1128/JVI.00694-10.

Sharma, U., et al., 2015. Biogenesis and function of tRNA fragments during sperm maturation and fertilization in mammals. Science 351, 391–396.

Shi, M., et al., 2016. Redefining the invertebrate RNA virosphere. Nature 540, 539–543. https://doi.org/10.1038/nature20167.

Shivaji, S., Chaturvedi, P., Begum, Z., et al., 2009. *Janibacter hoylei sp. nov., Bacillus isronensis sp. nov.* and *Bacillus aryabhattai sp. nov.*, isolated from cryotubes used for collecting air from the upper atmosphere. Int. J. Syst. Evol. Microbiol. 59, 2977 2986.

Smith, W.E., September 26, 2013. 2013. Life is a cosmic phenomenon: the "Search for Water" evolves into the "Search for Life". In: Hoover, R.B., Levin, G.V., Rozanov, A.Y., Wickramasinghe, N.C. (Eds.), Proc. SPIE 8865, Instruments, Methods, and Missions for Astrobiology XVI. San Diego, California, United States. https://doi.org/10.1117/12.2046862.

Snyder, D.P., 2015. The origins of megacryometeors: troposphere or extraterrestrial? Cosmology 19, 70–86 (Cosmology.com).

Spadafora, C., 2008. Sperm-mediated "reverse" gene transfer: a role of reverse transcriptase in the generation of new genetic information. Hum. Reprod. 23, 735–740. https://doi.org/10.1093/humrep/dem425.

Steele, E.J., 1979. Somatic Selection and Adaptive Evolution : on the Inheritance of Acquired Characters, first ed. University of Chicago Press, Chicago. Williams-Wallace, Toronto, 1979; 2nd Edit.

Steele, E.J., 2014. Reflections on ancestral haplotypes: medical genomics, evolution and human individuality. Perspect. Biol. Med. 57, 179–197.

Steele, E.J., 2015. Ancestral Haplotypes: Our Genomes Have Been Shaped in the Deep Past. Nearurban Dallas,Tx, ISBN 978-0-9864115-0-2.

Steele, E.J., 2016a. Origin of congenital defects: stable inheritance through the male line via maternal antibodies against eye lens antigens inducing autoimmune eye defects in developing rabbits in utero. In: Levin, M., Adams, D.S. (Eds.), Ahead of the Curve -Hidden Breakthroughs in the Biosciences Chapter 3. Michael Levin and Dany Spencer Adams IOP Publishing Ltd 2016, Bristol, UK.

Steele, E.J., 2016b. Somatic hypermutation in immunity and cancer: critical analysis of strand-biased and codon-context mutation signatures. DNA Repair 45, 1–24. https://doi.org/10.1016/j.dnarep.2016.07.001.

Steele, E.J., Dawkins, R.L., 2016. New Theory of HIV Diversification : Why it May Never Be Possible to Make a Protective Vaccine viXra.org 1612.0346. http://viXra.org/abs/1612.0346.

Steele, E.J., Lindley, R.A., 2017. ADAR deaminase A-to-I editing of DNA and RNA moieties of RNA: DNA hybrids has implications for the mechanism of Ig somatic hypermutation. DNA Repair 55, 1–6.

Steele, E.J., Lloyd, S.S., 2015. Soma-to-germline feedback is implied by the extreme polymorphism at IGHV relative to MHC. Bioessays 37, 557–569.

Steele, E.J., Gorczynski, R.M., Pollard, J.W., 1984. The somatic selection of acquired characters. In: Pollard, J.W. (Ed.), Evolutionary Theory: Paths into the Future. John Wiley, London, pp. 217–237.

Steele, E.J., Lindley, R.A., Blanden, R.V., 1998. In: Davies, Paul (Ed.), Lamarck's Signature : How Retrogenes Are Changing Darwin's Natural Selection Paradigm. Allen & Unwin, Frontiers of Science: Series. Sydney, Australia, 1998.

Strugnell, J., Nishiguchi, M.K., 2007. Molecular phylogeny of coleoid cephalopods (Mollusca: cephalopoda) inferred from three mitochondrial and six nuclear loci: a comparison of alignment, implied alignment and analysis methods. J. Molluscan Stud. 73, 399–410.

Strugnell, J., et al., 2005. Molecular phylogeny of coleoid cephalopods (Mollusca: cephalopoda) using a multigene approach: the effect of data partitioning on resolving phylogenies in a Bayesian framework. Mol. Phylogenet. Evol. 37, 426–441.

Strugnell, J., et al., 2006. Divergence time estimates for major cephalopod groups:

E.J. Steele et al. / Progress in Biophysics and Molecular Biology 136 (2018) 3–23   23

evidence from multiple genes. Cladistics 22, 89–96.

Telesnitsky, A., Wolin, S.L., 2016. The host RNAs in retroviral articles. Viruses 8, 235. https://doi.org/10.3390/v8080235, 15 pages.

Temin, H.M., 1974. On the origin of the RNA tumor viruses. Annu. Rev. Genet. 8, 155–177.

Tepfer, D., Leach, S., 2017. Survival and DNA damage in plant seeds exposed for 558 and 682 Days outside the international space station. Astrobiology 17, 205–215.

Tegmark, M., 2014. Our Mathematical Universe. Random House, New York.

Tian, C., et al., 2007. Virion packaging determinants and reverse transcription of SRP RNA in HIV-1 particles. Nucleic Acids Res. 35, 7288–7302. https://doi.org/10.1093/nar/gkm816.

Vanysek, V., Wickramasinghe, N.C., 1975. Formaldehyde polymers in comets. Astrophys. Space Sci. 33, L19–L28.

Villarreal, L.P., 2004. Can viruses make us human? Proc. Am. Phil. Soc. 148, 296–323.

Wainwright, M., Wickramasinghe, N., Narlikar, J., Rajaratnam, P., 2003. Microorganisms cultured from stratospheric air samples obtained at 41km. FEMS Microbiol. Lett. 218, 161–165.

Wainwright, M., et al., 2014. Recovery of cometary microorganisms from the stratosphere. Astrobiol Outreach 2 (1). https://doi.org/10.4172/2332-2519.1000110.

Wainwright, M., et al., 2015a. Biological entities isolated from two stratosphere launches-continued evidence for a space origin J. Astrobiol Outreach 3 (2). https://doi.org/10.4172/2332-2519.1000129.

Wainwright, M., et al., 2015b. Masses staining positive for DNA-isolated from the stratosphere at a height of 41 km. Astrobiol Outreach 3 (2). https://doi.org/10.4172/2332-2519.1000130.

Walker Jr., J., Wickramasinghe, C., 2015. Big Bang and God - an Astro-theology. Palgrave Macmillan, US.

Wallis, M.K., 2007. Exotic amino acids across the K/T boundary — cometary origin and relevance for species extinction. Int. J. Astrobiol. 6, 303–306.

Wallis, J., et al., 2013. The Polonnaruwa meteorite — oxygen isotope, crystalline and biological composition. J. Cosmol. 21, 10004–10011.

Wallis, M.K., Wickramasinghe, N.C., 2015. Rosetta images of Comet 67P/Churyumov-Gerasimenko: inferences from its terrain and structure. J. Astrobiol Outreach 3 (1). https://doi.org/10.4172/2332-2519.1000127.

Wesson, P., 2011. Necropanspermia. Observatory 131, 63–66.

Wickramasinghe, N.C., 1974. Formaldehyde polymers in interstellar space. Nature 252, 462–463.

Wickramasinghe, N.C., 2010. The astrobiological case for our cosmic ancestry. Int. J. Astrobiol. 9, 119–129.

Wickramasinghe, C., 2011. Viva panspermia. Observatory 131, 130–134.

Wickramasinghe, N.C., 2012. DNA sequencing and predictions of the cosmic theory of life. Astrophys. Space Sci. 343, 1–5.

Wickramasinghe, N.C., et al., 2012. Life-bearing primordial planets in the solar vicinity. Astrophys. Space Sci 341, 295–299.

Wickramasinghe, Chandra, 2015a. The Search for Our Cosmic Ancestry. World Scientific, Singapore.

Wickramasinghe, Chandra, 2015b. Vindication of Cosmic Biology. Tribute to Sir Fred Hoyle (1915-2001). Edit. Chandra Wickramasinghe, World Scientific, Singapore.

Wickramasinghe, N.C., Rycroft, M., 2018. Transport of submicron dust including bacteria from the Earth's surface to the high ionosphere. Adv. Astrophys. In press.

Wickramasinghe, D.T., Allen, D.A., 1986. Discovery of organic grains in Comet Halley. Nature 323, 44–46.

Wickramasinghe, C., Smith, W.E., 2014. Convergence to panspermia. Hypothesis 12 (1), e9,. https://doi.org/10.5779/hypothesis.v12i1.358.

Wickramasinghe, N.C., Steele, E.J., 2016. Dangers of adhering to an obsolete paradigm: could Zika virus lead to a reversal of human evolution? J. Astrobiol. Outreach 4 (1). https://doi.org/10.4172/2332-2519.1000147.

Wickramasinghe, N.C., Tokoro, G., 2014a. Life as a cosmic phenomenon: 1 the socioeconomic control of a scientific paradigm. J. Astrobiol.Outreach 2 (2). https://doi.org/10.4172/2332-2519.1000113.

Wickramasinghe, N.C., Tokoro, G., 2014b. Life as a cosmic phenomenon: 2.The panspermia trajectory of Homo sapiens. J. Astrobiol Outreach 2 (2). https://doi.org/10.4172/2332-2519.1000115.

Wickramasinghe, N.C., et al., 1996. Eruptions of comet hale-bopp at 6.5AU. Astrophys. Space Sci. 240, 161–165.

Wickramasinghe, J.T., et al., 2009. Liquid water and organics in Comets: implications for exobiology. Int. J. Astrobiol. 8, 281–290.

Wickramasinghe, J.T., et al., 2010. Comets and the Origin of Life. World Scientific, Singapore.

Wickramasinghe, N.C., et al., 2015. Rosetta studies of Comet 67P/Churyumov–Gerasimenko: prospects for establishing cometary biology. J. Astrobiol. Outreach 3 (1). https://doi.org/10.4172/2332-2519.1000126.

Wickramasinghe, N.C., et al., 2017. Sunspot cycle minima and pandemics: the case for vigilance? ? J. Astrobiol. Outreach 5 (2). https://doi.org/10.4172/2332-2519.1000159.

Yohn, C.T., Jiang, Z., McGrath, S.D., Hayden, K.E., Khaitovich, P., et al., 2005. Lineage-specific expansions of retroviral insertions within the genomes of african great apes but not humans and orangutans. PLoS Biol. 3, e110.

Contents lists available at ScienceDirect

Progress in Biophysics and Molecular Biology

journal homepage: www.elsevier.com/locate/pbiomolbio

Lamarck and Panspermia - On the Efficient Spread of Living Systems Throughout the Cosmos

Edward J. Steele [a, b, c, *], Reginald M. Gorczynski [d], Robyn A. Lindley [e, f], Yongsheng Liu [g], Robert Temple [h], Gensuke Tokoro [b, i], Dayal T. Wickramasinghe [b, j], N. Chandra Wickramasinghe [b, i, k]

[a] C.Y.O'Connor ERADE Village Foundation, Piara Waters, Perth, 6112, WA, Australia
[b] Centre for Astrobiology, University of Ruhuna, Matara, Sri Lanka
[c] Melville Analytics Pty Ltd, Melbourne, Vic, Australia
[d] Department of Surgery & Immunology, University of Toronto, Toronto, Ontario, Canada
[e] Department of Clinical Pathology, Faculty of Medicine, Dentistry & Health Sciences, University of MelbourneVic, Australia
[f] GMDx Group Ltd, Melbourne, Vic, Australia
[g] Henan Collaborative Innovation Center of Modern Biological Breeding, Henan Institute of Science and Technology, Xinxiang, 453003, China
[h] The History of Chinese Science and Culture Foundation, Conway Hall, London, UK
[i] Institute for the Study of Panspermia and Astrobiology, Gifu, Japan
[j] College of Physical and Mathematical Sciences, Australian National University, Canberra, Australia
[k] Buckingham Centre for Astrobiology, University of Buckingham, UK

ARTICLE INFO

Article history:
Received 18 May 2019
Received in revised form
14 August 2019
Accepted 21 August 2019
Available online 22 August 2019

Keywords:
Panspermia
Interstellar dust
Comets
Lamarckian inheritance
Neo-Darwinism
Epigenetic-genetic coupling
Reverse transcription-linked somatic hypermutation

ABSTRACT

We review the main lines of evidence (molecular, cellular and whole organism) published since the 1970s demonstrating Lamarckian Inheritance in animals, plants and microorganisms viz. the transgenerational inheritance of environmentally-induced acquired characteristics. The studies in animals demonstrate the genetic permeability of the soma-germline *Weismann Barrier*. The widespread nature of environmentally-directed inheritance phenomena reviewed here contradicts a key pillar of neo-Darwinism which affirms the rigidity of the *Weismann Barrier*. These developments suggest that neo-Darwinian evolutionary theory is in need of significant revision. We argue that Lamarckian inheritance strategies involving environmentally-induced rapid directional genetic adaptations make biological sense in the context of cosmic Panspermia allowing the efficient spread of living systems and genetic innovation throughout the Universe. The Hoyle-Wickramasinghe Panspermia paradigm also developed since the 1970s, unlike strictly geocentric neo-Darwinism provides a cogent biological rationale for the *actual widespread existence* of Lamarckian modes of inheritance - it provides its *raison d'être*. Under a terrestrially confined neo-Darwinian viewpoint such an association may have been thought spurious in the past. Our aim is to outline the conceptual links between rapid Lamarckian-based evolutionary hypermutation processes dependent on reverse transcription-coupled mechanisms among others and the effective cosmic spread of living systems. For example, a viable, or cryo-preserved, living system travelling through space in a protective matrix will need of necessity to *rapidly adapt and proliferate* on landing in a new cosmic niche. Lamarckian mechanisms thus come to the fore and supersede the slow (blind and random) genetic processes expected under a traditional neo-Darwinian evolutionary paradigm.

© 2019 The Authors. Published by Elsevier Ltd. This is an open access article under the CC BY-NC-ND license (http://creativecommons.org/licenses/by-nc-nd/4.0/).

Contents

* Corresponding author. Centre for Astrobiology, University of Ruhuna, Matara, Sri Lanka.
   E-mail address: ejsteele@cyo.edu.au (E.J. Steele).

https://doi.org/10.1016/j.pbiomolbio.2019.08.010

E.J. Steele et al. / Progress in Biophysics and Molecular Biology 149 (2019) 10–32   11

Preamble - purpose of this article

All of us have contributed these past 50 years to the assembly of biological, biophysical and astrophysical data consistent with both Lamarckian modes of evolution and the conclusion that life itself is not specifically restricted to Earth but is a cosmic phenomenon (Panspermia). Our purpose then in writing this speculative review is to assemble the relevant molecular, cellular, evolutionary and astrobiological data in a coherent new evolutionary synthesis. We make the scientific case for the efficient spread and further evolution of *pre-existing* diverse living systems, unicellular or multicellular, prokaryote, archaea and eukaryote, throughout the observable universe. While we discuss the problems of the odds against the emergence of life from non-living chemistry on Earth our pragmatic position leaves the mechanisms for the ultimate cosmological origin of life in the Universe an open question. We make this clear at the outset - this article is *not* about the origin of

life *per se*. However our article is concerned with how life has been continuously seeded to Earth from the Cosmos, and how terrestrial life has evolved as we recently discussed in this journal (Steele et al., 2018, 2019). Obviously, all our discussions on Lamarckian modes of inheritance are derived from observations and experiments about living systems in habitats here on Earth. This provides valuable insight, in our opinion, of how life can spread throughout the Cosmos and literally infect and colonize every available niche in which evolution proceeds as a cosmologically defined and connected process. The whole universe is thus a single connected biosphere.

1. Summary of terrestrial neo-Darwinism

The widely accepted traditional view of the origin of Life and its further evolution on Earth, in the period after the Hadean Epoch (~4 billion years ago) can be summarised by the following dot-points:

12   *E.J. Steele et al. / Progress in Biophysics and Molecular Biology 149 (2019) 10–32*

• Life emerged as the first free-living cell on Earth from non-living chemistry (Abiogenesis), perhaps via an RNA World, 3—4 billion years ago in one of Darwin's hypothetical "warm little ponds" or the canonical "primordial soup." The current consensus is that hydrothermal deep sea vents are a plausible location for the origin of terrestrial life (Martin et al., 2008; Baross, 2018; Ménez et al., 2018).

• The first primitive free-living cells then replicated and flourished by Darwinian evolution.

• These early cells repeatedly duplicated their genomes and genes, slowly mutating their DNA sequences and further rearranging their genomes. This allowed progression from the archaeal and prokaryotic bacterial worlds, thence to diversify into a vast range of new and diverse cellular species. At the inception the multiplication and production of viruses by most cells further aided cell-cell genetic communication.

• All these evolutionary genetic steps arose by random events which were then preserved by natural selection.

• The emergence of the first free-living eukaryotic cells occurred by cell-cell fusions and symbiosis events providing the evolutionary path prior to the emergence of the metazoans, multicellular plant and animal life.

• Many of these evolutionary phases were ponderously slow, taking millions if not hundreds of millions of years. However the fossil record, as well as phylogenetic nucleic acid and protein sequence analyses, show that most novel species and life forms emerge suddenly in a "punctuated" way either persisting to the present or going to extinction (termed "punctuated equilibrium" by Eldridge and Gould).

• Since the explosive events of the Cambrian adaptive radiation (~542 million years ago), two further major extinctions and adaptive radiations have been recorded in the fossil record, at the Permian/Triassic (P/T) boundary (~252 million years ago) and the Cretaceous/Paleocene (K/T) boundary (~65.5 million years ago).

• The time intervals between such apocalyptic events, roughly about every 200—300 hundred million years, suggests a cosmic orbiting cycle of our Sun and Solar System around the galactic centre of the Milky Way; and shorter 30 million year cycles as our star system oscillates through the galactic plane (Clube et al., 1996, Wickramasinghe, J.T. et a., 2010).

This dot-point summary accurately describes the widely held scientific view of Life under the umbrella term "neo-Darwinism", on which the analytical discipline of "Population Genetics" is firmly based. This conventional schema is scientifically valuable because its "big data" statistical methods have allowed the navigation of the genomes of thousands of diverse organisms made possible by next generation sequencing. However, we ourselves and many others over the years have considered neo-Darwinism itself as being in need of major conceptual reform. While it unquestionably deserves respect as the over-arching foundation theory of biology it no longer reflects the actual state of affairs concerning the totality of life, its history and how it may have emerged and evolved both on Earth and throughout the Cosmos (Steele, 1979; Hoyle and Wickramasinghe, 1981, 1982; Bateson et al., 2017; Noble, 2013, 2017, 2019).

Since the 1970s many key lines of scientific investigation have produced evidence contradicting this comfortable view of Life on Earth. We shall discuss some of that key evidence below as it pertains to inheritance and genetic mechanisms (Sections 2 and 3). Recently we ourselves and many colleagues have reviewed most of this salient contradictory evidence in the context of the data supporting Panspermia (Steele et al., 2018, 2019). The clear conclusion is that the restricted neo-Darwinian view of terrestrial evolution is untenable and no longer scientifically credible. It is not denied that evolutionary developments have occurred in the terrestrial setting. However at key junctures widely accepted observations do not fit the actually observed data which allows the plausible conclusion that " … living organisms such as space-resistant and space-hardy bacteria, viruses, more complex eukaryotic cells, and on very rare occasions, even fertilized ova and seeds have been continuously delivered … to Earth so being one important driver of further terrestrial evolution which has resulted in considerable genetic diversity and which has led to the emergence of mankind" (Steele et al., 2018). Thus life on Earth in all its astonishing variety appears to have been seeded from the wider Cosmos with the further terrestrial evolution of these space-derived "varieties" occurring over hundreds of millions and billions of years on Earth (marked, as it were, by major cosmic bolide "seeding" events caused by passing star systems and the passage of our solar system through giant molecular clouds (e.g. see Hoyle and Wickramasinghe, 1993, Wickramasinghe, J.T. et al., 2010). We will return to this evidence and the critical arguments in Sections 4,5 and 6.

2. The evidence for Lamarck

2.1. The rise of neo-Lamarckian acquired inheritance and the collapse of traditional neo-Darwinian thinking on evolution

A simplified overview of the main evidence gathered since the 1970s is summarised in Table 1. This will be expanded on further in Section 3. The data collected in this period have firmly established the validity of the neo-Lamarckian evolutionary paradigm. This 50 year period documents the rise of neo-Lamarckian acquired inheritance and the collapse of traditional neo-Darwinian thinking on evolution. These environmentally-induced cellular and molecular processes can now be considered the *primary evolutionary driver mechanisms* for the evolution and ongoing diversification of life on Earth. We then further argue the case (Section 5) that these DNA and RNA inheritance mechanisms are likely to be general throughout the Cosmos (e.g. see Wickramasinghe et al., 2018a) and will likely operate in the efficient Panspermic dispersal of living systems throughout the Universe. That is, they allow the immediate proliferation, rapid adaptation and genetic diversification on landing of the cosmically-derived organisms surviving impact in their new cosmic niche.

2.2. Environmental stimulation as the directional mutational driver

Tangible signals from the environment in their broadest sense, play the key driving role in the origins of "directed" physiological adaptations and mutations which emerge in the "somatic" body of the organism. For example, by induced stresses such as pathogen-inducing innate and adaptive immune responses (deaminase-mediated mutagenesis at Transcription Bubbles, Fig. 1) but there are others as discussed in Section 3.

Table 1
Evidence consistent with Lamarckian evolutionary processes.

1	Environmental Stimulation as the Directional Mutational Driver
2	Role of Epigenetic Gene Targeting
3	Rapid Genetic Adaptation
4	Penetration of the *Weismann Barrier*
5	Horizontal Gene Transfer (HGT)
6	Central Role of Reverse Transcription

The summaries of evidence for Horizontal Gene Transfer phenomena are well covered at the Wikipedia site https://en.wikipedia.org/wiki/Horizontal_gene_transfer.

E.J. Steele et al. / Progress in Biophysics and Molecular Biology 149 (2019) 10–32   13

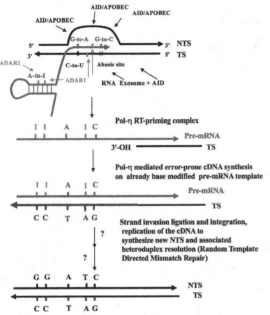

Fig. 1. The key features of the reverse transcriptase mechanism of somatic hypermutation (SHM) at Transcription Bubbles - a type of representation of the deaminase-based "Universal Mutator" likely to operate in many kingdoms of life (Lindley, 2018; Krishnan et al., 2018). Some elements of this figure have appeared before, and this figure is a modified combination of parts from (Steele, 2017), Lindley and Steele (2013), as well as from mechanism figures in Steele (2009, 2016a) and Steele and Lindley (2017). This is also an adaptation of the target site reverse transcription process reported in Luan et al. (1993). Shown is an RNA Polymerase II-generated Transcription Bubble with C-site and A-site substrate deamination events by AID, APOBEC and ADAR deaminase enzymes, which generates the strand-biased transition mutation signatures - A-to-G, G-to-A, G-to-T, and G-to-C. DNA strands shown by **black lines**; pre-mRNA as **red lines**; cDNA strands as thick **blue lines** due to DNA polymerase η acting in its reverse transcriptase mode (Franklin et al., 2004; the RT activity of DNA Polymerase η has been independently confirmed recently by Su et al., 2019). **Green bars** are Inosines. Shown also is the action of the RNA exosome (Basu et al., 2011) allowing access of AID deaminase to cytosines on the transcribed strand (TS). The ssDNA regions on the displaced non-transcribed strand (NTS) are established targets of AID action. Note that DNA mutations are first introduced as AID/APOBEC-mediated C-to-U, followed by excision of uracils by DNA glycosylase (UNG), which creates Abasic sites in the TS (these can mature into single strand nicks with 3'-OH ends via the action of AP endonuclease, Zanotti et al., 2019). These template Uracil and Abasic sites can be copied into pre-mRNA by RNA Pol II generating G-to-A and G-to-C modifications as shown (Kuraoka et al., 2003). Following target site reverse transcription (Luan et al., 1993), this results in G-to-A and G-to-C mutations in the NTS, in a strand biased manner. Separately at W<u>A</u> targets in nascent dsRNA substrates, adenosine-to-inosine (A-to-I) RNA editing events, mediated by ADAR1 deaminase, are copied back into DNA by reverse transcription via Pol-η (Franklin et al., 2004; Steele et al., 2006). In theory, ADARs can also deaminate the RNA and DNA moieties in the RNA: DNA hybrid (Zheng et al., 2017; Steele and Lindley, 2017). The strand invasion and integration of the newly synthesized cDNA transcribed strand, as well as random-template mismatch repair (MacPhee, 1995) are hypothesized additional steps (not shown here). In short, RNA Pol II introduces modifications in the Ig pre-mRNA as it copies the TS DNA with AID/APOBEC lesions (Uracils, Abasic sites) and this is coupled to A-to-I editing in dsRNA stem-loops near the transcription bubble (Steele et al., 2006) as well as in RNA:DNA hybrids within the bubble (Steele and Lindley, 2017). Next, a RT-priming substrate is formed when the nicked TS strand with an exposed 3'-OH end anneals with the base modified pre-mRNA copying template allowing cDNA synthesis by Y Family translesion DNA polymerase-η, now acting in its reverse transcriptase mode (Franklin et al., 2004). These 3'-OH annealed priming sites could arise due to excisions at previous AID/APOBEC-mediated Abasic sites. Alternatively, they could arise due to an endonuclease excision associated with the MSH2-MSH6 heterodimer engaging a U:G mispaired lesion (Wilson et al., 2005; Zanotti et al., 2019). Shown is an A-to-T transversion generated at the RT step at a template Inosine. ADAR, Adenosine Deaminase that acts on RNA; AP, an Abasic, or apurinic/apyrimidinic, site; APOBEC family, generic abbreviation for the C-to-U DNA/RNA deaminase family of which AID is a

2.3. Role of epigenetic gene targeting

This environmentally-induced phase "lights up" or "targets" expressed genes for the adaptive regulation of gene expression in progeny cells and organisms (Fig. 2). The main epigenetic modifications are the methylation of targeted cytosines (at CpG sites) via methyltransferases and their subsequent demethylation of such sites by AID/APOBEC deaminases and/or TET oxidase enzymes (reviewed in Guo et al., 2011a,b; Nabel et al., 2012). Demethylations of this type can thus allow reactivation of gene expression in previously suppressed genes. During the demethylation process such genes are vulnerable to cytosine to uracil and 5me cytosine to thymine deaminase mutations via the AID/APOBEC family of deaminases causing C-to-U and 5MeC-to-T primary somatic mutations (at DNA and RNA substrates generated at Transcription Bubbles (Steele and Lindley, 2017, Fig. 1). This first phase of an induced adaptive response thus involves "soft" Lamarckian inheritance, popularly known as "epigenetic inheritance" as it is reversible, see Skinner 2015, Skinner et al., 2015 for a recent comprehensive view (and Fig. 2).

2.4. Rapid genetic adaptation

Evolutionary adaptive change can be very fast and directional - immediately adaptive to a changing environment within one or two progeny generations. There is rapid genetic update of genomic DNA sequences being passed on to progeny organisms. Matic (2019) has recently reviewed these hypermutation rate strategies allowing survival of populations of living systems in unpredictable environments.

2.5. Penetration of the Weismann Barrier

There are numerous instances showing the genetic permeability of the Soma-Germline *Weismann Barrier* in higher animals. This actually requires the resurrection (Liu, 2008; Liu and Li, 2016) of the ancient idea of Pangenesis employed by Charles Darwin, to paraphrase Democritus " …. that the seed is formed continuously from all parts of the body". The published work now describes the molecular-vesicle variety of Darwin's "gemmules". There is now a solid foundation for the concept of Pangenesis as a molecular, cellular and physiological explanation for the inheritance of environmentally-induced acquired characters in higher animals (with a *Weismann Barrier*) and plants (with no traditional *Weismann Barrier*), see Fig. 2 and legend, and the review by Noble (2019).

2.6. Horizontal gene transfer (HGT)

Facilitating these genetic diversification and adaptation processes are the ubiquitous phenomena associated with horizontal gene transfer (HGT) involving genetic exchanges between cells (and their viruses) involving all levels of life, prokaryote, archaea, eukaryote.

2.7. Central role of reverse transcription

Apart from horizontal gene transfer, the next widespread and mutagenic phase is the *vertical transmissions of Lamarckian acquired adaptations* which involves somatic mutation, somatic selection

---

member (e.g., APOBEC1; APOBEC3 A, B, C, D, F, G, H); AID, activation induced cytidine deaminase causing C-to-U lesions at WRC<u>Y</u>/R<u>G</u>YW C-site motifs in ssDNA; W, A, or U/T; W<u>A</u>-site, target motif for ADAR deaminase including DNA polymerase-η error prone incorporation *in vitro* (Rogozin et al., 2001); Y, pyrimidines T/U or C.; R, purine A or G.

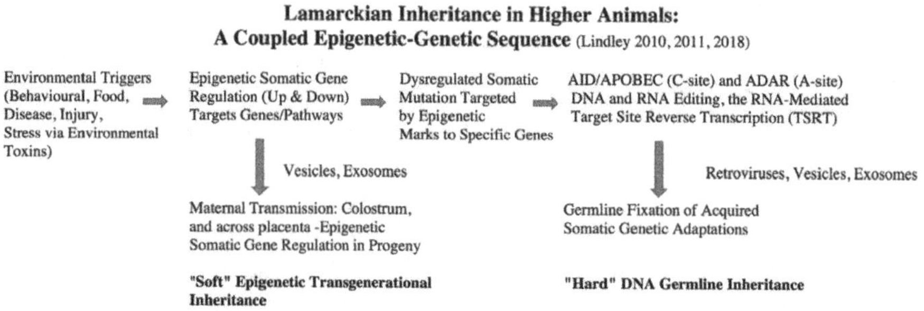

14   *E.J. Steele et al. / Progress in Biophysics and Molecular Biology 149 (2019) 10–32*

Lamarckian Inheritance in Higher Animals:
A Coupled Epigenetic-Genetic Sequence (Lindley 2010, 2011, 2018)

Environmental Triggers (Behavioural, Food, Disease, Injury, Stress via Environmental Toxins) ⟹ Epigenetic Somatic Gene Regulation (Up & Down) Targets Genes/Pathways ⟹ Dysregulated Somatic Mutation Targeted by Epigenetic Marks to Specific Genes ⟹ AID/APOBEC (C-site) and ADAR (A-site) DNA and RNA Editing, the RNA-Mediated Target Site Reverse Transcription (TSRT)

Vesicles, Exosomes

Retroviruses, Vesicles, Exosomes

Maternal Transmission: Colostrum, and across placenta -Epigenetic Somatic Gene Regulation in Progeny

Germline Fixation of Acquired Somatic Genetic Adaptations

"Soft" Epigenetic Transgenerational Inheritance

"Hard" DNA Germline Inheritance

Fig. 2. Coupled Epigenetic-Genetic Mechanisms of Lamarckian Inheritance with the Penetration of the *Weismann Barrier* in Higher Animals. The point of the sequence is to show that genes targeted first for epigenetic transgenerational regulation can mature via a reverse transcription step targeting the same genes causing hard genetic (DNA) inheritance. The key epigenetic-genetic concepts are discussed at length in Lindley (2010, 2011) and specifically in Lindley (2018). The properties of cytosine modifications play a key role in the plasticity of the Epigenetic-Genetic coupling (see Guo et al., 2011a,b, Nabel et al., 2012). The distinction between "soft" and "hard" Lamarckian inheritance is discussed explicitly in Steele (2016b). The often confused distinction between the *Central Dogma of Molecular Biology* and the *Weismann Barrier* (Steele, 1979; 2016b) is discussed and further clarified in Noble (2018). In the first phase after stimulation, the environmentally-induced "epigenetic" gene regulatory factors (e.g. methylation-demethylation at CpG sites and other modifications at cytosines; synthesis of small 21 nt-24nt sRNAs such as miRNAs etc. and guided by other non-coding regulatory RNAs) light up and target specific genes and gene pathways for regulated gene expression. The epigenetic role of long non-coding RNAs (>200 nt) targeting regulatory portions flanking protein-coding genes is covered in conceptual detail by Mattick (2003, 2018). The recent review by Kulski (2019) shows the functional importance of locus-wide lncRNAs in conserving long ancestral haplotypes at the human Major Histocompatibility Complex locus - where they act as genomic anchor points for binding transcription factors, enhancers, and chromatin remodeling enzymes thus regulating transcription and chromatin folding. LncRNAs specifically target DNA sequences usually via RNA-DNA triple helix interactions involving the weaker yet biologically significant Hoogsteen hydrogen bonding. Hoogsteen base pairing, considerably weaker than Watson-Crick base pairing is varied, in both parallel and anti-parallel configurations with the RNA sequence aligned in the major groove of the DNA duplex (Li et al., 2016). These allow multiple points of hydrogen bonding over significant sequence lengths (e.g. Enhancer or Promoter regions) thus allowing gene-specific recognition. RNA-DNA triple helix interactions thus allow targeted delivery of chromatin modifications resulting in either active transcription (activation via acetyltransferase-associated complexes) or gene silencing (chromatin compaction via methyltransferase -associated complexes). These data and the analytical methodology are reviewed in detail in Smith et al. (2013, 2017), Buske et al., (2011, 2012) and in Li et al. (2016). Such lncRNA epigenetic regulators are ubiquitously found in secreted extracellular vesicles and exosomes, particularly in tumours and tumour cell microenvironments (Xie et al., 2019; Chen et al., 2019). Epigenetically "marked" genes can become targets for AID/APOBEC-deaminase mediated cytosine to uracil (C-to-U) and cytosine to thymine (C-to-T) mutations (at 5Me CpG sites, Morgan et al., 2004), which result in G•U and G•T mispairs. Then as shown in part in Fig. 1 these can progress through further error-prone steps of DNA repair following base excision resulting in Abasic sites and then single stranded DNA nicks in the transcribed strand with 3′OH ends that can prime both DNA and RNA-dependent cDNA synthesis (off homologous newly transcribed RNA sequence templates). These downstream nicks resulting from ncRNA regulatory targeting therefore "open" the DNA in that genomic region to invasion and targeting of previously base-modified and mutated mRNA sequence templates which can be reverse transcribed and their specific cDNA fragments integrated at these C-sites (and surrounding sequence) into the genomic DNA, by target site reverse transcription,TSRT (Luan et al., 1993) as discussed at length elsewhere (e.g. Steele, 2016a. Steele and Lindley, 2017) and shown in Fig. 1. This is a variant of AID/APOBEC deaminase-mediated dysregulated immunoglobulin somatic hypermutation-like responses initiated at C-sites across the cancer genome (Lindley, 2013; Lindley and Steele, 2013; Lindley et al., 2016). ADAR deaminases causing adenosine to inosine modifications in RNA and DNA are also part of this dysregulated Ig SHM-like response scheme (A-to-I, read out as A-to-G transitions, Lindley, 2013; Lindley and Steele, 2013; Steele and Lindley, 2017). The enzymatic deaminase targeting specific C-sites and A-sites in DNA and RNA substrates occurs in protein-coding regions in codon context (Lindley, 2013) most plausibly in the 3D environment of stalled Transcription Bubbles (Lindley, 2013; Steele and Lindley, 2017). There is evidence that deamination of 5-methylcytosine (5 mC) and 5-hydroxymethylcytosine (5hmC) and generation of mutagenic C-to-T mutations directly by the activity of AID/APOBEC complexes is an alternative path to successive oxidation reactions by TET enzymes for the initiation and regulation of DNA demethylation (Guo et al., 2011a,b, Nabel et al., 2012, Pastor et al., 2013, Scourzic et al., 2015). The role of extracellular secreted vesicles and exosomes is discussed in Fig. 1 of Steele and Lloyd (2015) based on the seminal vesicle/exosome data published in Cossetti et al. (2014) (mice) and later in Sharma et al. (2016) (humans). B lymphocytes themselves when activated by mitogens secrete large numbers of endogenous retroviruses (Moroni and Schumann, 1975; Moroni et al., 1980). The significance of the very high concentrations (>10¹¹ per ml) of endogenous retroviruses in seminal fluid, surrounding the placenta and actually bound to the heads of spermatozoa (Keissling et al., 1987) challenges the widely held belief *that only one successful sperm* affects the internalized genetic cargo at fertilization. The questioning of this commonly held belief is justified given the huge number of spermatozoa attached to a given ovum. Finally, apoptotic vesicles have also been invoked as DNA/RNA soma-to-germline transmission vehicles (Steele et al., 2002). Indeed there are many formal similarities between retroviruses and secreted extracellular vesicles (Hoena et al., 2016). The properties of extracellular extruded vesicles and exosomes has been extensively reviewed (van der Pol et al., 2012) and extracellular membrane vesicles with exported cargos appear across the three domains of life and form a intercellular communication system (Gill et al., 2018). All this has been recently highlighted by Noble (2019) in the context of Darwin's Pangenesis.

and then reverse transcription at the RNA level into germline genomes of multicellular animals and plants (Steele, 1979). In many cases this begins via cytosine and adenosine deaminase action during gene expression - as represented by the key mutagenic events at Transcription Bubbles as shown in Fig. 1.Thus RNA modifications brought about by deaminase action are locked into the genomic DNA by the process of Target Site Reverse Transcription, TSRT (Fig. 1 and see specifically Luan et al., 1993). The coupling of the "soft" inheritance of the "epigenetic" first phase with the second "hard" germline or DNA inheritance phase, leads to the stable transmission of the acquired character(s) to cells and progeny organisms. Lamarckian inheritance can be envisaged therefore as a two-step process involving Epigenetic-Genetic coupling (Fig. 2).

In Section 3 we select representative examples where each one is a type of conceptual and/or evidential 'Demarcation Data' point in its own right - forcing us to choose between the traditional "slow, random and blind " neo-Darwinian view of Life to the now rapid, directional and far more accurate Lamarckian-Panspermic coupled paradigm of biological evolution.

3. Acquired inheritance phenomena

The development of the main conceptual and experimental steps are outlined here more or less in chronological order as the field(s) infolded since 1970 when Temin and Baltimore first reported the discovery of reverse transcriptase in RNA tumour viruses (Temin and Mizutani, 1970; Baltimore, 1970). The implications of reverse transcriptase for the inheritance of some acquired characters was made explicit by Howard Temin at this time if not earlier (Temin, 1970, 1971). These examples are selective and illustrative of the diversity and thus generality of Lamarckian acquired inheritance phenomena. More detailed technical information and references are confined to figure legends for the interested reader to further explore in depth.

3.1. Somatic Selection Hypothesis (1979): origin, maintenance, diversification of antibody V genes

The variable (V) genes of higher vertebrate antibodies, or

E.J. Steele et al. / Progress in Biophysics and Molecular Biology 149 (2019) 10–32 15

immunoglobulins (Ig), exist as large arrays in the germline DNA of very similar V sequences ($\geq$50–100 V gene segments). In the germline they are inactive V segments (coding for about 100 amino acids) but in a mature somatic B lymphocyte in the lymphoid and blood circulation they rearrange at the DNA level to join with shorter D and J elements forming transcriptionally active somatic genes encoding rearranged heavy (VDJ) and light (VJ) chains of the HL heterodimers of antibody proteins. A viable antigen combining site is formed from a heterodimer of one heavy (H)) and one light (L) chain, essentially by a combinatorial protein association sorting process in any given B cell. In this "somatic configuration" the V[D]J genes hypermutate following antigenic stimulation. This is a typical "Darwinian" process of rapid mutation, proliferation of antigen-selected B cell survivors with large cellular apoptotic death factors (in so called "Germinal Centres" in peripheral lymphoid organs, such as spleen, lymph nodes).

Thus many B cells are destined to die (>90%) in Germinal Centres. The successful antigen-selected mutants, bearing an antigen-specific receptor on their surface membrane survive to become affinity-improved, clonally expanded, memory B lymphocytes (clonal selection). The daughter cells then enter the vascular circulation and seed other lymphoid organs. All the extant *in vivo* molecular and cellular evidence indicates the mechanism of Ig somatic hypermutation (SHM) is driven by antigenic stimulation via an AID (APOBEC) and ADAR deaminase-coupled Reverse Transcription process (RNA/RT), as shown in outline in Fig. 1 (Steele et al., 2006; Steele 2016a; Steele and Lindley, 2017). The first iteration of the RNA/RT-Ig SHM model was by Steele and Pollard (1987), and the demonstration that the key error-prone DNA polymerase-Eta (η) involved in Ig SHM is a very efficient reverse transcriptase was first demonstrated by Franklin et al. (2004) and independently confirmed recently by Su et al. (2019).

The Somatic Selection Hypothesis (Steele, 1979) was created to explain the origin, maintenance and diversification of the germline V gene arrays via the agency of somatic mutation and clonal selection (Burnet, 1957, 1959) utilizing Temin's harmless endogenous retroviruses acting as somatic gene vectors transducing somatic V mutant sequences at the mRNA level and shuttling them into the germline of immunized animals. Rothenfluh (1995) vastly improved the model by invoking mobile mutant B lymphocytes interpenetrating reproductive tissue and delivering the endogenous V-transducing vectors more or less directly to germ cells (later apoptotic B cell-derived vesicles were also invoked as transport vehicles, Steele et al., 2002). Rothenfluh (1995) also reviewed the evidence that endogenous retroviruses are secreted in large numbers from B lymphocytes stimulated by antigens and mitogens of foreign pathogens (Moroni and Schumann, 1975; Moroni et al., 1980).

The Somatic Selection Hypothesis was the first attempt, post the Lysenko era, to build a viable Lamarckian genetic model for the penetration of the *Weismann Barrier* - that was at the same time consistent with all the known facts of development, molecular genetics, virology and Mendelian inheritance. As far as the genetic structure of higher vertebrate germline V gene arrays are concerned it is still the most economical explanation for the origin, maintenance and further diversification of all the current published germline V segment data (Steele and Lindley, 2018) which always bear the hallmark signatures of intense somatic mutation and selection implying regular soma-to- germline V gene feedback during life and across generations (Blanden et al., 1998; Steele et al., 1998; Steele and Lloyd, 2015).

3.2. Inheritance of acquired neonatal tolerance to foreign histocompatibility antigens in mice

These experiments showed that the deep tolerance of immune reactivity at the level of cytotoxic T lymphocytes (CTL) measured in *in vitro* assay systems which was induced in neonatal male mice, could, after mating those males as adults to females of the same inbred stain, be passed on to first and second generation progeny (appearing in the second generation without exposure to the foreign histocompatibility (H-2) antigens used to set up specific tolerance in the original father (Gorczynski and Steele 1980, 1981). In later experiments the specific H-2 tolerance in progeny generations correlated with specific delayed skin graft rejection (Gorczynski et al., 1983). Experiments in the Brent-Medawar laboratory claimed these acquired paternal transmission experiments could not be repeated (Brent et al., 1981). The controversy surrounding these differences in the two studies initially focused on significant differences in the way the CTL assay was performed in the Toronto/Canada and Harrow/UK laboratories. However, the Brent et al. (1981) progeny clearly showed significant numbers of delayed skin graft rejectors (Steele, 1981) later confirmed by Gorczynski et al. (1983). In subsequent follow-up studies the same group again claimed negative paternal transmission results (Brent et al., 1982) when they set up a smaller number of breeding males than the original experiments - four neonatally treated males, down from ten in the original protocols (Gorczynski and Steele, 1980; Brent et al., 1981). This exposed this work to the further criticism that these investigators had reduced the odds of observing paternal transmission given that previous observations had shown that only ~ two out of ten neonatally H-2 tolerant males routinely documented high transmission of H-2 specific hyporesponsiveness (Gorczynski and Steele, 1980). Indeed, Mullbacher and colleagues, conducting breeding experiments at the same time and in the same laboratory as Brent et al., with inactive *Bebaru* virus antigens, demonstrated a positive non-antigen specific paternal transmission of induced neonatal hypo-responsiveness at the CTL level with *in vitro* cytotoxicity assays (Mullbacher et al. 1983). Later, positive paternal transmission was demonstrated in experiments in inbred mice to foreign (rat) erythrocytes, using both repeated high dose neonatal male tolerance (Steele et al., 1984) or single shot immunity to the erythrocytes in adult males prior to breeding to normal females (Steele, 1984). So these acquired inheritance immune system effects induced in male inbred mice were certainly controversial 30–40 years ago, but they were real, yet complex with respect to mechanism, involving most likely, in retrospect, all the epigenetic and genetic dimensions summarised in Fig. 2.

3.3. The sire effect, telegony and subsequent maternal influence

The acquired inheritance phenomena and history associated with what is called the "Sire Effect" have been reviewed (Lindley, 2010 pp. 22–29). The phenomenon was reported by Gorczynski et al. (1983) when they tested the normal inbred female mice who had raised offspring to male mice of the same inbred strain made neonatally tolerant to repeated doses of foreign lymphoid cells expressing specific H-2 histocompatibility antigens as just described (Gorczynski and Steele, 1980, 1981). When these mothers were bred to normal males of the same inbred strain they produced tolerant or hyporesponsive progeny to the *same H-2 antigens* as used in the original neonatal tolerance regime in the original breeding male.

This was a surprising result. Such mothers also passed on the effect when fostering normal pups, identifying causal factors in the colostrum and milk (Gorczynski et al., 1983). This is a striking and important result with implications resurrecting the old observations surrounding the non-Mendelian breeding results caused by male sperm and thus phenomena associated with "Telegony" (Watson et al., 1983). The "Sire Effect" thus opens a Pandora's Box with wide implications for pure-line animal breeding and wider societal implications (Lindley, 2010 pp. 22).

16   *E.J. Steele et al. / Progress in Biophysics and Molecular Biology 149 (2019) 10–32*

The "Sire Effect", whatever the detailed transmission mechanism, has real-world practical implications (Lindley, 2010 pp.26–27). Wild rabbits in rural Australia were in plague proportions in the 1940s and 1950s causing great damage to agriculture, particularly the sheep and cattle industries. To control these wild rabbit populations the Commonwealth Scientific and Industrial Research Organization (CSIRO) released rabbits infected with lethal *Myxomatosis* virus. The virus was very effective initially in controlling wild rabbit numbers. But the speed with which immunological resistance developed caused further investigations. At first sight it seemed much faster than simple "Darwinian" recovery of a resistant residual population after such a large kill ($\geq$90%). Indeed careful follow up controlled breeding experimental work by Bill Sobey and Dorothy Conolly discovered a significant factor in the rapid spread of resistance (Sobey and Conolly, 1986): bucks which had recovered from *Myxomatosis* virus when mated to a doe who had not previously been exposed to *Myxomatosis* virus produced litters that were resistant to the lethal effects of the virus- a clear paternal transmission or "Sire Effect" as described by Gorczynski et al. (1983). Thus when a non-immune buck was mated with a doe that had previously been mated to an immune buck a significant number of progeny were born with immunity to *Myxomatosis* virus. Sobey and Conolly concluded that an unknown factor transmitted via the semen of the *Myxomatosis* virus recovered bucks to the normal females which could be further transferred in other matings to normal non-exposed males.

The molecular-cellular mechanisms of the *Myxomatosis* virus sire effect in rabbits, as well as the H-2 antigen-specific maternal influence in the mother's milk acquired by the mother from the original neonatally tolerant male have not been analysed. However obvious candidates for study can be drawn from an array of epigenetic and genetic transmission effects discussed above and in Fig. 2. For example they could be related to the small regulatory RNA-mediated spermatozoa non-Mendelian inheritance effects described by Rassoulzadegan and colleagues (Rassoulzadegan et al., 2006; Kiani et al., 2013; Liebers et al., 2014) and other foreign RNA and DNA in semen and associated with spermatozoa reported by Spadafora and colleagues (Lavitrano et al., 1989, Zoraqi and Spadafora, 1997, Cossetti et al., 2014, Smith and Spadafora, 2005, Spadafora, 1998, 2008, 2018). These effects are also consistent with the functional role of sperm-associated RNA reviewed in Ostermeier et al. (2004). Indeed the oocyte during the fertilization process has many attached spermatozoa, and it is difficult not to believe that all the unsuccessful non-fertilizing sperm cells have not left a functional nucleic acid signature behind in the oocyte. These could be small regulatory RNAs, specific mRNAs as discussed, or via genetic information in endogenous somatic retroviruses (Steele, 1979) attached to sperm heads (Keissling et al., 1987; Rothenfluh, 1995). Indeed it is hard not to think that the specific nucleic acid cargoes in the seminal fluid vesicles described by Cossetti et al. (2014) and Sharma et al. (2016) are also not playing a functional inheritance role.

3.4. Pavlovian conditioning, coupled maternal influence: brain, behaviour, immunity

There have been numerous studies published on behavioural traits associated with Pavlovian conditioned immune phenomena (Ader and Cohen, 1982, 1993; Moynihan and Ader, 1996). The implications of these experiments and observations are far reaching for understanding the emergence of specific instincts in higher animals. In some specific conditioning experiments in mice, in which cyclophosphamide induced immune suppression was coupled with saccharin in the drinking water as the conditioning regime, Gorczynski and colleagues subsequently showed not

merely a saccharin-mediated conditioned recall of immune suppression, as initially described by Ader and Cohen (1982) but the propagation to progeny through several breeding generations of that conditioned immunosuppression. Gorczynski and colleagues localised the transmissible entity by a maternal cross-fostering design to characteristics of the nursing mother (Gorczynski and Kennedy, 1987). In other experiments they localised these causal effects to regulation by factors in the colostrum/foetal-placental unit modified by conditioning phenomena (Gorczynski, 1992). This conclusion is the same as the maternal immune factors transferred in the acquired sire effect described earlier by Gorczynski et al. (1983).

In a subsequent review Gorczynski et al. (2011) argued "there is now compelling evidence to suggest that a variety of perceived environmental "insults" to pregnant females, and even to nursing females in the post delivery period, in the form of physical, pathogen-related or emotional stressors, can produce significant perturbations in the immune responses seen in their offspring." The mechanisms involved are ill-understood, but at least in part may depend upon altered activation of the HPA axis, and of altered cytokine, neurohormone and neutrotransmitter production within the CNS. Other data imply an evolutionary balance is struck between changes in maternal behaviour sacrificing some aspects of maternal innate immunity at the expense of improved immunity in offspring. It is now acknowledged that even effects as subtle as an altered dietary behaviour change in the mother can itself produce profound changes in the microbiome of both mother and offspring, and this also can potentially have important implications for subsequent immune development. Since these interactions between behaviour and immune response potential in mothers and their offspring are reciprocal in nature, an altered immune activation in the mother may in turn thus evoke altered behaviour in the offspring, the "loop" essentially becoming closed.

Indeed at this juncture we can ask: How do instincts arise in evolution? If one studies the range of these strong and lifesaving reflex actions in humans and animals, logic implies an ultimate adaptive Lamarckian cause in ancestors. Strong survival instincts based on prior learnt fear responses must have arisen in our ancestors not by random chance events that were selected, but in a Lamarckian manner, which were then passed on to their progeny *en masse* providing a survival value to the small familial and interbreeding groups of mammals in the wild. The recent report by Dias and Ressler (2014) shows that parental mice subjected to Pavlovian odour fear conditioning before conception produced progeny generations with specific behavioural sensitivity to the specific chemical odour used to condition the parents. Unrelated chemical odours did not trigger a conditioned fear response. Other breeding experiments established that these specific acquired transgenerational effects are indeed inherited via parental gametes. Thus, both direct genomic and indirect epigenetic odorant receptor gene targeting appear to act together to establish what we now recognize as specific instinctual responses involving odorant receptor genes and behaviour. This is consistent with a coupling of both "soft" and "hard" inheritance schemes summarised in Fig. 2.

3.5. Transgenerational "epigenetic" experiments in endocrine metabolic systems in rodents

The maternally-mediated transgenerational effects just described in the immune and behavioural systems have traditionally been interpreted under the general "Above the Genes" or "Soft" acquired inheritance or "Epigenetics" paradigm (Jablonka and Lamb, 1995; Lindley, 2010; Skinner, 2015). This is indeed the first phase of environmental stimulation as summarised in Fig. 2. Definitive induced-transgenerational effects have been described

E.J. Steele et al. / Progress in Biophysics and Molecular Biology 149 (2019) 10–32   17

in the endocrine and metabolic physiological systems as reviewed by Campbell and Perkins (1988). The most well known are the studies showing the paternal and maternal transmission of chemically-induced acquired diabetes in rodents (Okamoto, 1965; Goldner and Spergel, 1972; Steele, 1988), passed down many breeding generations via male and female parents without any further exposure to the diabetogenic inducing agent (Goldner and Spergel, 1972). Clearly we are dealing here with a complex interactive epigenetic and genetic transmission system. In these studies the strategies described above (Gorczynski et al., 1983) of testing the potential of mothers mated to affected males for *in utero*/foetal effects by subsequent mating of such mothers to normal males or cross fostering effects via the colostrum and milk were not conducted.

3.6. The Dutch Famine

The epigenetic transgenerational phenomena described are not just of academic interest but impact human health. The famous after effects of the extreme starvation episodes at the end of World War II, the "Dutch Famine", underscore the long term inherited effects (Painter et al., 2008). Indeed Pembrey and colleagues have reviewed the induction by environmental conditions of grand parents and parents, such as nutritional deprivation, exposure to endocrine disruptors, and traumatic stresses, which can lead to disease susceptibility and altered immunity in the progeny and descendants (Pembrey et al., 2014).

Isabell Mansuy and colleagues have shown in mouse models of maternally-induced stress that unpredictable maternal separation combined with unpredictable maternal stress (MSUS) can lead to multiple effects in offspring transmitted via the male line up to three generations. The progeny phenotypes include depressive-like syndromes, aberrant social recognition, glucose (insulin) dysregulation and deficits in memory. In recent studies their results demonstrate both metabolic and behavioural symptoms in progeny mice into the 4th generation. They conclude that their MSUS induced transgenerational model produces solid and reproducible transmission effects initiated in the mother of early life adversity of male offspring (van Steenwyk et al., 2018).

In all these cases in humans and rodents the phenomena are interpreted as phase 1 "soft" epigenetic effects (Fig. 2) and thus potentially reversible via epigenetic reprogramming effects. It is difficult not to think, given the transmission through to four generations, that there are no associated "hard" DNA changes, related to the regulated expression of the relevant targeted gene pathways as outlined and predicted in phase 2 in Fig. 2. It has not escaped our notice that the phase 1 to phase 2 or soft-to-hard" acquired inheritance outlined in Fig. 2 has similarities to the simulated Lamarckian process described earlier (in 1896) referred to as the "Baldwin Effect" (Simpson, 1953).

3.7. Uptake of foreign DNA by spermatozoa and inherited effects in progeny

Corrado Spadafora and colleagues in Rome from the late 1980s (Lavitrano et al., 1989) to the present have published a series of important papers showing sperm uptake of foreign nucleic acid molecules and transmission of the genetic information to progeny organisms. Thus mouse spermatozoa clearly can take up foreign DNA/RNA molecules and express the genetic information in their progeny organisms. In some cases they show that a LINE-1-derived reverse transcription step can execute the copying of the RNA into DNA. In ≤ 10% of cases the DNA sequences are integrated into the germline genome. In most cases the sperm-absorbed DNA/RNA exists as extrachromosomal episomes which replicate along with

the host somatic cells during development displaying mosaic tissue expression (see reviews in Smith and Spadafora, 2005; Spadafora, 2008). Recent work in mice by Cossetti et al. (2014) suggests a role for exosomes vesicles released into the bloodstream from human tumour xenografts transferring somatic RNA to spermatozoa.

This work clearly shows there is no physical barrier in spermatozoa to the uptake of DNA or RNA, although developmental stages in spermatogenesis may be more susceptible to foreign nucleic acid uptake (Zoraqi and Spadafora, 1997).

In his most recent review of all his group's data Spadafora (2018) has arrived at an important generalisation:

" I propose that RNA-containing nanovesicles, predominantly small regulatory RNAs, are released from somatic tissues in the bloodstream, cross the *Weismann Barrier*, reach the epididymis, and are eventually taken up by spermatozoa; henceforth the information is delivered to oocytes at fertilization. In the model, a LINE-1-encoded reverse transcriptase activity, present in spermatozoa and early embryos, plays a key role in amplifying and propagating these RNAs as extrachromosomal structures. ".

This is among the most precise descriptions of Darwin's "gemmules" in animals published, and is a mode of transfer which is also utilised in genetic information transfer in plant graft-hybridization, described below (Liu, 2018) and consistent with the current way we now view Lamarckian inheritance, Fig. 2.

Finally in 2002 Patrick Fogarty reported a striking result of simple intraperitoneal injection of DNA into adult male or female mice. Employing a technique based on P-element transposons and delivering DNA transgenes intravenously in simple vesicles, Fogarty has shown that 50% of progeny from such male mice inherit the gene sequence (Fogarty, 2002). The critical integration event requires a transposase enzyme. Thus non-cellular DNA can readily transverse the testes tissue barriers, that normally quarantine the production of sperm, be integrated into the germline and be transmitted to progeny. This was a clear demonstration of the genetic penetration of the *Weismann Barrier* in mammals in a Lamarckian mode typical of what may take place in the wild in a now familiar Horizontal Gene Transfer event.

3.8. Adaptive mutations in bacteria and other micro-organisms

Somewhat separate from the above developments involving the *Weismann Barrier* in multi-cellular sexually differentiated vertebrates, the work in bacteria and other rapidly multiplying unicellular organisms (such as yeast) are less definitive conceptually. This is because simple Darwinian selection of rare population variants could never be ruled out. However very challenging demonstrations of substrate-induced adaptive evolution phenomena in bacteria and yeast have been described (Cairns et al., 1988; Hall, 1988; Rosenberg, 2001). The data focus thinking on the possibility of rapid mutator mechanisms in microorganisms during the stationary phase (slower replication) and this somehow increases the odds of 'selecting' an adaptive mutant. Thus Cairns et al. (1988) published data suggesting "directional" mutation phenomena in bacteria. Mutants of *E. coli* requiring lactose for growth (lac-) can be "directed" under certain conditions to produce lac+ (wild-type) revertants if cultured in the presence of lactose. They interpreted this phenomenon as being consistent with a Lamarckian process of adaptive evolutionary genetic change and they provided a reverse transcriptase-coupled mechanism for the inheritance of acquired characteristics, much like that proposed earlier (Steele and Pollard, 1987) for the somatic hypermutation process summarised and now updated in Fig. 1.

So their work then raised the unexpected and exciting possibility that environmentally induced, non-random mutator processes dependent on a reverse transcriptase step also occur in

18   *E.J. Steele et al. / Progress in Biophysics and Molecular Biology 149 (2019) 10–32*

bacteria. This was rapidly confirmed a few months later by the timely report of Lampson et al. (1989) demonstrating reverse transcriptase activity in *E. coli*. Temin dubbed them all "retrons" in bacteria (Temin, 1989) and many different reverse transcriptase activities have now been described throughout prokaryotes and archaea (Liu et al., 2002; Guo H et al., 2011, 2014; Paul et al., 2015). Indeed Radman (1999) had earlier predicted such polymerase enzymes of evolutionary change (Radman, 1974) as part of the now familiar adaptive "SOS response" in bacteria to a range of environmental stress signals (Tippin et al., 2004). What is very intriguing about all these developments is that the Y family DNA Polymerases that figure prominently in the SOS response are all error-prone polymerases and are indeed related by their DNA encoded sequence to the human Y family DNA repair polymerases eta, kappa, iota (Ohmori et al., 2001) all of which have been shown to be efficient reverse transcriptases (Franklin et al., 2004). However none of the other bacterial Y family DNA polymerase members have yet to be examined for their RT activity.

So all these different RT activities in bacteria associated with adaptive mutator responses such as the diversity-generating retroelements (DGR) (Guo H et al., 2011, Guo H et al., 2014; Paul et al., 2015) in bacteriophage, bacterial and archaeal genomes provide a unity with the RNA/RT process developed for the Ig SHM in the higher vertebrate and mammalian immune system. Mammalian systems seem to be employing an ancient hypermutation strategy - a targeted RNA template-directed and reverse transcriptase-mediated hypermutation process (estimated minimum age given archaeal systems - 3–4 billion years on Earth). Guo et al. (2014) also comment on the conserved protein folds of Ig domains in the DGR reverse transcriptases: "These observations suggest that DGR target proteins and antigen receptors may have evolved different solutions to accommodate sequence diversity in the context of Ig folds."

3.9. Deaminases, cancer progression and next generation sequencing analyses

The summary in Fig. 1 showing deaminase-mediated attack on DNA and RNA substrates in the context of the Transcription Bubble (ssDNA, RNA:DNA hybrids and nascent dsRNA stem loops) is very relevant to understanding the somatic mutator processes in progressing cancer genomes (Lindley, 2013; Lindley et al., 2016; Steele and Lindley, 2017). What is intriguing is the deaminase substrate analysis of the clinically relevant single nucleotide polymorphisms (SNPs) in the human germline - the OMIM data base (Online Mendelian Inheritance in Man) - and in the wider dbSNP itself (Lindley and Hall, 2018). The first point to note is that 30–40% of all the SNPs occur at deaminase sequence motifs typical of AID, APO-BEC3G, APOBEC3B and ADAR deaminase action in somatic cells during Innate and Adaptive Immunity to pathogens (see glossary legend Fig. 1). The next points are that >99% of the far larger number of millions of SNPs in the NCBI dbSNP are mild or benign (not associated with overt inherited diseases) and in the protein-coding regions are in typical C-sites and A-sites specifically targeted in codon-context as observed in somatic cancer genomes (Lindley, 2013; Lindley et al., 2016). Thus deaminase -mediated non-random mutation patterns appear written into human germlines over evolutionary time. Given the specificity of the targeted somatic mutation (TSM) signatures of the deaminases, and their coincidence with many common established C-site and A-site deamination motifs this suggests a causal direct role for the AID/APOBEC and ADAR deaminases mutating human germlines, triggered perhaps by innate immune responses to viral infections. But this speculation implies that human germline DNA is not quarantined from such pathogen-driven SHM-like processes. Currently some APOBEC deaminases are known to have low level expression

in normal human ovary but not testes (Refsland et al., 2010), and some ADAR isoforms are significantly expressed in normal human testes (Picardi et al., 2015). The deaminases could be acting directly on transcribed regions of the human germline; alternatively they act first in the tissues which are somatically selected and thus become physiologically "benign" (somatic polymorphic variant), then followed up by a soma-to-germline feedback step to deliver portions of the mutated somatic sequences into their homologous genomic sites in germline loci. It seems most unlikely that viral pathogens would be allowed, under normal circumstances, to stimulate dysregulated AID/APOBEC and ADAR deaminases to go on a "mutator spree" in oocytes or during spermatogenesis. Clearly future human studies should focus on these questions. The point of discussing all this is to raise the possibility that the current DNA sequencing and Bioinformatics technologies will soon provide definitive answers to a more accurate understanding of the true origins of human genetic variation.

3.10. Inheritance of characters acquired by plant grafting

Plant grafting is an ancient agricultural and horticultural practice that combines the shoot (scion) of one plant with the root system (stock) of another. Historically graft-induced variations were recorded to occur in ancient China. Charles Darwin (1868) however was the first to use the term "graft hybridization". He noted that the formation of breeding hybrids through plant grafting between distinct species or varieties (without the intervention of the sexual organs). Many such cases of "graft hybrids" were described by Darwin where shoots produced from grafted plants exhibited a combination of characters of both stock and scion. It was understandable that he would explain their formation by his theory of Pangenesis involving transmissible and transported "gemmules" in the phloem. Darwin's concept of graft hybridization was supported by Ivan Michurin, Lucien Daniel, Luther Burbank and many practical breeders. But there has been a reluctance to accept the existence of graft hybrids among some geneticists (Liu, 2018).

Trofim Lysenko was a keen supporter of the Lamarckian inheritance of acquired characters, and demonstrated experimentally the conversion of spring wheat into winter wheat and *vice versa*. He also accepted the existence of graft hybrids, and led large-scale experiments on graft-induced heritable changes. A German geneticist, Hans Stubbe, failed to confirm Lysenko's results, thus he regarded graft hybridization as part of Lysenko's fraud (Hagemann, 2002). However many epigenetic phenomena are now recognized in plants (reviewed in Sano, 2010) which would be equivalent to the first "Soft" inheritance phase in Fig. 2. Yet other studies in flax demonstrate "hard" inheritance following environmentally induced adaptive DNA changes (Cullis, 1984).

Over the past few decades, the existence of graft hybrids has been widely documented, and the results are clear and striking and regularly reproduced by many plant breeders and horticulturists. For example, Yosita Shinoto, the former president of the Genetics Society of Japan, a serious scientist and a man of the highest integrity, claimed to have obtained graft hybrids in eggplant and confirmed Lysenko's results (Shinoto, 1955). A similar example of such a graft hybrid is shown in eggplant by Zu and Zhao (1957) (see Fig. 3). There has also been increasing evidence for graft-induced heritable changes in pepper and other plants (Ohta, 1991; Taller et al., 1998). The key to success is the use of the so-called "mentor-grafting" method invented by Michurin.

Graft hybridization is now mainly explained by horizontal gene transfer and genetic transformation (Ohta, 1991). This is supported by recent experimental evidence that DNA and entire nuclear genomes can be transferred between plant cells (Fuentes et al., 2014;

E.J. Steele et al. / Progress in Biophysics and Molecular Biology 149 (2019) 10–32

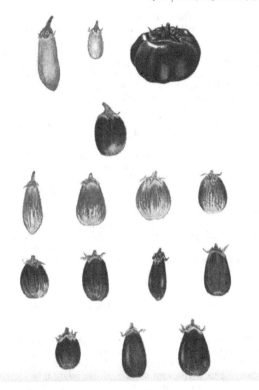

Fig. 3. Graft-induced variations in eggplant, in which 9-leaf eggplant was grafted onto white eggplant. **First row**: left; fruit of white eggplant; Right: fruit of 9-leaf eggplant; Middle: fruit in the stock of the immediate generation. **Second row**: Variant fruit in F1 generation. **Third-Fifth row**: Variant fruits in the F2 generation. Reproduced with permission from Zu, D.-M., Zhao, Y.-S. (1957) A study on the vegetative hybridization of some Solanaceous plants. Scientia Sinica, 6, 889–903. From Fig. 5 in Liu (2018).

Gurdon et al., 2016). In addition, the long-distance transport of mRNA and small RNAs is also considered to be involved in the formation of graft hybrids. Indeed plant hybrid transmission of small regulatory RNAs, mRNAs and other reporter sequences are standard experimental tools in plant molecular genetics and development (Ham and Lucas, 2017). We should now add a reverse transcription step to lock in such transported RNA phloem information into the hybrid seed genomes. Liu (2006) proposed that "the stock (or scion) mRNA molecules being transferred into the scion (or stock) — then reverse-transcribed into cDNA that can be integrated into the genome of the scion's (or stock's) germ cells, embryonic cells, callus cells, as well as the somatic cells of juvenile plants — and thus may be the main mechanism for graft hybridization".

3.11. Complexity of epigenetic and induced transgenerational inheritance

Despite more than several decades of studying induced epigenetic effects in animals and plants there are large areas of ignorance due to the complexity and variety of the phenomena. A recent balanced and sceptical review of the field by Panzeri et al. (2016) of non-coding RNA directed epigenetic regulation of gene expression is necessary corrective reading, despite the considerable molecular

detail on non-coding RNAs short and long now accrued (see legend Fig. 2). The large number of "above the genes" biochemical modifications to various regulated chromatin states justifies their conclusion: " Histone modifications comprise methylation, acetylation, acylation, phosphorylation, ubiquitination, sumoylation, proline isomerization, citrullination, and ADP ribosilation, but also more recently identified (and less represented) crotonylation, butyrylation, propionylation, succinylation, malonylation, hydroxylation, formylation, O-GlcNAcylation, and likely many others yet to be discovered". Furthermore, while gene silencing by methylation at CpGs and the actions of small regulatory 21 nt-24nt RNAs are the best studied transgenerational modes (e.g. see Kiani et al., 2013; Liebers et al., 2014) there are also clear cases of active gene *upregulation* by small RNAs (Portnoy et al., 2011). All these varied findings that are ongoing suggest that protein-coding genes and intervening genomic regions are targeted first by base sequence homologies (e.g. in the small miRNA stem loop structures, and see Fig. 2 legend) which then direct the epigenetic methylation and demethylation mechanisms (e.g. Bayne and Allshire, 2005; Molnar et al., 2010; He et al., 2011; Matzke and Mosher, 2014). It is our considered view, following Panzeri et al. (2016), that current investigations on the plethora of epigenetic-genetic couplings as summarised in Fig. 2 are just the tip of the iceberg, and that many genetic surprizes will be revealed in the research of coming years.

3.12. 100 years ago? - Experiments of Paul Kammerer, Guyer and Smith

One hundred years ago, both before, during and after the first world war there were serious attempts to demonstrate Lamarckian inheritance in higher animals by Paul Kammerer (Koestler, 1971; Vargas, 2009; Vargas et al., 2017) and by Michael Guyer and Elizabeth Smith at the University of Wisconsin (one of their key papers is republished with a modern interpretation in Steele, 2016c). In our view the definitive Lamarckian inheritance experiments in rabbits by Guyer and Smith in 1918–1924 on the transmission via the male line (up to 9 breeding generations) of maternal autoantibody-induced eye defects are on a level with the foundation work in genetics by Gregor Mendel. Yet these experiments were performed and reported in an earlier age antithetical to Lamarck. This was the time of the emergence of Mendel's rediscovery, and the rolling destructive controversies (Koestler, 1971) around the mid-wife toad and salamander experiments of Paul Kammerer — now given a modern interpretation in terms of current epigenetic concepts (Vargas, 2009; Vargas et al., 2017).

This period also heralded the birth of modern neo-Darwinism which became, with RA Fisher's statistical-based 'Population Genetics' with free recombination at and between all loci across the higher plant and animal genome (Hill, 2014), the dominant genetic paradigm for biology in the 20th century. We do not have space to deal fully with the RA Fisher paradigm which tacitly guides all Population Genetics thinking and analysis (Hill, 2014). However we point out that the prominent and genome-wide existence of long "ancestral haplotypes" in man and domestic livestock both structurally and functionally, are *profoundly non-Darwinian genetic phenomena*, in contradiction of the main assumptions of RA Fisher's free-recombination paradigm (Dawkins et al., 1999; Williamson et al., 2011; Dawkins, 2015; Steele, 2014; Steele and Lloyd, 2015). The existence of numerous and diverse functional long non-coding RNAs which display functional conservation (Mattick, 2003, 2018; Smith et al., 2013, 2017; Li et al., 2016) is consistent with the prior ancestral haplotype concepts (Steele, 2014) discovered by Roger Dawkins and colleagues at the Major Histocompatibility Complex (MHC). Indeed Yurek Kulski, who spent many years working on the long MHC haplotypes described by Dawkins et al.

20   *E.J. Steele et al. / Progress in Biophysics and Molecular Biology 149 (2019) 10–32*

(1999), recently reviewed the evidence for involvement of evolutionary conserved lncRNAs in the ancestral haplotype phenomena associated with the MHC region (Kulski, 2019). Indeed some of us have also published the possibility of reverse transcriptase-coupled generation of lncRNAs defining the origin and regulatory integration of long ancestral haplotypes (Steele et al., 2011).

3.13. Summary and conclusion- Definition of a "gemmule"

The general conclusion from our review of some of the main extant relevant data seems clear: the traditional *Weismann Barrier*, assumed for many years as the bedrock and protective foundation pillar of modern neo-Darwinism (the past 100 years at least) is *very permeable* to somatic DNAs and RNAs with inherited influences on subsequent generations. Thus a Darwinian "gemmule" or "pangene" can be defined as a somatically-derived vesicle loaded with a functional cargo - amongst other molecules (proteins, lipids, transcription factors) - of specific regulatory or specific coding nucleic acid information (small regulatory RNAs, mRNAs, lncRNAs and even DNAs). It is satisfying that the conceptual wheel has now come full circle (Noble, 2019) such that we are now able to coolly accept such an important conclusion on how extant life may be evolving on Earth (Fig. 2).

4. Pragmatic position: Demarcation Data and the statistical odds of abiogenesis

There are now solid grounds for believing in the reality of the inheritance of acquired characters as a widespread biological process, albeit with different molecular and cellular details in different living systems, whether unicellular or multicellular. There are also now good scientific grounds for believing in the in-fall of living systems from space continuously "seeding" various life forms on Earth over the past 4 billion years (Steele et al., 2018, 2019) and Section 5. However the question of the *actual* of origins of life whether on Earth or the wider Universe is clouded in mystery — with roots stretching into the deepest depths of cosmic antiquity. Here we outline, as we have done before (Hoyle and Wickramasinghe, 1981, 1993, 1999a, Steele et al., 2018), our philosophical or, if you will, our pragmatic position.

4.1. Eukaryotic and prokaryotic microfossils in carbonaceous meteorites dated at > 4.5 billions years

In our view the hard evidence *already exists* distinguishing terrestrial neo-Darwinism from the evidence for Cosmic Panspermia (Steele et al., 2019). We refer to this key evidence as the "Demarcation Data".The accrual of this and other multifactorial evidence has been comprehensively covered in successive books since the 1970s as the data and observations unfolded by Fred Hoyle and N. Chandra Wickramasinghe (1978a, 1979, 1981, 1985, 1991, 1993, 2000 with references to all peer-reviewed papers). A recent detailed summary of all the key evidence covering the terrestrial atmosphere, bacteria and other micro-organisms, the comets as protective incubators and amplifiers of living systems, the infra-red (IR) analyses of interstellar dust and cometary ejecta among other central issues can be found in Wickramasinghe (2015a, 2015b, 2018).

The "Demarcation Data", or data that has a defining interpretation, distinguishing neo-Darwinism from Cosmic Panspermia have been recently highlighted by us (Steele et al., 2019).

A key focus is on the internal structure of carbonaceous meteorites showing clear microfossils of both eukaryotic and prokaryotic organisms. These published observations have been secured from *independently curated and examined* carbonaceous meteorites,

dated at > 4.5 billion years old. The data have been confirmed by experts in four well curated and characterised carbonaceous meteorites: Murchison (Pflug and Heinz, 1997; Hoover, 2005, 2011), Murchison, Orgueil, Mighei (Rozanov and Hoover, 2013), Polonnaruwa (Wallis et al., 2013; Wickramasinghe et al., 2013). Terrestrial contamination has been ruled out e.g. the scanning analytical EM technology now allows confirmation that the mineralised fossil has the same chemical composition as the surrounding matrix in which it is embedded.

As scientists we must critically evaluate these four different and independent "experiments of nature "on their own terms. Eukaryotic fossils with silica-based hard shells, are prominent in these fossils. Certainly in the Polonnaruwa meteorite (Wickramasinghe et al., 2013) the frustules of clear diatoms are evident and not considered to be contaminants (Fig. 4). Striking eukaryotic microfossils like this are also evident in the other carbonaceous meteorites (Rozanov and Hoover, 2013). Clearly these are features of mature cell biology in astrophysical phenomena that require a coherent explanation. "They strongly imply that complex cell-based life, now immortalised as fossils in carbonaceous meteorites, pre-dates the age of the Earth (and solar system). An explanation based on Panspermia seems unavoidable to us." (Steele et al., 2019).

4.2. Abiogenesis: life arose from non-living chemistry on earth - what are the statistical odds ?

The question of the actual origins of life should, in our view, be considered in terms of the information content of life as we know it and thus in terms of pragmatic statistical probabilities. Thus the actual origins of Life with its near infinite information content, enshrouded in the deep recesses of Cosmic antiquity are, for all practical purposes, scientifically unknowable. Our view on this is unabashedly pragmatic, which forces a philosophical position on priorities on where research funds should be deployed in the scientific investigation of both the origins of life, e.g. laboratory 'abiogenetic' experiments, and in searches where it might exist or arise across the Universe.

What are the main claims of Abiogenesis? What are their weaknesses in supporting a localised chemical origin of life? The summary in the excellent and comprehensive Wikipedia article

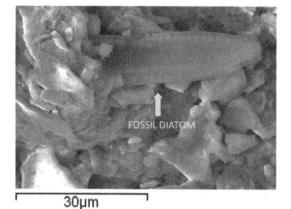

Fig. 4. Eukaryotic microfossil in Carbonaceous meteorite. voidal-shaped ribbed structure embedded in the rock matrix of the Polonnaruwa carbonaceous meteorite, Wickramasinghe et al. (2013), see also other chemical analyses in Wallis et al. (2013).

E.J. Steele et al. / Progress in Biophysics and Molecular Biology 149 (2019) 10–32   21

needs to be read in association with our analysis here (https://en. wikipedia.org/wiki/Abiogenesis) — it clearly shows that apart from the type of laboratory experiments in the Miller-Urey tradition of the 1950s (showing that many organic molecules can be created by electrical discharge processes that may have existed on the early Earth) the whole discussion in this area is built entirely on hypothesis, assumption and speculation with *no evidence* anywhere documenting the emergence of a living cell from non-living chemistry. This is not surprizing on reflection —the scientific enterprise investigating Abiogenesis is built (to quote the Wikipedia article) on "the prevailing scientific hypothesis ... that the transition from non-living to living entities was not a single event, but an evolutionary process of increasing complexity that involved molecular self replication, self assembly, autocatalysis, and the emergence of cell membranes." There is a great enthusiasm (Martin et al., 2008; Lane, 2015) and much inspired laboratory and theoretical research for the first RNA replicator (Szostak et al., 2001; McFadden, 2016) that would have flourished in the hypothesized RNA world some 3–4 billion years ago. Such a brief summary is not to downgrade the importance of the question of the likelihood of Abiogenesis. We have to be cautious, re. contaminations by all pervasive living systems here on Earth (cf. observations on tryptophan abiosynthesis at shallow subterranean levels at deep sea hydrothermal vents as in Menez et al., 2018 — which need critical evaluation given the known all pervasive existence of the deep hot microbiological biosphere, Gold, 1992, 1999). And we need to be aware there have also been some spectacular claims (RNA self replicators) that turned out to be based on experimental artifacts,so skepticism and caution are warranted (Litovchick and Szostak, 2008, retracted 2017; and see https://retractionwatch.com/2017/ 12/05/definitely-embarrassing-nobel-laureate-retracts-non-reproducible-paper-nature-journal/).

Omission of key information in science is not helpful in any investigation. Nor should we turn a blind eye to certain overriding philosophical and epistemological difficulties that have been recognized. The philosopher of science Karl Popper (1974) expressed a huge problem for abiogenesis theories thus:

"What makes the origin of life and of the genetic code a disturbing riddle is this: the genetic code is without any biological function unless it is translated; that is, unless it leads to the synthesis of the proteins whose structure is laid out by the code. But .... the machinery by which the cell (or at least the non-primitive cell, which is the only one we know) translates the code consists of at least fifty macromolecular components which are themselves coded in the DNA. This constitutes a baffling cycle; a really vicious circle, it seems, for any attempt to form a model or theory of the genesis of the genetic code ... ...Thus we may be faced with the possibility that the origin of life (like the origin of physics) becomes an impenetrable barrier to science ... ..."

Certainly the 'sin' of omission applies to the Abiogenesis field. Thus the pragmatic statistical probabilities we discuss below are rarely mentioned at all in the Abiogenesis research literature nor at the Abiogenesis Wikipedia site (but see the interesting work by McFadden, 2016, below).

The paucity of supportive direct scientific evidence for Abiogenesis is in stark contrast with our own efforts to review here all the extant concrete and positive evidence demonstrating the reality of Lamarckian modes of inheritance in nature (Sections 2, 3) and the direct positive biophysical and astrobiological evidence (Fig. 4, Section 5) consistent with the extraterrestrial origins of life on Earth (Steele et al., 2018, 2019).

As indicated in our Preamble we are not at all pretending to provide an explanation for the *actual origins of life* in the Universe. We have discussed this again recently (Steele et al., 2018 and Appendix A in that paper). Many commentators, public and private,

consider we are just shifting the problem — "kicking the can down the road"- and not solving the actual origin of life itself. However our pragmatic view is that conventional hypothetical explanations for Abiogenesis - as an explanation for the emergence of life on Earth - are mathematically and statistically improbable. Indeed the odds against successful "Abiogenesis" events popping up all the time around the Cosmos as implied by regular NASA Press releases and fuelled by conventional thinking (Walker, 2017) are also not scientifically supported in any way, and are moreover super-astronomically improbable. This is based on what we know of the information content of the simplest minimal cell capable of an independent self-replicating existence. The odds of bootstrap self-assembly are formidable (despite the argument that the odds are sequentially reduced by the emergence of "self replication, self assembly, autocatalysis, and the emergence of cell membranes."

Thus the odds against a successful Abiogenesis event are formidable. For the emergence of the first independent free living bacterial-like cell using a minimal number of essential 256 protein-coding genes (Mushegian and Koonin, 1996), we can expect one successful abiogenic trial in $10^{5,120}$ trials (Hoyle and Wickramasinghe, 1999a) an improbable event anywhere in the currently known universe, as this number far exceeds by many orders of magnitude the known atomic and molecular resources of the observable universe (below). It is thus baffling to continue with the insistence that this event took place in the infinitesimal locales that could ever have become available on a primitive Earth. If we invoke an intermediary RNA world hypothesis as a way of reducing the odds, then the advocation of a successful "first RNA self-replicator" is also highly improbable at 4^{100} (McFadden, 2016). McFadden is an expert and concedes the improbabilities as advanced by Hoyle and Wickramasinghe based on the "Koonin" number of minimal essential genes. Thus he considers that 4^{100} is an impossible number. He tries to reduce the odds by his Quantum computing Life Search model, but he compounds the problem (in our view) by further assuming highly improbable intermediate steps. The invocation of improbable intermediate steps is a common feature of all experimental modelling of Abiogenesis.

The enormity of these super-astronomical numbers we consider is not often fully appreciated (Hoyle and Wickramasinghe, 1999b). They can be made somewhat clearer by reference to other large familiar numbers such as the number electrons, protons, and neutrons in the known Universe, at 10^{80} to 10^{90}. The magnitude of these truly vast improbability factors against abiogenesis is such that their full impact is not being fully appreciated by the mainstream scientific community. To repeat ourselves, the figure of $10^{5,120}$ for a minimal number of trials far exceeds by many orders of magnitude the known molecular as well as probabilistic resources of the observable universe.

So this is our pragmatic and philosophical position, much like the pragmatic Copenhagen interpretation in Quantum Mechanics. Yet we realise that it leads to the following, and to many, unpalatable conclusions: *Abiogenesis is unlikely anywhere in the known Universe but would be possible in an "Infinite" Universe or one approaching infinite size where "Big Bangs" need to be considered as local space-time expansion-contraction phenomena* (which we termed "rolling Big Bangs", in Appendix A in Steele et al. (2018). Indeed a powerful *raison d'etre* for our continuing insistence to present an alternative cosmological/panspermic viewpoint is that every avenue of research in laboratory simulations of localised abiogenesis have led thus far to an impasse.

Craig Venter's recent success in transplanting a synthetically manipulated genome in an existing bacterial cell has been hailed by some as a significant step forward in the quest to create artificial life *de novo* (Gibson et al., 2010). This claim, however, is in our view seriously flawed because what was achieved, using the entire

22   *E.J. Steele et al. / Progress in Biophysics and Molecular Biology 149 (2019) 10–32*

biochemical machinery of a living cell, was to modify or engineer an *existing* genome in a fully functioning living cell. Manifestly this is a far cry from synthesising life. A digitally modified DNA sequence alone is a world apart from generating a living bacterium.

To move forward scientifically we suggest we adapt and embrace a realistic and pragmatic position in the scientific search for extraterrestrial life. We show below that what is knowable can be gleaned from the evidence already available from Earth-based observation and experiment, as well as careful observation and experiment of relevant astrophysical/biophysical phenomena in our near-Earth neighbourhood (as discussed in Steele et al., 2018, 2019, and see the data of Allen and DT Wickramasinghe, 1981, DT Wickramasinghe and Allen, 1983, 1986, NC Wickramasinghe Hoyle, 1998, Wainwright et al., 2015, Grebennikova et al., 2018, Wickramasinghe et al., 2018b, Shatilovich et al., 2018).

We expand on the implications in Sections 5 and 6 in relation to the spread of pre-existing living systems throughout the cosmos via rapid and directional Lamarckian inheritance.

5. Lamarck and Panspermia

5.1. Panspermia provides the raison d'etre for Lamarckian Inheritance

Here we strengthen the association between Lamarck and Panspermia that we began to assert a few years ago. To us it is plausible to consider a strong conceptual link between rapid Lamarckian-based evolutionary processes dependent on reverse transcription-coupled mechanisms among others (Wickramasinghe and Steele, 2016) and the effective cosmic spread of living systems via Panspermia. Thus our position is embodied in the answer to the following key question:

"Why, in contrast to the erroneous fundamental assumptions of neo-Darwinism, should there be widespread evidence for the existence on Earth for environmentally-driven (non-random, directional) Lamarckian modes of inheritance in all the kingdoms of life?"

Indeed one main purpose in writing this review is to be able to conclude that H–W Panspermia provides the *raison d'etre* for the existence of Lamarckian Inheritance *per se*; a conclusion quite apart from any controversial engagement with the limitations of neo-Darwinism itself. Yet we also agree with the reviewer who made the following important points:

"..In the manuscript, the rapid adaptation processes that are inherent in the Lamarckian view of evolution (Section 2, 3) are the sole conceptual links with Panspermia (Section 5 of the manuscript). The authors provide no additional evidence to strengthen this correlation. This is a critical aspect that requires a more stringent discussion and conceptual justification."

Our re-joiner to this type of criticism is this – we are advancing a conceptual position based on the critical review of the extant evidence from the Lamarckian Evolution and Panspermia scientific fields. The new synthesis thus provides the basis for research programs in space research. Our conceptual position advances a hypothesized causal link between "Lamarck" and "Panspermia" which can advance knowledge in a positive conceptual way, greater than either one alone. As we discuss below, this allows rational evaluation of data and speculations of outcomes from current research programs for the search for extraterrestrial life in the near-Earth neighbourhood. e.g. orbiting biological laboratories on the ISS, or other similar platforms, to detect potential space-derived pathogens, incoming eukaryotic microorganisms, bacteria and viruses (a research program that can be considered part of the "Hoyle Shield", Smith, 2013). .

Further to this, it allows us to understand why adaptive

evolution strategies *always involve* hypermutation and clonal diversification (Rosenberg, 2001; Matic, 2019), very much like the antigen-driven somatic hypermutation process in vertebrate immune responses (Steele, 2016a, 2017). We expect this "survival" strategy to be implemented by all surviving incoming living systems from space – so the genetic signature of a surviving population of progeny organisms (after an in-fall) will *always be one of hypermutation and adaptive diversity.* This is an important insight that can be applied to the epidemiological and genetic analyses of all incoming (read "rapidly emerging") diseases from space (Hoyle and Wickramasinghe, 1979). And it is an insight that supports our conclusion that Panspermia provides the *raison d'etre* for Lamarckian evolution which is independent of any other criticism of traditional neo-Darwinian theory.

We also try here to make quantitative estimates and predictions, and discuss how living systems may survive in long term space journeys. Thus on the basis of available evidence *Archaea* enmeshed and protected from lethal radiation in salt crystals may survive space conditions and be revived after at least 100 million years (Vreeland et al., 2007). The revival of a spore-forming bacterium *Virgibacillus sp* from brine inclusions in halite crystals has been discovered after 250 million years during which time exposure to the Earth's natural radioactivity may have delivered radiation doses exceeding those encountered in the typical transit time between two exoplanetary systems in space (Satterfield et al., 2005). Perhaps such long-term survivability of bacteria, their spores and archaea is not surprising. But what about more complex multicellular animals? For example, a viable, or cryo-preserved, complex multicellular living system (fertilized egg or plant seed) travelling through space buried deep within an icy bolide or large meteorite could be transferred to another habitable planet and will need to rapidly adapt and proliferate on a landing and thawing in a new cosmic niche. Within more finely dispersed ejecta arising from an impact of an asteroid on an inhabited planet, DNA from locally evolved life could similarly be transferred to other distant habitable planets. Lamarckian mechanisms of environmentally-driven inherited rapid adaptation discussed above would come to the fore in such situations and supersede the infinitesimally slow (blind and random) genetic processes that are expected under the traditional neo-Darwinian evolutionary paradigm.

5.2. Growing astronomical evidence from interstellar dust and comets

With the advent of infrared and ultraviolet astronomy through the 1970's the evidence for organic molecules existing on a vast galactic scale became incontrovertible (e.g. Hoyle and Wickramasinghe, 2000). There is no easy way by which one could argue that the discovery of vast quantities of complex organic molecules in the universe could be unconnected with life. As in the case of the Earth the overwhelming bulk ($\gg$99.99 ... %) of organic molecules present on a cosmic scale could most plausibly have a biological connotation. Although a trend emerged to assert without proof that pre-biotic chemistry or even pre-biotic chemical evolution was taking place on an astronomical/cosmological scale, the only correct line of argument in our view is to accept that biology is a galactic, even cosmological, process (see references in Wickramasinghe, 2015a; b, 2018). Biological genetic transfers were clearly taking place over astronomical distance scales. Thus *de novo* origination of improbable events for life (Abiogenesis) on the Earth or on other galactic habitats becomes unnecessary. Panspermia, modulated and augmented by Lamarckian inheritance processes now becomes an inescapable cosmic imperative.

The current biophysical and astrophysical evidence strongly suggests that the dust grains in the interstellar medium have an

E.J. Steele et al. / Progress in Biophysics and Molecular Biology 149 (2019) 10—32 23

infrared (IR) absorption spectrum typical of desiccated (freeze-dried) *E. coli* bacteria (secured in the laboratory by PhD student Shirwan Al-Mufti). These data, following age-old standard procedures in Astronomy, were predicted by Hoyle and Wickramasinghe *in advance* of the interstellar dust observations by DT Wickramasinghe and DA Allen, is shown in Fig. 5 (from Steele et al., 2018 Fig. 1 insert). This figure shows the normalised IR extinction (absorption) flux for two independent data sets. The IR absorption spectrum in the wavelength range 2.9—4.0 (μm) for desiccated (freeze dried) *E. coli* bacterial cells (solid line). This is an intricate and complex IR absorption spectrum of living, albeit dried and dormant, living cells. The observational data points were secured at each wavelength indicated for IR electromagnetic radiation emitted 23,000 light years away near the centre of the Milky Way. As this IR light traverses through clouds of the dust grains it is absorbed in a similar fashion to the IR absorption by dry *E. coli* cells in the laboratory experiment on Earth.

The data shown in Fig. 5, was confirmed independently by the team of Okuda et al. (1990) (and see Fig. 4.3b page 43 in Hoyle and Wickramasinghe, 1993). The Pearson correlation of this paired comparison data gives r as 0.9324 for N = 77 pairs. For Okuda et al. (1990) the r value is 0.9275 for N = 35 pairs. The P values for both are <10^{-9}. That is, we would expect to see such an exact spectral match by chance alone in more than one billion similar trials (DT Wickramasinghe, G Briggs, NC Wickramasinghe, EJ Steele unpublished calculations).

The simplest option is to concede that the dust grains in the interstellar medium have infrared absorption properties over the entire continuum from 2.8 to 4.0 μm that are identical to desiccated bacterial cells. After 1983 many other spectral features of interstellar dust over other wavebands have also found ready explanations in terms of dust particles of biological origin. We note in particular the IR absorption spectral matches of larger eukaryotic cells such as diatoms (algae) for the 8—13 μm infrared range (e.g. Hoyle et al., 1982; Hoover et al., 1986; Majeed et al., 1988, and see Wickramasinghe and Hoyle, 1998).

To the best of our knowledge no artificial modelling of compound organic mixtures will produce such invariant and exact matches to astronomical data with any reasonable set of assumptions. It is difficult therefore to provide an interpretation for these data that avoids Panspermia.

The idea of biology connected with comets also moved swiftly from speculation to serious science following the last perihelion passage of Comet P/Halley in 1986. The first investigation of a comet in the Space Age (ESA's Giotto mission) thus marked a

turning point in the history of cometary science. A dark organic comet surface (darker than the darkest coal) was vindicated by the Giotto photometry. More importantly, in our view, D.T. Wickramasinghe was the first to obtain the first 2—4 μm spectrum of the dust from an outburst of the comet on 31st March 1986 (D.T. Wickramasinghe and Allen, 1986), Fig. 6. This spectrum showed unequivocal evidence of C—H rotational/vibrational stretching indicating complex aromatic/aliphatic hydrocarbon structures, which moreover was consistent with a calculated spectrum for bacterial dust. Similar data have been published since by others (e.g. Capaccione et al., 2015).

Another significant correspondence with a putative biology emerged in the *Stardust Mission* which captured high speed cometary dust in blocks of aerogel that were later brought back to laboratories on the Earth. Amongst the minute fraction of surviving molecular residues found was the most common of amino acids Glycine together with a complex mixture of hydrocarbons (Elsila et al., 2009).

The most recent Rosetta Mission to comet 67P/C-G yielded data that satisfy consistency checks for biology. Fig. 7 shows a close consistency between the surface properties of the comet and the spectrum of a desiccated bacterial sample.

The presence of complex organic molecules including the building blocks of life in comets is amply confirmed, suggesting fully-fledged microbial life in comets, or the chemical components of life (Altwegg et al., 2016) that through coincidence match exactly the spectra of bacteria. The latter more "conservative" view is that such molecules could be formed by ion-molecule reactions including surface chemistry on the surfaces of pre-solar or interstellar grains.

Biological catalytic transformations are of course the most efficient processes by which simple organic and inorganic molecules can be turned into complex biochemistry of the type seen in astrophysical phenomena (Steele et al., 2019). Once biology gets started the conversion of non-biological molecules to biomolecules (Figs. 5—7) proceeds with an unparalleled efficiency as is indeed evident from our terrestrial experience. Over 99.9 percent of all the organic material found on Earth is biologically produced. If biology is permitted to exist and spread on a galactic/intergalactic scale a

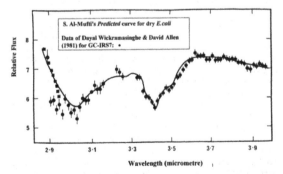

Fig. 5. Comparison of the infrared flux (arbitrary units) from the astronomical source GC-IRS7 near the galactic centre, with the curve predicted for freeze dried *E. coli* cells (Allen D.A. and D T Wickramasinghe, 1981). Also see Wickramasinghe, D.T. and Allen, D.A. (1983). This is a blow up of the inset in Fig. 1 Steele et al., 2018.

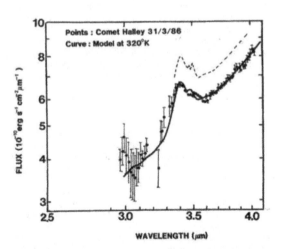

Fig. 6. Comparison of the infrared flux (arbitrary units) from the astronomical source GC-IRS7 near the galactic centre, with the curve predicted for freeze dried *E. coli* cells (Allen D.A. and D T Wickramasinghe 1981). Also see Wickramasinghe, D.T., Allen, D.A., 1983. This is a blow up of the inset in Fig. 1 Steele et al., 2018.

24   *E.J. Steele et al. / Progress in Biophysics and Molecular Biology 149 (2019) 10–32*

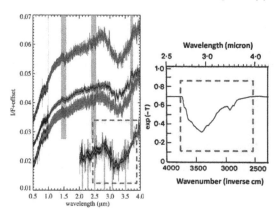

Fig. 7. The surface reflectivity spectra of comet 67P/C-G (left panel, Capaccione et al., 2015; taken at different times) compared with the transmittance spectrum of desiccated E-coli (cf. Figs. 5 and 6) over approximately the same wavelength range for comparison. Also from Wickramasinghe et al., 2018a,b).

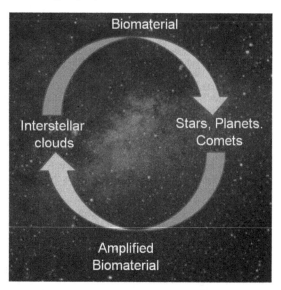

Fig. 8. Amplification cycle of cosmic life. Within our galaxy alone about 100 billion circuits have been completed, one for every sun-like star.

similar outcome is to be expected astronomically, consistent with the data in Figs. 5–7. It is useful to point out that the IR and other specific spectral signatures of complex and specific biochemical molecules in the interstellar medium - commonly assumed to be a rich supply of building blocks for cosmic Abiogenesis events - have a simple explanation: they are the molecular detritus of dead, broken and dying cells released into the interstellar medium.

5.3. Space survivability of microbiota, and habitable planets

The requirements for an astronomical source of bacteria-like cosmic dust and complex organic molecules is (a) the operation of biological replication in a large class of astronomical bodies, and (b) the assumption that a non-zero fraction of microbiology so generated survives the transit between such astronomical habitats, at any rate between nearest neighbours. Both these pre-conditions have been established over the past several decades. Survival properties of bacteria under the most hostile space conditions have been amply demonstrated both in the laboratory and by means of direct space experiments. Furthermore, over a hundred billion icy comets that are known to surround our planetary system (the Oort cloud of comets) have been convincingly shown to be likely habitats for microbiology — microbial viability and replication being accomplished within their radioactively heated interiors (Wickramasinghe et al., 2012). A fraction of the microbes amplified in comets are returned into interstellar clouds from which new stars, comets and planets can form. The feedback loop of cosmic biology is schematically shown in Fig. 8. In addition to the well-attested survival attributes of bacteria, particularly of extremophiles (to which we refer later), it should be stressed here that only a minuscule survival fraction of interstellar bacteria, $\ll 10^{-20}$ is required for every circuit in this loop for panspermic transfers to the maintained (Hoyle and Wickramasinghe, 2000).

Evidence of bacteria has also been discovered recently in geological sediments (rocks) that formed 4.1–4.3 by ago during the Hadean Epoch at a time when the Earth suffered an episode of heavy bombardment by comets and asteroids (Bell et al., 2015). This new geological evidence also supports the point of view that impacting comets brought living entities to the Earth, and by extension similar impacts on other planetary bodies could establish life elsewhere in the galaxy.

Perhaps most relevant to the ideas of Panspermia and

Lamarckian inheritance are the recent discoveries of habitable exoplanets occupying the so-called "Goldilocks zone". The Orbiting Kepler telescope launched in 2009 has to date reported the discovery of over 3000 exoplanets in a small sampling volume of the galaxy. Extrapolating from these discoveries the current estimate of the total number of habitable planets in the galaxy exceeds 100 billion — approximately one habitable planet for every sun-like star (Kopparapu, 2013). The estimated mean separation between such planets can be estimated to be a few light years. In view of all such recent discoveries it will be foolish to maintain a pre-Copernican idea that biology is necessarily confined to our planet, and more importantly that it originated here against manifestly impossible odds.

5.4. Transfer of evolved living systems across the galaxy

Whilst amplification of microorganisms within primordial comets could supply a steady source of primitive life (archaea, bacteria, unicellular eukaryotes and their viruses) to interstellar clouds and thence to new planetary systems via comets, the genetic products of evolved life could also be disseminated on a galaxy-wide scale. Transportation of entire ecologies of evolved aquatic life on much rarer occasions could also be possible if life-laden watery worlds (or large frozen fragments thereof) could occasionally collide with new habitats in the "Goldilocks zones" of stellar systems. It is tempting to speculate that the Cambrian explosion of "adaptive radiation" on a grand scale was indeed the product of such a cosmic seeding of "life-laden watery worlds (or large frozen planetoid fragments thereof)" as discussed (Steele et al., 2018).

Our present-day solar system with its extended halo of ~100 billion comets (the Oort Cloud) moves around the centre of the galaxy with a period of 240My. Every 40 million years, on the average, this comet cloud becomes perturbed due to the close passage of an interstellar molecular cloud (e.g. the Orion Nebula). Gravitational interaction then leads to hundreds of comets from the Oort Cloud being injected into the inner planetary system, some to collide with the Earth. Such collisions can not only cause

E.J. Steele et al. / Progress in Biophysics and Molecular Biology 149 (2019) 10–32

extinctions of species (as one impact surely did 65 million years ago, killing the dinosaurs), but they could also result in the expulsion of surface material back into space. A fraction of the Earth-debris so expelled survives shock-heating and could be laden with viable microbial ecologies of all types as well as genes and viruses of evolved life. Such life-bearing material could reach newly forming planetary systems in the passing molecular cloud within a few hundred million years of the ejection event. A fledgling planetary system thus comes to be infected with terrestrial microbes - terrestrial genes that can contribute, via horizontal gene transfer, to an ongoing process of local biological evolution. If every life-bearing planet transfers genes (bacteria, viruses, somatic cells and in rare instances deep frozen seeds and even fertilized eggs) in this way to more than one other planetary system, life throughout the galaxy on this picture will inevitably constitute a single connected biosphere.

5.5. Some quantitative estimates - cosmic distribution and numbers of living systems

There are thus several key factors to consider in the largely plausible yet speculative scenarios below on the Panspermic dispersal of living systems. All are based on known hard data (Hoyle and Wickramasinghe, 1979; 1981; Wickramasinghe, 2015a,b) that have recently been reviewed (Wickramasinghe, 2018; Steele et al., 2018, 2019).

5.5.1. Space Hardiness

The "space hardy" features of bacteria are legendary, displaying un-Earthly properties unlikely to be selected for survival on Earth but certainly in varied space environments (Hoyle and Wickramasinghe, 1993). A typical example illustrating such resistance properties to radiation, cold, dehydration, vacuum, acid is the extremophile *Deinococcus radiodurans*. Thus bacteria and their spores, other micro-organisms and eukaryotic cells, and some exemplar microscopic animals (Tardigrades) are by now well recognized for these space survival properties. For example the space survival of algae cultures outside the International Space Station (Leya et al., 2017), of plant seeds (Tepfer and Leach, 2017) as well as species of bacteria detected by their DNA sequences in the cosmic dust on the external surface of the ISS (Grebennikova et al., 2018). This is quite apart from the >100 million year survival times of bacteria and archaea in terrestrial salt crystals that we have already discussed (Vreeland et al., 2007; Satterfield et al., 2005).

5.5.2. Effective seeding population sizes

The population size, N, of a living system within an impacting bolide that has been ejected from another inhabited planetary or cometary body must be sufficiently large to permit viable transfer. The transfer could take the form of viral particles, bacteria, spores and plant seeds. In some instances even fertilized eggs of insects and higher animals cannot be excluded. When N is very large $\geq 10^6$ it is obvious that a 90% or 99% kill on impact still leaves a significant number of survivors to rapidly proliferate in a Lamarckian manner in a congenial niche. This obviously automatically applies to impacting populations of viruses, bacteria, many microorganisms and their spores, large populations of plant seeds, and even the highly contentious suggestion (Steele et al., 2018, 2019) of cryopreserved fertilized Cephalopod eggs which could arrive on impact given large $N \geq 10^6$ (below).

5.5.3. Protection radiation damage

Encasement in a protective matrix or deep burial is important both during space travel and on impact. While many organisms display "space hardy" features, long term survival during space travel (100 million to billions of years) requires a living system to be buried or cryopreserved *within* cometary or planetoid bodies. We have argued elsewhere that such vehicles as comets or larger planetoids may act as both protective incubators (active amplifiers) of living systems and post impact allow significant percentages to survive and proliferate.

5.5.4. Cryopreservation

In this scenario cryopreservation is a key consideration, particularly for mature complex multicellular differentiated organisms. We note the recent observations on the viable recovery of nematode worms from 42,000 year old Late Pleistocene Siberian permafrost (Shatilovich et al., 2018). Such findings need to be replicated at other locations and with other species. The data we have currently available leads to the obvious question: if 42,000 years, why not a billion years of cryopreservation? The discovery relevant to our argument is that soma-to-germline transfer of genetic information (penetration of the *Weisman Barrier*) has been recently demonstrated in *C. elegans*, a nematode (regulatory double stranded RNA triggering RNA interference phenomena Devanapally et al., 2015). This result is of potential importance to the Lamarckian adaptability of thawed nematodes adapting after arrival in a new cosmic niche.

All these discoveries have been of crucial importance for the Hoyle-Wickramasinghe Panspermia paradigm which can include the transportation of cryopreserved plant seeds and animal embryos within protective matrices (e.g. comets, moons and planets) or minimally their genes encoded in viruses via undisturbed space travel extending to hundreds of millions if not billions of years is not just possible but inevitable. Indeed we would not find it beyond the realm of possibility that populations of mature microscopic life forms for example Tardigrades and nematode spp. have a wide cosmic prevalence and can on occasion be transferred between suitable cosmic habitats. This would involve a process that merits being called cosmic Lamarckian evolution. We speculated on such a scenario for the "sudden" emergence of Cephalopods on Earth 275 mya viz. cryopreserved Octopus eggs (Steele et al., 2018). The same scenario could apply to a whole range of populations of fertilized insect eggs of many species as well as plant seeds.

5.5.5. Exoplanets

The number of exoplanetary systems possessing orbiting eco-systems within habitable zones (comets, moons, planets), with available water, surface or subterranean, will determine the total tally of potential cosmic habitats that can be infected. The current estimates of exo-planets in the habitable zones is $> 10^{10}$ (Kopparapu, 2013) and possibly much larger if we consider all types of extreme habits, say, $> 10^{11}$. The range of the types of terrestrial microorganisms existing in the "deep hot biosphere" as first described by Tommy Gold (1992, 1999) is an indication of the extraordinary range of extreme habitats that can support life. Indeed in our Solar System alone there may be an unknown number of extreme habitats in the form of moons and planetoids on which large populations of sub-surface living systems could exist (moons such as Europa, Enceladus, are obvious examples).

We are thus led from many different directions to admit a convergence to the concept of a genuine "Cosmic Gene Pool" based on common DNA/RNA/Protein biochemistry (Wickramasinghe et al., 2018a). Indeed the vast variety of living species on Earth would be a minuscule subset, albeit a significant sub-set, of an almost infinite pool.

In terms of magnitudes of incidence of living systems throughout the Cosmos we might be tempted to rank organisms (see Table 2) as follows based on a known "Earth equivalent" multiplied by 10^{22} as an educated guess of the number of Earth-like

26   *E.J. Steele et al. / Progress in Biophysics and Molecular Biology 149 (2019) 10–32*

habitats in the universe (100 billion in every galaxy and 100 billion galaxies).

Table 2
Cosmic distribution and numbers of living systems.

• Viruses − terrestrial number 10^{31}	10^{53}
• Bacteria/Archaea - terrestrial number $\geq 10^{30}$	10^{52}
• Single cell eukaryotes - terrestrial number 10^{20}-10^{30}	10^{32}–10^{52}
• Complex Metazoans - terrestrial number $\geq 10^{20}$	10^{42}
• Higher plants, terrestrial number $\geq 10^7$ species	10^{29}
• Higher animals, terrestrial number $\geq 10^7$ species	10^{29}

Thus the *potential* cumulative incidence of complex orbiting ecosystems (on planets, moons, comets) around each observable star in our galaxy alone begins to approach super-astronomical magnitudes when these are multiplied by the estimated number of stars in the observable Universe ∼ 10^{22}. We should stress at this point that all the numbers listed above are highly conservative *underestimates* according to current thinking in cosmology. Even within the framework of the currently accepted Big Bang model of the universe (with early inflation), the observable universe would only be a minute fraction of what would be a very much larger, initially causally connected, region that *inflated* and would thus be out there, out of contact, but within which Lamarckian transfers would occur.

5.6. Evidence from the near-earth environment

With some 50–100 tonnes of cometary debris entering the Earth's atmosphere on a daily basis the collection and testing of this material for signs of life should in principle at least be straightforward. Some such projects have been carried out from 2001 onwards. The first serious project was carried out with the support of the Indian Space Research Organisation (ISRO) in partnership with a group of scientists in the UK including one of us (NCW). Samples of stratospheric aerosols collected using balloon-borne cryosamplers were investigated independently in the UK and India and revealed evidence of microbial life (Harris et al., 2002). A particularly interesting component of the collected samples was in the form of 10 μm clumps that were identified by SEM and fluorescence tests as being viable but not culturable microorganisms. Fig. 9 shows putative biological entities discovered in stratospheric samples by electron microscopy; and the left panel of Fig. 9 shows a clump of putative cocci and a bacillus. The right panel of Fig. 9 shows evidence of viable microorganisms which did not prove to be culturable.

Because such large aggregates are virtually impossible to loft to

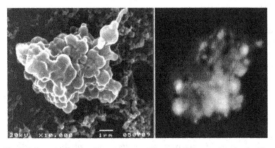

Fig. 9. Left: a clump of carbonacesous particles resembling cocci and a bacillus Right: A clump of viable but non-culturable bacteria fluorescing under the application of a carbocyanine dye which tests for electric potential across cell walls. Harris et al., 2002.

41 km a *prima facie* case for their extraterrestrial cometary origin has been made. A similar experiment to that conducted in 2001 was repeated by ISRO in 2009 (Shivaji et al., 2009) and 3 new microorganisms were discovered, including one named in honour of Fred Hoyle as *Janibacter hoylei*.

The genetic similarities of the new stratospheric bacteria to existing terrestrial genera have been cited by some as an argument to discount their possible space origin. However, in our view, terrestrial bacterial genera all have a space origin, so homologies of the type found are to be expected and do indeed corroborate a space origin of all bacteria on Earth (Hoyle and Wickramasinghe, 1979; 1981). In order to take the matter further, and hopefully reach a decisive conclusion, further tests of the collected microbial samples would be desirable. One such test involves the deployment of a rather rare laboratory resource − a Nanosims machine. This will determine the isotopic composition of carbon, oxygen and other constituent elements within the individual bacterial cells, and if the composition turns out to be non-terrestrial (Tokoro G, Wickramasinghe NC, Temple R and colleagues, experiments underway).

Experiments can also be conducted on the International Space Station (ISS) to sample the zodiacal cometary dust trails through which the Earth continuously passes in its orbit around the Sun. Such initial experiments are reported (Grebennikova et al., 2018; Wickramasinghe et al., 2018b). Bacteria in the cosmic dust have been detected by standard PCR techniques on the external surface of the ISS. Uplifting of micro-organisms has been ruled out. These are ground breaking experiments and contamination has been ruled out. Uplifting of micro-organisms to 360–400 km seem quite improbable on physical grounds (Wickramasinghe and Rycroft, 2018). These data offer the promise that such ISS microbiological phenomena can be confirmed or refuted by independent teams of scientists. We can imagine ISS real-time biological laboratories conducting routine genetic analyses and tissue cultures using the portable Next Generation Sequencing (NGS) machines now available. The range of microbial life, prokaryotic and eukaryotic, in the near Earth cosmic environment can become, as discussed already, part of the proposed "Hoyle Shield", predicting potential pandemics from space (Hoyle and Wickramasinghe, 1979; Smith, 2013).

Such studies may allow confirmation that Darwinian-Lamarckian evolution takes place not just within a closed biosphere on Earth but extends over a large and connected volume of the cosmos (Wickramasinghe et al., 2018a).

5.7. Scientific pragmatism: the near earth neighbourhood?

In our view pragmatic research on extraterrestrial life is now required. The research budgets directed to the search for extant and living extra-terrestrial life needs to be far more focused on the near Earth neighbourhood. The experiments are relatively cheap and can be definitive and unequivocal. They offer real-time experimentation in standard biological laboratories. We have discussed some of the promising data emerging and there are more recent findings.

Microorganisms have been detected by Milton Wainwright and colleagues in-falling from space at 41 Km in the Stratosphere (Wainwright et al., 2015). These data were secured in balloon-lofted experiments and conducted to avoid terrestrial contamination. They were set up technically to establish that the microorganisms and other cellular and viral aggregates *were observed following in-fall not by upwelling*. Critics may conclude it is all due to terrestrial contamination, but the data need to be dispassionately evaluated in their own terms. Many of the eukaryotic species detected can be classed as unassigned Acritarch, and appear viable on impact with the collection medium. The data more readily fit with Panspermia theory (Wainwright et al., 2015).

E.J. Steele et al. / Progress in Biophysics and Molecular Biology 149 (2019) 10–32 27

5.8. Cosmic octopus?

We have tried to discuss throughout this article the "Demarcation Data" which allows distinction between conventional terrestrial neo-Darwinism (Section 1) and the Cosmic Lamarckian - Panspermia paradigm. Thus there are a plethora of multifactorial awkward facts and observations, biological and biophysical, which fit neatly into the Hoyle-Wickramasinghe Panspermia paradigm but are often puzzling or inexplicable under a pure neo-Darwinian terrestrial evolution paradigm - anchored to a super-astronomically improbable and unproven Abiogenesis event producing the first cell here on Earth about 4 billion years ago. Most of the relevant problems and contradictions in this viewpoint are covered in our recent papers (Steele et al., 2018, 2019). In the same vein a similar set of awkward facts and observations fall neatly under a Lamarckian world view but not so easily under neo-Darwinism.

Thus we note again the recent observations on the viable recovery of nematodes from 42,000 year old Late Pleistocene Siberian permafrost (Shatilovich et al., 2018). Such findings need to be replicated at other locations and with other species. Nevertheless the implications under the Hoyle-Wickramasinghe paradigm suggest that the transportation of cryopreserved complex mature animals within protective matrices (e.g. comets, moons and planets) or minimally their genes encoded in viruses via undisturbed space travel extending to hundreds of millions if not billions of years is the favoured "cross infection" mode across the Cosmos. This would remain true even if survival probabilities remain minuscule – with massive death rates during catastrophic ejection events (e.g. comet collisions), followed by further attrition upon re-entry onto receiving host planets. The hundreds of billions of habitable planets in our galaxy alone would make exchanges of mature biological entities a virtual certainty – no matter how ridiculous such a proposition might appear at first sight. The situation is similar to the sowing of seeds in the wind – most of them are lost, but so very many are the seeds that some among them are destined to survive. It is in a similar way that mature animals can albeit exceedingly rarely land, thaw out in a favourable cosmic habitat for growth, and thus undergo further cosmic Lamarckian evolution.

We speculated on precisely such a scenario for the emergence of Cephalopods on Earth 275 mya viz. cryopreserved Octopus eggs (Steele et al., 2018). This possibility has provoked much discussion and some ridicule in our circle of private discussions. However there is no logic whatsoever by which it can be excluded given the current data. The whole point of our discussion was to show a 250 million year gap between nautiloid precursors and squid/octopus. That is the whole point of the discussion in Steele et al., 2018. All the phylogenetic analyses points that out-all experts agree on this gap in the molluscian evolutionary record. But such huge punctuated equilibrium-type gaps permeate the fossil/phylogenetic emergence record, not just the molluscian evolutionary record. That is why Eldridge-Gould is discussed at length – it is a major unexplained conundrum (see Fig. 6 in our paper Steele et al., 2018).

6. Panspermia and Lamarckian inheritance are no longer mere "Hypotheses"

It is reasonable to assert that a scientific theory is a "mature hypothesis" surviving rigorous critical analyses and hard observation and experiment. However, it is still in essence Popperian and thus vulnerable. It can, in principle, be refuted or modified from its original form, as for instance Einstein's modification/generalisation of Newtonian mechanics. On the other hand, a hypothesis is usually the first tentative public utterance of a provisional explanation of a given set of natural phenomena. It will only mature into a "theory" if it survives refutation by severe demarcation tests involving

further critical analyses, observation and experiment. By these criteria the modern field of Cosmic Biology/Panspermia, first clearly advanced by Hoyle and Wickramasinghe, can be deemed a mature scientific theory. It provides a coherent explanation for both the origin of life on Earth and its further non-linear progress of terrestrial evolution and adaptation as reviewed recently by Steele et al. (2018).

The H–W thesis has thus survived numerous demarcation tests, and it has offered many predictions that have been subsequently fulfilled and furthermore has strong explanatory and predictive power. For example, a key prediction concerns the distribution and number of living systems in the known Universe. This distribution is dictated *solely by* the "habitability" or otherwise of available viable Cosmic niches (comets, moons, planets - both orbiting or wandering) and the DNA/RNA/Protein paradigm for life will hold across the Cosmos (Wickramasinghe et al., 2018a). This is an important and definite prediction.

H–W Panspermia theory thus brings together a range of multifactorial biological facts and phenomena, at first sight unrelated, providing a coherent explanation for their existence, their biological form and their ongoing evolutionary features (Steele et al., 2018). It therefore provides a general mechanism for the widely accepted evolutionary pattern of "Punctuated Equilibrium" described clearly by Eldredge and Gould (1972), then Gould and Eldredge (1977) but which otherwise remains a semantic description of the known facts. It also predicts and qualifies the 'genetic' boundaries of H–W theory. Thus extraterrestrial life is expected, as just discussed, to possess the same biochemistry, genetic code, the same DNA and RNA as life on Earth. A radically different life form discovered would be significant evidence against a universal Galactic panspermia and the H–W theory would require modification (Wickramasinghe et al., 2018a). Yet Galactic-wide panspermia,as we outline here, is now being widely accepted by the mainstream astronomical community. Thus the Harvard group of Ginsburg et al. (2018) have recently developed a mathematical model of Galactic-wide panspermia in which icy comets or rocky asteroids carrying microbiota could be widely distributed in the galaxy and exchanged between planetary systems. Their calculations lend further support to the H–W model of cosmic biology and our present thesis of Lamarckian transfer in which the galaxy and the wider universe become a single connected biosphere.

We have also discussed above the vast amount of new evidence that has accumulated since the 1970s consistent with Lamarckian Acquired Inheritance phenomena from bacteria through to plants and animals. Indeed the "Hypothesis of Lamarck" has now survived some stringent and severe tests earning recognition as a maturing "Theory" of biological evolution. Our discussion here has focused where possible on the molecular mechanisms which are now much clearer in many cases than they were 40 years ago. And our discussion here has also been on much of the key "Demarcation Evidence" which, as with Cosmic Panspermia, needs to be confronted by the scientific mainstream. Lamarckian inheritance of acquired characteristics, based, at their core, on RNA and reverse transcriptase steps, has successfully run the gauntlet of numerous "Popperian" tests during the past 40 years. In our considered opinion the effective spread of living systems throughout the Cosmos is both by Lamarckian and Darwinian mechanisms - with the emphasis on Lamarckian evolutionary processes as these provide rapid and "directional' adaptations to new Cosmic niches immediately after the organisms have landed.

Authors' Note

In addition to the well attested mechanisms for particle transport discussed it is worth considering other modes assisting the

28   *E.J. Steele et al. / Progress in Biophysics and Molecular Biology 149 (2019) 10–32*

panspermic dispersal of living systems throughout the Cosmos.

Appendix by Robert Temple: *On the Panspermia of the Ancients, Cosmic Spermata and Speculation on Birkeland Currents and Mechanisms of Space Journeys*

It is a challenging task to write an appendix to the above paper which would meet some of the standards we have set for the wide range of evidence for Lamarckian Panspermia. Although I have some additional scientific observations to make, I will start with an update to the situation regarding the *Prehistory of Panspermia*, which is a scholarly matter relating to early pre-scientific thinking by ancient peoples of panspermic notions.

In 2006 I delivered a paper entitled 'The Prehistory of Panspermia: Astrophysical or Metaphysical?', which was published in 2007 (Temple, 2007). In this paper I surveyed proto-panspermia ideas in a variety of ancient cultures, commencing with the ancient Egyptians. Amongst the ancient Egyptian texts which I discussed were the Pyramid Texts, written in what is known as 'Old Egyptian', and which date from the 5th Dynasty (early 25th century BC to mid 24th century BC) but include much earlier archaic material. During 2018, this paper came to the attention of Professor Joanna Popielska-Grzbowska of the Institute of Mediterranean and Oriental Cultures, Polish Academy of Sciences, in Warsaw. She is an expert in Old Egyptian and she informed me that in her studies of the terminology and concepts embodied in the Pyramid Texts my comments about them had been confirmed. She also said that she had found much more evidence in those texts expressing proto-panspermia ideas. She and I will be producing a joint paper on this subject during 2019, which will considerably enlarge the discussion of the prehistory of Panspermia.

I would like also to mention that since my 2007 paper, I have come to know and appreciate the particular interest of Professor Otto Rössler in the same crucial passage by the ancient Greek philosopher Anaxagoras (510-428 BC) which I had discussed. He and I are in frequent contact and it is interesting that we both found the Anaxagoras passage astonishing, though from two separate, albeit probably compatible, perspectives. Rössler's interest relates to his seminal work in chaos theory (he is for example the discoverer of the Rössler Attractor), and he did not consider this passage from the point of view of Panspermia at all. But as his views on the same passage are so important, I feel that I should mention them and refer readers to the remarkable volume of scientific dialogue with him, 'Chaotic Harmony' (Sanayei and Rössler, 2014), which contains non-mathematical accounts of what he saw in that passage of Anaxagoras. In the meantime Rossler and I have published a joint paper in 2019 entitled 'Early Einstein Completed', concerning the equivalence principle and global-c.

I return now to our present task. There are several aspects of the Panspermia field which in my opinion have scarcely been touched. I shall address these in a succession of headings.

Transport through space of the microbiota

The part of this subject which we understand very well is the dispersal of dust and microbiota into the Earth's atmosphere and its slow drifting down to the surface, namely the 50–100 tonnes per day of cosmic dust and debris which reaches the surface of our planet daily, which is referred to in the main text above. We can also understand the transport of much of this material by comets and its dispersal from the comet tails. There is nothing about either of these processes which is really unusual or indeed unexpected, once they have been suggested and brought to our attention, as they first were by Fred Hoyle and Chandra Wickramasinghe in numerous publications (which has founded the Science of

Panspermia as we now understand it).

The long life of the microbiota, or should we say cosmic spermata (to use the ancient Greek word), is a more than plausible concept, as witness the main text above. Thus we know from available evidence that it is possible for cryopreserved cosmic spermata to survive interplanetary, interstellar, and even inter-Galactic distances of travel and still be viable entities.

But what is lacking is a full understanding of all the available means of transport of spermata in those regions where there are no comets, or where radiation pressure is somehow ineffective. What then? How do they get around? So far the thinking seems to be of a slow drifting through space and a tediously ponderous passive dispersal, mostly by pressure from light rays from stars (radiation pressure).

My idea is 'a better design', and provides for rapid transport through space of vast quantities of cosmic spermata, so that the slow part of the transport process would not be across the vast interstellar and inter-Galactic distances, but would be when the particles of dust and biota reach a more cluttered region such as our solar system, where the entire transportation process would significantly *slow down*, like a plane coming in for a landing. Charged dust entering a protoplanetary or planetary environment with denser plasmas and higher values of magnetic field might be magnetically braked with charge repulsion rather than collisions playing a dominant role.

The hypothesis here is that the means of transporting the cosmic spermata could be through the moving of sheathed and internally structured plasmoids within gigantic Birkeland Currents on a cosmic scale (Peratt, 1992). They would be hurtled through vast distances at nearly relativistic speeds between star systems and even between galaxies. These Birkeland Currents would be super-highways full not only of the charged particles which we know them to contain but of opportunistic cosmic spermata hitching a ride. And lest we think this unlikely, we only need to understand enough about plasma in space to realise that it is always full of dust particles, not only grains, and frankly plasma is not particularly bothered about what kind of dust, since essentially 'any old dust will do, and if some of it is "alive", well what the hell, jump in for the ride'. And the other thing is that all dust particles are *charged*, which thus most likely helps lock them in the cosmic streams of the Currents.

Chandra Wickramasinghe and I are currently exploring the details of how this process works, and the evidence of the Birkeland Currents in space. It provides an additional mechanism for meaningful and effective cosmic transport of the cosmic spermata anywhere and everywhere in the Universe.

Dust clouds

We all know that the Universe is full of gigantic dust clouds, some 100 light years or more across - so full of them in fact that it might be asked 'Does God smoke?' and is the Universe really a smoke-filled room? There is much more to be said about cosmic dust clouds and their relationship to Panspermia. Chandra Wickramasinghe and I will also be revisiting this question in a future more detailed investigation (Temple and Wickramasinghe, 2019). A key factor in what we have to relate is that *all cosmic dust clouds are charged*. The charges can be positive or negative, and even if an entire cloud appears to have zero net charge in total, the internal structures within the cloud can be so complicated that isolated and ensheathed regions within the cloud can have opposite charges which are isolated, and a vast variety of different regions containing different things. Within the clouds, as within the Birkeland Currents, pockets of living things can be isolated from barren regions. The key to understanding this is to understand complex dusty

E.J. Steele et al. / Progress in Biophysics and Molecular Biology 149 (2019) 10–32   29

plasmas. We should try now to think of cosmic dust clouds not as just a lot of stuff floating around at random and see them for what they possibly are, highly structured and immensely complex genuine entities having a biological provenance. This will all be further explained in a forthcoming paper.

References

Ader, R., Cohen, N., 1982. Behaviorally conditioned immunosuppression and murine systemic lupus erythematosus. Science 215, 1534–1536.

Ader, R., Cohen, N., 1993. Psychoneuroimmunology: conditioning stress. Annu. Rev. Psychol. 44, 53–55.

Allen, D.A., Wickramasinghe, D.T., 1981. Diffuse interstellar absorption bands between 2.9 and 4.0 mm. Nature 294, 239–240.

Altwegg, K., Balsiger, H., Bar-Nun, A., et al., 2016. Prebiotic chemical – amino acid and phosphorus in the coma of comet 67P/Churyumov-Gerasimenko. Sci.Adv. 2016 2, e1600285, 27 May.

Baltimore, D., 1970. RNA-dependent DNA polymerase in virions of RNA tumor virus. Nature 226, 1209–1211.

Baross, J.A., 2018. The rocky road to biomolecules. Nature 564, 42–43. https://doi.org/10.1038/d41586-018-07262-8.

Basu, U., Meng, F.L., Keim, C., Grinstein, V., Pefanis, E., et al., 2011. The RNA exosome targets the AID cytidine deaminase to both strands of transcribed duplex DNA substrates. Cell 144, 353–363. https://doi.org/10.1016/j.cell. 2011.01.001.

In: Bateson, P., Cartwright, N., Dupre, J., Laland, K., Noble, D. (Eds.), 2017. New trends in evolutionary biology: biological, philosophical and social science perspectives. Interface Focus, 7, 20170051. https://doi.org/10.1098/rsfs.2017.0051.

Bayne, E.H., Allshire, R.C., 2005. RNA-directed transcriptional gene silencing in mammals. Trends Genet. 21, 370–373.

Bell, E.A., Boehnke, P., Harrison, T., Mao, W.L., 2015. Potentially biogenic carbon preserved in a 4.1 billion-year-old zircon. Proc. Natl. Acad. Sci. U.S.A. 112, 14518–14521.

Blanden, R.V., Rothenfluh, H.S., Zylstra, P., Weiller, G.F., Steele, E.J., 1998. The signature of somatic hypermutation appears to be written into the germline IgV segment repertoire. Immunol. Rev. 162, 117–132.

Brent, L., Chandler, P., Fiertz, W., Medawar, P.B., Rayfield, L.S., Simpson, E., 1982. Further studies on supposed Lamarckian inheritance of immunological tolerance. Nature 295, 242–244.

Brent, L., Rayfield, L.S., Chandler, P., Fiertz, W., Medawar, P.B., Simpson, E., 1981. Supposed Lamarckian inheritance of immunological tolerance. Nature 290, 508–512.

Burnet, F.M., 1957. A modification of Jerne's theory of antibody production using the concept of clonal selection. Aust. J. Sci. 20, 67–69.

Burne, F.M., 1959. Clonal Selection Theory of Acquired Immunity. Cambridge: Cambridge University Press.

Buske, F.A., Mattick, J.S., Bailey, T.L., 2011. Potential in vivo roles of nucleic acid triple-helices. RNA Biol. 8, 427–439. PMC3218511.

Buske, F.A., Bauer, D.C., Mattick, J.S., Bailey, T.L., 2012. Triplexator: detecting nucleic acid triple helices in genomic and transcriptomic data. Genome Res. 22, 1372–1381. https://doi.org/10.1101/gr.130237.111.

Cairns, J., Overbaugh, J., Miller, S., 1988. The origin of mutants. Nature 335, 142–145.

Campbell, J.H., Perkins, P., 1988. Transgenerational effects of drug and hormonal treatments in mammals: a review of observations and ideas. In: Boer, G.J., Feenstra, M.G.P., Mirmiran, M., Swaab, D.F., van Haaren, F. (Eds.), Progress in Brain Research, vol. 73, pp. 535–553.

Capaccione, F., Coradini, A., Filacchione, G., Erard, S., Arnoldf, G., et al., 2015. The organic-rich surface of comet 67P/Churyumov- Gerasimenko as seen by VIRTIS/Rosetta. Science 347 (6220).

Chen, F., Wang, N., Tan, H.Y., Guo, W., Zhang, C., Feng, Y., 2019. The functional roles of exosomes-derived long non-coding RNA in human cancer. Cancer Biol. Ther. 20 (5), 583–592. https://doi.org/10.1080/15384047.2018.1564562, 2019.

Clube, S.V.M., Hoyle, F., Napier, W.M., Wickramasinghe, N.C., 1996. Giant comets, evolution and civilization. Astrophys. Space Sci. 245, 43–60.

Cossetti, C., Lugini, L., Astrologo, L., Saggio, I., Fais, S., Spadafora, C., 2014. Soma-to-Germline transmission of RNA in mice xenografted with human tumour cells: possible transport by exosomes. PLoS One 9 (7), e101629. https://doi.org/10.1371/journal.pone.0101629.

Cullis, C.A., 1984. Environmentally induced DNA changes. In: Pollard, J.W. (Ed.), Evolutionary Theory: Paths into the Future. John Wiley, London, pp. 217–237.

Darwin, C., 1868. The Variation of Plants and Animals under Domestication. John Murray, London.

Dawkins, R.L., 2015. Adapting Genetics: Quantal Evolution after Natural Selection – Surviving the Changes to Come. Nearurban Publishing, Dallas, TX, ISBN 978-0-9864115-1-9.

Dawkins, R.L., Leelayuwat, C., Gaudieri, S., Tay, G., Hui, J., Cattley, S., et al., 1999. Genomics of the major histocompatibility complex: haplotypes, duplication, retroviruses and disease. Immunol. Rev. 167, 275–304.

Devanapally, S., Ravikumar, S., Jose, A.M., 2015. Double-stranded RNA made in C. elegans neurons can enter the germline and cause transgenerational gene silencing. Proc. Natl. Acad. Sci. U.S.A. 112, 2133–2138. https://doi.org/10.1073/pnas. 1423333112.

Dias, B.G., Ressler, K.J., 2014. Parental olfactory experience influences behavior and

neural structure in subsequent generations. Nat. Neurosci. 17, 89–96.

Eldredge, N., Gould, S.J., 1972. Punctuated equilibria : an alternative to phyletic gradualism. In: Schopf, T.J.M. (Ed.), Models in Paleobiology. Freeman Cooper, San Francisco, pp. 82–115.

Elsila, J., Glavin, D.P., Dworkin, J.P., 2009. Cometary glycine detected in samples returned by Stardust. Meteorit. Planet. Sci. 44, 1323–1330.

Fogarty, P., 2002. Optimizing the production of animal models for target and lead validation. Targets 1 (3), 109–116. https://doi.org/10.1016/S1477-3627(02)02198-0.

Franklin, A., Milburn, P.J., Blanden, R.V., Steele, E.J., 2004. Human DNA polymerase-η an A-T mutator in somatic hypermutation of rearranged immunoglobulin genes, is a reverse transcriptase. Immunol. Cell Biol. 82, 219–225. https://doi.org/10.1046/j.0818-9641.2004.01221.x.

Fuentes, I., Stegemann, S., Golczyk, H., Karcher, D., Bock, R., 2014. Horizontal genome transfer as an asexual path to the formation of new species. Nature 511, 232–235.

Gibson, D., Glass, J., Lartigue, C., Noskov, V., Chuang, R., et al., 2010. Creation of a bacterial cell controlled by a chemically synthesized genome. Science 329, 52–56. https://doi.org/10.1126/science.1190719.

Gill, S., Catchpole, R., Forterre, P., 2018. Extracellular membrane vesicles (EVs) in the three domains of life and beyond, 2018 Nov 21 FEMS Microbiol. Rev.. https://doi.org/10.1093/femsre/fuy042 ([Epub ahead of print]).

Ginsburg, I., Lingam, M., Loeb, A., 2018. Galactic panspermia. Astrophys. J. Lett. 868, L12 arXiv:1810.04307.

Gold, T., 1992. The deep hot biosphere. Proc. Natl. Acad. Sci. U.S.A. 89, 6045–6049.

Gold, T., 1999. The Deep Hot Biosphere: the Myth of Fossil Fuels. Copernicus. Springer Verlag, New York.

Goldner, M.G., Spergel, G., 1972. On the transmission of alloxan diabetes and other diabetogenic influences. Adv. Metab. Disord. 60, 57–72.

Gorczynski, R.M., 1992. Conditioned stress responses by pregnant and/or lactating mice reduce immune responses of their offspring after weaning. Brain Behav. Immmun. 6, 87–95.

Gorczynski, R.M., Kennedy, M., 1987. Behaviour trait associated with conditioned immunity. Brain Behav. Immun. 1, 72–80.

Gorczynski, R.M., Kennedy, M., MacRae, S., Ciampi, A., 1983. A possible maternal effect in the abnormal hyporesponsiveness to specific alloantigens in offspring born to neonatally tolerant fathers. J. Immunol. 131, 1115–1100.

Gorczynski, R.M., Steele, E.J., 1980. Inheritance of acquired immunologic tolerance to foreign histocompatibility antigens in mice. Proc. Natl. Acad. Sci. U.S.A. 77, 2871–2875.

Gorczynski, R.M., Steele, E.J., 1981. Simultaneous yet independent inheritance of somatically acquired tolerance to two distinct H-2 antigenic haplotype determinants in mice. Nature 289, 678–681. https://doi.org/10.1038/289678a0.

Gorczynski, L.Y., Gorczynski, C.P., Terzioglu, T., Gorczynski, R.M., 2011. Pre-and post-natal influences of neurohormonal triggering and behaviour on the immune response of offspring. Adv. Neuroimmune Biol. 1, 39–51.

Gould, S.J., Eldredge, N., 1977. Punctuated equilibria: the tempo and mode of evolution reconsidered. Paleobiology 3, 115–151.

Grebennikova, T.V., Syroeshkin, A.V., Shubralova, E.V., Eliseeva, O.V., Kostina, L.V., et al., 2018. The DNA of bacteria of the world ocean and the Earth in cosmic dust at the international space station. Sci. World J. 2018, Article ID 7360147, 7 pp https://doi.org/10.1155/2018/7360147.

Guo, H., Arambula, D., Ghosh, P., Miller, J.F., 2014. Diversity- generating retroelements in phage and bacterial genomes. Microbiol. Spectr. 2 (6) https://doi.org/10.1128/microbiolspec.MDNA3-0029-2014. MDNA3-0029-2014.

Guo, H., Tse, L.V., Nieh, A.W., Czornyj, E., Williams, S., et al., 2011. Target site recognition by a diversity-generating retroelement. PLoS Genet. 7 (12), e1002414 https://doi.org/10.1371/journal.pgen.1002414.

Guo, J.U., Su, Y., Zhong, C., Guo-li Ming, G.-l., Song, H., 2011a. Emerging roles of TET proteins and 5-Hydroxymethylcytosines in active DNA demethylation and beyond. Cell Cycle 10, 2662–2668.

Guo, J.U., Su, Y., Zhong, C., Ming, G.L., Song, H., 2011b. Hydroxylation of 5- methylcytosine by TET1 promotes active DNA demethylation in the adult brain. Cell 145 (3), 423–434. https://doi.org/10.1016/j.cell.2011.03.022.

Gurdon, C., Svab, Z., Feng, Y., Kumar, D., Maliga, P., 2016. Cell-to-cell movement of mitochondria in plants. Proc. Natl. Acad. Sci. U.S.A. 113, 3395–3400.

Hagemann, R., 2002. How did East German genetics avoid Lysenkoism? Trends Genet. 18, 320–324.

Hall, G.H., 1988. Adaptive evolution that requires multiple spontaneous mutations. 1.Mutations involving an insertion sequence. Genetics 120, 887–897.

Ham, B.-K., Lucas, W.J., 2017. Phloem-mobile RNAs as systemic signaling agents. Annu. Rev. Plant Biol. 68, 173–195, 2017. https://doi.org/10.1146/annurev-arplant-042916-041139.

Harris, M.J., Wickramasinghe, N.C., Lloyd, D., Narlikar, J.V., Rajaratnam, P., et al., 2002. Detection of living cells in stratosphere samples. Proc. SPIE 4495, 192. https://doi.org/10.1117/12.454758.

He, Y.F., Li, B.Z., Li, Z., Liu, P., Wang, Y., et al., 2011. Tet-mediated formation of 5-carboxylcytosine and its excision by TDG in mammalian DNA. Science 333, 1303–1307. https://doi.org/10.1126/science.1210944.

Hill, W.G., 2014. Applications of population genetics to animal breeding, from Wright, Fisher and Lush to genomic prediction. Genetics 196, 1–16.

Hoena, N-t.E., Cremera, T., Gallo, R.C., Margolisc, L.B., 2016. Extracellular vesicles and viruses: are they close relatives? Proc. Natl. Acad. Sci. 113, 9155–9161. www.pnas.org/cgi/doi/10.1073/pnas.1605146113.

Hoover, R.B., 2005. Microfossils, biominerals, and chemical biomarkers in meteorites. In: Hoover, R.B., Rozanov, A.Y., Paepe (Eds.), Perspectives in Astrobiology. RR IOS Press, Amsterdam, pp. 43–65.

Hoover, R.B., 2011. Fossils of cyanobacteria in CI1 carbonaceous meteorites: implications to life on comets, Europa and Enceladus. J. Cosmol. 16, 7070–7111.

Hoover, R.B., Hoyle, F., Wickramasinghe, N.C., Hoover, M., Al-Mufti, S., 1986. Diatoms on Earth, comets, Europa and in interstellar space. Earth Moon Planets 35, 19–45.

Hoyle, F., Wickramasinghe, N.C., 1978. Life Cloud. J.M. Dent Ltd, London.

Hoyle, F., Wickramasinghe, N.C., 1979. Diseases from Space. J.M. Dent Ltd, London.

Hoyle, F., Wickramasinghe, N.C., 1981. Evolution from Space. J.M. Dent Ltd, London.

Hoyle, F., Wickramasinghe, C., 1982. Why Neo-Darwinism Does Not Work. University College Cardiff Press, ISBN 0 906449 50 2.

Hoyle, F., Wickramasinghe, N.C., 1985. Living Comets. Univ. College, Cardiff Press, Cardiff.

Hoyle, F., Wickramasinghe, N.C., 1991. The Theory of Cosmic Grains. Kluwer, Dordrecht.

Hoyle, F., Wickramasinghe, N.C., 1993. Our Place in the Cosmos : the Unfinished Revolution. J.M. Dent Ltd, London.

Hoyle, F., Wickramasinghe, N.C., Al-Mufti, S., et al., 1982. Infrared spectroscopy over the 2.9-3.9μm waveband in biochemistry and astronomy. Astrophys. Space Sci. 83, 405–409.

Hoyle, F., Wickramasinghe, N.C., 1999a. Panspermia 2000. Astrophys. Space Sci. 268, 1–17.

Hoyle, F., Wickramasinghe, N.C., 1999b. The Universe and Life: deductions from the weak anthropic principle. Astrophys. Space Sci. 268, 89–102.

Hoyle, F., Wickramasinghe, N.C., 2000. Astronomical Origins of Life : Steps towards Panspermia. Reprints from *Astrophys*. Space Sci 268. Kluwer Academic Publishers, Dordrecht, The Netherlands, pp. 1–3, 1999.

Jablonka, E., Lamb, M.J., 1995. Epigenetic Inheritance and Evolution:The Lamarckian Dimension. Oxford University Press, Oxford.

Kopparapu, R.K., 2013. A revised estimate of the occurrence rate of terrestrial planets in habitable zones around Kepler M-Dwarf. Astrophys. J. 767, L8.

Keissling, A.A., Crowell, R.C., Connell, R.S., 1987. Sperm- associated retroviruses in the mouse epididymis. Proc. Natl. Acad. Sci. U.S.A. 84, 8667-8571.

Kiani, J., Grandjean, V., Liebers, R., Tuorto, F., Ghanbarian, H., et al., 2013. RNA–mediated epigenetic heredity requires the cytosine methyltransferase Dnmt2. PLoS Genet. 9 (5) https://doi.org/10.1371/journal.pgen.1003498 e1003498.

Koestler, A., 1971. The Case of the Midwife Toad. Pan Books, London.

Krishnan, A., Iyer, L.M., Holland, S.J., Boehm, T., Aravind, L., 2018. Diversification of AID/APOBEC-like deaminases in metazoa: multiplicity of clades and widespread roles in immunity. Proc. Natl. Acad. Sci. U.S.A. 115, E3201–E3210.

Kulski, J.K., 2019. Long noncoding RNA HCP5, a hybrid HLA Class I endogenous retroviral gene: structure, expression, and disease associations. Cells 8 (5), 480. https://doi.org/10.3390/cells8050480.

Kuraoka, I., Endou, M., Yamaguchi, Y., Wada, Y., Handa, H., Tanaka, K., 2003. Effects of endogenous DNA base lesions on transcription elongation by mammalian RNA polymerase II. J. Biol. Chem. 278, 7294–7299. https://doi.org/10.1074/jbc.M208102200.

Lampson, B.C., Sun, J., Hsu, M.-Y., Vallejo-Ramirez, J., Inouye, S., Inouye, M., 1989. Reverse transcriptase in a clinical strain of Escherichia coli: production of branched RNA-linked msDNA. Science 243, 1033–1038.

Lavitrano, M., Camaioni, A., Fazio, V.M., Dolci, S., Farace, M.G., Spadafora, C., 1989. Sperm cells as vectors for introducing foreign DNA into eggs: genetic transformation of mice. Cell 57, 717–723.

Lane, N., 2015. The Vital Question: Energy, Evolution, and the Origins of Complex Life. W.W. Norton & Company, London.

Leya, T., et al., 2017. Algae Survive outside Space Station. AlgaeIndustryMagazine.Com, 7th February, 2017. http://www.algaeindustrymagazine.com/algae-survive-outside-space-station/.

Li, Y., Syed, J., Sugiyama, H., 2016. RNA-DNA triplex formation by long noncoding RNAs. Cell. Chem. Biol. 23, 1325–1333. https://doi.org/10.1016/j.chembiol.2016.09.011.

Liebers, R., Rassoulzadegan, M., Lyko, F., 2014. Epigenetic regulation by heritable RNA. PLoS Genet. 10, e1004296. https://doi.org/10.1371/journal.pgen.1004296.

Lindley, R., 2010. The Soma: How Our Genes Really Work and How that Changes Everything! CYO Foundation. POD book. CreateSpace, Amazon.com, ISBN 1451525648.

Lindley, R.A., 2011. How evolution occurs: was Lamarck also right? EdgeScience #8, 6–9. https://www.scientificexploration.org/edgescience/8.

Lindley, R.A., 2013. The importance of codon context for understanding the Ig-like somatic hypermutation strand-biased patterns in TP53 mutations in breast cancer. Cancer Genet. 206, 222–226. https://doi.org/10.1016/j.cancergen.2013.05.016.

Lindley, R.A., 2018. A new treaty between disease and evolution - are deaminases the "universal mutators" responsible for our own evolution? EdgeScience #36, 16–20. http://www.scientificexploration.org/edgescience/edgescience-issue-36.

Lindley, R.A., Hall, N.A., 2018. APOBEC and ADAR deaminases may cause many single nucleotide polymorphisms curated in the OMIM database. Mutat. Res. Fundam. Mol. Mech. Mutagen. 810, 33–38. https://doi.org/10.1016/j.mrfmmm.2018.03.008.

Lindley, R.A., Steele, E.J., 2013. Critical analysis of strand-biased somatic mutation signatures in TP53 versus Ig genes, in genome-wide data and the etiology of cancer ISRN Genomics, 2013 Article ID 921418, 18 pages. https://www.hindawi.com/journals/isrn/2013/921418/.

Lindley, R.A., Humbert, P., Larmer, C., Akmeemana, E.H., Pendlebury, C.R.R., 2016. Association between targeted somatic mutation (TSM) signatures and HGS-OvCa progression. Cancer Med. 5, 2629–2640. https://doi.org/10.1002/cam4.825.

Litovchick, A., Szostak, J.W., 2008. Selection of cyclic peptide aptamers to HCV IRES RNA using mRNA display. Proc. Natl. Acad. Sci. U.S.A. 105, 15293–15298. https://doi.org/10.1073/pnas.0805837105.

Liu, Y., 2006. Historical and modern genetics of plant graft hybridization. Adv. Genet. 56, 101–129. https://doi.org/10.1016/S0065-2660(06)56003-1.

Liu, Y., 2008. A new perspective on Darwin's Pangenesis. Biol. Res. 83, 141–149. https://doi.org/10.1111/j.1469-185X.2008.00036.x.

Liu, Y., 2018. Darwin's Pangenesis and graft hybridization. Adv. Genet. 102, 27–66. https://doi.org/10.1016/bs.adgen.2018.05.007.

Liu, M., Deora, R., Doulatov, S.R., Gingery, M., Eiserling, F.A., et al., 2002. Reverse transcriptase-mediated tropism switching in Bordetella bacteriophage. Science 295, 2091–2094.

Liu, Y., Li, X., 2016. Darwin's Pangenesis as a molecular theory of inherited diseases. Gene 582, 19–22. https://doi.org/10.1016/j.gene.2016.01.051.

Luan, D.D., Korman, M.H., Jakubczak, J.L., Eichbush, T.H., 1993. Reverse transcription of R2B mRNA is primed by a nick at the chromosomal target site; A mechanism for non-LTR retrotransposition. Cell 72, 595–605. PMID: 7679954.

MacPhee, D.G., 1995. Mismatch repair, somatic mutations and the origins of cancer. Cancer Res. 55, 5489–5492.

Martin, W., Baross, J., Kelley, D., Russell, M.J., 2008. Hydrothermal vents and the origin of life. Nat. Rev. Microbiol. 6, 805–814. https://doi.org/10.1038/nrmicro1991.

Matic, I., 2019. Mutation rate heterogeneity increases odds of survival in unpredictable environments. Mol. Cell 75, 421–425. https://doi.org/10.1016/j.molcel.2019.06.029.

Mattick, J.S., 2003. Challenging the dogma: the hidden layer of non-protein-coding RNAs in complex organisms. Bioessays 25, 930–939.

Mattick, J.S., 2018. The State of long non-coding RNA biology. Noncoding RNA 4 (3), E17. https://doi.org/10.3390/ncrna4030017.

McFadden, J., 2016. Quantum leap: could quantum mechanics hold the secret of (alien) life ? In: Al-Khalili, J. (Ed.), Aliens: Science Asks: Is There Anyone Out There? Profile Books Ltd, London, pp. 137–146.

Majeed, Q., Wickramasinghe, N.C., Hoyle, F., Al-Mufti, S., 1988. A diatom model of dust in the Trapezium Nebula. Astrophys. Space Sci. 140, 205–207.

Matzke, M.A., Mosher, R.A., 2014. RNA-directed DNA methylation: an epigenetic pathway of increasing complexity. Nat. Rev. Genet. 15, 394–408.

Ménez, B., Pisapia, C., Andreani, M., Jamme, F., Vanbellingen, Q.P., Brunelle, A., Richard, L., et al., 2018. Nature 564, 59–63. https://doi.org/10.1038/s41586-018-0684-z.

Molnar, A., Melnyk, C.W., Bassett, A., Hardcastle, T.J., Dunn, R., Baulcombe, D.C., 2010. Small silencing RNAs in plants are mobile and direct epigenetic modifications in recipient cells. Science 328, 872–875. https://doi.org/10.1126/science.1187959.

Morgan, H.D., Dean, W., Coker, H.A., Reik, W., Petersen-Mahrt, S.K., 2004. Activation-induced cytidine deaminase deaminates 5-methylcytosine in DNA and is expressed in pluripotent tissues: implications for epigenetic reprogramming. J. Biol. Chem. 279, 52353–52360. https://doi.org/10.1074/jbc.M407695200.

Moroni, C., Schumann, G., 1975. Lipopolysaceharide induces C-type virus in short term cultures of BALB/c spleen cells. Nature 254, 60–61.

Moroni, C., Stoye, J.P., DeLamarter, J.F., Erb, P., Jay, F.A., et al., 1980. Normal B-cell activation involves endogenous retroviral antigen expression: implications for leukemogenesis. Cold Spring Harbor Symp. Quant. Biol. 44, 1205–1210.

Moynihan, J.A., Ader, R., 1996. Psychoneuroimunology: animal models of disease. Psychosom. Med. 58, 546–558.

Mullbacher, A., Ashman, R.B., Blanden, R.V., 1983. Induction of T-cell hyporesponsiveness to Bebaru and abnormalities in the immune responses in progeny of unresponsive males. Aust. J. Exp. Biol. Med. Sci. 61, 187–191 (now Immunol. Cell Biol.).

Mushegian, A.R., Koonin, E.V., 1996. A minimal gene set for cellular life derived by comparison of complete bacterial genomes. Proc. Natl. Acad. Sci. U.S.A. 96, 10268–10273.

Nabel, C.S., Manning, S.A., Kohli, R.M., 2012. The curious chemical biology of cytosine: deamination, methylation and oxidation as modulators of genomic potential. ACS Chem. Biol. 7, 20–30. https://doi.org/10.1021/cb2002895, 2012.

Noble, D., 2013. Physiology is rocking the foundations of evolutionary biology. Exp. Physiol. 98, 1235–1243.

Noble, D., 2017. Dance to the Tune of Life. Cambridge University Press. ISBN 1-107-17624-9.

Noble, D., 2018. Central dogma or central debate? Physiology 33, 246–249. https://doi.org/10.1152/physiol.00017.2018.

Noble, D., 2019. Exosomes, Gemmules, Pangenesis and Darwin to Be Published in Exosomes in Health and Disease. Elsevier, 2019.

Ohmori, H., Friedberg, E.C., Fuchs, R.P.P., Goodman, M.F., Hanaoka, F., Hinkle, D., et al., 2001. The Y-family of DNA polymerases. Mol. Cell 8, 7–8.

Ohta, Y., 1991. Graft-transformation, the mechanism for graft-induced genetic changes in higher plants. Euphytica 55, 91–99.

Okamoto, K., 1965. Apparent transmittance of factors to offspring by animals with experimental diabetes". In: Wrenshall, G.A. (Ed.), On the Nature and Treatment of Diabetes Liebe BS, Exerpta Med, Amsterdam, vol. 6, pp. 627–637.

Okuda, H., Shibai, H., Nakagawa, T., Matsuhara, H., Kobayashi, Y., et al., 1990. An infrared quintuplet near the galactic center. Astrophys. J. 351, 89–97.

E.J. Steele et al. / Progress in Biophysics and Molecular Biology 149 (2019) 10–32

Ostermeier, G.C., Miller, D., Huntriss, J.D., Diamond, M.P., Krawetz, S.A., 2004. Reproductive biology: delivering spermatozoan RNA to the oocyte. Nature 429, 154.

Painter, R., Osmond, C., Gluckman, P., Hanson, M., Phillips, D., Roseboom, T., 2008. Transgenerational effects of prenatal exposure to the Dutch famine on neonatal adiposity and health in later life. BJOG 115, 1243–1249.

Panzeri, I., Rossetti, G., Pagani, M., 2016. Basic principles of noncoding RNAs in epigenetics in: medical epigenetics (Chapter 4). https://doi.org/10.1016/B978-0-12-803239-8.00004-1.

Pastor, W.A., Aravind, A., Rao, A., 2013. TETonic shift: biological roles of TET proteins in DNA demethylation and transcription. Nat. Rev. Mol. Cell Biol. 14, 341–356. https://doi.org/10.1038/nrm3589.

Paul, B.G., Bagb, S.C., Czornyj, E., Arambula, D., Sumit Handa, S., et al., 2015. Targeted diversity generation by intraterrestrial archaea and archaeal viruses. Nat. Commun. 6, 6585]. https://doi.org/10.1038/ncomms7585.

Pembrey, M., Saffery, R., Bygren, L.O., 2014. Human transgenerational responses to early-life experience: potential impact on development, health and biomedical research. J. Med. Genet. 51, 563–572.

Pflug, H.D., Heinz, B., 1997. Analysis of fossil organic nanostructures: terrestrial and extraterrestrial. SPIE Proc. Instrum. Methods Missions Invest. Extraterr. Microorg. 86, 3111, 1997. https://doi.org/10.1117/12.278814.July11.

Picardi, E.C., Manzari, C., Mastropasqua, F., Aiello, I., D'Erchia, A.M., Pesole, G., 2015. Profiling RNA editing in human tissues: towards the inosinome Atlas. Sci. Rep. 5, 14941.

Popper, K.R., 1974. Scientific reduction and the essential incompleteness of all science. In: Ayala, F., Dobzhansky, T. (Eds.), Studies in the Philosophy of Biology. Univ. of California Press, p. 270, 1974.

Portnoy, V., Huang, V., Place, R.F., Li, L.-C., 2011. Small RNA and transcriptional upregulation. WIREs RNA 2, 748–760. https://doi.org/10.1002/wrna.90.

Radman, M., 1999. Enzymes of evolutionary change. Nature 401, 866–869.

Radman, M., 1974. In: Molecular and Environmental Aspects of Mutagenesis (eds Prakash, L. et al.). C. C. Thomas, Springfield, Illinois, pp. 128–142.

Rassoulzadegan, M., Grandjean, V., Gounon, P., Vincent, S., Gillot, I., et al., 2006. RNA-mediated non-mendelian inheritance of an epigenetic change in the mouse. Nature 441, 469–474.

Refsland, E.W., Stenglein, M.D., Shindo, K., Albin, J.S., Brown, W.L., Harris, R.S., 2010. Quantitative profiling of the full APOBEC3 mRNA repertoire in lymphocytes and tissues: implications for HIV-1 restriction. Nucleic Acids Res. 38, 4274–4284.

Rogozin, I.B., Pavlov, Y.I., Bebenek, K., Matsuda, T., Kunkel, T.A., 2001. Somatic mutation hotspots correlate with DNA polymerase eta error spectrum. Nat. Immunol. 2, 530–536. https://doi.org/10.1038/88732.

Rosenberg, S.M., 2001. Evolving responsively: adaptive mutation. Nat. Rev. Genet. 2, 805–815.

Rothenfluh, H.S., 1995. Hypothesis: a memory lymphocyte specific soma-to-germline genetic feedback loop. Immunol. Cell Biol. 73, 174–180.

Rozanov, A.Y., Hoover, R.B., 2013. Acritarchs in carbonaceous meteorites and terrestrial rocks instruments, methods, and missions for astrobiology XVI. In: Hoover, Richard B., Levin, Gilbert V., Rozanov, Alexei Yu, Wickramasinghe, Nalin C. (Eds.), Proc of SPIE, vol. 8855. https://doi.org/10.1117/12.2029608, 886507-7.

Sano, H., 2010. Inheritance of acquired traits in plants Reinstatement of Lamarck. Plant Signal. Behav. 5, 346–348.

Satterfield, C.L., Lowenstein, T.K., Vreeland, R.H., Rosenzweig, W.D., Powers, D.W., 2005. New evidence for 250 Ma age of halotolerant bacterium from a Permian salt crystal. Geology 33, 265–268. https://doi.org/10.1130/G21106.1.

Scourzic, L., Mouly, E., Bernard, O.A., 2015. TET proteins and the control of cytosine demethylation in cancer. Genome Med. 7, 9. https://doi.org/10.1186/s13073-015-0134-6.

Sharma, U., Conine, C.C., Shea, J.M., Boskovic, A., Derr, A.G., Bing, X.Y., et al., 2016. Biogenesis and function of tRNA fragments during sperm maturation and fertilization in mammals. Science 351, 391–396. https://doi.org/10.1126/science.aad6780.

Shatilovich, A.V., Tchesunov, A.V., Neretinal, T.V., Grabarnik, I.P., Gubin, S.V., Vishnivetskaya, T.A., et al., 2018. Viable nematodes from late Pleistocene permafrost of the Kolyma river lowland. Dokl. Biol. Sci. 480, 100–102. https://doi.org/10.1134/S0012496618030079.

Shinoto, Y., 1955. Graft experiments in eggplant. Kagaku 25, 602–607.

Shivaji, S., Chaturvedi, P., Begum, Z., Pindi, P.K., Manorama, R., et al., 2009. Janibacter hoylei sp. nov., Bacillus isronensis sp. nov. and Bacillus aryabhattai sp. nov., isolated from cryotubes used for collecting air from the upper atmosphere. Int. J. Syst. Evol. Microbiol. 59, 2977–2986.

Simpson, G.G., 1953. The Baldwin Effect. Evolution 7, 110–117.

Skinner, M.K., 2015. Environmental epigenetics and a unified theory of the molecular aspects of evolution: a neo-Lamarckian concept that facilitates neo-Darwinian evolution. Genome Biol. Evol. 7, 1296–1302. https://doi.org/10.1093/gbe/evv073.

Skinner, M.K., Guerrero-Bosagna, C., Muksitul Haque, M., 2015. Environmentally induced epigenetic transgenerational inheritance of sperm epimutations promote genetic mutations. Epigenetics 10, 762–771. https://doi.org/10.1080/15592294.2015.1062207.

Smith, M.A., Gesell, T., Stadler, P.F., Mattick, J.S., 2013. Widespread purifying selection on RNA structure in mammals. Nucleic Acids Res. 41, 8220–8236. https://doi.org/10.1093/nar/gkt596.

Smith, M.A., Seemann, S.E., Quek, X.C., Mattick, J.S., 2017. DotAligner: identification and clustering of RNA structure motifs. Genome Biol. 18, 244. https://doi.org/10.1186/s13059-017-1371-3.

Smith, W.E., 2013. September 26, 2013. Life is a cosmic phenomenon: the "search for water" evolves into the "search for life". In: Hoover, R.B., Levin, G.V., Rozanov, A.Y., Wickramasinghe, N.C. (Eds.), Proc. SPIE 8865, Instruments, Methods, and Missions for Astrobiology XVI. San Diego, California, United States. https://doi.org/10.1117/12.2046862.

Smith, K., Spadafora, C., 2005. Sperm-mediated gene transfer: implications and applications. Bioessays 27, 551–562.

Sobey, W.R., Conolly, D., 1986. Myxomatosis; nongenetic aspects of resistance to myxomatosis in rabbits, Oryctogagus cuniculus aust. Wildlife Res. CSIRO 13, 177–187.

Spadafora, C., 1998. Sperm cells and foreign DNA: a controversial relation. Bioessays 20, 955–964.

Spadafora, C., 2008. Sperm-mediated "reverse" gene transfer: a role of reverse transcriptase in the generation of new genetic information. Hum. Reprod. 23, 735–740. https://doi.org/10.1093/humrep/dem425.

Spadafora, C., 2018. The "evolutionary field" hypothesis. Non-Mendelian transgenerational inheritance mediates diversification and evolution. Prog. Biophys. Mol. Biol. 134, 27–37. https://doi.org/10.1016/j.pbiomolbio.2017.12.001.

Steele, E.J., 1979. Somatic Selection and Adaptive Evolution : on the Inheritance of Acquired Characters, first ed. Williams- Wallace, Toronto, 1979; 2nd Edi University of Chicago Press, Chicago.

Steele, T., 1981. Lamarck and immunity; a conflict resolved. New Sci. 90, 360–361.

Steele, E.J., 1984. Acquired paternal influence in mice. Altered serum antibody response in the progeny population of immunized CBA/H males. Immunol. Cell Biol. 62, 253–268.

Steele, E.J., 1988. Observations on offspring of mice made diabetic with streptozocin. Diabetes 37, 1035–1043.

Steele, E.J., 2014. Reflections on ancestral haplotypes – medical genomics, evolution and human individuality. Perspect. Biol. Med. 57, 179–197.

Steele, E.J., 2009. Mechanism of somatic hypermutation: critical analysis of strand biased mutation signatures on A:T and G:C base pairs. Mol. Immunol. 46, 305–320.

Steele, E.J., 2016a. Somatic hypermutation in immunity and cancer: critical analysis of strand-biased and codon-context mutation signatures. DNA Repair 45, 1–24. https://doi.org/10.1016/j.dnarep.2016.07.001.

Steele, E.J., 2016b. Commentary: past, present, and future of epigenetics applied to livestock breeding — hard versus soft Lamarckian inheritance mechanisms. Front. Genet. 7, 29. https://doi.org/10.3389/fgene.2016.00029.

Steele, E.J., 2016c. Origin of congenital defects: stable inheritance through the male line via maternal antibodies specific for eye lens antigens inducing autoimmune eye defects in developing rabbits in utero. In: Levin, M., Adams, D.S. (Eds.), Ahead of the Curve -Hidden Breakthroughs in the Biosciences Chapter 3. Michael Levin and Dany Spencer Adams IOP Publishing Ltd 2016, Bristol, UK.

Steele, E.J., 2017. Reverse transcriptase mechanism of somatic hypermutation: 60 years of clonal selection theory. Front. Immunol. 8, 1611. https://doi.org/10.3389/fimmu.2017.01611. eCollection 2017, 2017 Nov 23

Steele, E.J., Al-Mufti, S., Augustyn, K.A., Chandrajith, R., Coghlan, J.P., Coulson, S.G., et al., 2018. Cause of Cambrian explosion - terrestrial or cosmic? Prog. Biophys. Mol. Biol. 136, 3–23. https://doi.org/10.1016/j.pbiomolbio.2018.03.004.

Steele, E.J., Al-Mufti, S., Augustyn, K.A., Chandrajith, R., Coghlan, J.P., Coulson, S.G., et al., 2019. Cause of Cambrian explosion - terrestrial or cosmic? – reply to commentary by R Duggleby. Prog. Biophys. Mol. Biol. 136. https://doi.org/10.1016/j.pbiomolbio.2018.11.002.

Steele, E.J., Hapel, A.J., Blanden, R.V., 2002. How can DNA patterns of somatically acquired immunity be imprinted on the germline of immunoglobulin variable (V) genes ? IUBMB Life 54, 305–307.

Steele, E.J., Gorczynski, R.M., Pollard, J.W., 1984. The somatic selection of acquired characters. In: Pollard, J.W. (Ed.), Evolutionary Theory: Paths into the Future. John Wiley, London, pp. 217–237.

Steele, E.J., Lloyd, S.S., 2015. Soma-to-germline feedback is implied by the extreme polymorphism at IGHV relative to MHC. Bioessays 37, 557–569.

Steele, E.J., Lindley, R.A., 2018. ADAR deaminase A-to-I editing of DNA and RNA moieties of RNA:DNA hybrids has implications for the mechanism of Ig somatic hypermutation. DNA Repair 55, 1–6. https://doi.org/10.1016/j.dnarep.2017.04.004.

Steele, E.J., Lindley, R.A., 2018. Germline V repertoires: origin, maintenance, diversification. Scand. J. Immunol. 87 e12670. https://doi.org/10.1111/sji.

Steele, E.J., Lindley, R.A., Blanden, R.V., 1998. Lamarck's Signature: How Retrogenes Are Changing Darwin's Natural Selection Paradigm. Allen & Unwin, Sydney, Australia.

Steele, E.J., Lindley, R.A., Wen, J., Weiler, G.F., 2006. Computational analyses show A-to-G mutations correlate with nascent mRNA hairpins at somatic hypermutation hotspots. DNA Repair 5, 1346–1363. https://doi.org/10.1016/j.dnarep.2006.06.002.

Steele, E.J., Pollard, J.W., 1987. Hypothesis: somatic hypermutation by gene conversion via the error-prone DNA->RNA->DNA information loop. Mol. Immunol. 24, 667–673. https://doi.org/10.1016/0161-5890(87)90049-6.

Steele, E.J., Williamson, J.F., Lester, S., Stewart, B.J., Millman, J.A., Carnegie, P., Lindley, R.A., Pain, G.N., Dawkins, R.L., 2011. Genesis of ancestral haplotypes: RNA modifications and RT-mediated polymorphism. Hum. Immunol. 72, 283–293.

Su, Y., Ghodke, P.P., Egli, M., Li, L, Wang, Y., Guengerich, F.P., 2019. Human DNA polymerase η has reverse transcriptase activity in cellular environments. J. Biol. Chem. 294, 6073–6081. https://doi.org/10.1074/jbc.RA119.007925.

Szostak, J.W., Bartel, D.P., Luisi, P.L., 2001. Synthesizing life. Nature 409, 387–390.

Taller, J., Hirata, Y., Yagishita, N., Kita, M., Ogata, S., 1998. Graft-induced changes and the inheritance of several characteristics in pepper (Capsicum annuum L.).

Theor. Appl. Genet. 97, 705–713.

Tepfer, D., Leach, S., 2017. Survival and DNA damage in plant seeds exposed for 558 and 682 Days outside the international space station. Astrobiology 17, 205–215.

Temin, H.M., 1970. Malignant transformation of cells by viruses. Perspect. Biol. Med. 14, 11–26. https://doi.org/10.1353/pbm.1970.0006.

Temin, H.M., 1971. The protovirus hypothesis: speculations on the significance of RNA directed DNA synthesis for normal development and for carcinogenesis. J. Natl. Cancer Inst. 46, 3–7.

Temin, H.M., 1989. Reverse trancriptases- retrons in bacteria. Nature 339, 254–255.

Temin, H.M., Mizutani, S., 1970. RNA-dependent DNA polymerase in virions of rous sarcoma virus. Nature 226, 1211–1213. https://doi.org/10.1038/2261211a0.

Tippin, B., Phuong Pham, P., Goodman, M.F., 2004. Error-prone replication for better or worse. Trends Microbiol. 12, 2988–2995. https://doi.org/10.1016/j.tim.2004.04.004.

van der Pol, E., Boing, A.N., Harrison, P., Sturk, A., Nieuwland, R., 2012. Classification, functions, and clinical relevance of extracellular vesicles. Pharm. Rev. 64, 676–705. https://doi.org/10.1124/pr.112.005983.

van Steenwyk, G., Roszkowski, M., Manuella, F., Franklin, T.B., Mansuy, I.M., 2018. Transgenerational inheritance of behavioral and metabolic effects of paternal exposure to traumatic stress in early postnatal life: evidence in the 4th generation. Environ. Epigenet. 1–8. https://doi.org/10.1093/eep/dvy023.

Vargas, A.O., 2009. Did Paul Kammerer discover epigenetic inheritance? a modern look at the controversial midwife toad experiments. J. Exp. Zool. B Mol. Dev. Evol. 312, 667–678. https://doi.org/10.1002/jez.b.21319.

Vargas, A.O., Krabichler, Q., Guerrero-Bosagna, C., 2017. An epigenetic perspective on the midwife toad experiments of Paul Kammerer (1880-1926). J. Exp. Zool. B Mol. Dev. Evol. 328 (1–2), 179–192. https://doi.org/10.1002/jez.b.22708.

Vreeland, R.H., Jones, J., Monson, A., Rosenzweig, W.D., Lowenstein, T.K., Timofeeff, M., et al., 2007. Isolation of live Cretaceous (121–112 million years old) halophilic Archaea from primary salt crystals. Geomicrobiol. J. 24, 275–282. https://doi.org/10.1080/01490450701456917, 2007.

Wainwright, M., Rose, C.E., Baker, A.J., Wickramasinghe, N.C., Omairi, T., 2015. Biological entities isolated from two stratosphere launches-continued evidence for a space origin. J. Astrobiol. Outreach 3 (2). https://doi.org/10.4172/2332-2519.1000129.

Walker, S.I., 2017. Origins of life: a problem for physics, a key issues review. Rep. Prog. Phys. 80, 092601 (21pp). https://doi.org/10.1088/1361-6633/aa7804.

Wallis, J., Miyake, N., Hoover, R.B., Oldroyd, A., Wallis, D.H., Samaranayake, A., et al., 2013. The Polonnaruwa meteorite ; Oxygen isotope, crystalline and biological composition. J. Cosmol. 22 (2) published, 5 March 2013.

Watson, J.G., Carroll, J., Chaykin, S., 1983. Reproduction in mice: the fate of sperm cells not involved in fertilization. Gamete Res. 7, 75–84. https://doi.org/10.1002/mrd.1120070107.

Wickramasinghe, Chandra, 2015a. The Search for Our Cosmic Ancestry. World Scientific, Scientific, Singapore.

Wickramasinghe, Chandra, 2015b. In: Wickramasinghe, Chandra (Ed.), Vindication of Cosmic Biology. Tribute to Sir Fred Hoyle, 1915-2001 Hoyle (1915-2001). World Scientific, Singapore.

Wickramasinghe, Chandra, 2018. Proofs that Life Is Cosmic. World Scientific Publishing Co, Singapore, ISBN 978-981-3233-10-2.

Wickramasinghe, D.T., Allen, D.A., 1983. Three components of 3-4 um absorption bands. Astrophys. Space Sci. 97, 369–378.

Wickramasinghe, D.T., Allen, D.A., 1986. Discovery of organic grains in Comet Halley. Nature 323, 44–46.

Wickramasinghe, N.C., Hoyle, F., 1998. Infrared evidence for Panspermia: an update. Astrophys. Space Sci. 259, 385–401.

Wickramasinghe, N.C., Rycroft, M., 2018. On the difficulty of the transport of

electrically charged submicron dust, including bacteria, from the Earth's surface to the high ionosphere. Adv. Astrophys. 3 (3), 150–153. August 2018. https://dx.doi.org/10.22606/adap.2018.33003.

Wickramasinghe, N.C., Steele, E.J., 2016. Dangers of adhering to an obsolete paradigm: could Zika virus lead to a reversal of human evolution? J. Astrobiol.Outreach 4 (1). https://doi.org/10.4172/2332-2519.1000147.

Wickramasinghe, N.C., Wallis, J., Wallis, D.H., Schild, R.E., Gibson, C.H., 2012. Life-bearing primordial planets in the solar vicinity. Astrophys. Space Sci. 341, 295–299.

Wickramasinghe, N.C., Wallis, J., Wallis, D.H., Samaranayake, A., 2013. Fossil diatoms in a new carbonaceous meteorite. J. Cosmol. 21 (37) published, 10 January 2013.

Wickramasinghe, J.T., Wickramasinghe, N.C., Napier, W.M., 2010. Comets and the Origin of Life (WSPC).

Wickramasinghe, N.C., Wickramasinghe, D.T., Tout, C.A., Lattanzio, J.C., Steele, E.J., 2018a. Cosmic biology in perspective. https://arxiv.org/abs/1805.10126.

Wickramasinghe, N.C., Rycroft, M., Wickramasinghe, D.T., Steele, E.J., Wallis, D.H., Temple, R., Tokoro, G., Syroeshkin, A.V., Grebennikova, T.V., Tsygankon, O.S., 2018b. Confirmation of microbial ingress from space. Adv. Astrophys. 3, 266–270.

Williamson, J.F., Steele, E.J., Lester, S., Kalai, O., Millman, J.A., Wolrige, L., et al., 2011. Genomic evolution in domestic cattle: ancestral haplotypes and healthy beef. Genomics 97, 304–312. https://doi.org/10.1016/j.ygeno.2011.02.006.

Wilson, T.M., Vaisman, A., Martomo, S.A., Sullivan, P., Lan, L., Hanaoka, F., et al., 2005. MSH2-MSH6 stimulates DNA polymerase eta, suggesting a role for A:T mutations in antibody genes. J. Exp. Med. 201, 637–645. https://doi.org/10.1084/jem.20042066.

Xie, Y., Dang, W., Zhang, S., Yue, W., Yang, L., Zhai, X., Yan, Q., Lu, J., 2019. The role of exosomal noncoding RNAs in cancer. Mol. Cancer 18 (1), 37. https://doi.org/10.1186/s12943-019-0984-4. Review, 2019 Mar 9.

Zanotti, K.J., Maul, R.W., Yang, W., Gearhart, P.J., 2019. DNA Breaks in Ig V Regions are predominantly single stranded and are generated by UNG and MSH6 DNA Repair Pathways. J Immunol. published online 21 January 2019. http://www.jimmunol.content/early/2019/01/18/jimmunol.1801183.

Zheng, Y.C., Lorenzo, C., Beal, P.A., 2017. DNA editing in DNA/RNA hybrids by adenosine deaminases that act on RNA. Nucleic Acids Res. 45, 3369–3377. https://doi.org/10.1093/nar/gkx050.

Zoraqi, G., Spadafora, C., 1997. Integration of foreign DNA sequences into mouse sperm genome. DNA Cell Biol. 16, 291–300. https://doi.org/10.1089/dna.1997.16.291.

Zu, D.-M., Zhao, Y.-S., 1957. A study on the vegetative hybridization of some Solanaceous plants. Sci. Sin. 6, 889–903.

Appendix References

Rossler, O.E., Temple, R., 2019. Early Einstein completed. In: Lasker, George E., Hiwaki, Kensei (Eds.), Personal and Spiritual Development in the World of Cultural Diversity, The International Institute for Advanced Studies in Systems Research and Cybernetics (IIAS), vol. 16, pp. 35–37. Tecumseh, Ontario, Canada.

Sanayei, Ali., Rössler, Otto E., 2014. Chaotic Harmony: A Dialog about Physics, Complexity and Life. Springer Verlag, Heidelberg, 2014.

Temple, Robert, 2007. The prehistory of panspermia: astrophysical or metaphysical? Int. J. Astrobiol. 6, 169–180.

Temple, Robert., Wickramasinghe, N. Chandra., 2019. In Preparation.

Peratt, Anthony, 1992. Birkeland currents in cosmic plasma. In: Physics of the Plasma Universe, XII, Springer-Verlag, Berlin Heidelberg New York, ISBN 3-540-97575-6, pp. 43–92, 0-387-97575-6.

SECTION 3

Early Months: Origin Through to April–May 2020

Comments on the Origin and Spread of the 2019 Coronavirus

N Chandra Wickramasinghe[1,2,3,4*], Edward J Steele[2,5], Reginald M Gorczynski[6], Robert Temple[7], Gensuke Tokoro[2,4], Jiangwen Qu[8], Daryl H Wallis[2,4] and Brig Klyce[9]

[1]Buckingham Centre for Astrobiology, University of Buckingham, MK18 1EG, England, UK

[2]Centre for Astrobiology, University of Ruhuna, Matara, Sri Lanka

[3]National Institute of Fundamental Studies, Kandy, Sri Lanka

[4]Institute for the Study of Panspermia and Astroeconomics, Gifu, Japan

[5]C Y O'Connor, ERADE Village, Foundation, Piara Waters, Perth 6112 WA, Australia

[6]University Toronto Health Network, Toronto General Hospital, University of Toronto, Canada

[7]History of Chinese Science and Culture Foundation, Conway Hall, London, UK

[8]Department of Infectious Disease Control, Tianjin Centers for Disease Control and Prevention, Hedong Qu, Tianjin Shi, China

[9]Astrobiology Research Trust, Memphis, TN, USA

Abstract

We propose that the new coronavirus which first appeared in the Hubei province of China was probably linked to the arrival of a pure culture of the virus contained in cometary debris that was dispersed over a localised area of the planet namely China. The sighting of a fireball some 2000 kilometers north of Wuhan on 11 October 2019 followed shortly after with the first recorded cases in Hubei is suggestive of a causal link. Gene sequencing data of the virus that show little or no genetic variations between isolates, combined with available epidemiological data point to the predominance of a transmission process directly from an "infected" environment, with person-to-person transmission playing a comparatively weaker secondary role. The facts relating to this epidemic are discussed and placed in the context of other pandemics that have been recorded throughout history.

Keywords: Coronavirus • Epidemiology • Comets • Panspermia

Introduction

With a new coronavirus (COVID-19) that has affected tens of thousands of people in mainland China, including many hundreds of deaths, approaching 1700 at time of proof correction and with its consequences wreaking havoc in the financial and business world, the truest cause of this and other similar pandemics needs to be urgently and honestly explored. All the epidemiological, genetic, geophysical and astrophysical data appear to be consistent with a primary cause associated with the deposition of dust carrying the virus that was transported through the troposphere and deposited in the wider environs of China including parts of the China Sea.

The first cases of COVID-19 infection in the human population were reported during November 2019 localised in Wuhan in the Hubei province of China. It is interesting that this followed remarkably close on the heels of a cometary bolide that exploded on 11 October 2019 lighting up the skies above north-east China over Sonjyan City in the province of Jilan. The bolide may have been part of the Orionid meteor stream that contains the debris of comet P/Halley.

Although the sighting of the fireball itself was some 2000 km distant from the epicentre of the coronavirus outbreak in Wuhan, a loosely held cometary bolide carrying the virus may have fragmented in the atmosphere prior to the fireball event. Micron-sized dust including bacteria and viruses released from such a fragment may then have become dispersed over a wide area and this material could fall non-destructively to the ground. Such a scheme of events, although representing an unorthodox point of view, has been discussed extensively by the late Sir Fred Hoyle and one of us close upon 4 decades ago [1-3]. Over this period support for the astronomical and biological ideas underlying the contingent theory of cosmic life – panspermia-has grown to the point to being compelling [4,5].

In the case of the new coronavirus (COVID-19) we note that conventional theories of infection are being strained to the limit in

*Corresponding author: Dr N Chandra Wickramasinghe, Buckingham Centre for Astrobiology, University of Buckingham MK18 1EG, England, UK, Tel: +44 (0)2920752146/+44 (0)7778389243; E-mail: ncwick@gmail.com

Received: February 14, 2020; Accepted: February 28, 2020; Published: March 06, 2020

NC Wickramasinghe et al.   Virol Curr Res, Volume 4: 1, 2020

their capacity to account for the unfolding facts. In our view, the virus itself became dispersed in the troposphere and was transported to ground level being first incorporated as the nucleation centres of rain and mist, the first cases showing up during November 2019 in Wuhan. Infective dust/droplets might still (in February 2020) be falling over a wide region of China, even possibly affecting ships at sea.

It is also entirely likely in our view that other virus-carrying fragments that became more widely dispersed in the stratosphere might still lead to smaller clusters of disease – for instance at the Ski resort in Mont Blanc as might well have happened. Thus a continual world-wide vigilance is therefore not out of place and the monumental efforts of Governments and Health authorities worldwide must be praised. Hoyle and Wickramasinghe [1-4] have argued that the draining out of a viral sized inoculant once it became widely distributed in the stratosphere could take several years. This happens with a distinct seasonal bias for viruses like influenza and indeed also for the smallest dust particles uplifted during powerful volcanic eruptions. Whether the October/November 2019 event leading to COVID-19 was entirely localised over China and therefore largely containable still remains to be seen. At the time of proofs independent clusters of COVID-19 have shown up in several places distant from China, including northern Italy, and a Global Pandemic has been discussed.

Data from Epidemiology and Sequencing

A recent paper by Huang et al. [5] and commentary by Cohen [6] highlights many unusual aspects of the outbreak of COVID-19. The evidence clearly demonstrates that many cases of disease (about 30%) arose in locations unconnected with the Wuhan seafood and meat market. The speculation that bats were an intermediary reservoir for the virus isolated in humans has not been confirmed, and it is possible to argue that all the animals currently harbouring the virus may often have been infected from the same external source. The "lethality" or "death rate" from this epidemic appears to increase in older patients with pre-existing conditions with of overall death rate estimated at 1-2%.

Phylogenetic analyses of COVID-19 sequences show little by way of sequence variation across a wide range of samples thus indicating low mutation rates approximating closely to what would be expected for a pure culture [5-7]. (See also: http://virological.org/t/clock-and-tmrca-based-on-27-genomes/347). This fact combined with the available epidemiological data points to little or no human-to-human transmission except from instances of close proximity with high doses of virus delivered at very close quarters. A contact transfer interpretation is also confounded by the fact that intimate social units may often have shared or sampled the same infected space, so transfer and "co-infection" cannot always be distinguished. In instances where a group of people who shared a confined geographical space become affected, but with one individual case appearing ahead of others (which we would expect statistically) the concept of "the super spreader" has been introduced, but this is not based on any independent scientific evidence.

Whilst the number of reported cases (as of mid-February) keeps soaring in China it is comforting to note that spread in more distant locations around the world has been largely contained, being confined in the main to persons who have contracted the disease from visiting China or neighbouring East Asian locations – the regions where the virus was deposited from its primary cosmic source. We predict that over a few weeks the entire population of China, and possibly its environs, would have been sub-clinically affected and thus acquired "herd" immunity when the epidemic in China would come to an end. Whether other foci of infection (from independent "fall out") develops around the world remains to be seen.

A Comparison with SARS

In an earlier communication, the possibility was discussed that the 2003 SARS outbreak (also caused by a corona virus), which started in China may similarly have been triggered by a space event [8]. In this case the virus may have been introduced into the troposphere from a disintegrating fragment of a carbonaceous meteorite at a location east of the Himalayan mountain range. Prevailing winds from the West might then have transported the virus eastwards to make a first deposition in China, a situation consistent with the first appearance of SARS. The subsequent course of its global distribution, however, depended on stratospheric transport and mixing, thus leading to a global fall-out continuing seasonally over a few years, eventually coming to an end due to a combination of factors including exhaustion of a primary source and the development of immunity.

Evidence of Viruses Reaching the Ground

It is only relatively recently that scientists have been able to fully grasp the enormous magnitude of the microbial and viral content of the terrestrial biosphere. We now know that a typical litre of surface seawater contains at least 10 billion microbes as well as some 100 billion viruses-the vast majority of which remain unidentified and uncharacterized to date. Recently an international group of scientists collected bacteria and viruses that fell through the rarefied atmosphere near the 4000 metre peaks of the Sierra Nevada Mountains of Spain [9]. They arrived at an astonishing tally of some 800 million viruses falling per square metre per day with an associated smaller tally of bacteria-all of which would ultimately fall upon the Earth's surface.

The assumption normally made is that all such viruses and bacteria necessarily originate on the Earth's surface itself, swept upwards in air currents, and then fall down; but in such a model many difficulties associated with upward transport processes are ignored. In our view, some fraction of this vast number of falling microbes must originate outside the terrestrial biosphere – viruses and bacteria that are actually expelled from comets.

Independent evidence can be obtained from sampling the stratosphere for its bacterial content. By analysing samples of the stratosphere from a height of 41 km using balloon-borne equipment we had already obtained in 2001 an estimated input of 20-200 million bacteria per square metre per day, as well as 10 to 100 times more in the form of viruses, falling downwards to the Earth [10].

If we take into account all the facts available to date we cannot avoid the conclusion that vast numbers of bacteria and viruses

NC Wickramasinghe et al.   Virol Curr Res, Volume 4: 1, 2020

continue to fall through the Earth's atmosphere, and it seems inevitable that a significant fraction is of external origin. We are also beginning to obtain further evidence pointing to the first signs of bacterial life being lodged in ancient rocks that formed 4.2-4.3 billion years ago at a time when the Earth was being relentlessly bombarded by comets. The strong indications are that comets carried the first bacteria to our planet at this time, and moreover that the entire subsequent evolution of life on Earth took may have taken place against the backdrop of comets regularly introducing new genes in the form of bacteria and viruses [3,11].

Organic structures identifiable with bacteria and viruses have been reported in carbonaceous meteorites over several decades, including studies by Pflug [12]. Figure 1 shows one of many carbonaceous structures in the Murchison meteorite that were identified with fossilised microbiota including a virus resembling the corona virus.

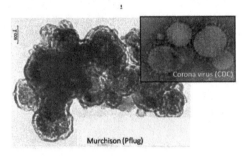

Figure 1. Electron micrograph of organic structure within the Murchison meteorite compared with the structure of the coronavirus [12].

Relation to Historical Evidence

Reports of the sudden spread of plagues and pestilences punctuate human history throughout the millennia [2,3]. The various epidemics, scattered through history often bear little or no resemblance one to another. However, they generally share a common property of suddenly afflicting entire cities, countries or even widely separated parts of the Earth in a matter of days or weeks. The Greek Historian Thucydides describes one such event-the plague of Athens of 429BC thus:

"It is said to have begun in that part of Ethiopia above Egypt....On the city of Athens it fell suddenly, and first attacked the men in Piraeus; so that it was even reported by them that the Peloponnesians had thrown poison into the cisterns....."

This event from Classical Greece bears striking similarities to the modern unfolding events in China relating to the new coronavirus. Thucydides writes that many families were simultaneously struck by a disease with a combination of symptoms hitherto unknown in more recent epidemics. The idea of an enemy (the Peloponnesians) poisoning the drinking water bears a striking similarity to what has happened in the Corona virus outbreak in China.

The orthodox point of view, that is by no means well-proven, is that major pandemics, such as the present coronavirus and indeed pandemic influenza, start by a random mutation or genetic recombination of a virus which then spreads across a susceptible population by direct person-to-person contact. If this were the case, it is somewhat surprising that all major pandemics tend to be self-limiting. In general, they are relatively short-lived, usually lasting about a year, and that they do not eventually affect the entire human population which would not be expected to have any prior immunity to a totally new pathogen. We would argue alternatively that a primary cometary dust infection is potentially the most lethal, and that secondary person-to-person transmissions can progressively reduce virulence thus resulting in a diminishing incidence of the disease over a limited period.

Many recent pandemics of viral disease, including influenza, are known to have followed a similar pattern of behaviour and a number have first appeared in China [2,8]. Following the initial deposition in a small localised region (eg: Wuhan, Hubei province, China) particles that have already become dispersed through the troposphere will fall to ground in a higgledy-piggledy manner, and this process could be extended over a typical timescale of 1-2 years until an initial inoculant of the infective agent (embedded in submicron cometary dust) would be seasonally drained.

Conclusion

In conclusion we affirm that it is prudent for Governments and Public Health Authorities around the world to maintain their state of high alert until more is discovered. At the same time assertions of false knowledge, such as the existence of "superspreaders", are probably a hindrance to understanding truest causes and thereby in dealing constructively and indeed compassionately with an unfolding crisis. In our view, it will also be prudent to put in place a programme of regular stratospheric sampling, using the most modern gene sampling techniques, essentially expanding what was begun in 2001. By such a program we could be forewarned of incoming offending bacteria and viruses before they fall to the troposphere and eventually to the Earth. We have a typical lead time of 1-2 years (time of fall through the stratosphere) during which time appropriate public health measures including production of vaccines could be put in place.

References

1. Hoyle, F and Wickramasinghe NC. Lifecloud JM Dent Ltd, London (1978b).

2. Hoyle, F and Wickramasinghe NC. Diseases from Space JM Dent Ltd, London (1979).

3. Hoyle, F and Wickramasinghe NC. Evolution from Space JM Dent Ltd, London (1981).

4. Hoyle, F and Wickramasinghe NC. "The Case for Life as a Cosmic Phenomenon." Nature 322(1986): 509e511.

5. Huang, C, Wang Y, Li X and Ren, et al. "Clinical Features of Patients Infected with 2019 Novel Coronavirus in Wuhan." China(2019) Lancet, Published online January24,2020 https://doi.org/10.1016/S0140-6736(20)30183-5

6. Cohen, Wuhan. "Seafood Market may not be Source of Novel Virus Spreading Globally Science." Jan 26 (2020). doi:10.1126/science.abb0611

7. Lu, R, Zhao X, Li J and Niu P, et al. "Genomic Characterisation and Epidemiology of 2019 Novel Coronavirus: Implications for Virus Origins and Receptor Binding." The Lancet published Online January 29 (2020) https://doi.org/10.1016/ S0140-6736(20)30251-8

8. Wickramasinghe, C, Wainwright M, Narlikar J. "SARS: A Clue to its Origins?" Lancet 361(2003): 1832.

9. Reche, I, D Orta G and Mladenov N, et al. The ISME Journal (2018). https://doi.org/10.1038/s41396-017-0042-4

NC Wickramasinghe et al.

Virol Curr Res, Volume 4: 1, 2020

10. Harris, MJ, Wickramasinghe NC, Lloyd D and Narlikar JV et al. "Detection of living cells in stratospheric samples." Proceedings of SPIE Conference 4495(2002): 192-198.

11. Steele, EJ, Gorczynski RM, Lindley RA and Liu Y, et al. "Lamarck and Panspermia: On the Efficient Spread of Living Systems Throughout the Cosmos." Prog Biophys Mol Biol 149(2019): 10-32.

12. Pflug, HD. "In Fundamental Studies and the Future of Science." University College Cardiff Press, UK(1983).

How to cite this article: N Chandra Wickramasinghe, EJ Steele, Reginald M Gorczynski and Robert Temple et al. "Comments on the Origin and Spread of the 2019 Coronavirus". *Virol Curr Res* 4 (2020) doi:10.37421/Virol Curr Res. 2020.4.109

Commentary   Open Access

Growing Evidence against Global Infection-Driven by Person-to-Person Transfer of COVID-19

N Chandra Wickramasinghe[1,2,3,4*], Edward J Steele[2,5], Reginald M Gorczynski[6], Robert Temple[7], Gensuke Tokoro[2,4], Daryl H Wallis[2,4] and Brig Klyce[8]

[1]Buckingham Centre for Astrobiology, University of Buckingham, MK18 1EG England, UK

[2]Centre for Astrobiology, University of Ruhuna, Matara, Sri Lanka

[3]National Institute of Fundamental Studies, Kandy, Sri Lanka

[4]Institute for the Study of Panspermia and Astroeconomics, Gifu, Japan

[5]C Y O'Connor, ERADE Village, Foundation, Piara Waters,Perth 6112 WA, Australia

[6]University Toronto Health Network, Toronto General Hospital, University of Toronto, Canada

[7]History of Chinese Science and Culture Foundation, Conway Hall, London, UK

[8]Astrobiology Research Trust, Memphis, TN, USA

Abstract

Examining a sample of still unfolding epidemiological data relating to the world-wide epidemic of Covid-19, we conclude that a connection with an atmospheric in fall appears increasingly probable.

Keywords: Coronavirus • Epidemiology • Panspermia

Introduction

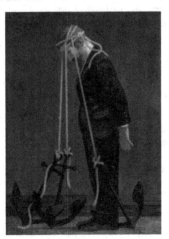

Figure 1. Thinking straight is hard if one is anchored on a shore of ignorance– (Painting by Gerart DuBois)

Events that are unfolding in relation to the COVID-19 outbreak appear to question the validity of many of our normal assumptions that relate to airborne infectious diseases, epidemics and pandemics Figure 1.

"A pathogenic virus must always pass from one infected animal (or carrier) to another animal in a causal chain in order to cause an epidemic disease"

This is a sacred dogma of medical science that has been firmly held and rigorously defended for decades. In the normal conduct of science and philosophy it takes only one decisive contradiction to disprove and dislodge a reigning dogma or theory. We have already argued in an earlier communication that the standard theory is hard pressed to account for many of the emerging facts [1].

Cases Reported at End of February, 2020

In the past several weeks new cases of coronavirus (COVID-19) seem to have appeared in their thousands in a region of China (Wuhan) and then spread within China as well as sporadically to

*Corresponding author: Dr. N Chandra Wickramasinghe, Buckingham Centre for Astrobiology, University of Buckingham MK18 1EG, England, UK, Tel: +44 (0)2920752146/+44 (0)7778389243; E-mail: ncwick@gmail.com

Received: February 28, 2020; Accepted: March 13, 2020; Published: March 20, 2020

Wickramasinghe NC, et al.   Virol Curr Res, Volume 4: 1, 2020

distant locations in the world. The question still baffling everyone is how did it all start and who was case zero [2]?

A summary (necessarily incomplete) of the reported case numbers/statistics as on 27 February 2020 in many countries are as follows:

o China: 78,514 cases; 2,744 deaths

o Asia and Oceania: 3,020 cases; 25 deaths (Philippines, Hong Kong (2), Japan (4), Taiwan, Diamond Princess (4), South Korea (13), India (3), Pakistan (2), Sri Lanka (1))

o Europe: 810 cases; 19 deaths (France (2), Italy (17))

o Middle East: 358 cases; 26 deaths (Iran)

o Africa: 2 cases

o South America: 1 case

o North America: United States (60 cases), Canada (13 cases)

Whilst the escalation in the number of COVID-19 cases globally is a reason for legitimate public health concern, it is prudent to keep in mind the fact that this disease has a lower rate of morbidity (death rate) than seasonal influenza, which is about 2 percent globally. The average death rate from COVID-19 has a similar value in Wuhan, but it is much lower, about 0.7% globally outside China. It also wise to keep our concerns in perspective by noting that this is generally a mild and self-limiting disease and that serious complications are confined to older people with underlying health problems.

The presumption is that the spread occurs only by direct contact with an infected person. That this may not be the entire story has become increasingly apparent when links between individual cases and geographical foci of infection are often difficult to establish. Over a wide region of China around the "epicentre" in Wuhan large numbers of positive detections of COVID-19 were reported throughout November and December 2019 and January and February 2020. We have already highlighted the fact that the several isolates of the virus distantly placed in time and space appear to have little or no genetic variations, implying a "pure culture" of the virus of external origin being maintained over several weeks [2-4]. This situation is difficult to reconcile with a brisk replication of the virus in hundreds of thousands of individuals who are infecting one another - as the viruses will often mutate in transit, however slightly. In this section, we highlight a few instances of the disease (positive COVID-19) that have been brought to our notice where no connection to another infected individual can be traced. It is thus predicted that when sequencing of the RNA genomes of the COVID-19 isolates is performed (from these widely distributed global samples) the sequences will show little or no variation, thus indicative of a common source.

France

The day after the announcement of the death of the first French coronavirus case on February 26th 2020 investigations were conducted to determine the "conditions of contamination" in the Paris hospital of Pitié-Salpêtrière to which the patient was admitted as an emergency. The victim, a 60-year-old teacher, came from Oise. A second patient, also from Oise, was a 55-year-old civilian working on the Creil air base. He was in a serious condition when he was

admitted to the intensive care unit at the University Hospital Centre (CHU) of Amiens. According to the sources neither of these two victims had visited China or northern Italy which had become the main epidemic centre in Europe [3].

According to the Director of the Hauts-de-France regional health agency Etienne Champion:

"The two patients from the Oise did not go to high-risk exposure areas. And that is why, at first, they were not identified as possible cases of coronavirus. Investigations are underway to determine the source of the two infections..." (Reported on February 26, 2020).

United States of America

A case of COVID-19 has been confirmed in a Northern California resident in Solano County, (northeast of San Francisco) who had no travel history to an affected area and no known contact with any person previously diagnosed with COVID-19, the Centers for Disease Control and Prevention (CDC) announced today (February 26, 2020).

"At this time, the patient's exposure is unknown. It's possible this could be an instance of community spread of COVID-19, which would be the first time this has happened in the United States," the CDC said in a statement. "Community spread means spread of an illness for which the source of infection is unknown. It's also possible, however, that the patient may have been exposed to a returned traveler who was infected."

Our comment is that "Community spread" is the trope of ignorance being widely deployed by health authorities the world over. Like "punctuated equilibrium" in biology it describes a phenomenon without attempting to understand it in any way.

Japan

Headline: None of Japan's new coronavirus patients had direct China links [4].

• February 13th, 2020: "A Kanagawa Prefecture woman in her 80s died from the coronavirus. Her son-in-law also tested positive for the disease. A doctor in Wakayama Prefecture and a man in Chiba Prefecture are confirmed to have the virus. None of them travelled to China recently or had contact with people who visited Hubei Province, the epicentre of the outbreak. ..... The 80 year old woman's symptoms began Jan. 22 when she felt fatigue, the health ministry said. Symptoms worsened on Jan. 25, prompting her to see a doctor three days later. She was placed under observation. .... The victim was hospitalized Feb. 1, diagnosed with pneumonia. She underwent screening for the coronavirus Wednesday. The test results came back positive Thursday, the day she died. Her son-in-law also tested positive for the coronavirus. The man, a taxi driver in his 70s living in Tokyo, has been hospitalized since February 6, but the symptoms are reportedly mild. He developed a fever Jan 29.

• "A doctor in Wakayama Prefecture south of Osaka has been infected with the virus, prefectural officials said Thursday. The man, in his 50s, has been hospitalized with symptoms of pneumonia, but is otherwise in stable condition. The doctor did not travel outside the country in the 14 days prior to the onset of symptoms, nor can any contact with people coming from China be confirmed. Wakayama officials suspect the infection had domestic origins."

Wickramasinghe NC, et al.   Virol Curr Res, Volume 4: 1, 2020

• "Elsewhere, a man in his 20s from Chiba Prefecture near Tokyo is also confirmed to have the virus. He developed a fever and other symptoms February. 2. The man reportedly has neither travelled overseas nor had contact with other infected individuals. "

• "Besides the outbreak on the Diamond Princess cruise ship, which has infected over 200 people aboard the vessel quarantined in Yokohama, 29 cases of coronavirus had been confirmed inside Japan through Wednesday. "

• "These cases raise new challenges for health officials, who until now had been trying to contain the virus by closely monitoring people with the possibility of contracting the disease. If more people with no direct links to China become sick, determining infection routes will become impossible."

Source: Yusuke Kurabe, Nikkei staff writer, in Nikkei Asian Review

February 13 13, 2020 22:37 JST Updated on February 14, 2020 04:52 JST

Italy

In the Italian outbreak of CORONA2019 the search for the first patient goes on with little success:

"…As for the alleged 'zero patient' the manager returning from China, it turned out that he had not had the coronavirus. From tests carried out on the friend of the 38-year-old Codogno (patient 1) who had been to dinner with him after having returned from China, "it emerged that he did not develop antibodies," explained Deputy Health Minister Pierpaolo Sileri in the evening. "The man had already tested negative for the first coronavirus test. Therefore, he did not start spreading the virus in the Lodi area [5]."

United Kingdom

A man from Surrey has been taken to a hospital isolation unit after becoming the UK's 20th confirmed case of coronavirus.

He is allegedly the first patient in England to catch the illness in the UK. It appears to be unclear whether he contracted it directly or indirectly from someone who had recently returned from abroad.....

"This is being investigated and contact tracing has begun……"

From Guardian 29 February 2020 [6].

Worldwide Spread of the Virus

As we keep searching for case zero in many instances where a sudden development of COVID-19 clusters are seen, the global distribution of cases as it unfolds is worthy of comment. As of 29 February the situation world-wide is displayed in Figure 2.

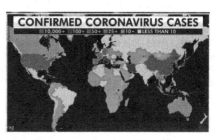

Figure 2. The distribution of COVID-19 cases as on 29 February 2020 [7].

The distribution of cases can be accommodated within a stratospheric deposition model of the kind first discussed by Hoyle and Wickramasinghe [8]. It is of interest to note that the early disposition of cases reported in the USA is uncannily similar to the distribution of cases recorded in case of the H3N2 (Hong Kong flu) pandemic which started in 1968 [9]. In Figure 3a we compare the current picture of COVID-19 in the USA with the progress of the spread of the 1968 Hong Kong flu pandemic. The development of cases from weeks 40-45 (top two frames) is beginning to look uncannily similar to the early phases of the COVID-19 epidemic as it is first making its tentative entry into the United States. Whether later spread of COVID-19 follows the trend shown in Figure 3b is left to be seen.

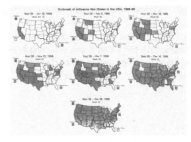

Figure 3a. The spread of influenza H3N2 in 1968 in the USA [8,9].

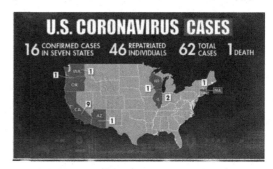

Figure 3b. The distribution of COVID-19 cases as on 29 February 2020 [7].

A fast changing scene

The data that we have discussed in this communication is necessarily in a state of rapid flux, and eventually it may become more difficult to disentangle competing processes and the modes of spread of the disease. As of 29 February 2020 it seems fairly clear

Wickramasinghe NC, et al.   Virol Curr Res, Volume 4: 1, 2020

that a primary infall process that is both geographically and temporally patchy is followed by varying degrees of efficacy of person-to-person spread. It is tempting to speculate that the latter could be contingent on the variations in habits of greeting around the world – eg Namaste (hands together) in the Indian subcontinent, embrace and hugging through the middle East, and the predominantly western handshake.

Note added in proofs

The proposal to rename COVID-19 to SARS-CoV-2 could fortuitously fit in with our arguments for a putative space origin of both SARS-CoV-1 and SARS-CoV-2. Wickramasinghe et al. [10] had already argued that the 2003 SARS outbreak first appearing in China may have been linked to the dispersal of viruses into the stratosphere from a cometary bolide. We note that the first cases of SARS-CoV-1 recorded in November 2002 appeared a few weeks after a bright cometary bolide exploded in the Ikutsk region of Siberia [11]. It was suggested that the SARS-virus-dust could have been deposited in the stratosphere and subsequently carried by Westerlies to fall first over China. The events of 2002 bear an uncanny similarity to the events that followed the sighting of the Jilin fireball in October 2019 [1].

Conclusion

The case against person-to-person transmission as the sole mode of transmission of the new virus is beginning to grow by the day. Whenever a long-held belief system fails to account for emerging new facts humans have had a long history of turning away from facts or even resorting to deception and falsehood. Let's hope this will not happen in the present case! Should we not honestly declare that we simply do not know?

Acknowledgement

We are grateful to Drs. R. Equem and M. Vitaly for alerting us to news about France and Italy.

References

1. Wickramasinghe, N.C., Steele, E.J., Gorczynkski, R.M.. Temple, R. et al. "Comments on the Origin and Spread of the 2019 Coronavirus." Virol Curr Res (2020), 4:1.
2. Duarte, Fernando. "Who is 'patient zero' in the coronavirus outbreak?" BBC Future, 24th February (2020).
3. Mandard, Stephane. "Coronavirus : A la recherche de « la source des contaminations » des deux patients de l'Oise." Le Monde, 27th February, (2020).
4. KURABE, YOSUKE. "None of Japan's new coronavirus patients had direct China links." Nikkei Asian Review. 14th February, (2020).
5. "Coronavirus: Salgono a due le vittime italiane, 76 contagiati, casi a Milano e Torino." La Repubblica, 22nd February, (2020).
6. "UK's 20th coronavirus case is first to catch illness in Britain." Support The Guardian, February, (2020).
7. Adams, Jerome. "US surgeon general details coronavirus response on 'Justice'." Fox News, March (2020).
8. Hoyle, F and Wickramasinghe C. "Diseases from Space." J M. Dent Lond, (1978).
9. Selby, P. "Influenza Virus, Vaccines and Strategy" Academic Press, (1976).
10. Wickramasinghe, C, Wainwright Narlikar and Narlikar JV. "SARS a clue to its origins." The Lancet (2003), 361: 1832.
11. "Bodaybo event is believed to be an impact by a bolide (fireball) in the Vitim River basin." Vitim event wikipedia, 25th September, (2002).

How to cite this article: Wickramasinghe, N Chandra, Edward J Steele, Reginald M Gorczynski and Robert Temple et al. "Growing Evidence against Global Infection-Driven by Person-to-Person Transfer of COVID-19." *Virol Curr Res* 4 (2020) doi: 10.37421/Virol Curr Res.2020.4.110

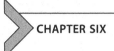

CHAPTER SIX

Origin of new emergent Coronavirus and Candida fungal diseases—Terrestrial or cosmic?

Edward J. Steele[a,b,c,]*, Reginald M. Gorczynski[d], Robyn A. Lindley[e,f], Gensuke Tokoro[g], Robert Temple[h], and N. Chandra Wickramasinghe[c,g,i,j,]*

[a]C.Y.O'Connor ERADE Village Foundation, Piara Waters, Perth, WA, Australia
[b]Melville Analytics Pty Ltd, Melbourne, VIC, Australia
[c]Centre for Astrobiology, University of Ruhuna, Matara, Sri Lanka
[d]University Toronto Health Network, Toronto General Hospital, University of Toronto, Toronto, ON, Canada
[e]Department of Clinical Pathology, Faculty of Medicine, Dentistry & Health Sciences, University of Melbourne, Melbourne, VIC, Australia
[f]GMDx Group Ltd, Melbourne, VIC, Australia
[g]Institute for the Study of Panspermia and Astroeconomics, Gifu, Japan
[h]The History of Chinese Science and Culture Foundation, Conway Hall, London, United Kingdom
[i]University of Buckingham, Buckingham, United Kingdom
[j]National Institute of Fundamental Studies, Kandy, Sri Lanka
*Corresponding authors: e-mail address: e.j.steele@bigpond.com; ncwick@gmail.com

Contents

Advances in Genetics, Volume 106
ISSN 0065-2660
https://doi.org/10.1016/bs.adgen.2020.04.002

Abstract

The origins and global spread of two recent, yet quite different, pandemic diseases is discussed and reviewed in depth: *Candida auris*, a eukaryotic fungal disease, and COVID-19 (SARS-CoV-2), a positive strand RNA viral respiratory disease. Both these diseases display highly distinctive patterns of sudden emergence and global spread, which are not easy to understand by conventional epidemiological analysis based on simple infection-driven human- to-human spread of an infectious disease (assumed to jump suddenly and thus genetically, from an animal reservoir). Both these enigmatic diseases make sense however under a Panspermia in-fall model and the evidence consistent with such a model is critically reviewed.

1. Introduction

In the past 40 years there have been a number of suddenly emerging epidemic viral diseases. Many were self-limiting and "went away" or "disappeared" almost as quickly as they appeared (SARS, MERS, ZIKAV). The origins in all cases were a mystery, and very controversial. Others such as the far more deadly HIV retrovirus has finally succumbed to highly effective antiretroviral therapy (HAART) making life bearable for infected HIV+ people. However it has integrated into the human germline in many cases and is likely to be a permanent "endogenized retroviral signature" in the human germline, joining the many thousands of other HERVS, human endogenous retrovirus sequences that litter the human genome as fragments or potentially active retroviruses (Wickramasinghe, 2012; Wickramasinghe & Steele, 2016).

However the great exemplar of the emergence of a new pandemic disease of considerable virulence and pathogenicity was the Spanish Flu Pandemic 1918–1919. That pandemic has been analyzed in great detail by Hoyle and Wickramasinghe (1979), and the astute and engaged reader of all that evidence is left *with only one conclusion*—the Spanish Flu disease came from Space on a massive scale, and killed tens of millions before the advent of air travel.

We do not intend here to discuss these earlier epidemics and pandemics—which have been covered in previous papers (some cited here). We focus our analysis on the actual origins of two recently emergent epidemics: a fungal disease caused by *Candida auris* and the current coronavirus "common cold-type" epidemic caused by the COVID-19 virus. These two epidemics display distinctive features and clear evidence that they may have come from a space in-fall of infectious viruses and micro-organisms in cometary dust or meteorite-derived dust particles.

2. Sudden simultaneous emergence of *Candida auris* infections in separate global regions

Candida species are well-known yeasts that can cause a variety of cutaneous and invasive infections; however, they had never been considered a serious global health threat until the recent emergence of *Candida auris*. This was first reported in the ear canal of a patient in Japan in 2009. Since then, cases have been recorded on all continents except Antarctica (Rhodes & Fisher, 2019). It can cause a variety of invasive infections with a mortality rate of up to 60%, typically infecting susceptible hosts, namely those with long hospitalizations, many illnesses and impaired immunity (Bradley, 2019). In addition, it can be resistant to multiple antifungals and has the capacity to cause outbreaks within healthcare facilities (Chow et al., 2018). Its ability to colonize and persist for a long time on human skin, tolerate some disinfectants that are commonly used in healthcare settings, and to survive on inanimate surfaces for many weeks, all contribute to its effectiveness as an outbreak agent (Jackson et al., 2019).

Even more remarkable though is its emergence. An analysis of whole genomic sequencing from 54 isolates of *C. auris* from four regions around the world revealed four major clades or genetically distinct populations. This finding supports the hypothesis of the nearly simultaneous and independent emergence of these clades in geographically separate human populations The SENTRY Antifungal Surveillance Program is a global system that has continued for 20 years (1997–2016). It collects consecutive invasive *Candida* isolates from medical centers located in four regions during each calendar year, namely: North America, Europe, Latin America, and the Asia-Pacific (Pfaller, Diekema, Turnidge, Castanheira, & Jones, 2019). Despite going back to 1997, the SENTRY data did not identify *C. auris* until 2009 (Jackson et al., 2019). In fact, the earliest *C. auris* isolates were found in South Korea in 1996 and Japan in 1997 (Forsberg et al., 2018).

Although it is a Candida species, *C. auris* is quite distinct from its Candidal relatives. The genus consists of > 500 species, many of which greatly differ from each other. *C. auris* comes from the Clavispora clade of the Metschnikowiaceae family. It has not been identified from any natural environments (Jackson et al., 2019). It is relatively thermotolerant in that it can grow at temperatures as high as 42 °C. Such thermotolerance could potentially allow it to infect avian hosts (Chatterjee et al., 2015).

Thus, infections caused by the fungus *Candida* spp. have been recognized for many years. However, of interest here is the abrupt emergence of a new strain *Candida auris* which presents a profound puzzle (Lockhart et al., 2017). This new strain which is multi-drug resistant has emerged as a major cause of mortality and is posing a serious challenge for health officials the world over (Chowdhary, Sharma, & Meis, 2017; Cortegiani et al., 2018; Jeffery-Smith et al., 2018; Lockhart et al., 2017). While *Candida auris* was reported for the first time in Japan in 2009 it appears to have been *isolated more or less simultaneously* in many widely separated locations across the world.

Phylogenetic analysis by Lockhart et al. (2017) has identified four distinct clades separated by tens of thousands of single nucleotide polymorphisms (SNPs) each of which is geographically localized. A large number of SNPs have been discovered in isolates that were recovered from four widely separated locations (South Asia, East Asia, South America, and South Africa). Whole genome sequencing of these isolates has revealed an exceedingly low genetic diversity within individual regions even across the largest clade involving some 36 isolates from as wide a field as India and Pakistan. The conclusion by Lockhart et al. (2017) is that *C. auris* must have arisen almost simultaneously in multiple four different global locations. Further, from isolates of *Candida* from four continents Lockhart et al. (2017) did not find *C. auris* before 2009 confirming that this pathogen was not simply misidentified previously. While there have been claims that earlier isolates of Candida species may also have been *Candida auris* which were incorrectly identified, these assertions have not been confirmed. Thus, it seems reasonable to conclude that a 2009 date for the origin *Candida auris* is fairly secure (Cortegiani et al., 2018).

Since global cross-infection over a short timescale (<1 year) appears very unlikely one possibility is of independent multiple origins of *Candida auris* from some widely present *Candida* ancestor. A fungicide driver model has been advanced to explain the phenomenon. However this vague model does not fit the available data. We thus argue here that a panspermic in-fall model should be considered as a plausible and better alternative.

Thus, in our explanation (from all the available data) it could be concluded that *C. auris* first arose in 2009 from several environmentally-induced hypermutation events that occurred after in-fall from cosmic (cometary) dust clouds through which the Earth had traversed sometime during or before 2009. Thus this new *C. auris* would appear simultaneously in many widely separated places on the Earth. Alternatively, a genetic hybridization event may have taken place at this time involving a globally distributed set of comet-borne gene segments that were themselves genetically diverse.

How could this have occurred? We critically evaluate the data from a genetic point of view. The data demands that there are at least four pre-existing clades ($\geq$10,000 SNP differences) in an external non-terrestrial source (cometary dust tails) and these came down separately in separate regions and thereafter spread clonally (Lockhart et al., 2017). The other alternative is to consider the existence of a single "mother" or "parent" *C. auris* clade in the cometary dust source, which upon landing and infection of susceptible hosts is induced into a hypermutation-adaptation sequence via a fast, essentially Lamarckian, Adaptive Mutation strategy (Rosenberg, 2001; Chapter "The Efficient Lamarckian Spread of Life in the Cosmos" by Steele et al.) thereby generating in excess of 10,000 new SNP differences from the parent orbiting cosmic strain. The final step that can be envisaged is the dispersal of a successful adaptive variant in a particular region to other hospitals in that region. Thus on the basis of a Panspermic model there are two possible explanations for the strange and striking *C. auris* patterns of genome diversity. The Lamarckian hypermutation strategy at each separate in-fall location (susceptible hospital patients) from a pure line "mother" strain is, on parsimony grounds, preferred.

We have previously argued that a sudden emergence of new pathogenic variants of circulating viruses could be linked to cosmic events related to the well-known 11-year sunspot cycle (Qu & Wickramasinghe, 2017, 2018; Wickramasinghe et al., 2017, 2019). The Earth's magnetosphere, and the interplanetary magnetic field in its vicinity, are both modulated by the solar wind that controls the flow of charged particles onto the Earth. During times of sunspot minima, a general weakening of magnetic field occurs and this would be accompanied by an increase in the flux of galactic cosmic rays (GCR's) and also of charged interstellar and interplanetary dust particles. Evidence for such periodic increases linked to solar activity is evident in the high frequency of noctilucent clouds (as at present, in 2019–2020) and also in the increase of particulate deposits in polar ice cores. Since the latter could, in our view, include biological entities such as bacteria, viruses and other eukaryotic microorganisms like *C. auris*, an increase in their incidence on the Earth will therefore be expected at such times. It is interesting to note that in 2008–2009 (the solar minimum under discussion) the interplanetary magnetic field was the lowest on record since the beginning of the space age. We would therefore expect a significantly enhanced flux of both cosmic rays as well as electrically charged biological entities at this time, so the arrival of a new clade of *C. auris* from a space source should not be ignored.

A crucial fact relating to the first appearance of *Candia auris* in 2009 is that this time marks not merely a solar minimum but *the lowest minimum* of the sunspot cycle in 100 years (see Figs. 1 and 2). This particular minimum was all the more remarkable because the sun was spotless (devoid of spots) for more than 70% of the time. The opportunity of the transference of both Galactic Cosmic Rays (GCR's) and charged molecular structures (e.g., *C. auris*) thus remained continuously optimal over extended periods. At the present time (February 2020) as we approach a new sunspot minimum the sun continues to be exceedingly "quiet" and the expectations are that we are heading for an even deeper minimum than before. The case for epidemiological vigilance for new microbial and viral pathogens cannot be greater than at the present time.

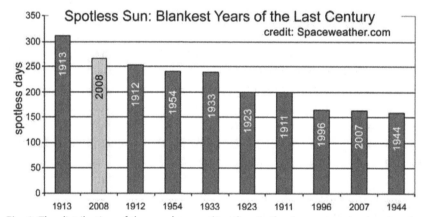

Fig. 1 The distribution of the number spotless days in the Sunspot cycle, showing the period 2008/2009 to be the lowest on record for a century. Exceptionally low sunspot activity in solar minima open the floodgate to interstellar and comet dust.

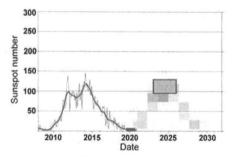

Fig. 2 Current sunspot cycle 24 and predicted cycle 25 (Wickramasinghe et al., 2019). From term solar observations-world data center, Royal observatory of Belgium, Brussels (http:/www.sidc.be/silso/home).

3. Sudden emergence new Coronavirus (COVID-19) causing respiratory infections in Wuhan, China and neighboring regions

We now turn to our critical analysis of the origin of the COVID-19 epidemic underway as we draft this chapter.

3.1 Overview of the COVID-19 epidemic

The global extent of the emotion around this epidemic in the mainstream popular media, and even the scientific press (*Science* magazine) is disturbing. It is without parallel in our experience in this social media internet age. However, it does approach the justified hysteria around the far more serious, and initially more lethal, HIV epidemic/pandemic that suddenly emerged 40 years ago.

The actual COVID-19 viral disease itself causes respiratory "common cold-like" illness in most people diagnosed with symptoms (but many potential carriers of the disease are asymptomatic). The infection can progress to severe pneumonia in elderly and already medically-compromised patients with other conditions (diabetes, coronary disease, etc.). About 2% of all COVD-19 cases have died due to the pneumonia (Fig. 4). Vaccine and antivirals will not help the latter group, but standard well trusted medical care will—to help patients through the respiratory crisis of the life-threatening pneumonia and dangerous inflammatory bronchitis symptoms. Such care will allow recovery of most patients. The fact that "Recoveries" far exceed "Deaths" (Fig. 4) indicates that timely medical care for this otherwise "common cold" respiratory illness must be the medical priority in the epicenter of the infection in Wuhan and nearby regions in China. We believe this medical care is being implemented throughout China.

But it is the origin of this new emergent virus disease which has raised the most angst. It is literally explosively centred on Wuhan, which appears to be the epicenter. And it appeared suddenly without warning. The theory that it jumped from bats via snakes to humans is implausible (below). The same angst over viral origins was also evident when HIV, SARS, MERS, Ebola, and ZIKAV suddenly appeared on the scene. We will not deal with these earlier diseases as their origins, in our considered opinion, are far less clear cut than COVID-19.

However sorting out what is true from what is untrue is a challenge. The current distribution and case numbers as February 14, 2020 are shown in Figs. 3 and 4. The epidemic is centred on the city of Wuhan, in the central Hubei province of China (for an update on our analyses since drafting of this chapter, see Appendix C).

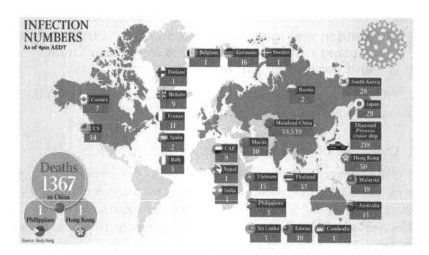

Fig. 3 *The Australian* newspaper as February 14, 2020, p. 8. Illustrative of newspaper reports on the early phase of the COVID-19 pandemic at time of writing in mid-February 2020—infection numbers February 14 2020 are: Canada, 7; US, 14; Finland, 1; Britain, 9; France, 11; Spain, 2; Italy, 3; Belgium, 1; Germany, 16, Sweden, 1; UAE, 8, Nepal, 1; India 3; Macao, 10; Vietnam, 15; Philippines, 3; Sri Lanka, 1; Mainland China, 59,539; Russia, 2; Thailand, 33; Taiwan, 18; Cambodia, 1; South Korea, 28; Japan, 29; Diamond Princes cruise ship, 218; Hong Kong, 50; Malaysia, 18; Australia, 15. Deaths: 1367 China, 1 Philippines, 1 Hong Kong. An update on the total toll of the pandemic, now approaching a global total of 9 million confirmed cases as June 22, 2020 is in Appendix C.

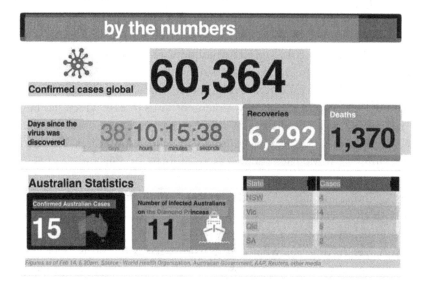

Fig. 4 COVID-19 by numbers, in the Australian newspaper February 14, 2010, p. 8. Figures as of February 14, 6.30 a.m. Source—World Health Organization, Australian Government, AAP, Reuters, other media.

From about mid-January the Chinese government ordered the complete quarantine and lock-down of Wuhan and wider region around the city in Hubei province, affecting 50–100 million people. *ABC News* in Australia estimates Coronavirus (COVID-19) has affected 500 million people in China under lock-down (Updated February 15, 2020, 1:29 a.m.). A problem with all these reports is the lack of detailed information that led officials to such an extraordinary quarantine decision. We speculate later on this.

At the time of writing, the case incidence of this newly discovered Coronavirus is passing through 60,000 and >99.99% of all cases, almost exclusively, are Chinese. From reports of cases that exited Wuhan by aircraft in late January to other countries, say to Australia, the disease does not spread in a sustained way easily person-to-person. But there are clearly apparent cases of person-to-person spread elsewhere (say in United Kingdom and Europe, Box 1). But there is no doubt this disease is centred on China. The Johns Hopkins University COVID-19 case density maps are extremely informative. These are in Figs. 5–7.

To put one interpretation on the striking case patterns in Figs. 5–7, particularly the symmetrical pattern in Fig. 7 it actually looks like a huge viral bomb explosion took place near or over Wuhan and then the radial fall-out of the disease causing viral particles to land on the millions of people either laterally or from above—some of those infected would be susceptible and who then have succumbed to the respiratory illness (in Appendix A, in relation to the expected fall of viruses through the stratosphere is an analysis by way of quantitative analogy, of the expectation of radioactive fall-out patterns from an atmospheric nuclear test in 1958).

Moreover, and paradoxically, asymptomatic patients can be efficient "spreaders" of the disease. This is contrary to normal expectations as usually the infected potential spreader would display overt and full blown disease (and the coughed-up aerosols from such a patient would be dense with viral particles). Indeed, there are wide reports in the media that incubation times can range from 1 to 28 days. But once a potentially infective virus successfully navigates the Innate Immune response (see table 1, Chapter "The Efficient Lamarckian Spread of Life in the Cosmos" by Steele et al.) it would be expected to rapidly multiply within cells and spread peaking in virion numbers 5–7 days later. The actual size of the infective dose is also an important variable. So these wide-range estimates of incubation time reflect, in our view, the variable depth and extent of the *actual physical viral contamination* in the immediate environment of a susceptible subject viz. potentially all objects in the family home environment as well as cars, bicycles, and on their bodies—hair, clothes—and other personal effects, clothes, money, keys, etc. Indeed, the external

**BOX 1 Summary of United Kingdom cases
(N.C. Wickramasinghe email report to Edward J. Steele).**

- January 21, 2020

CDC confirms 1 case of transmission between person who returned from Wuhan, and a person who shared accommodation in the United States.

Via a ski resort in the French Alpine town of Les Contamines-Montjoie, near Switzerland, late last month,

- January 28, 2020

A cluster linked to an Alpine chalet

A British man (Mr. Walsh) from Brighton, was found to have the virus when he returned to the UK (London Gatwick Airport) from Geneva on January 28 on an EasyJet flight. A total of six people in Britain, including Mr. Walsh, and Britons in France who have the virus have been staying in two apartments in a ski chalet in the Alpine resort area near Mont Blanc when they were visited by Mr. Walsh on January 24 *who had attended a* business *conference at the Grand Hyatt Hotel Singapore, where he is believed to have contracted the virus.*

Mr. Walsh is *thought* to have passed the virus onto eleven confirmed cases while he was at the Ski resort. But he is thought to have come into contact with scores of people after leaving Singapore and no others have yet succumbed.

All the supposed transmissions of the virus from Mr. Walsh to the others were while they occupied the Chalets in France.

Four are from Brighton and Hove. They are Dr. Greenwood and three men, one of whom is a healthcare worker. He also passed it to one other person in the United Kingdom, one person who is now in Mallorca and five United Kingdom nationals in France—one of which is Dr. Greenwood's husband Bob Saynor and another their 9-year-old son. None are said to be in a serious condition.

So far, the places in Brighton and Hove being quarantined are:

- County Oak Medical Centre, where Dr. Catriona Greenwood worked one admin day last week, and its branch surgery at Deneway.
- Grenadier Pub in Hangleton, which was visited by Steve Walsh on February 1.
- Cornerstone Community Centre, where a yoga teacher came into contact with Steve Walsh on February 3. No other people have been advised to self-isolate.
- Easyjet flight EZS8481 to Gatwick from Geneva on January 28, which is believed to be the flight Mr. Walsh took back to the United Kingdom.
- Bevendean Primary School, where a staff member has been in close contact with someone who has been advised to self-isolate (but is not themselves diagnosed).
- Portslade Academy, which told parents on Friday one of its pupils has been advised to self-isolate for a fortnight after coming into contact with the Hove father. It's believed pupils at other schools have been given the same advice.
- Patcham Nursing Home, which has closed its doors to all visitors after being visited by one of the medics now confirmed as having the virus.

The cluster associated with Mr. Walsh could have been coinfected from a common source, with Mr. Walsh showing symptoms first.

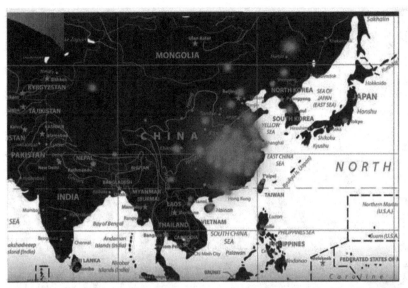

Fig. 5 Case density map—South East Asia region wide. Johns Hopkins University as February 7, 2020. Johns Hopkins University's Centre for Systems Science and Engineering.

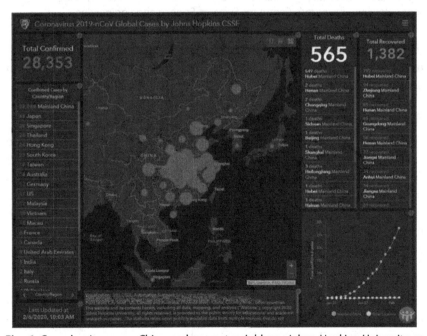

Fig. 6 Case density map—China and nearest neighbors. Johns Hopkins University as February 7, 2020. Johns Hopkins University's Centre for Systems Science and Engineering.

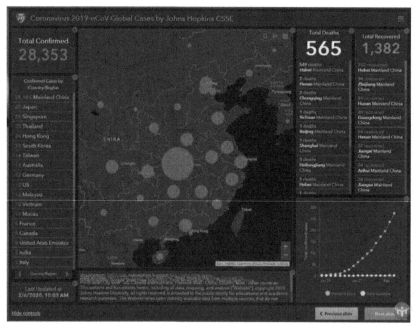

Fig. 7 Case density map—China itself. Johns Hopkins University as February 7, 2020. Johns Hopkins University's Centre for Systems Science and Engineering.

surface of the face mask may be the main carrier of the physical contamination. We explore the extent of viral environmental contamination further below.

3.2 Detailed analysis of COVID-19 epidemic

We now analyze all reliable genetic, epidemiological and geophysical and astrophysical data. This leads to the alternate hypothesis that COVID-19 arrived via a meteorite, a presumed relatively fragile and loose carbonaceous meteorite, that struck North East China on October 11, 2019. This is at odds with the main stream expert "Infectious Disease" opinion of traditional person-to-person spread of an infectious endemic disease such as, for example, Cholera (*Vibrio cholerae*).

We then assume the viral debris and particles then made land fall in the Wuhan and related regions about a month to 6 weeks later resulting in first cases of the viral pneumonia caused by COVID-19 emerging in Wuhan regions late November 2019-early December 2019 (Cohen, 2020; Huang et al., 2020). Such an hypothesis is indeed consistent with the striking patterns shown in Fig. 7. And it makes, therefore, an extraordinary set of predictions, that we will explore at some length in our conclusions.

It suggests, first, massive region-wide physical contamination with potentially trillions of infective COVID-19 viral particles in central China-contaminating buildings, roadways, cars and factory equipment, vegetation, surface water pools, people (and their clothes, body parts such as hair, skin, personal affects, mobile phone, keys, wallets, etc.) as well as wild and domestic animals, etc. This would explain the actions of the Chinese Government who are acting to appear to be in receipt of such presumed knowledge (or information) from region-wide sampling to detect COVID-19 RNA sequences in swabs from physical objects, people and animals (via real time PCR).

The recent paper by Huang et al. (2020) and the extremely important news commentary by Cohen in *Science* (Cohen, 2020) highlights many unusual aspects of the outbreak of COVID-19. The evidence demonstrates that many cases of disease (about 30% of case reports) arose in locations unconnected with the Wuhan seafood and meat market, and the total tally continues to increase. Phylogenetic analyses of COVID-19 (previously named nCov-2019) sequences show little by way of sequence variation thus indicating low mutation rates thus approximating closely to what would be expected for a pure culture, of a single infecting and replicating sequence affecting disease cases (Andersen, 2020; Lu et al., 2020). These facts are now combined with the global epidemiological data, that points in the main to little or no really sustained human-to-human transmission thus far (e.g., latest reports by the Australian Department of Health). We are aware there are apparent exceptions, e.g., the "super-spreader" from Singapore, via the French Alps, and then to a United Kingdom GP surgery reporting mild symptoms, resulting in the GPs also getting the disease (Box 1). We interpret that spread by viral contamination of physical objects in the main rather than direct "cough in your face" human to human spread.

In any case, current data suggest that the human-to-human spread rate is unusually low, and may be dependent on proximity and dose of virus delivered at very close quarters. The "lethality" or "death rate" from this or any other epidemic disease increases in older patients with pre-existing conditions so wider global estimates yield a death rate at 2% of infected (Fig. 4). All these basic facts now appear agreed.

The initial traditional explanation of the new epidemic of COVID-19 is that it jumped from bats (possibly via snakes) to humans and then spread by human-to-human infection contact mutating at a high rate. This explanation is at odds with the data at present. Indeed Jon Cohen the respected *Science* magazine journalist reports that the head of the Huang et al. (2020) study when interviewed said:

> *Bin Cao of Capital Medical University, the corresponding author of* The Lancet *article and a pulmonary specialist, wrote in an email to* ScienceInsider *that he and his co-authors "appreciate the criticism" from Lucey (Daniel Lucey, an infectious disease specialist at Georgetown University confirmed the epidemic could not possibly be caused by visits to the Wuham seafood and meat market).*
>
> *"Now It seems clear that [the] seafood market is not the only origin of the virus," he wrote. "But to be honest, we still do not know where the virus came from now." (our italics)*

Indeed Dr. Bin Cao speaks for all mainstream medical and epidemiological professionals around the world—no formal traditional explanation can be provided for the origins of COVID-19. Thus Andrew Rambaut, Professor of Molecular Evolution at the University of Edinburgh tweeted: "Don't think any epidemiologist is still thinking that a non-human animal reservoir has had anything to do with the nCoV-2019 epidemic since December.

Certainly the genome data doesn't support that." (Reported in Heidi Han and Kieran Gair, Associated Press, *The Australian* newspaper January 27, 2020.)

Thus, when we combine all the available facts we cannot rule out a viral in-fall event targeting the Wuhan province and the wider region around it as an explanation as a first cause of the epidemic. This would fit with the admittedly heterodox view of viral pandemics first proposed by Hoyle and Wickramasinghe as far back as 1978 (Hoyle & Wickramasinghe, 1979, 1990; Wickramasinghe et al., 2019; Wickramasinghe, Wainwright, & Narlikar, 2003). This concept accords with the theory of cosmic biology for which growing evidence have recently been presented in the Chapters of this book and in recent peer-reviewed papers where all the main extant evidence has been reviewed and is consistent with the Hoyle-Wickramsinghe thesis (Steele et al., 2018; Steele, Al-Mufti, et al., 2019; Steele, Gorczynski, et al., 2019). Our theory thus posits a sporadic input of cosmic bacteria, viruses and other micro-organisms that has the potential to interact with evolving terrestrial life forms, causing terrestrial diseases and further adaptive evolution on Earth.

3.3 Link with a direct strike of meteorite over central-North East China, October 11, 2019

In the case of the current coronavirus epidemic in China it is interesting to note that an exceptionally bright fireball event was seen on October 11, 2019 over Sonjyan City in the Jilin Province of NE China (see Fig. 8). It is tempting to speculate that this event (although it happened hundreds of kilometers distant from Hubei) had a crucial role to play in what is now unfolding in and

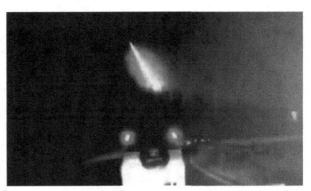

Fig. 8 The public record of this meteorite strike can be found at the Space.com website in an article by Tariq Malik, on October 13, 2019 "Brilliant Midnight Fireball Lights Up Sky Over Northeast China". The October event is described at: https://www.space.com/china-midnight-meteor-brilliant-fireball-october-2019.html.

throughout China. Indeed, the match with the Johns Hopkins University case incidence patterns is so striking it is difficult to easily dismiss this as a chance correspondence of patterns, in both time and place (e.g., Fig. 7).

If a fragment of a fragile and loosely held carbonaceous meteorite carrying a cargo of trillions of viruses/bacteria and other primary source cells (for the cosmic replication of the COVID-19 virus), may have entered the mesosphere and stratosphere at high speed ~30 km/s, its outer, loosely-held envelope carrying a biological cargo may have got dispersed in the mesosphere stratosphere and troposphere. Indeed, a much larger original meteoroid could easily have been fragmenting and dispersing its contents before the ignition of the fireball event. A reasonable assumption is that the fireball which struck 2000 km N of Wuhan may have been part of a wide tube of debris the bulk of which was deposited in the stratosphere to fall over Wuhan. The fall time through the atmosphere of 1–10 μm-sized solid particles could range from a few months to well over a year on the basis of straightforward calculations (e.g., in the Appendix of Hoyle & Wickramasinghe, 1979 "Diseases from space"). Because dispersal at ground level depends on the vagaries of meteorology and precipitation the deposition of virus at ground level is expected to be patchy in regard to both time and place. This is certainly consistent (thus far) with what has happened in relation to the new COVID-19 coronavirus epidemic between November 2019 and the present day (February 15, 2020). Following the initial deposition of infective particles in a small localized region (e.g., Wuhan, Hubei province, China) particles that have already become dispersed over a wider area in the troposphere will fall to ground in a higgledy-piggledy manner, and this process could be extended over a typical timescale of 1–2 years until an initial inoculant of the infective agent would be drained. This accords well with many new strains of viruses including influenza that have appeared in recent years (Wickramasinghe et al., 2019).

The possible link of sunspots with pandemics has been discussed over many years (Qu & Wickramasinghe, 2017, 2018; Wickramasinghe et al., 2017, 2019) and is worthy of brief further discussion. The present cycle (interface between cycles 24 and 25, Fig. 2) has seen the lowest minimum for well over a century with many sunspot free days recorded in the last months of 2019. Sunspot minima are associated with a weakening of the interplanetary magnetic field near the Earth, which in turn allows easy ingress of Galactic Cosmic Rays (GCRs) and electrically charged bacteria and viruses to the Earth. The mutagenic role of GCRs can cause genetic changes in already circulating viruses, but it is primarily to an enhanced flux of new infective particles released by the exploding meteoroid that we turn. Indeed a perfect storm over China is paying out before our eyes, a meteorite delivering COVID-19 particles corresponding with a very significant Sunspot Minimum cycle. It raises the important issue: How would other densely populated countries have reacted to, and handled, this event involving COVID-19? It was only the vagaries of chance that it exploded over China.

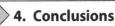

4. Conclusions

We conclude by noting some predictions and expectations:

- We expect the pattern of further spread of the new Coronavirus (COVID-19) to be dictated mostly by primary in-fall until a high level of person-to-person infectivity might *possibly* be achieved and the virus then acquires the status of an endemic virus.

- Viral contamination of the "environment" in the most general sense explains most of the apparent contagion, e.g., news reports like in Box 1.

- Thus, the possibility cannot be ruled out that the *Diamond Princess* cruise ship (and the more recent Westerdam cruiseship) in the South China Sea was contaminated by a fragment of the main COVID-19 dust cloud. Similar inexplicable events appeared to happen for ships at sea during the 1918–1919 Spanish Flu Pandemic (Hoyle & Wickramasinghe, 1979).

- And, further to this, other drifting COVID-19 smaller dust clouds that have not as yet made land fall may target remote island and other communities, as was also the case during the 1918–1919 Spanish Flu Pandemic (Hoyle & Wickramasinghe, 1979).

- Given the low mutation rate, the very wide apparent in-fall infectivity pattern (Fig. 7) the expectation is this pure viral culture has inoculated millions of Chinese citizens (as well as potentially millions of wild and domestic animals in China) inducing protective adaptive immune responses (Acquired Herd Immunity) on a very large scale.
- Thus, development of a so called "COVID-19 vaccine" which is much in the news at the time of writing would be a waste of public tax-payer funds if mounted on the scale envisaged by governments and national centers for disease control.
- We thus expect the decline of the epidemic (peaking and declining at time of writing) to be driven by this mass natural vaccination process now underway in China. So, the suddenly emerging COVID-19 epidemic, like many similar suddenly emerging human epidemics in the past (SARs, MERs, ZIKAV), is expected to rapidly end by the self-limiting processes of wide spread herd immunity (a pattern likely to be repeated in other countries, Appendix C).
- We thus expect that the incidence of serum antibodies specific for COVID-19 to be wide-spread in the Chinese population in the coming months. So, millions will be potentially immunized for life against future infections with COVID-19.
- How long will COVID-19 remain potentially infective in the physical environment? Clearly for some time—given that over the space of a month or so many cases appeared rapidly, spread by environmental contamination in our view, and not by traditional person-to-person generated aerosols at the height of the donor's infection. This is consistent with those news reports out of China "As the death toll rose to 80, China said, increasing concerns about the potential the virus was infectious even before symptoms were visible rapidity of its spread." (Heidi Han and Kieran Gair, Associated Press, *The Australian* newspaper January 27, 2020.)

5. Postscript

As this chapter was submitted to the publisher an authoritative news despatch from Japan reports sporadic outbreaks across the country with *no direct link* with China (Appendix B). Further, in early February we tried to alert the world on our interpretation of the origins of COVID-19 with many of the same arguments and analyses listed in this chapter. One succinct letter was sent to *The Lancet*, and the other was a more general article for a wider lay readership, to *The Australian* newspaper—both articles were rejected by the editors. The archived PDFs of both articles can be found at the viXra.

org site under accession numbers URLs http://viXra.org/abs/2002.0039? ref=11076818, and https://vixra.org/abs/2002.0118. However an expanded comments on the origin and spread of the 2019 Coronavirus (COVID-19) has now been published in Wickramasinghe et al. (2020a, 2020b, 2020c), and see Steele and Lindley (2020) also in discussion in Appendix C.

Acknowledgment

We thank Professor Sanjaya Senanayake for bringing the *Candida auris* data to our attention and for discussions.

Appendix A
On the fall of viruses through the stratosphere

The defining feature of infectious diseases which are caused by biological entities that arrive from space relates to the manner in which they come to be distributed over the Earth's surface. If such microbial agents are introduced via the agency of cometary bolides that survive frictional heating in the mesosphere, their fragmentation and dispersal as clouds of particles in the stratosphere will determine the way in which they finally arrive at the surface of the Earth.

The falling speed of spherical particles of various sizes (with a notional density $1\,\mathrm{g\,cm^{-3}}$) through the atmosphere can be calculated as a function of height (y-axis) was calculated from formulae and data given by Kasten (1968). The results are shown in Fig. A1. We note from the extreme right curve of Fig. A1 that a particle of radius $10\,\mu\mathrm{m}$ falls through the lowest $10\,\mathrm{km}$ of the stratosphere at a speed of $\sim 1\,\mathrm{cm/s}$ and so takes only a few days to cover what for smaller particles is the slowest part of their downward journey. All such particles fall comparatively rapidly through the mesosphere ($z = 80$–$50\,\mathrm{km}$), and then more and more slowly down through the stratosphere below $z = 50\,\mathrm{km}$. A particle with the size of a typical bacterium $\sim 1\,\mu\mathrm{m}$, falls through the lowest $10\,\mathrm{km}$ of the stratosphere at a speed of about $2 \times 10^{-2}\,\mathrm{cm/s}$ and thus falls to ground in a time-scale of $\sim 5 \times 10^{7}\,s$, that is about 2 years. Because there is more of the stratosphere through which such a particle must fall at high latitudes than in the tropics (the troposphere being higher in the tropics) the slow part of the journey is more extended the higher the latitude. A bacterium falling in ~ 1 year in the tropics would fall in ~ 2 years in temperate latitudes and in 2–3 years towards the poles.

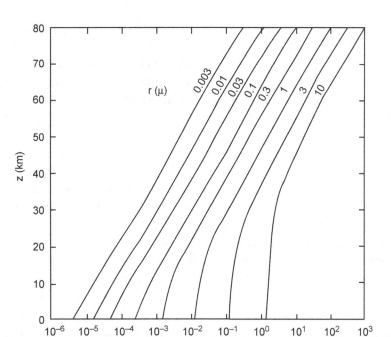

Fig. A1 Falling speed of spherical dust particles as a function of height in the atmosphere. *Reproduced from Hoyle & Wickramasinghe. 1982, Proofs that life is cosmic, Mem. Inst. Fund. Studies, Sri Lanka. Copyright Chandra Wickramasinghe.*

If a particle of the size of a typical virus, a particle say with a diameter of ~0.03 μm, fell under gravity through still air the timescale for the slowest part of the journey through the bottom 10 km of the stratosphere ($z = 20$–10 km) will be ~10^9 s, that is about 30 years (see Fig. A1). This is so slow that other means of descent involving large-scale air movements in the stratosphere have to be considered. Further, the possibility of large clumps of viruses encased in cosmic dust particles will also change the relative effective sizes of infective particles and consequently their speeds of entry. We say this because ... "The sophistication of viral infectivity and their *modus operandi* of cell-cell spreading does not end here ... viral genomes ... can be propagated almost indefinitely (Combe, Garijo, Geller, Cuevas, & Sanjuan, 2015) as 'virion clusters' of mixtures of infective and crippled genomes with significant numbers of newly minted virus particles enwrapped in protective membrane vesicles—a type of multiunit nanoparticle. This then constitutes the actual infective dose (or *unit*) rather than just a single exported virion entering a nearby target cell to cause a productive infection as is commonly believed (Chen et al., 2015; Combe et al., 2015)." Text and references from Steele et al. (2018).

Thus, although in general vertical mass movements of air are feeble compared to those in the troposphere, some vertical stratospheric movement takes place despite the inhibiting effect of an inverted temperature gradient. The physical mechanism for mass stratospheric movements is the equator-to-pole temperature difference which acts as a heat engine across parallels of latitude, a heat engine that operates more strongly the larger the temperature difference—i.e., much more strongly in winter than in the summer. A similar mechanism applies also to the troposphere, where an engine crossing parallels of latitude transfers heat from tropical regions towards the poles, again more in winter than in the summer.

Ozone measurements can be used to trace the mass movements of air in the stratosphere. Such measurements show a winter downdraft that is strongest over the latitude range 40–60 degrees. Taking advantage of this annual downdraft, individual virus particles (or dust-encased clumps) incident on the atmosphere from space would therefore reach ground-level generally in temperate latitudes, which therefore emerge from these considerations as the regions of the Earth where upper respiratory infections are likely to be most prevalent. This is true on the supposition that the Earth is smooth, which of course it is not. The exceptionally high mountains of the Himalayas on the North India-China boundary rearing up through most of the height range to the stratosphere, introduce a large perturbation to the smooth condition, which may be expected to affect adversely this particular region of the Earth, particularly China. In effect the Himalayan peaks, higher than 8 km, could act as a drain plug for most of the viruses incident on the atmosphere at latitude about 30 degrees N. The vast 1.4 billion population of China will thus be inundated by this drainage effect making China the quickest and worst affected region of the planet for cosmic pathogen-particle in-falls. As a consequence other parts of the Earth at about 30 degrees N could fortunately be largely free of incoming viral particles, unless it happens that such particles are incident as components within larger particles.

A direct proof that the winter downdraft effect in the stratosphere occurs overwhelmingly over the latitude range 40–60 degrees was demonstrated by Kalkstein (1961). In the last of the series of nuclear bombs that were tested in the atmosphere, a radioactive tracer element Rh-102 was introduced into the atmosphere at a height above 100 km and the fall out of the tracer was measured month by month through airplane and balloon sampling at altitudes of ~20 km. The radioactive tracer Rh-102 took more than a decade to clear itself through repeated seasonal downdrafts of the kind we

Origin of new emergent Coronavirus and Candida fungal diseases   95

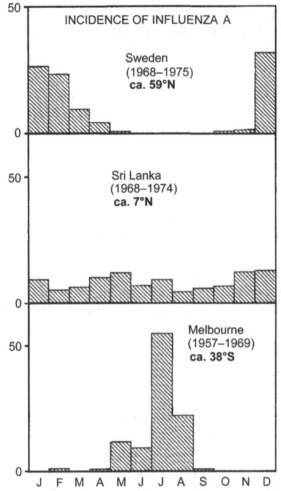

Fig. B1 Incidence of seasonal influenza A in three countries. *Reproduced from Hoyle & Wickramasinghe. (1982). Proofs that life is cosmic. Figure copyright Chandra Wickramasinghe.*

have described. The fall out was found to be much greater at temperate latitudes than elsewhere with the period January to March being the dominant months for the Northern Hemisphere. This is exactly similar to the pattern of incidence of influenza and other seasonal respiratory viral diseases in Northern temperate latitudes, a situation that is well-known to every medical practitioner and health authority. In the Southern hemisphere the situation is similar but 6 months displaced. This is clearly evident in Fig. B1. Note that in a tropical location such as Sri Lanka no discernible seasonal effect can be detected in the data between 1968 and 1974.

Appendix B as February 15, 2020

Headline: None of Japan's new coronavirus patients had direct China links

First death raises fear that virus is quietly spreading

By Yusuke Kurabe, Nikkei staff writer, in Nikkei Asian Revie

February 13, 2020 22:37 JST Updated on February 14, 2020 04:52 JST

https://asia.nikkei.com/Spotlight/Coronavirus/None-of-Japan-s-new-coronavirus-patients-had-direct-China-links

- A Kanagawa Prefecture woman in her 80s died from the coronavirus. Her son-in-law also tested positive for the disease. A doctor in Wakayama Prefecture and a man in Chiba Prefecture are confirmed to have the virus. None of them traveled to China recently or had contact with people who visited Hubei Province, the epicenter of the outbreak. The 80 year old woman's symptoms began January 22 when she felt fatigue, the health ministry said. Symptoms worsened on January 25, prompting her to see a doctor 3 days later. She was placed under observation. The victim was hospitalized February 1, diagnosed with pneumonia. She underwent screening for the coronavirus Wednesday. The test results came back positive Thursday, the day she died. Her son-in-law also tested positive for the coronavirus. The man, a taxi driver in his 70s living in Tokyo, has been hospitalized since February 6, but the symptoms are reportedly mild. He developed a fever January 29.

- A doctor in Wakayama Prefecture south of Osaka has been infected with the virus, prefectural officials said Thursday. The man, in his 50s, has been hospitalized with symptoms of pneumonia, but is otherwise in stable condition. The doctor did not travel outside the country in the 14 days prior to the onset of symptoms, nor can any contact with people coming from China be confirmed. Wakayama officials suspect the infection had domestic origins.

- Elsewhere, a man in his 20s from Chiba Prefecture near Tokyo is also confirmed to have the virus. He developed a fever and other symptoms February 2. The man reportedly has not travelled overseas or had contact with other infected individuals.

- Besides the outbreak on the Diamond Princess cruise ship, which has infected over 200 people aboard the vessel quarantined in Yokohama, 29 cases of coronavirus had been confirmed inside Japan through Wednesday.

- These cases raise new challenges for health officials, who until now had been trying to contain the virus by closely monitoring people with the possibility of contracting the disease. If more people with no direct links to China become sick, determining infection routes will become impossible. Instead of containment, treating seriously sick people may have to become the priority.

Appendix C

An update on published and submitted work by the group as June 22, 2020

The COVID-19 pandemic has now engulfed almost all parts of the globe inhabited by human beings. Confirmed cases are approaching 9 million and confirmed global deaths as June 22 are 468,589. We have updated our analysis here as the pandemic further unfolded. These analyses are now in several papers which have been published (or under-submission) since this paper was drafted. The most important developments are covered in the new citations in the reference list (and below), particularly our discussion on the progress of the major explosive outbreaks following the original epidemic in Wuhan through December-January 2020. Initially, in February, this appeared to go from China across the Pacific to the US West Coast (Wickramasinghe et al., 2020b), but it then became apparent the putative viral-laden meteorite dust clouds moved along the north 40° latitude band heading in a westerly direction from China towards Europe (Wickramasinghe et al., 2020c). We speculate this transportation took place mainly in the Stratosphere and upper Troposphere, and this helps explain in part the major explosive outbreaks of COVID-19 in the temporal order, Tehran/Qom, Italy/Lombardy, Spain then New York City all on the north 40° latitude band. The genetic sequence of the virus has been analyzed where available in each of the major explosive locations, particularly Wuhan and New York City (Steele & Lindley, 2020). Contrary to a widely held perception that the COVID-19 is a hypermutating contagious virus it is still the case, at the time of writing, that the most vulnerable at risk of death through respiratory complications are the co-morbid elderly. Further, the virus does not hypermutate, it appears to a use a riboswitch-mediated haplotype variation strategy which could be associated with the ethnic-genetic background of the subjects infected. Thus the genetic sequence of the virus in Wuhan/China, West Coast USA (February, 2020), Spain and New York City is essentially ≥99.98% identical apart from a small set of key variant putative riboswitch sites (ranging from 2 to 5 on average across the length of the 29,903 nt RNA genome) which define a given haplotype. Thus, there is much haplotype homogeneity in China, but considerable haplotype diversity in New York City. The virus appears to adapt to new host genetic backgrounds by switching putative haplotype presumably allowing superior RNA replication in that cellular environment. The only factor we cannot explain then is why the super explosions of the viral epidemics in certain locations and not others. One likely factor would be the infective dose of the virus which we predict was far greater at these epicentre locations because it came in as a high dose in-fall in meteorite dust from the upper atmosphere.

References

Andersen, K. (2020). *Clock and TMRCA based on 27 genomes Novel 2019 coronavirus*. http://virological.org/t/clock-and-tmrca-based-on-27-genomes/347.

Bradley, S. F. (2019). Candida auris infection. *JAMA, 322*, 1526.

Chatterjee, S., Alampalli, S. V., Nageshan, R. K., Chettiar, S. T., Joshi, S., & Tatu, U. S. (2015). Draft genome of a commonly misdiagnosed multidrug resistant pathogen Candida auris. *BMC Genomics, 16*, 686.

Chen, Y.-H., Du, W.-L., Hagemeijer, M. C., Takvorian, P. M., Pau, C., et al. (2015). Phosphatidylserine vesicles enable efficient en bloc transmission of enteroviruses. *Cell, 160*, 619–630. https://doi.org/10.1016/j.cell.2015.01.032.

Chow, N. A., Gade, L., Tsay, S. V., Forsberg, K., Greenko, J. A., Southwick, K. L., et al. (2018). Multiple introductions and subsequent transmission of multidrug-resistant Candida auris in the USA: A molecular epidemiological survey. *Lancet Infectious Diseases, 18*, 1377–1384.

Chowdhary, A., Sharma, C., & Meis, J. F. (2017). Candida auris: A rapidly emerging cause of hospital-acquired multidrug-resistant fungal infections globally. *PLoS Pathogens, 13*(5), e1006290. https://doi.org/10.1371/journal.ppat.1006290.

Cohen, J. (2020). Wuhan seafood market may not be source of novel virus spreading globally. *Science,* January 26. https://doi.org/10.1126/science.abb0611.

Combe, M., Garijo, R., Geller, R., Cuevas, J. M., & Sanjuan, R. (2015). Single-cell analysis of RNA virus infection identifies multiple genetically diverse viral genomes within single infectious units. *Cell Host Microbe, 18*, 424–432. https://doi.org/10.1016/j.chom.2015.09.009.

Cortegiani, A., Misseri, G., Fasciana, T., Giammanco, A., Giarratano, A., & Chowdhary, A. (2018). Epidemiology, clinical characteristics, resistance, and treatment of infections by Candida auris. *Journal of Intensive Care, 6*, 69. https://doi.org/10.1186/s40560-018-0342-4.

Forsberg, K., Woodworth, K., Walters, M., Berkow, E. L., Jackson, B., Chiller, T., et al. (2018). Candida auris: The recent emergence of a multidrug-resistant fungal pathogen. *Medical Mycology, 57*, 1–12.

Hoyle, F., & Wickramasinghe, N. C. (1979). *Diseases from space*. London: J.M. Dent & Sons, Ltd.

Hoyle, F., & Wickramasinghe, N. C. (1990). Influenza—Evidence against contagion: Discussion paper. *Journal of the Royal Society of Medicine, 83*(4), 258–261.

Huang, C., Wang, Y., Li, X., Ren, L., Zhao, J., Hu, Y., et al. (2020). Clinical features of patients infected with 2019 novel coronavirus in Wuhan, China. *The Lancet*, *395*, 497–506. Published online January 24,2020. https://doi.org/10.1016/S0140-6736(20)30183-5.

Jackson, B. R., Chow, N., Forsberg, K., Litvintseva, A. P., Lockhart, S. R., & Welsh, R. (2019). On the origins of a species: What might explain the rise of Candida auris? *Journal of Fungi*, *5*, 58.

Jeffery-Smith, A., Taori, S. K., Schelenz, S., Jeffery, K., Johnson, E. M., Borman, A., et al. (2018). Candida auris: A Review of the Literature. *Clinical Microbiology Reviews*, *31*(1), pii: e00029-17. https://doi.org/10.1128/CMR.00029-17.

Kalkstein, M. I. (1961). Rhodium-102 high altitude tracer experiment. *Science*, *137*, 645.

Kasten, F. (1968). Falling speed of aerosol particles. *Journal of Applied Meteorology*, 7, 944.

Lockhart, S. R., Etienne, K. A., Vallabhaneni, S., Farooqi, J., Chowdhary, A., Govender, N. P., et al. (2017). Simultaneous emergence of multidrug-resistant Candida auris on 3 continents confirmed by whole-genome sequencing and epidemiological analyses. *Clinical Infectious Diseases*, *64*, 134–140. https://doi.org/10.1093/cid/ciw691.

Lu, R., Zhao, X., Li, J., Niu, P., Yang, B., Wu, H., et al. (2020). Genomic characterisation and epidemiology of 2019 novel coronavirus: Implications for virus origins and receptor binding. *The Lancet*, *395*, 565–574. published Online January 29, 2020. https://doi.org/10.1016/S0140-6736(20)30251-8.

Pfaller, M. A., Diekema, D. J., Turnidge, J. T., Castanheira, M., & Jones, R. N. (2019). Twenty years of the SENTRY antifungal surveillance program: Results for Candida species from 1997–2016. *Open Forum Infectious Diseases*, *6*(S1), S79–S94.

Qu, J., & Wickramasinghe, C. (2017). SARS, MERS and the sunspot cycle. *Current science*, *113*(8), 1501–1502.

Qu, J., & Wickramasinghe, C. (2018). Weakened magnetic field, cosmic rays and the Zikavirus outbreak. *Current science*, *115*(3), 382–383.

Rhodes, J., & Fisher, M. C. (2019). Global epidemiology of emerging Candida auris. *Current Opinion in Microbiology*, *52*, 84–89.

Rosenberg, S. M. (2001). Evolving responsively: Adaptive mutation. *Nature Reviews Genetics*, 2, 805–815.

Steele, E. J., Al-Mufti, S., Augustyn, K. A., Chandrajith, R., Coghlan, J. P., Coulson, S. G., et al. (2018). Cause of Cambrian explosion—Terrestrial or cosmic? *Progress in Biophysics and Molecular Biology*, *136*, 3–23. https://doi.org/10.1016/j.pbiomolbio.2018.03.004.

Steele, E. J., Al-Mufti, S., Augustyn, K. A., Chandrajith, R., Coghlan, J. P., Coulson, S. G., et al. (2019). Cause of Cambrian explosion—Terrestrial or cosmic?—Reply to commentary by R Duggleby. *Progress in Biophysics and Molecular Biology*, *141*, 74–78.

Steele, E. J., Gorczynski, R. M., Lindley, R. A., Liu, Y., Temple, R., Tokoro, G., et al. (2019). Lamarck and Panspermia—On the efficient spread of living systems throughout the cosmos. *Progress in Biophysics and Molecular Biology*, *149*, 10–32. pii: S0079-6107(19)30112-9. https://doi.org/10.1016/j.pbiomolbio.2019.08.010.

Steele, E. J., & Lindley, R. A. (2020). Analysis of APOBEC and ADAR deaminase-driven Riboswitch Haplotypes in COVID-19 RNA strain variants and the implications for vaccine design. Accepted for publication in *Research Reports*, June 22, 2020, under Quantitative Biology. https://vixra.org/abs/2006.0011?ref=11360015.

Wickramasinghe, N. C. (2012). DNA sequencing and predictions of the cosmic theory of life. *Astrophysics and Space Science*, *343*, 1–5.

Wickramasinghe, N. C., & Steele, E. J. (2016). Dangers of adhering to an obsolete paradigm: Could Zika virus lead to a reversal of human evolution? *Journal of Astrobiology & Outreach*, *4*(1). https://doi.org/10.4172/2332-2519.1000147.

Wickramasinghe, N. C., Steele, E. J., Gorczynski, R. M., Temple, R., Tokoro, G., Qu, J., et al. (2020a). Comments on the origin and spread of the 2019 Coronavirus. *Virology: Current Research, 4*(1). https://doi.org/10.37421/Virol Curr Res.2020.4.109.

Wickramasinghe, N. C., Steele, E. J., Gorczynski, R. M., Temple, R., Tokoro, G., Wallis, D. H., et al. (2020b). Growing evidence against global infection-driven by person-to-person transfer of COVID-19. *Virology: Current Research, 4*(1). https://doi.org/10.37421/Virol Curr Res.2020.4.110.

Wickramasinghe, N. C., Steele, E. J., Gorczynski, R. M., Temple, R., Tokoro, G., Kondakov, A., et al. (2020c). Predicting the future trajectory of COVID-19. *Virology: Current Research, 4*(1). https://doi.org/10.37421/Virol Curr Res.2020.4.111.

Wickramasinghe, N. C., Steele, E. J., Wainwright, M., Tokoro, G., Fernando, M., & Qu, J. (2017). Sunspot cycle minima and pandemics: The case for vigilance. *Journal Astrobiology and Outreach, 5*, 2. https://doi.org/10.4172/2332-2519.1000159.

Wickramasinghe, C., Wainwright, M., & Narlikar, J. (2003). SARS—A clue to its origins? *The Lancet, 361*, 1832.

Wickramasinghe, N. C., Wickramsinghe, D. T., Senananyake, J., Qu, J., Tokoros, G., Temple, R., et al. (2019). Space weather and pandemic warnings? *Current Science, 117*(10), 1554 (25 Nov 2019).

Review article   Open Access

Predicting the Future Trajectory of COVID-19

N Chandra Wickramasinghe[1,2,3,4*], Edward J Steele[2,5], Reginald M Gorczynski[6], Robert Temple[7], Gensuke Tokoro[4], Alexander Kondakov[8], Daryl H. Wallis[4], Brig Klyce[9] and D T Wickramasinghe[10]

[1]Buckingham Centre for Astrobiology, University of Buckingham, MK18 1EG England, UK

[2]Centre for Astrobiology, University of Ruhuna, Matara, Sri Lanka

[3]National Institute of Fundamental Studies, Kandy, Sri Lanka

[4]Institute for the Study of Panspermia and Astroeconomics, Gifu, Japan

[5]C Y O'Connor, ERADE Village, Foundation, Piara Waters, Perth 6112 WA, Australia

[6]University Toronto Health Network, Toronto General Hospital, University of Toronto, Canada

[7]History of Chinese Science and Culture Foundation, Conway Hall, London, UK

[8]193/ Sinyavinskaya str 16/11, Moscow, Russia

[9]Astrobiology Research Trust, Memphis, TN, USA

[10]College of Physical and Mathematical Sciences, Australian National University, Canberra, Australia

Abstract

We argue that the new coronavirus COVID-19 was probably linked to the arrival of a pure culture of the virus in cometary debris that was deposited in the stratosphere, and first came down in the Hubei province of China. The subsequent worldwide spread of the virus has taken place by a combination of two effects: the deposition of further large quantities of virus at several locations – Iran, North Italy, South Korea – combined with much slower spread through person-to-person infection (itself enhanced largely by contaminated surfaces and personal affects). The location of the foci outside China all lie close to latitude 40 degrees N, consistent with the transport of aerosols by cyclonic winds in the stratosphere. It is also remarkably consistent with observations in the 1960's of the fall-out of radioactive dust deposited in the stratosphere in the last of the atmospheric atom bomb tests. On this basis, we conclude that a stratospheric loading of the Coronavirus that happened in October/November 2019 could take a few winter seasons to be fully drained. A clearer understanding of the causal events that led to the COVID-19 pandemic could help planning future strategy.

Keywords: Coronavirus • Epidemiology • Comets • Panspermia

Introduction

In our earlier papers [1,2] we have discussed the possibility that the onset of the 2019-COVID-19 pandemic in Wuhan in China was triggered by the in-fall of a cloud of virus-laden dust deposited by a cometary bolide. We suggested that the cometary bolide may have been linked to a spectacular fireball event that was witnessed in the province of Jilin on 11 October 2019. The proposal to rename COVID-19 to SARS-CoV-2 could fortuitously fit in with the case for space origin of both SARS-CoV-1 AND SARS-CoV-2. The first cases of SARS-CoV-1 recorded in November 2002 actually appeared a few weeks after a bright cometary meteoroid exploded in the Ikutsk region of Siberia [2]. This suggesting that the SARS-virus-dust may have been deposited as a dispersed fragment of the same bolide in the stratosphere and subsequently carried by air currents to fall first over China. The events of 2002 bear an uncanny resemblance to the events that followed the sighting of the Jilin fireball in October 2019 [1].

Both bolides of 2002 and 2019 most probably belonged to the Orionid meteor stream which is associated with the historic Comet P/Halley. Comet P/Halley in pursuing its orbit around the sun ejects fragments of all sizes from dust to bolides that eventually separate from the parent body and pursue similar highly elliptic orbits with a period of 76 years. The last perihelion passage was in 1986 and at this time the Giotto space mission combined with ground-based telescope observations began a new era of cometary studies. Halley's comet itself is about 10 km in diameter and the material ejected from its pitch-black surface in 1986 was found to have an infrared spectrum consistent with biological dust [3].The stream of dust and debris of all sizes ejected throughout the entire life of Comet Halley continues to orbit within a broad stream constituting the Orionid meteor stream. The Earth crosses this stream of debris every year in late October/early November. The events in Ikutsk and Jilin,

*Corresponding author: Dr N Chandra Wickramasinghe, Buckingham Centre for Astrobiology, University of Buckingham MK18 1EG, England, UK, Tel: +44 (0)2920752146/+44 (0)7778389243; E-mail: ncwick@gmail.com

Received: March 16, 2020; Accepted: April 06, 2020; Published: April 13, 2020

Wickramasinghe NC, et al.

Virol Curr Res, Volume 4: 1, 2020

which are exactly 17 years apart, could represent encounters of the Earth with two large frozen lumps that had broken off from the comet which contained clonal variants of the Corona virus [4].

The unfolding global pandemic of COVID-19 as time proceeds becomes increasingly difficult to unravel given both a possible continuing in-fall of the now-dispersed virus-laden dust cloud fragments combined with a slow contagion or person to person spread (itself contributed largely derived, in our view, from contaminated surfaces and personal affects [5]. The various measures being taken to "contain" or "delay" the progress of this pandemic, although taken in good faith, fall short of planning for resurgences caused by a continuing sequence of further in-fall episodes of this viral-dust.

Critical Summary of Main Facts and Popular Assumptions

Some of the following main facts appear to be undeniable, yet some need a critical reappraisal:

(a) An initial "in-fall" of trillions of virions in bolide dust particles (acting as protective matrices) from outside the human population took place leading to a huge number of COVID-19 cases in the region of incidence (Hubei) and its environs, particularly Wuhan city. Our informed view is that many people were almost simultaneously infected and naturally inoculated with the same COVID-19 virus strain. This happened in a matter of days after the first cases were recorded in early November 2019 [1,6].

(b) The claim that the virus was transferred to humans from bats through an intermediary animal has been widely claimed, but there is no direct supporting evidence for such a hypothesis, and it is not generally supported by the phylogenetic analyses. These analyses themselves rest on the false premise of circular logic – the evolutionary model [7] at their heart actually assumes a progression of viral evolution through two animal species then to human as its first unwavering principle. It is also based on highly questionable analyses of gene sequence data involving two intermediate, and unlikely, animal jumps, first from bats to an intermediary animal "X" (= pangolins) then to humans who acquire infection from eating that animal (Steele EJ and colleagues In preparation). For example in Tang et al. [7] the two linked single nucleotide substitutions (the basis of the two circulating haplotypes, L and S) appear at APOBEC and ADAR deaminase motif sites that appear to be hotspots for C-to-U and A-to-I deaminations and thus are part of the expected quasi viral sequence species pool *in vivo* during the early acute phase of infection i.e. part and parcel of natural viral "evolution" *in vivo* [8]. The claim that the minor S variant evolved in two steps in animals (bats -> pangolins?) and then mutated at these sites to produce the major L haplotypes, thus producing both the SARS-CoV-1 and SARS-CoV-2 variants, is pure conjecture with no hard evidence Tang et al. [7]. It could equally be that on in-fall in 2002 by SARS-CoV-1 the naturally occurring or *in vivo* generated S variant thrived best in the animals studied, while the L variant was best suited for human replication.

The fact that the second of the two linked SNV variants is a T>C at a clear ADAR deamination motif site (..GTTTACCTTT..) in the 5'UTR, a region known for regulating viral replication [9], implies that replication rates could be controlled at a alternative secondary RNA structure ("riboswitch") by T>C (ADAR) and/or C>T (APOBEC) deaminations at this site. None of this biological insight is evident in the Tang et al. [7] analysis nor in any other coronavirus phylogenetic analyses we have seen recently.

(c) A worldwide spread solely from an initial case or cluster of cases in Wuhan is generally claimed but evidence for this is still lacking. A simultaneous or near simultaneous attack of thousands of people from an external source/reservoir appears in our view a more likely explanation for the available data.

(d) Transmissions (contagion) must certainly have contributed to spread within Wuhan and surroundings, but transmissions outwards from Wuhan across the wider world based on contagion alone proceeds at a much slower rate depending on movement of infected persons and would in general be overwhelmed by secondary infall events.

Global Dissemination

We have discussed earlier [1,2] the many unsuccessful searches for a case zero that may have triggered secondary foci of infection that exploded several months after the original outbreak in Wuhan. Tracing index cases has been a frustratingly difficult endeavour, and an alternative model of independent origins or secondary in-fall events from the stratosphere, characterised by high attack rates, is strongly suggested as an alternate explanation of the epidemiological data. This appears to be relevant to the cases in Iran and Italy where an almost uncanny simultaneous exponential initial rise in case numbers is to be seen at clear epicentres (Figure 1) at highly specific locations in the country (Lombardy in Italy; Tehran-Qom in Iran), in the analogous fashion to the specific epicentre location at Wuhan in China (Figure 2).

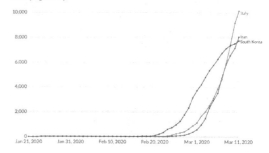

Figure 1. Total cases of COVID-19 to March 11, 2020 from data in [10].

The slower spread out from an initial focus of in-fall is clearly evident from the diminishing attack rates seen in Figure 2 outside of the Lombardy valley which suddenly acquired thousands of cases, and similarly in the case of foci in South Korea and Iran.

Wickramasinghe NC, et al.

Virol Curr Res, Volume 4: 1, 2020

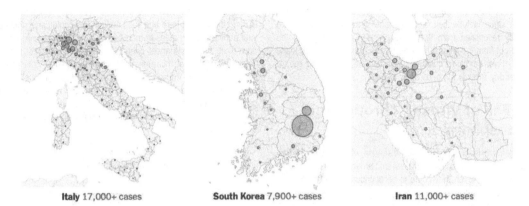

Italy 17,000+ cases   **South Korea** 7,900+ cases   **Iran** 11,000+ cases

Figure 2. Gross inequalities of the attack rates Italy, Iran and South Korea. These are from New York Times 12 March 2020 [11].

Similar patterns were seen outside the other main foci world-wide until contagion began to even out the numbers to some extent. In this connection, we should stress that the case numbers thus far recorded everywhere, although large enough to cause concern, are certainly underestimates of case incidence. Considering the manner in which the samples are chosen the total numbers of seropositive COVID-19 cases may be higher everywhere by factors in excess of 10 or 100. We await the COVID-19 serology data, or presence/absence of COVID-19 specific antibodies, with great interest Figure 3.

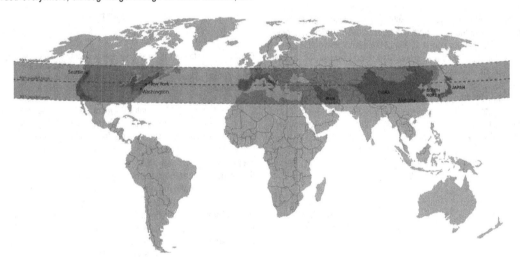

Figure 3. Chain of foci of COVID-19 straddling latitude belt 30-50 degrees N (prepared by Alexander Kondakov, assisted by Chandra Wickramasinghe).

Perhaps the most remarkable feature of the foci of infection outside China is that they are all located close to latitude 30-50 degrees N. These foci seem to have developed more or less in sequence moving westward from in China, South Korea, Iran and the Lombardy valley of Italy in mid-February 2020, and thence to North America along more or less the same belt of latitude. The times of descent to ground from such a belt of dispersed material depends, however, on local tropospheric weather conditions, and the early outbreaks in the west coast of the USA could be explained as the result of dust clouds carried by winds moving in an easterly direction from Wuhan [1]. It should be noted that the same general belt of latitude (30-50 degrees N) is implicated in many seasonal respiratory diseases including seasonal influenza and respiratory syncitial virus, RSV. The incidence of the latter is shown in Figure 4.

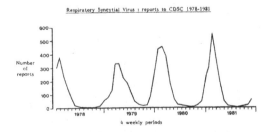

Figure 4. Incidence of RSV- virus in the UK from 1977-1982. (Data from Communicable Disease Surveillance Centre, UK).

Wickramasinghe NC, et al.   Virol Curr Res, Volume 4: 1, 2020

This could be interpreted as evidence of a seasonal in-fall pattern over the same latitude belt of a common virus that may well be constantly resupplied from the stratosphere. Considering that the daily fall-out from the atmosphere of viruses above the atmospheric boundary layer has been measured at billions of viruses per square metre per day, this would not be a surprise [12].

The Fall of Viruses Through the Stratosphere

The defining feature of infectious diseases which are caused by biological entities (bacteria and viruses) that arrive from space relates to the manner in which they come to be distributed over the Earth's surface. If such microbial agents are introduced *via* the agency of cometary bolides (e.g. fragments of the Jilin meteor) that survive frictional heating in the mesosphere, their fragmentation first as smaller bolides and then as dispersed clouds of particles in the stratosphere will determine the way in which they finally arrive at the surface of the Earth.

The falling speed of spherical particles of various sizes (with a notional density 1 g cm^{-3}) through the atmosphere can be calculated as a function of height (y-axis) and was calculated from formulae and data given by Kasten [13]. The results are shown in Figure 5. We note from the extreme right curve of Figure 5 that a particle of radius 10 μm falls through the lowest 10 km of the stratosphere at a speed of ~ 1 cm/s and so takes only a few days to cover what, for smaller particles, is the slowest part of their downward journey. All such particles fall comparatively rapidly through the mesosphere (z = 80-50 km), and then more and more slowly down through the stratosphere below z=50 km. A particle with the size of a ~ 3 μm appropriate for a clump of viruses, falls through the lowest ten kilometers of the stratosphere at a speed of about 2×10^{-1} cm s-1 and thus falls to ground in a time-scale of ~ 5×10^7 sec, that is about 2 months – consistent with the delay time between sighting of the Jilin meteor and the first cases in Wuhan.

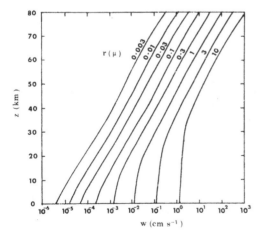

Figure 5. Falling speed of spherical dust particles as a function of height in the atmosphere (reproduced from Hoyle and Wickramasinghe [14], Proofs that Life is Cosmic, Mem. Inst.Fund.Studies, Sri Lanka, 1982) (copyright Chandra Wickramasinghe).

Ozone measurements can be used to trace the mass movements of air in the stratosphere and such movements could carry clusters of viral particles. Such measurements have consistently shown a winter downdraft that is strongest over the latitude range 40-60 degrees. Taking advantage of this annual downdraft, individual virus particles (or significant dust encased in 10 micrometre sized clumps) incident on the atmosphere from space would therefore reach ground-level generally in temperate latitudes. These latitudes therefore emerge as the location where upper respiratory infections would be predicted to be most prevalent.

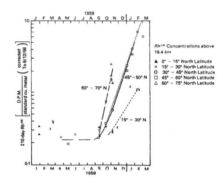

Figure 6. The fall out of Rh-102 at various latitude intervals from the HARDACK atmospheric nuclear bomb test exploded on 11 August 1958 (Kalskstein, 1962; Ref 15) (reproduced from Hoyle & Wickramasinghe: Proofs that Life is Cosmic, 1982; Ref 14).

A direct proof that the winter downdraft effect in the stratosphere occurs overwhelmingly over the latitude range 40-60 degrees was given by Kalkstein [15]. In the last of the series of nuclear bombs that were tested in the atmosphere, a radioactive tracer element Rh-102 was introduced into the atmosphere at a height above 100 km and the fall out of the tracer was measured year by year through airplane and balloon sampling at altitudes of ~ 20 km. The tracer took more than a decade to clear itself through repeated seasonal downdrafts of the kind we have described. This is shown in Figure 6 where we should note that the y-axis is on a logarithmic scale. Here the fall out of the radioactive tracer Rh-102 can be seen to be much greater at temperate latitudes than elsewhere, with the period January to March being the dominant months for the Northern Hemisphere. In correlating this data with the COVID-19 pandemic we might predict that the in-fall in temperate latitudes may wane after April. However, if smaller clumps of viruses still remain in the stratosphere, the repeated flushing occurring seasonally over the winter months could nevertheless lead to persistent risk for a few years to come. Off-setting this ongoing risk is that following a first wave of pathogen exposure, herd immunity is predicted to develop, with subsequent incursions of the virus representing no more a challenge than season influenza or the RSV virus.

Seasonal Recurrence

The distinct seasonality of respiratory viruses, including influenza and the common cold, which more or less disappear with the advent of Spring, is traditionally attributed (without proof) to warm weather,

Wickramasinghe NC, et al.   Virol Curr Res, Volume 4: 1, 2020

ultraviolet light acting as a sterilizer, and to changing social behaviour. Much more likely, in our view, is that a primary source of the virus from the troposphere declines in late spring due to well-attested atmospheric circulation patterns. A reservoir of viruses deposited in the troposphere will thus have a cyclical seasonal turn over – coming down more vigorously in the winter months. Likewise, a new virus deposited in the stratosphere over the northern temperate latitude belt shown in Figure 3 will be largely confined Northern latitudes until it diffuses to the southern hemisphere and is thereafter deposited to the ground 6 months later.

If our model is valid the epidemic behaviour of COVID-19 from January to March in the Northern and Southern hemispheres should be dramatically different. Cases of COVID-19 in the southern hemisphere (e.g. Australia) during the months January-March would be more or less exclusively determined by the movement of infected people from foci of disease in the Northern hemisphere. Precisely this type of difference between the two categories is clearly to be seen in Figures 7 and 8 compiled by Macintyre [16].

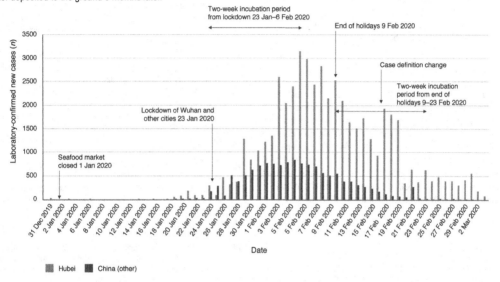

Figure 7. Epidemic in China – exponential rise, peak and decline.

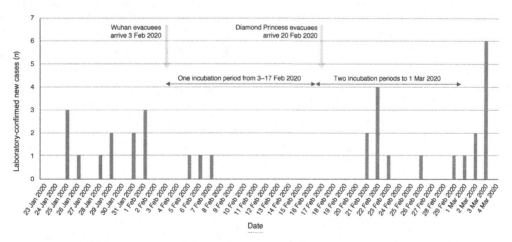

Figure 8. Australian cases of COVID19 – slow spread from random injections of infected people and goods during the period January – March 2020 [15].

With the draconian measures including restrictions of travel and social gatherings that are being put in force in several countries, and hospital resources stretched to full capacity, the most positive outcome to anticipate is the eventual development of natural herd immunity. This has acted as a major driver of rapid declines in similar emerging diseases like SARS and MERS. A decline attributable to

the production and clinical introduction of an effective vaccine, given past experience, is likely some 12-18 months away. In the longer term, it seems to us imperative that we should explore methods for predicting such events ahead of their occurrence with a view to making appropriate plans for alleviating disaster. We have already suggested a few general criteria that could be looked for – e.g. the

Wickramasinghe NC, et al.   Virol Curr Res, Volume 4: 1, 2020

phase of the sunspot cycle and cosmic ray flux [17-19]. More important, however, is to recognise the emerging irrefutable fact that the Earth is not an isolated biological system and that bacteria and viruses may be arriving more or less steadily from a wider cosmic biosphere. Some 800 million viruses per square metre per day that have recently been estimated to be falling through the atmospheric boundary layer from altitudes of 4 km in the Sierra Nevada Mountains [12]. Most, though not all of this flux can be attributed to a terrestrial origin and recycling of uplifted material, but a significant number are not accounted for. Furthermore, collections of stratospheric material over the past decade have consistently revealed the presence of bacteria, including new bacterial species, at height of 41 km [20-22] and the presence of bacteria on the exterior of the International Space Station at 400 km has also been reported [23].

Conclusion

These developments give added credence to microbiota of external origin arriving steadily at the Earth. Because the descent through the atmosphere of viral and bacterial-sized particles from heights above 40 km could take several months the desirability of monitoring the stratosphere is amply clear. Aircraft, balloons and rockets could be deployed for this purpose along with next generation gene sampling technologies to give us advanced warning of future pandemic-causing pathogens before they fall to Earth. Not to do so is an abrogation of our duty as members of the species *Homo sapiens sapiens* in the year 2020.

References

1. Wickramasinghe, NC and Steele EJ, Gorczynski RM and Temple R et al. "Comments on the Origin and Spread of the 2019 Coronavirus." VirolCurr Res (2020) 4:1.

2. Wickramasinghe, NC and Steele EJ, Gorczynski RM and Temple R et al. "Growing Evidence against Global Infection-Driven by Person-to-Person Transfer of COVID19 ." VirolCurr Res (2020) 4:1.

3. Wickramasinghe, DT and Allen DA. "Discovery of organic grains in Comet Halley." Nature (1986) 323: 44-46.

4. "Bodaybo event is believed to be an impact by a bolide (fireball) in the Vitim River basin." Vitim event wikipedia, (2002).

5. Cai, J, Sun W, Huang J and Gamber M et al. "He G Indirect Virus Transmission in Cluster of COVID-19 Cases, Wenzhou, China." Centers for Disease Control and Prevention June Research Letter (2020) Vol 26: 6.

6. "Coronavirus Disease (COVID-19) – Statistics and Research By Max Roser, Hannah Ritchie and Esteban Ortiz-Ospina". Our world in Data (2020).

7. Tang, X, Wu C, Li X, Song Y et al. "On the origin and continuing evolution of SARS-CoV-2." National Science Review (2020).

8. Lindley, RA and Steele EJ. "ADAR and APOBEC editing signatures in viral RNA during acute- phase Innate Immune responses of the host-parasite relationship to Flaviviruses." Research Reports (2018) vol 2:e1-e22.

9. Yang, D and Leibowitz JL. "The structure and functions of coronavirus genomic 3' and 5' ends." Virus Research (2015) 206 :120–133.

10. "Guidance for health system contingency planning during widespread transmission of SARS-CoV-2 with high impact on healthcare services." European Centre for Disease Prevention and Control.]

11. Anjali, Singhvi, Allison McCann, Jin Wu and Blacki Migliozzi. "How the World's Largest Coronavirus Outbreaks Are Growing." 12 March (2020).

12. Reche, I, Orta DG, Mladenov N. "Deposition rates of viruses and bacteria above the atmospheric boundary layer Deposition rates of viruses and bacteria above the atmospheric boundary layer." The ISME Journal (2018).

13. Kasten, F. "Falling speed of aerosol particles." J App Met (1961) 7: 944.

14. Hoyle, F and Wickramasinghe NC. "Proofs that Life is Cosmic, Mem." Inst.Fund.Studies, Sri Lanka (1982).

15. Kalkstein, MI. "Rhodium-102 high altitude tracer experiment science." (1961) 137,645.

16. Macintyre, CR. "On a knife's edge of a COVID-19 pandemic: is containment still possible?" Public Health Res Pract (2020) 30: 1.

17. Qu, J and Wickramasinghe C. "SARS, MERS and the sunspot cycle." Current Science (2017) 113: 8.

18. Qu, J and Wickramasinghe C. "Weakened magnetic field, Cosmic rays and the Zikavirus outbreak." Current Science (2018) 115: 3.

19. Wickramasinghe, NC and Steele EJ. "Dangers of adhering to an obsolete paradigm: could Zika virus lead to a reversal of human evolution?" J Astrobiol Outreach (2016) 4:1.

20. Harris, MJ, Wickramasinghe NC and Lloyd D. "Detection of living cells in stratospheric samples." Proceedings of SPIE (2002) 4495:192-198.

21. Shivaji, S, Chaturvedi P and Suresh K. "Bacillus aerius sp. nov., Bacillus aerophilus sp. nov., Bacillus stratosphericus sp. nov. and Bacillus altitudinis sp. nov., isolated from cryogenic tubes used for collecting air samples from high altitudes." Int J Syst Evol Microbiol (2006) 56: 7.

22. Shivaji, S, Chaturvedi P and Begum Z. "Janibacter hoylei sp. nov., Bacillus isronensis sp. nov. and Bacillus aryabhattai sp. nov., isolated from cryotubes used for collecting air from the upper atmosphere." Int J Syst Evol Microbiol (2009) 59: 12.

23. Grebennikova, TV, Syroeshkin AV and Shubralova EV. "The DNA of Bacteria of the World Ocean and the Earth in Cosmic Dust at the International Space Station." Scientific World Journal (2018) 7360147.

How to cite this article: N Chandra Wickramasinghe, Daryl H. Wallis, Edward J Steele and Reginald M Gorczynski et al. "Predicting the future Trajectory of Trajectory of COVID-19". *Virol Curr Res* 4 (2020) doi:10.37421/*Virol Curr Res*.2020.4.11

Review Article Open Access

Intercontinental Spread of COVID-19 on Global Wind Systems

N Chandra Wickramasinghe[1,2,3,4*], Max K. Wallis[2], Stephen G. Coulson[2], Alexander Kondakov[2], Edward J. Steele[3,5], Reginald M. Gorczynski[6], Robert Temple[7], Gensuke Tokoro[2], Brig Klyce[8] and Predrag Slijepcevic [9]

[1]Buckingham Centre for Astrobiology, University of Buckingham, MK18 1EG, UK

[2]Institute for the Study of Panspermia and Astroeconomics, Gifu, Japan

[3]Centre for Astrobiology, University of Ruhuna, Matara, Sri Lanka

[4]National Institute of Fundamental Studies, Kandy, Sri Lanka

[5]C Y O'Connor, ERADE Village, Foundation, Piara Waters, Perth 6112 WA, Australia

[6]University Toronto Health Network, Toronto General Hospital, University of Toronto, ON M5G 2C4, Canada

[7]History of Chinese Science and Culture Foundation, Conway Hall, London, UK

[8]Astrobiology Research Trust, Memphis, TN, USA

[9]School of Health Sciences, Brunel University, London, UK

Abstract

The pattern of the SARS-CoV-2 incidence concentrated in the 30-50N latitude zone suggests dust carrying the virus is spread by a circum-global jet-stream, specifically the northern sub-tropical jet-stream that blows in the high-altitude troposphere over northern China in early spring-time. It is known that the agent of the Kawasaki disease is carried by long-range winds to Japan and California from north-east China. We hypothesize that dust carrying the virus SARS-CoV-2 was similarly transported from the huge virus reservoir generated in Wuhan province to southern USA, thence across the Atlantic to Portugal and further states to the east. On this model the primary in fall of the dust/virus-carrier depends on the jet-stream interaction with regional weather systems, causing incidence of SARS-CoV-2 cases in various countries/states along this latitude belt. The notable case of Brazil on 31 March 2020-exceptionally outside the 30-50N belt-is proposed to be due to the Azores cyclonic system entraining part of the jet-stream west of Portugal into the south-westerly trade winds, when these winds penetrate to Brazil during spring-time.

Keywords: Coronavirus • Epidemiology • Jet-stream • Dust-vector • Global winds

Introduction

In earlier communications [1-3] we suggested that the primary infall of the SARS-CoV-2 virus probably occurred as a result of an inoculant contained in a cometary bolide that first came down into the troposphere in Wuhan in October/November 2019. It did not significantly spill out around the world until January-February 2020 when the virus spread to locations defining the striking pattern of Figure 1, foci of infection being manly distributed within a latitude belt 30-50N. The delays of incidence within this belt can be put down to auspicious wind conditions, primarily the requirement that local winds coincided with the Hadley cell turnover carrying the virus into the east-Asian subtropical jet-stream lying to the north of Wuhan's 30N latitude. Once the jet-stream is loaded, transport along a belt 30-50N latitude led to subsequent deposits of the virus at various other locations. The jet-stream circles the globe in ~3 days (moving at speeds of ~150-200 km/hr) and deposits initial inoculants of the virus

relatively easily, being close to the down-welling flow at the convective Hadley-Ferrel cell boundaries. Deposits are close in time but can be well-spaced in longitude. Two or three episodes of lofting and deposition could occur on each occasion, but at different latitudes corresponding to the irregular N-S fluctuations.

The Hadley and Ferrel convective cells are driven by the temperature gradient between the tropics and the temperate zone, but ocean-continent temperature differences add strong irregularity. Research into the into the physics of H-F cells has so far been restricted to modelling of the East-Asian section, covering the relatively stable region over north China and the tracking of two branches across North America (Figure 2). Regular satellite probing was started in 2018 by the Isolus mission and updates to the modelling are to be expected.

Knowledge of global transport of infective agents is generally sparse. The Kawasaki disease is thought to cross the North Pacific Ocean on the jet-stream from north China. Bacteria and viruses travel

*Corresponding author: Dr N Chandra Wickramasinghe, Buckingham Centre for Astrobiology, University of Buckingham MK18 1EG, England, UK, Tel: +44 (0)2920752146/+44 (0)7778389243; E-mail: ncwick@gmail.com

Received: May 01, 2020; Accepted: May 22, 2020; Published: May 29, 2020

Wickramasinghe NC, et al.   Virol Curr Res, Volume 4: 1, 2020

the north Atlantic ocean, embedded in Saharan dust, the transcontinental transport of which long been known. Evidence of fall-out and rain-out of dust carrying viruses from south eastern USA and from the Sahara has also been described by Reche et al. [4] who found both dry and wet deposition of viruses in the Spanish Sierra Nevada.

We consider that a primary in-fall of virus at any particular locality would give rise to an almost simultaneous infection in large numbers of susceptible members of the population. After such an episode of initial infection further infections occur through a combination of person-to-person transmission within a community and wind-dependent transport of a virus-carrier (SARS-CoV-2 contaminated dust). It is the process of person-to-person infection that is being curtailed through the social distancing measures being taken, but subsequent deposits from the atmosphere remain possible as well as near-ground level transfers via incorporation in dust particles. We now set out to trace the global transport and deposition of virus-bearing micro-dust, whether as urban dust, agricultural dust or desert dust.

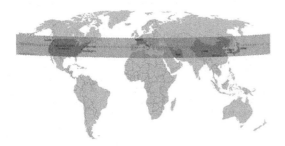

Figure 1. The 30-50N latitude band as the possible distribution of primary infall sites from an original source spread from China by the mid-latitude jet stream.

Transfer of Virus from one Ground Location to another

The idea of an infective agent – virus or bacterium – being transferred over long distances by meteorological processes is not new. Precisely this process was discussed at length by Fred Hoyle and one of the present authors (NCW) in their 1979 book Diseases from Space [5]. The same book considered the possibility that seasonal influenza and other respiratory viruses had a reservoir in the troposphere that was periodically released [5].

Discussions of long-range transfer of microscopic organisms through atmospheric processes can be traced back to the middle of the nineteenth century. Charles Darwin [6] long ago reported that dust landing on vessels far out in the Atlantic Ocean in the southern trade-wind zone carried microscopic biological matter. His diary quotation which is of historical interest is as follows:

"Many scattered accounts have appeared concerning the dust which has fallen in
considerable quantities on vessels on the African side of the Atlantic Ocean. It has appeared
to me desirable to collect these accounts, more especially since Professor Ehrenberg's

remarkable discovery that the dust consists in considerable part of Infusoria and
Phytolitharia. I have found fifteen distinct statements of dust having fallen; and several of
these refer to a period of more than one day, and some to a considerably longer time."

The transport of Saharan dust to the Amazon region carrying Darwin's organisms (single-cell protozoans, in the main) occurs episodically, February to April, with huge tonnages involved-in total of order 10 Mt/yr. From mid-summer, when the Saharan dust switches to land in the Caribbean and in Florida, it is linked to seasonal respiratory problems [7,8]. It is thought that micro-organisms within cracks and crevices in the dust grains are the main source of the respiratory irritations and asthma attacks.

More recently it is recognized that the dispersal of bacterial and viral pathogens via tropospheric winds is a real phenomenon. The studies of Reche et al. [4] showed bacteria and viruses land on the surface in the Sierra Nevada mountain range (at heights of ~ 3 km) in large numbers (~ 800 million/m^2/day). This flux was associated with winds from southern USA and winds from the Sahara on two separate days.

North-East China is recognised as the source of a fungal agent presumed to cause the Kawasaki disease and is carried in winds at 2-3 km altitude to reach Japan [9]. This unusual disease travels still further in winds across the Pacific Ocean to southern California at times that are seen to correlate with a phase of El Niño [10]. Intercontinental transport of bacteria and viruses associated with desert and agricultural dust by winds above 2 km altitude to the Sierra Nevada is also seen in Spanish studies [4].

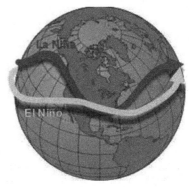

Figure 2. The Jet-stream from north China and Japan crosses the southern USA and over to Europe (source: NOAA).

Its route across the north Pacific varies with the ENSO (El Niño/La Niña) phase driven by periodic changes in the warm equatorial ocean current. This year's phase is not extreme; an El Niño Modoki (the yellow band), has been correlated with incidence of the Kawasaki disease in southern California. As the Kawasaki agent (perhaps a micro-fungus) makes this crossing, it is plausible that the SARS-CoV-2 virus carried on fine dust can similarly travel from NE China across the Pacific.

The ~10-wide jet-stream (Figure 2) varies in latitude and over days, with its mean location changing seasonally. Details of jet-stream linkage to lower altitude regional meteorology are little known,

Wickramasinghe NC, et al.   Virol Curr Res, Volume 4: 1, 2020

so we have to rely on plausibility arguments with clues derived from maps of the detailed low-altitude wind patterns. The East-Asian section of the Subtropical Westerly Jet Stream is more stable and has been modelled to fit satellite data [11]. We take its speed to be 180 km/hr (50 m/s) from the study of Huang and Liu "Simulation of the East Asian Subtropical Westerly Jet Stream" [11].

Corona-Virus Transport via Dust Pollutants

Corona viruses have a limited lifetime in the open air dependent on sunlight and humidity. Tests of virus particles emanating from a cough or sneeze have been simulated by aerosol deposition on wet-wiped surfaces, finding viruses are killed within minutes in sunlight. While aerial transmission of naked viruses could occur over short distances, it is when they are embedded in micron-sized dust particles that long-range transport can take place [8,12]. Bacteria too can arrive with the dust and this was found in transcontinental dust reaching the Sierra Nevada in Spain [4]. Analysis of dust trapped in filters of air-conditioning systems in north Italy shows the SARS-CoV-2 virus attached to urban dust particles. Martelletti and Martelletti [13] have reported the recovery of SARS-Cov-2 RNA in air filters in the north Italian city of Bergamo which was the centre of the major COVID-19 outbreak.

Survival on dust particles has also been known in the case of other single-stranded RNA viruses, including the virus causing Foot and Mouth Disease, as well as SARS-Cov-1 [14,15]. If the SARS-Cov-2 virus is likewise transported in viable form, the consequences for managing the current pandemic will be profoundly altered. A dust "vector" could well turn out to be a significant source of community spread of SARS-CoV-2, a process that has so far remained somewhat mysterious and difficult to track down. An investigation of this process will involve a systematic study of the lofting of dust by local winds and its modes of spread within the locality.

Data from Epidemiology

World Health Organization (WHO) reporting on 30 January initially showed 82 confirmed cases of COVID-19 in 18 countries outside of China. These cases were mostly in S-E Asia, the East and West Coasts of the US and some European centers.

Work by John Hopkins University's Corona Virus Resource Centre identified countries at risk from the virus by considering the large number of international flights originating from Wuhan before lockdown took effect in China. Their results suggested greater scatter than appeared in the actual distributions reported by the WHO, including a number of locations outside the 30-50N latitude band, such as the UK. It is possible that a large number of directly transmitted cases went undetected for a while and these were widely distributed over many areas.

Outside of China, the number of cases began to rise in several European countries, parts of the USA and Iran in late February and early March.

Figure 3 shows the statistics for states in the USA that were reporting to the WHO, most of which developed their epidemics after internal flights had been stopped. COVID-19 clearly took off just after the US declaration of National Emergency on 12 March. Washington state and New York already had ~100 new cases per day, but in most other states the numbers rose rather little till about 18 March. This is consistent with containment of their initial few cases, till a sudden external source from the troposphere doused them all on dramatically around 7 March for 2 or 3 days. With 5 days gestation [16] and diverse reporting times, that led to extra new cases from 14 March, with person-to-person transmission building up case numbers from 19 March onwards.

Date (March)	M13	M14	M15	M16	M17	M18	M19	M20	M21	M22	M23
New York	93	107	212	235	742	1342	2341	3052	1993	5440	5123
New Jersey	21	19	29	80	89	160	315	148	437	587	930
Massachusetts	15	15	26	33	21	38	72	85	112	121	131
California	45	57	67	132	150	141	161	198	184	364	378
Texas	16	13	16	12	25	87	87	110	79	125	208
Pennsylvania	19	0	19	13	33	43	52	96	88	88	165
Washington	126	74	127	135	108	175	189	148	269	203	225
Florida	15	26	39	45	57	111	89	146	96	348	220
Louisiana	17	41	25	34	64	80	112	145	48	252	335
Ohio	8	13	11	13	17	22	30	54	74	104	91

Figure 3. Daily Confirmed Cases in selected US States. Source: Worldometers [17].

Wickramasinghe NC, et al.   Virol Curr Res, Volume 4: 1, 2020

Massachusetts escaped, unlike adjacent New Jersey (and Pennsylvania), having its onset of new cases a few days later on 19 March (Figure 3). To the north, Canada (Figure 4) shows no event until 14 March. The southern states Texas and Florida show a stronger effect, consistent with the southerly location of the normal path of the jet-stream, while NE states show little impact. Like Texas and Florida, Mexico to the south shows growth around 14 March (Figure 4).

If an infectious cloud was carried in the jet-stream it might have doused the western states half a day earlier than the eastern states. In practice the cloud would be spread out along the jet-stream and its descent would be patchy, depending on large scale (km-depth) wind turnover. The half-day delay would not show up.

	Lat. °N	1st 10	F29	M1	M2	M3	M4	M5	M6	M7	M8	M9	M10	M11	M12	M13	M14	M15	M16	M17	M18	M19	M20	M21	M22	M23
Japan	36-45	J29	8	15	18	19	38	33	56	41	41	28	57	52	52	43	70	29	17	28	36	29	64	47	47	27
Germany	48-53	F2	5	51	35	38	59	283	125	130	240	184	341	401	779	930										
France	46	F8	43	30	61	21	73	138	230	296	260	203	372	497	595	785										
Iran	27-37	F21	305	385	523	825	586	591	1234	1076	743	595	881	958	1075	1289										
Italy	38-43	F22	239	573	335	466	587	769	778	1247	1492	1797	977	2313	2651	2547										
Spain	28-44	F26	25	26	36	45	63	54	119	124	149	557	464	582	869	2086										
UK	55	F23	3	13	3	12	36	29	48	47	69	43	62	77	130	208	342	251	152	407	676	643	714	1035	665	967
Canada	45	F24	5	4	3	3	4	3	17	6	6	11	18	15	32	56	54	89	100	157	129	146	214	241	142	621
Switz'land	47	F28	4	5	6	28	35	27	94	54	64	42	123	155	216	271	236	842	136	389	373	1107	1393	1248	611	1321
Austria	48	F29	3	4	4	6	5	14	23	15	23	27	51	64	115	143	151	205	158	314	314	533	470	343	590	892
Israel	31	M2	0	3	2	0	3	5	4	4	14	11	25	11	12	34	50	20	85	39	96	244	28	178	188	371
Nederland	52	M1	5	3	8	5	15	44	46	60	77	56	61	121	111	190	155	176	278	292	346	409	534	637	573	545
Belgium	51	M3		1	6	7	8	27	59	60	31	39	28	47	85	160	130	197	172	185	243	309	462	558	586	342
Denmark	56	M4	1	1	0	6	4	5	2	6	8	55	172	252	160	130	32	28	50	63	80	94	104	71	69	65
Portugal	39	M6				2	2	3	4	8	9	9	2	20	17	34	57	76	86	117	194	144	234	260	320	460
Egypt	22-31	M6		1					12	33	7	4	0	8	13	13	17	16	40	30	14	46	29	9	33	39
Russia	>42	M6			1	0	0	4	6	1	3	3	0	8	6	11	14	4	30	21	33	52	54	53	61	71
Romania	46	M7				1	2	0	3	4	2	2	12	18	12	36	28	16	29	49	43	17	31	59	66	143
Poland	50-54	M8						4	1	5	6	5	9	20	17	36	21	52	61	49	68	70	111	98	115	
Belarus	52-56	M11			3	2						3	0	12	6		0	0	9	0	15	0	18	7	0	5
Serbia	45	M11									1	3	13	6	11	11	2	9	15	17	14	32	36	51	27	
Mexico	18-30	M12	2	1	0	0	0	0	0	0	1	0	0	4	1	3	11	17	10	29	11	25	46	39	48	65
Afgh'stan	34	M14											2	0	0	4	5	5	1	1	0	2	0	16		
Turkey	41	M15												4	1	12	29	51	93	168	311	277	289	293		
Ukraine	48	M17											2	0	0	0	4	7	2	10	15	6	26	0		

Figure 4. Daily new cases. Countries included with over 10 000 cases at 28 May 2020 on [17] (excluding China and the USA) and within or close to the 30-50°N zone. The blank elements are where numbers were mounting quickly, not relevant here. F, M denote months February and March. Countries are roughly ordered according to the date he cumulative number of confirmed cases reached 10 (Col.3) [18].

In Europe, the steep raises in cumulative cases due to person-to-person contact spreading makes it hard to discern any additional increases in central European countries.

In central Europe, by late February the epidemic was well underway, 10 or more cumulative cases being observed in various countries (Figure 4, Col.3), likely to have been caused by person-to-person infections seeded by individuals who had travelled previously from infected areas. Figure 4 includes data for the 30 European and near Asian countries in or near the 30-50°N zone where the disease in early March had barely started, but exceeded 10,000 cumulative cases by the end of May. In Portugal, Israel, Egypt and Romania the numbers of new cases show a spurt about 14 March, whereas Turkey's case-numbers rose on 15 March. The onset there is similar to Mexico, lagging by a day, consistent with the delay of a day while the jet-stream crossed the Atlantic. Differing speed in reporting cases in these countries may underlie the difference of a couple of days. The onward track of the jet-stream across to E Asia is apparent in the Ukraine, possibly Afghanistan (statistics incomplete). Egypt and Israel lie on the 30°N margin, suggesting the jet-stream was aligned with the Mediterranean ocean. On the northern boundary of the zone Poland showed a not dissimilar rise, but not Belarus. Thus Figure 4's pattern of shaded-in countries does suggest effects from jet-stream deposition, but requires further study. Since person-to-person infection rates rise more in towns, while wind-borne dust infection impacts uniformly, geographically detailed studies could potentially distinguish the two.

Deviation from the Jet-Stream Belt

From the third week of March 2020 there was one country conspicuously located outside the 30-50N belt-Brazils. Brazil's case tally actually out-numbered some countries in 30-50N by the second week of April 2020.

Consider the statistics of new cases in Brazil (Figure 5) which show a similar pattern to the USA, with several days of sporadic new cases followed by rapid take-off. In Brazil's case, the pattern and surge (~31 March) lags still further behind Texas-Mexico-Florida and Portugal-Turkey.

Wickramasinghe NC, et al.   Virol Curr Res, Volume 4: 1, 2020

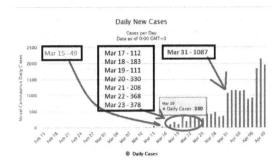

Figure 5. Daily new cases in Brazil [1].

To explain the case of Brazil, we envisage part of the jet stream being entrained in the Trade Winds where they turn south off Portugal in the north Atlantic circulation. Around the 7th March (Figure 6) there was a strong cyclonic circulation between the Azores and Portugal. It takes approximately 7-9 days from SARS-CoV-2 virus arrival to registration of a case [16], plus 13-15 days for it to cross from Portugal (8000 km at 30 km/hr, but slower and erratic over the land mass than over ocean).

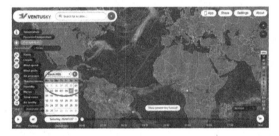

Figure 6. Wind pattern in Atlantic and South America on 7 March 2020 [20].

Figure 6 shows winds moving towards Brazil from the strong anticyclone near Portugal which lasted several days. We suggest this is how COVID-19 arrived so dramatically in Brazil. There was no effect in neighboring countries, Suriname and Guyana to the north, Uruguay and Argentina to the south, the latter two being in a different wind system.

The Trade Winds circulating in the North Atlantic have long been relied on by transatlantic sailors for both W-E and E-W crossing of the ocean. The southerly winds start from the Portuguese coast where the westerlies divide and cast off large-scale eddies and continue down the Saharan coast. They entrain Saharan dust, as was known to fall on southbound ships long before Charles Darwin's record above. Once entrained in the southerly Trade Winds, large tonnages of this dust reach northern Brazil in (northern) spring-time, when the winds tend to dissipate over the continent, some joining the anti-clockwise South Atlantic wind system down the Brazilian coast. We envisage that part of the higher-level jet stream over Portugal became entrained in these Trade Winds that carried the virus onwards to Brazil.

It is noteworthy that East-Asian countries near China have not been badly hit by the COVID-19 pandemic, South Korea successfully suppressing an outbreak of 20 February. The data reported on the website show that Italy had an isolated case on 31 January, but not

till 21 February did case numbers start to rise dramatically. Spain and France also had cases rising steeply from mid-February, likewise Iran, but not Afghanistan, Ukraine, Turkey and Greece (first cases only mid-March). West-coast USA had a first death 29 February and all US states had cases by mid-March. Brazil had its first case late (Sao Paulo, 26 February.) with person-to-person infection evidently starting up only from 11 March (Figure 5). While the first spreaders of the disease are expected to have been individuals from China or groups of Chinese travellers, the disease did not take off significantly in nearby countries, but did so strikingly in countries in the 30-50N belt. If carried by the mid-latitude jet-stream circling the globe in 4-5 days several kilometers high, the deposition will be patchy as it depends on entrainment of the jet stream in lower altitude weather systems. An infective dust cloud deposited/lofted above Wuhan in early February could drop the virus on Washington state, New York and N. Italy, France around 10 February. A second infective cloud may well have dropped virus-laden dust a month later around 7th March on the southern USA and Mexico as well as Portugal, Turkey, Ukraine etc. Part of this cloud was also entrained in the southerly Trade winds off the Portuguese coast, to be carried to Brazil (travel time around 14 days).

The SARS-CoV-2 virus was doubtless abundant in the urban and countryside environment around Wuhan in February-March. When the jet stream was positioned overhead and local winds favorable, virions attached to dust particles – as was the agent for the Kawasaki disease (section 3) – could even have been picked up from near ground level and transported around the globe. The lifetime within the surface of dust particles is presumed to be much longer than found in studies on metal or manufactured surfaces, so it would persist in infective state many times longer in the environment.

Conclusion

Previous studies have shown that long-distance intercontinental winds do indeed transport microorganisms around the globe, as free organisms or attached to dust particles. We hypothesize that dust plus virus transport on global winds could be an important element in the dynamics of the COVID-19 pandemic. This fits the patterns of global incidence, if we make the further assumption that the jet-stream is caught up in the stable trade wind system off Portugal, and then transported to northern South America and down the Brazilian coast. Differing densities of population in between and within countries naturally play a crucial role in determining the epidemiology but also the widely varying levels of airborne dust blown from areas where the epidemic has taken hold.

References

1. Wickramasinghe, NC, Steele EJ, Gorczynski RM and Temple R et al. "Predicting the Future Trajectory of COVID-19." Virol Curr Res (2020) 4:1.

2. Wickramasinghe, NC, Steele EJ, Gorczynski RM and Temple R et al. "Comments on the Origin and Spread of the 2019 Coronavirus." Virol Curr Res (2020) 4:1.

3. Wickramasinghe NC, Steele EJ, Gorczynski RM and Temple R et al. "Growing Evidence against Global Infection-Driven by Person-to-Person Transfer of COVID-19." Virol Curr Res (2020) 4:1.

4. Reche, I, D'Orta G Mladenov N, Winget DM and Suttle CA. "Deposition rates of viruses and bacteria above the atmospheric boundary layer." International Society for Microbial Ecology (2018) 42:4.

Wickramasinghe NC, et al.   Virol Curr Res, Volume 4: 1, 2020

5.   Hoyle, F and Wickramasinghe NC, " Diseases from Space." J M Dent London (1979).

6.   Darwin, C. "An account of the fine dust which often falls on vessels in the Atlantic Ocean." Q J Geol Soc London (1846) 2: 26–30.

7.   Griffin, DW, Garrison VH, Herman JR and Shinn EA. "African Desert Dust in the Caribbean Atmosphere: Microbiology and Public Health." Aerobiologia (2001) 17: 203–213.

8.   Griffin, DW. "Atmospheric Movement of microorganisms in clouds of desert dust and implications for human health." Clin Microbiol Rev (2007)20: 3.

9.   Rodo, X, Curcoll R, Robinson M et al. "Tropospheric winds from north eastern China carry the etiologic agent of Kawasaki disease from its source to Japan." PNAS (2014): 7952-7957.

10.   Ballesester, J, Burns, J., Cayan, D., et al. 2013. "Kawasaki disease and ENSO-driven wind circulation". Geophys. Res. Lett. 40(10):2284–2289.

11.   Huang, G. and Liu Y 2011."Simulation of the East Asian Subtropical Westerly Jet Stream with GFDL AGCM (AM2.1)" Atmos Ocean Sci Lett (2011) 4: 24-29.

12.   Martelletti, L and Martelletti P. 2020 "Air Pollution and the Novel Covid-19 Disease: a Putative Disease Risk Factor". SN Compr. Clin. Med. 2020 Apr 15 : 1–5.

13.   . Frazer, J. "Blowing in the wind." Nature (2012) 484: 21.

14.   Donaldson, AI and Alexandersen S. "Predicting the spread of foot and mouth disease by airborne virus." Rev Sc Tech Off int Epiz (2002) 21: 3.

15.   Chen, PS, Tsai, FT, Lin CK and Yang CY et al. "Ambient Influenza and Avian Influenza Virus during Dust Storm Days and Background Days." Environ. Health Perspect (2010)118: 9.

16.   Huang, C, Wang, Y and Xingwang L et al. "Clinical features of patients infected with 2019 novel coronavirus in Wuhan, China" Lancet (2020) 395: 497-506.

17.   Worldometers, coronavirus data by country, COVID-19 Pandemic.

18.   World Health Organization "Explore the data" May 31 2020.

19.   Worldometers, coronavirus data for Brazil, COVID-19 Pandemic.

20.   Ventusky map of global winds, marked by Alexander Kondakov.

How to cite this article: N Chandra Wickramasinghe, Max K. Wallis, Stephen G. Coulson and Alexander Kondakov et al. "Intercontinental Spread of COVID-19 on Global Wind Systems". *Virol Curr Res* 4 (2020) doi:10.37421/ Virol Curr Res.2020.4.113

SECTION 4

Strikes on Ships at Sea and Related Remote Regions

Short Communication Open Access

Mid-Ocean Outbreaks of COVID-19 with Tell-Tale Signs of Aerial Incidence

George A. Howard[1], N.Chandra Wickramasinghe[2,3,4,5*], Herbert Rebhan[6], Edward J. Steele[4,6], Reginald M. Gorczynski[7], Robert Temple[8], Gensuke Tokoro[3], Brig Klyce[9], Predrag Slijepcevic[10], Max K. Wallis[3] and Stephen J. Coulson[3]

[1]Restoration Systems, LLC, Raleigh, NC, USA

[2]Buckingham Centre for Astrobiology, University of Buckingham, UK

[3]Institute for the Study of Panspermia and Astroeconomics, Gifu, Japan

[4]Centre for Astrobiology, University of Ruhuna, Matara, Sri Lanka

[5]National Institute of Fundamental Studies, Kandy, Sri Lanka

[6]C. Y. O'Connor, ERADE Village, Foundation, Piara Waters, Perth 6112 WA, Australia

[7]University Toronto Health Network, Toronto General Hospital, University of Toronto, Toronto, ON M5S, Canada

[8]History of Chinese Science and Culture Foundation Conway Hall, London, UK

[9]Astrobiology Research Trust, Memphis, TN, USA

[10]School of Health Sciences, Brunel University, London, UK

Abstract

Outbreaks of COVID-19 in passengers and crew in ships at sea continue to pose a problem for conventional epidemiology. In one instance the crew of an Argentinian fishing trawler, who were quarantined and tested negative before sailing, contracted the disease after 35 days at sea. In another instance a livestock ship had crew that was isolated and confined becoming sick with presumed COVID-19 whilst sailing in mid-ocean.

Keywords: Pathogen • Virus • Bacterium • Airborne

Introduction

The conventional belief in epidemiology is that epidemics start and end with animals and humans on Earth, and that transmission occurs only by one infected individual transferring the infective pathogen – virus or bacterium – to another person. Airborne transfers are admitted to take place but these instances are universally believed to have a human or animal as an immediate aerosol source. These assumptions have been challenged for 40 years but the idea of a primary significant non-human or non-animal reservoir has been difficult for orthodox science to embrace.

Hoyle and Wickramasinghe's 1979 provocative classic "Diseases from Space" cited many examples of pandemics where person-to-person infection as the sole mode of origin and spread was shown difficult to defend [1,2]. The sudden onset of a pandemic, the speed and patchiness of its spread, and sudden termination were factors that were satisfactorily interpreted by atmospheric transfers of a viral or bacterial pathogen. The 1979 analysis documented the distribution of influenza in the 1977 H1N1 pandemic in boarding houses in schools in England and Wales; and the study of earlier epidemics as were reported in medical as well as media sources were also discussed [1]. An atmospheric mode of transport and transfer of the influenza virus was clearly described as the most parsimonious and arguably the only suitable interpretation of all the facts. In the 1918/1919 influenza pandemic the incidence was found to be both temporally and geographically patchy, strongly suggesting an atmospheric reservoir, albeit a transient one. For instance, communities in the most remote Alaskan regions succumbed to the virus -- as did ships at sea. Passenger liners arriving in Australia following weeks sailing in the high seas recorded attack rates that varied between four and forty-three percent.

Discussion of COVID-19

In the case of the current COVID-19 pandemic we have argued the case for an initial introduction of the virus from a non-terrestrial reservoir into the troposphere/stratosphere, and subsequent windborne spread and re-distribution across the globe [3-6]. Although

*Corresponding author: Dr N Chandra Wickramasinghe, Buckingham Centre for Astrobiology, University of Buckingham MK18 1EG, England, UK, Tel: +44 (0)2920752146/+44 (0)7778389243; E-mail: ncwick@gmail.com

Received: July 21, 2020; Accepted: August 05, 2020; Published: August 13, 2020

DOI: 10.37421/vcrh.2020.4.114

https://www.hilarispublisher.com/open-access/midocean-outbreaks-of-covid19-with-telltale-signs-of-aerial-incidence-47220.html

Wickramasinghe NC, et al.   Virol Curr Res, Volume 4: 2, 2020

spread in local areas was certainly the result of person-to-person transmission, large-scale initial deposition and distribution of the virus across the globe was postulated to occur mainly through the entrainment of micro-dust particles with embedded viruses in a circum-global jet-stream [5]. The arrival of the pandemic in Brazil and South America is explained in this way - the deposition from the mid-latitude jet stream over Portugal in early March, followed by transport *via* winds across the Atlantic [6].

In this context it should be recalled that recent counts of ambient viruses in the oceans as well as in the atmosphere is truly mind boggling [7,8]. Some 10 million virions are present in a single drop of surface ocean water and approximately 800 million are documented to settle on each square meter of terrestrial earth each day [8]. If this virus population included a recent fall of novel viruses such as COVID-19, then sea spray in mid ocean may be expected to be an anticipated route of infection for seagoing vessels.

Ships at Sea

There are currently several reports of COVID-19 outbreaks on ships at sea and most of these are rather poorly or incompletely explained by invoking contaminated materials/provisions that had been delivered to the ships.

One striking example is the livestock ship Al Kuwait that docked in Fremantle harbor on May 22, 2020, with 21 of its 48 crews testing positive for COVID-19. One of us (Herbert Rebhan, HR) who was the Veterinary surgeon on board, found nearly all of the ill crew members had displayed symptoms of a viral/bacterial infection (sore throat and sinusitis) whilst at sea. No ill crew member had complained of any problems with breathing or any other COVID indicative symptoms. HR did not expect a viral agent to be at work as all or crew who were ill improved 48 hours after starting antibiotic medication, with most being deemed fit for duty 96 hours after the start of antibiotics. HR was as surprised as anyone else when these crew members tested positive for COVID upon reaching Freemantle, as the crew had no outside contact since early March. The source of the infection and or the infecting agent still remains a mystery.

Although it is possible the virus could have entered the ship on supplies obtained from shore, the explanation of exposure whilst sailing through a "viral cloud" or several such clouds is more plausible in our view for several reasons. One is that the crew members who tested positive -- all fell ill within 48 hours of one another – a clear indication of near simultaneous exposure. There was no evidence of person-to-person transmission. The second is the well attested nature of the virus itself. Studies have shown that when this virus is exposed to environmental temperatures greater than 30 degrees C, viral viability is greatly reduced. The supplies taken aboard the Al Kuwait were exposed for many hours to environmental temperatures much greater than 30 degrees C. We find it hard to accept that the goods would have been contaminated with a great enough viral load to infect four people at the same time. Indeed, the crew members who tested positive for COVID were all deck workers and would not have any contact with the goods (provisions) brought

on the ship. The chef and galley help who did handle the goods brought onto the ship, and would have had maximum exposure to any viral contaminated supplies, all subsequently tested negative for COVID.

An equally strong case or even stronger case of direct incidence in mid-ocean has been reported for Argentinian fishing trawler Echizen Maru on which 57 sailors came down with the coronavirus after 35 days of isolation at sea. The reports of this event provide, in our view, a real-life proxy for a controlled clinical experiment of direct atmospheric transmission. The bare facts are as follows: The entire crew of the trawler was quarantined for two weeks in Ushuaia and tested negative before sailing. After 35 days at sea the trawler returned to port when 57 out of 61 crew members were diagnosed as infected with the virus.

Conclusion

All existing understanding concerning the incubation of COVID-19 is challenged by the length of the time between the initial negative test and symptoms appearing for the crew of the Echizen Maru. However, when examined against the predictions of the Hoyle-Wickramasinghe theory of over four decades ago they are entirely understandable. The incidents on both Al Kuwait and Echizen Maru could arguably be regarded as compelling a confirmation of atmospheric transport/survival of the virus that we might hope to get without a deliberately controlled investigation.

References

1. Hoyle, Fred and Wickramasinghe, NC. "Diseases from Space. J.M. Dent Ltd." London (1979).

2. Wickramasinghe, NC. "Diseases from Outer Space, World Scientific Publishing". Singapore (2020).

3. Wickramasinghe, NC, Steele EJ, Gorczynski RM and Temple R et al. "Comments on the origin and spread of the 2019 Coronavirus". Virology: Current Research 4(2020):1.

4. Wickramasinghe, NC, Steele EJ, Gorczynski, R. M and Temple, R. et al. "Growing evidence against global infection-driven by person-to-person transfer of COVID-19". Virology: Current Research 4(2020):1.

5. Wickramasinghe, NC, Steele EJ, Gorczynski RM and Temple R et al. "Predicting the future trajectory of COVID-19". Virology: Current Research 4(2020):1.

6. Wickramasinghe NC, Wallis MK, Coulson SG and Kondakov A et al. "Intercontinental spread of COVID-19 on global wind systems Virology" 4 (2020):1.

7. Gregory AC, Zayed AA and Conceic Na´ dia. "Marine DNA viral macro- and microdiversity from Pole to Pole Cell". 177(2019): 1109–1123.

8. Reche, Orta and Mladenov GN. "Deposition rates of viruses and bacteria above the atmospheric boundary layer". The ISME Journal(2018).

How to cite this article: George, A Howard, Wickramasinghe NC, Herbert Rebhan and Edward J. Steele et al.. "Mid-Ocean Outbreaks of COVID-19 with Tell-Tale Signs of Aevial Incidence". *Virol Curr Res* 4 (2020) : 114.

Review Article   Open Access

Seasonality of Respiratory Viruses Including SARS-CoV-2

N. Chandra Wickramasinghe [1,2,3,4*], Edward J. Steele [3,5,6], Ananda Nimalasuriya [7], Reginald M. Gorczynski [8], Gensuke Tokoro [2], Robert Temple [9] and Milton Wainwright [2,3]

[1]Buckingham Centre for Astrobiology, University of Buckingham, Buckingham MK18 1EG, United Kingdom

[2]Institute for the Study of Panspermia and Astroeconomics, Gifu, Japan

[3]Centre for Astrobiology, University of Ruhuna, Matara, Sri Lanka

[4]National Institute of Fundamental Studies, Kandy, Sri Lanka

[5]C. Y. O'Connor, ERADE Village, Foundation, Piara Waters, Perth 6112 WA, Australia

[6]Melville Analytics Pty Ltd , Melbourne, VIC 3000 Australia

[7]Kaiser Permanente Riverside Medical, 10800 Magnolia Ave # 1, Riverside, CA 92505, USA

[8]University Toronto Health Network, Toronto General Hospital, University of Toronto, Toronto, ON, Canada

[9]History of Chinese Science and Culture Foundation Conway Hall, London, UK

[10]Department of Molecular Biology and Biotechnology, University of Sheffield, Sheffield, UK

Abstract

We propose that a reservoir of respiratory viruses in clumps of micro-sized dust exists in tropospheric clouds from which virions can be seasonally released into the lower atmosphere and thence to ground level. Respiratory Syncytial Virus (RSV), Seasonal Influenza and Human Para Influenza Virus (HPIV) are all diseases that fall in this category, including SARS-CoV-2. The seasonal incidence of disease at ground level would appear to be patchy over distance scales that are largely dictated by viral-laden dust cloud size modulated by scales of atmospheric turbulence. This could produce clustering of cases in space and time that has given rise to 'contagion' concepts of community spread and of superspreaders.

Keywords: Seasonal respiratory viruses • Troposphere • COVID-19

Introduction

The presence of microorganisms in the troposphere (8-10 km), their role in the nucleation of ice crystals as well as the seeding of rain clouds has been known for many years [1]. However, the role they play in atmospheric physics and biological processes, more generally, still remains poorly understood. Recent studies by Rodriguez et al. [2] have shown that this region of the troposphere actually constitutes a substantial microbiome with a large fraction of micrometre-sized aerosols that are actually associated with bacteria. More recently Smith et al. [3] have reported the existence of a more or less homogeneous distribution of bacteria extending into the stratosphere up to 12 km so defining what can be described as an extended terrestrial biosphere. It is evident that a largely unknown and diverse microbial habitat including bacteria and viruses (possibly embedded in electrically charged clumps of dust) is present in the upper tropospheric clouds. This microbial ecology would inevitably have a continuing connection and interchange with regions of the atmosphere both above in the stratosphere and below through the troposphere closer to the surface. This connection would involve the periodic recycling of viruses between the tropospheric reservoir and the biosphere at ground level.

The most recent study by Reche et al. [4] does in fact show such a connection and implies a steady deposition and/or re-deposition of viruses numbering~10^9 m^{-2} day^{-1}. However, the work of Reche et al. [4] quantified the virus deposition using a previously used FACS algorithm [5] and not by direct analysis of infection. There are other independent studies [6] that show viruses being involved in atmospheric recycling that can remain viable and infective after long-range atmospheric transport and circulation. Against this backdrop the emergence from time to time of disease-causing viruses in the human population should occasion no surprise.

Seasonal Deposition of Atmospheric Viruses

It has been known for some time that many respiratory viruses have a distinctly seasonal pattern of incidence. These include RSV (Respiratory Syncytial Virus), seasonal influenza and HPIV (Human Para Influenza Virus), as well as a number of common cold viruses. The reason for their predominance in the winter seasons in both northern and southern temperate latitudes has remained a mystery from the time of the earliest discussions by Sir Andrewes C [7]. The current status of this dilemma is summarised in a recent paper by Price et al. [8]. Although social and behavioural causes, such as people tending to stay indoors in winter have been discussed, there is no compelling case for such causal associations. On the other hand, physical environmental factors such as ambient temperature, humidity and the flux of ultraviolet radiation that vary through the seasonal cycle have shown promising signs of a correlation. This is illustrated in the humidity-

Corresponding Author: *Dr. N Chandra Wickramasinghe, Buckingham Centre for Astrobiology, University of Buckingham MK181EG, England, UK, Tel: +44(0)2920752146/+44 (0)7778389243; E-mail: ncwick@gmail.com*

Copyright: *© 2020 Wickramasinghe NC, et al. This is an open-access article distributed under the terms of the creative commons attribution license which permits unrestricted use, distribution and reproduction in any medium, provided the original author and source are credited.*

Received: October 13, 2020; **Accepted:** November 06, 2020 ; **Published:** November 13, 2020

DOI: 10.37421/vcrh.2020.4.117

https://www.hilarispublisher.com/open-access/seasonality-of-respiratory-viruses-including-sarscov2-51923.html

Wickramasinghe NC, et al.   Virol Curr Res, Volume 4: 2, 2020

HPIV-3 virus correlation given by Price et al. [8], but decisive proof of a causal connection with any environmental factor has been much harder to establish (Figure 1).

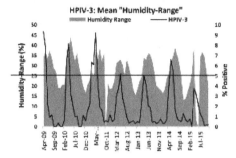

Figure 1. The seasonality of HPIV incidence compared with percent humidity (from Price et al. [8].

However, what happens during the winter months in both the northern and southern hemispheres, 6 months apart, is the phenomenon of large-scale atmospheric recycling and turbulence leading to mixing through different layers in the atmosphere. This is in remarkable correspondence with the worldwide seasonality of non-pandemic influenza as seen in the data collated in 1977 by Hoyle and Wickramasinghe [9] for two northern and southern latitude countries, as well as for an island in the tropics (Sri Lanka) where no distinct seasonality is seen Figure 2.

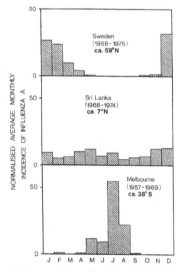

Figure 2. Normalised average influenza incidence showing seasonality – Sweden, Sri Lanka, Melbourne (from Hoyle and Wickramasinghe, Diseases from Space [7]).

Reche et al. [1] report that the viruses reaching the peaks of the Sierra Nevada mountain range were associated with organic aerosols of sizes less than <0.7 μm. In the case of respiratory viruses the aerosols could well have been contained in virus/cell aggregates. Within such aggregates it is possible that viruses may have remained viable in the upper tropospheric clouds over several months. In this way a circulation of viable virus of the type Ground <=>Troposphere [1] might be imagined, and the seasonality of certain respiratory viral diseases could thus be explained.

Evidence of seasonal deposition of micron-sized dust from the stratosphere

The evidence for the existence of a transient biosphere, capable of harbouring bacteria and viruses that extends even into stratospheric clouds,

can be linked to early studies by Kalkstein [10]. In the last of a series of atmospheric nuclear bomb tests on August 11, 1958 a radioactive tracer, Rh-102 was introduced into the stratosphere at a height above 50 km and the incidence of the tracer was measured annually thereafter by means of airplane flights at altitudes ~10 km. It was discovered that the tracer took nearly a decade to clear itself through repeated seasonal downdrafts as seen in Figure 3. Noting that the ordinate scale in Figure 3 is logarithmic, we find that the fall-out of Rh-102 is very much greater in temperate latitudes than elsewhere, with the period January to March showing up as the dominant months. The notion that a similar incidence would be seen in southern temperate latitudes with an expected 6-month time lag was unfortunately not investigated by Kalkstein [10].

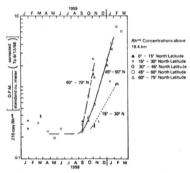

Figure 3. The fall out of Rh-102 at various latitude intervals from the HARDTACK atmospheric nuclear bomb that was exploded on 11 August 1958.

Since a large fraction of the viruses discovered by Reche et al. [1] At 3 km altitude was thought to be associated with wind-borne dust, the question arises as to whether during the COVID-19 pandemic a substantial population of suitably protected SARS-CoV-2 virions would have been lofted into the tropospheric reservoir. Tropospheric clouds may thus be regarded as a transitional inter-seasonal reservoir from which further depositions may occur in a seasonal cycle. This circuit requires a significant degree of survival of viruses in the stratosphere for ~6 months, and such survival within cryogenically preserved electrically charged dust clumps appears plausible. If this is indeed the manner by which seasonal influenza, the RSV and common cold viruses maintain their seasonal character it is not surprising to find SARS-CoV-2 behaving in a similar manner. The second wave of the COVID-19 pandemic can thus be understood in these terms with primary incidence at ground level displaying patchiness over scales of turbulence ranging from hundreds of kilometers to tens of meters. This is schematically illustrated in Figure 4, the shaded patches representing the scale of turbulence defining incidence at the ground.

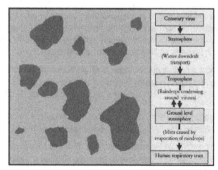

Figure 4. Schematic distribution of patches containing infective dust at ground level, and flow chart of presumed route from the atmosphere. The up-down arrows define the cycle leading to a transient tropospheric biosphere.

Wickramasinghe NC, et al.

Virol Curr Res, Volume 4: 2, 2020

Patchiness of incidence over diverse distance scales

This is the pattern of incidence that was seen in many of the pandemics and epidemics of influenza that were studied by Hoyle and Wickramasinghe [9] in the book *Diseases from Space*. One crucial study related to the H1N1 (Red Flu) pandemic of 1976. This subtype of influenza was not in circulation for over 20 years, so its re-emergence as a pandemic strain gave Hoyle and one of us (Wickramasinghe) an opportunity to consider school children with "virgin" immunities as detectors of the virus. This study revealed a pattern of exceedingly variable attack rates in schools across England and Wales showing a patchiness of incidence over distance scales ranging from tens of kilometres to hundreds of metres. At the time of the epidemic at Eton College (a famous English boarding school near Windsor) there were 1248 pupils residing in 25 houses. The total number of influenza cases at this school was 441 giving an average attack rate 35%. The disparities of attack rates from house to house were striking. College House which had a total of 70 pupils had only 1 case, whereas another house with a population of 51 pupils had 46 cases with the scale of separation between houses being typically hundreds of metres. The fluctuations from the mean attack rate in units of the sample standard deviation are shown in Figure 5.

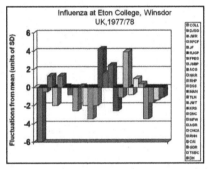

Figure 5. Fluctuation in attack rates from house to house, in terms of a sample standard deviation.

The probability of this distribution arising from a person-to-person infective process was estimated as 1 in 10^{10} (Hoyle and Wickramasinghe, [9]). Simultaneity of onset as displayed in the schematic patchiness in Figure 4, combined with the statistics of the type laid out in Figure 5 would give rise to a concept of a "superspreader" starting off each outbreak within a "patch", particularly evident in the school houses at Eton with attack rates that are 4 standard deviations above the mean.

Whereas an approximate simultaneity of initial outbreak within each patch (Figure 4) is to be expected by virtue of the cloud fragmentation/in fall process that we have considered, person-to-person spread would then take over as a secondary process of transmission that has the possibility of limitation through human interventions. Strong evidence for such a model of patchy incidence is to be found in the many instances of outbreaks of COVID-19 reported in ships at sea as documented in Howard et al. [11] (And reviewed further in detail in Steele et al. [12] and Supplementary File showing further recent evidence for patchy incidence COVID-19 outbreaks). While in some cases a shore connection of a primary infected source/ individual have been identified, very many cases still remain unexplained. These constitute examples akin to the cases of the two Eton school houses where the attack rate is 4 sample standard deviations above the mean. For our more detailed analysis of the COVID-19 pandemic based on a primary atmospheric infall followed by secondary person to person infection we refer the reader to our recent earlier publications [13-17]. In a forthcoming paper we shall discuss the largest scales of patchiness of incidence of COVID-19, across continents and specifically within Australia and individual states in the USA, that can at least partly be explained by the largest scales of patchiness such as displayed in Figure 4.

Clearly the new very large and localised cluster displayed in the data of Figure 6 can only be consistent with a patchiness of incidence in an infall process such as we have discussed. Unsurprisingly the authorities have been unable to identify the source of the outbreak, nor indeed a superspreader to account for this event.

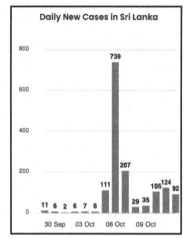

Figure 6. The Sri Lanka Health Department Covid 19 Live situational analysis dashboard of October 2020 give the data displayed above.

Conclusion

Turning to smaller scales of patchiness, we draw attention to breaking news of a new large cluster of COVID-19 that was reported recently in Sri Lanka. More than 1,000 workers out of a total 1700 in a garment factory in the island have tested positive for COVID-19 within a two-day period in October this year. Until this episode there had been no recently reported incidents of "community spread" (infective infall in our view) in Sri Lanka. The COVID 19 that was present was confined to only a few cases directly traceable to workers returning to the island from foreign countries.

References

1. Bigg, EK. "Particles in the upper atmosphere, in *Fundamental Studies and the Future of Science*." *University College Cardiff Press Cardiff* (1984).

2. Rodriguez, De Leon Natasha, Lathem Terry L, Rodriguez-R and Rodriguez R Luis M et al. "Microbiome of the Upper Troposphere: Species Composition and Prevalence, Effects of Tropical Storms, and Atmospheric Implications". *Proc Natl Acad Sci USA* (2013) 110: 2575–2580.

3. Smith, David J, Ravichandar Jayamary Divya, Jain Sunit and Griffin Dale W et al. "Airborne Bacteria in Earth's Lower Stratosphere Resemble Taxa Detected in the Troposphere: Results From a New NASA Aircraft Bioaerosol Collector (ABC)." *Front Microbiol* (2018) 9: 1752.

4. Reche, Isabel, D'Orta Gaetano, Mladenov Natalie and Winget Danielle M et al. "Deposition Rates of Viruses and Bacteria above the Atmospheric Boundary Layer." *The ISME Journal* (2018).

5. Brussaard, PD. "Optimization of Procedures for Counting Viruses by Flow Cytometry." *Appl Environ Microbiol* (2004) 70:1506–13

6. Sharoni, Shlomit, Trainic Miri, Schatz Daniella and Yoav Lehahn et al. "Infection of Phytoplankton by Aerosolized Marine Viruses." *Proc Natl Acad Sci USA* (2015)112:6643–6647.

7. Andrewes, C. "*The Common Cold. Weidenfeld & Nicolson*." (1965).

8. Macgregor Price, Rory Henry, Graham, Catriona and Sandeep Ramalingam. "Association between Viral Seasonality and Meteorological Factors." *Nature Research Journals* (2019) 9:929.

9. Hoyle, F, Wickramasinghe NC, Dent JM and Son Lond " (1977).

Wickramasinghe NC, et al.

Virol Curr Res, Volume 4: 2, 2020

10. Kalkstein, MI. "Rhodiem-102 high altitude tracer experiment." *Science* (1962) 137, 645.

11. Howard, George A, Wickramasinghe N Chandra, Rebhan Herbert and Steele Edward J et al. "Mid-Ocean Outbreaks of COVID-19 with Tell-Tale Signs of Aerial Incidence." *Virol Curr Res* (2020) 4:1.

12. Steele, Edward J, Reginald Gorczynski, Rebhan Herbert and Carnegie Patrick. "Implications of Haplotype Switching for the Origin and Global Spread of COVID 19." *Virol Curr Res* (2020) 4:2.

13. Steele, Edward J, Qu Jiangwen, Gorczynski Reginald M and Lindley Robyn A et al. "Origin of New Emergent Coronavirus and Candida Fungal Diseases—Terrestrial or Cosmic?" *Cosmic Genetic Evolution Adv Genet* (2020) 106.

14. Wickramasinghe, N Chandra, Steele Edward J, Gorczynski Reginald RM and Temple Robert et al. "Comments on the Origin and Spread of the 2019 Coronavirus." *Virol Curr Res* (2020)4:1.

15. Wickramasinghe, N Chandra, Steele Edward J, Gorczynski Reginald RM and Temple Robert et al. "Growing Evidence against Global Infection-Driven by Person-to-Person Transfer of COVID-19." *Virol Curr Res* (2020)4:1.

16. Wickramasinghe, N Chandra, Steele Edward J, Gorczynski Reginald RM and Temple Robert et al. "Predicting the Future Trajectory of COVID-19." *Virol Curr Res* (2020)4:1.

17. Wickramasinghe, N Chandra, Wallis Max K, Coulson Stephen G and Kondakov Alexander et al. "Intercontinental Spread of COVID-19 on Global Wind Systems." *Virol Curr Res* (2020)4:1.

How to cite this article: Wickramasinghe N Chandra, Steele Edward J, Nimalasuriya Ananda and Gorczynski Reginald M et al. "Seasonality OF Respiratory Viruses Including SARS-CoV-2. "*Virol Curr Res* 4 (2020): 117.

SECTION 5

The Adaptive Genetics of the Virus in First Half of 2020

Analysis of APOBEC and ADAR Deaminase-driven Riboswitch Haplotypes in COVID-19 RNA Strain Variants and the Implications for Vaccine Design

Edward J. Steele[1,2] and Robyn A. Lindley[2,3,4]

[1]CYO'Connor ERADE Village Foundation, 24 Genomics Rise, Piara Waters, 6112
[2]Melville Analytics Pty Ltd, Melbourne, Vic, AUSTRALIA
[3]GMDxCo Pty Ltd, Melbourne, Victoria, AUSTRALIA
[4]Department of Clinical Pathology, The Victorian Comprehensive Cancer Centre, Faculty of Medicine, Dentistry & Health Sciences, University of Melbourne, Victoria, AUSTRALIA

Correspondence: A/Professor Edward J. Steele, Melville Analytics Pty Ltd, 29 Scott St, Woods Point, Upper Yarra Ranges, 3723, Victoria, AUSTRALIA
email: e.j.steele@bigpond.com

Keywords: COVID-19 genomes; Coronavirus pandemic; Single Nucleotide Variations; Cytosine and Adenosine Deaminations; AID/APOBEC and ADAR Deamination Motifs

Author Information:
Edward J. Steele e.j.steele@bigpond.com
Robyn A. Lindley robyn.lindley@gmdxgroup.com

Abbreviations

ADAR, Adenosine Deaminase that act on RNA, two main isoforms, ADAR 1, ADAR 2 mediating adenosine-to-inosine **A-to-I**) mutation predominantly seen in RNA editing in Innate Immunity to viruses; **APOBEC family**, generic abbreviation for the deoxyribonucleic acid, or dC-to-dU, deaminase family (APOBECs 1, 2,4 and 3A/B/ C/D/F/G/H) similar in DNA sequence to the "apolipoprotein B RNA editor" APOBEC1, and known to activate mutagenic cytidine deamination during transcription in somatic tissues, particularly in cancer and Innate Immunity to viruses; **Deaminase**, zinc-containing catalytic domain in ADAR and APOBEC enzymes; **MC**, mutated codon; **MC1**, **MC2**, **MC3**, respectively refer to the first, second and third nucleotide mutation target position within a mutated codon read in the 5-prime to 3-prime direction; **R**, Adenosine (A) or Guanine (G), purines; **S**, strong base pair involving Cytosine (C) or Guanine (G); **SNV**, single nucleotide variation; **T**, Thymine; **TSM**, targeted somatic mutations: the process of targeting actively transcribed genes that results in a dominant type of mutation caused by a DBD or Inf-DBD targeting nucleotide sites at a particular codon position; **U**, uracil; **W**, weak base pair involving A or U/T; **Y**, pyrimidines T/U

Originally published in *Research Reports*, and access for all Supplementary data in the online version.
Steele EJ, Lindley RA (2020) Analysis of APOBEC and ADAR deaminase-driven Riboswitch Haplotypes in COVID-19 RNA strain variants and the implications for vaccine design. *Research Reports* DOI: 10.9777/rr.2020.10001
https://www.companyofscientists.com/index.php/rr

Abstract

This paper reports the results of our initial analysis of APOBEC and ADAR deaminase-mediated mutation signature patterns in complete COVID-19 genomes from informative locations and times in China, USA and Spain in the 2019–2020 pandemic. We have identified a unique set of 'new' putative coordinated Riboswitches in COVID-19 genomes not previously identified, and likely generating variants of the known common strain Haplotypes now in circulation. The results reveal that COVID-19 diversifies using switching of RNA Haplotypes with minimal alteration to protein structure (the normal targets for B and T cells in conventional vaccine development). The deaminase-driven RNA Haplotypes are most likely aligned with RNA secondary structures. Several studies already highlight how Riboswitches alter the ability of RNA to fold into intricate three-dimensional structures allowing them to execute their diverse cellular functions. The same functional outcomes are expected for viruses, particularly efficacy of RNA replication in new host cell environments. Thus, vaccine designs that assume that the main viral protein antigens will be the only putative protective targets could fail to produce effective and protective immunity. We conclude that understanding COVID-19 adaptation and survival strategy and identifying the host Haplotype, and which vaccine(s) is effective for each Haplotype group will be important for new vaccine design.

INTRODUCTION

There have been several recent reports that are attempting to understand the mode of transmission and pathogenesis of COVID-19 (Shi *et al.* 2020, Archaraya *et al.* 2020). However our purpose in this paper has been to analyse the genetic structure of COVID-19 genomes isolated early in the first two and a half months of 2019–2020 coronavirus pandemic: from its sudden explosive origins in China (Dec 2019–Jan 2020), through early spreading to the West Coast USA (through late Jan, then Feb-to early Mar 2020) to two other informative explosive epicenters of the pandemic in Spain and particularly New York, USA (through to March 14–22, 2020). In advance we decided the sequence data to be analysed had to be readily accessible online to other scientists, be authoritative, be curated by experts and thus accurate and reliable with GenBank linkage. We thus chose to focus exclusively on those COVID-19 sequences curated at the NIH, Bethesda, through its National Center for Bioinformatic Information, at their site *NCBI Virus*. In following this approach our aim has been to understand the adaptive genetic strategy of the virus through its deployment of putative riboswitch changes to its RNA sequence to generate robust RNA haplotypes able to replicate in the genetic background of the infected host.

Previously we applied our analyses of APOBEC (C>U) and ADAR (A>I) deaminase-mediated editing signatures in the viral RNA genomes of HCV and ZIKV during the acute-phase of innate immune responses of the host-parasite relationship (Lindley and Steele 2018); that is during the well-known host phase of the interferon-stimulated gene (or innate immune) response (Schoggins and Rice 2011, Schneider *et al.* 2014). We reported that the distinct signatures at known deamination motifs of cytosine to uracil (C>U read as C>T) and adenosine to inosine (A>I read as A>G) are written into the circulating viral genomes including the quasi-species of viral variants in an individual during *Flavivirus* infection (Stoddard *et al.* 2015). We also critically reviewed the literature showing that viral replicases themselves, the RNA-dependent RNA polymerases (RdRP), are of high replicative fidelity thus faithfully copying the deaminase-mediated mutation patterns into replicating viral progeny genomes. We concluded that this contributes to the production of the viral quasi-species observed during the acute phase of HCV disease *in vivo* (Stoddard *et al.* 2015).

Flaviviruses possess positive single stranded RNA genomes about two thirds smaller in length than COVID-19. We now apply this same targeted somatic mutation (TSM) codon-context methodology (Lindley 2013, Lindley and Steele 2018) to the analysis of the positive single stranded COVID-19 genomes collected from patients in China, USA and Spain during the acute phase of the infection. There is now a large amount of sequence data curated at the NIH website dedicated to this virus, "NCBI Virus" (particularly for the USA, lesser extent China and very little from other countries at time of initial writing). We have, by necessity, been focused and selective as our analyses are of a different type to conventional algorithm-dependent phylogenetics which focus on global strain features (Dorp *et al.* 2020a, b) and which may overlook some of the important features we report here. Indeed, in our analyses there is no algorithm interface between the patterns seen and the interpretation of the same data patterns (apart from the onscreen NCBI Virus alignment tool used). We concentrate on the mutational source of trusted, reliable widely accessible data viz. GenBank accessible NCBI-curated single nucleotide variants (SNVs) at the National Institutes of Health (NIH) creating the observed genetic patterns in isolated viral genomes from infected subjects during the innate immune response (which would be the first week of disease in most patients swabbed for the virus). Thus, we need to be selective so as to allow the maximum insight into the origin (source) and spread of this newly emergent viral disease (Table 1). Apart from region and country of origin, the NIH curated COVID-19 sequences lack detailed patient data, age, sex, racial origin, and clinical co-morbidities and clinical outcome. We thus chose to analyse sequence alignments for viral collections during the key early two and a half months of the pandemic at informative times and locations (Table 1). In the cases of Spain and New York we focused particularly on the mid-point of the exponential rising case curve from about March 14 to the end of the month in New York and March 6–10 in Spain *versus* the COVID-19 genetic patterns from the isolates in China in January 2020 (Figure S1). This report will thus focus on comparative Variable Site Diagram (VSD) patterns across full length COVID-19 genomes (29903 nt Hu-1 ref. seq) and will be very selective. A breakdown by critical time points and regions during the early periods of the global pandemic is displayed in Table 1 (and case incident statistics from online media sites with time in the Supplementary Information Figures S1–S6)). Future reports will analyse over 12,000 COVID-19 genomes (from non-NIH curations GISAID, Next Strain etc) to focus on a more detailed analysis to identify specific types of APOBEC and ADAR deaminases executing the observed mutational events and to provide further insights into riboswitch adaptions as a COVID-19 mechanism to evade host innate and adaptive immunity. Later papers will also deal with the further implications of these data for the origin and global spread of this suddenly emergent pandemic disease.

Table 1 Time-Line COVID-19 Patient Sample Collections and Locations

Location	Collection Dates	No. Complete COVID-19 Genomes Aligned v Hu-1 Ref.Seq.	Type of COVID-19 Outbreak
China -Wuhan and Regions	Dec 20-30 2019, Jan 2020, Feb 2-5 2020	47	Originating explosive epidemic in China centred om Wuhan, Hubei Province and immediate regions
California,USA	Jan 22- Feb 26 2020	10	Early sporadic reports and person-to-person (P-to-P) community spreads
Cruise Ship-at-Sea *Grand Princess* off CA coast,USA	Feb 17-25 2020	25	Localised yet explosive outbreak at-Sea
California,USA	Feb 27-Mar 4 2020	24	Local outbreaks and community P-to-P spreads
Washington State (Kirkland), USA	Feb 24-Mar 1	10	Local outbreak in nursing home
Spain	Feb 26- Mar5 2020,	8	Local outbreak just prior to explosive increase in Spanish cases
Spain	Mar 6- Mar 10 2020	13 +	Exponential increase phase of Spanish epidemic
New York , USA	Mar 5 - 9 2020	18	Local outbreaks and community P-to-P spreads just prior to explosive NYC outbreak
New York (overwhelmingly NYC), USA	Mar 14 - 22 2020	97	Explosive exponential phase of NYC epidemic

MATERIALS AND METHODS

Data Source and Acquisition

The National Centre for Biotechnology Information (NCBI) at the National Institutes of Health (NIH) curates as they come available all current complete and partial SARS-CoV-2 sequences at https://www.ncbi.nlm.nih.gov/genbank/sars-cov-2-seqs/#nucleotide-sequences particularly at the NCBI Virus site for this virus (at URL https://www.ncbi.nlm.nih.gov/labs/virus/vssi/#/virus?SeqTypes=Nucleotide&VirusLineage_ss=SARS-CoV-2,%20taxid:2697049). Complete genome COVID-19 sequences isolated during the phases of the epidemic can be selected and aligned with tools provided at the NCBI Virus site.

Details on Sample Access, Time Points and Regions

The collection time, for each sequence identified by GenBank Accession number is provided in the detailed major tabulated curations in Table 1 and online supplementary information Tables S1, S2, S3, S4. In some latter stages of the analyses we resorted to a screen shot record of key alignments and manual tabulation, reporting only key VSD patterns in those figures and tables discussed.

To summarise Table 1: for China, collections were from December 20 through February 5, but the great bulk of collections were through January (Table S1, Figures S1, S2). For West Coast USA during early sporadic outbreaks in that country, mainly California and the off-coast cruise ship (*Grand Princess*) collections were from January 22 through February 24, then February 27 through March 4 (Table S2, Figures S3, S4). An outbreak in an old person's hospital facility Washington State (Kirkland) were collections February 24–March 1 (Table S3, see Figure S5). For Spain there were two periods of collections examined February 26–March 5, then March 6–March 10. For New York sequence alignments were conducted on pre-epidemic collections March 5–9, then at the midpoint of the exponential rising case curve for March 14–22 in the USA which was almost exclusively due to the exponential increases of COVID-19 cases in New York City (Figures S1, S3, S5).

The analyses of data in **RESULTS and DISCUSSION** follows this chronology, to reflect more or less the order of reported key early outbreaks across the world in January, February to March 14–22, 2020. However, it is likely that both Spain and USA (which is overwhelmingly data from NYC, Supplementary Information) show very similar and overlapping case increase curves both in time and slope for March (Figure S1). The order of Spain before New York reflects the temporal order of the outbreaks reported in the mass media (following the slightly earlier explosive occurring outbreaks in Tehran/ Qom and Lombardy in Italy — the latter not analysed as no significant numbers of complete genome data from these locations had been uploaded to NCBI Virus site at time of data analysis and writing of this paper).

NCBI Virus Genome Sequence Alignment and Analysis

Our data analyses involve the following steps:

1. At the NCBI Virus site for SARS-CoV-2, all selected sequences were analysed while recording the sample country, region and time period of collection in the pandemic.

2. An alignment of the selected sequence set, including the original Wuhan Hu-1 reference sequence (NC_045512.2) was made using the on-screen tools at the NCBI Virus site.

3. In the Tabulation into the excel spread sheets (Tables S1, S2, S3, S4), each sequence is linked to Sequence ID or Accession Number (to GenBank), its Collection date, its Release date, on occasion the Length of the curated complete sequence (although that is in GenBank), and the Country of origin, and region where possible.

4. Each single nucleotide variation (SNV) from the Wuhan Ref. Seq. (Hu-1, NC_045512.2) was curated by position in the Multiple Alignment — viz. position in the

5' untranslated region (UTR), the protein coding (CDS), non-CDS gaps, and the 3' UTR. Most alignments gave exact sequence positions for key SNV sites, although the China alignment (Table S1) sequence positions at S Haplotype defining sites p.8782 and p.28144 are advanced by three to p.8785, and p.28147. Other adjustments, in our analysis, for in-frame whole codon deletions in the aligned collection were noted at times for p.11080/83 and p.25563/60. Suspect sequences in the 5' UTR or 3' UTR possibly due to sequencing technical artefacts were noted, and SNVs adjudged as genuine or not in those and other ambiguous regions (N). N runs and sequence quality were noted and reported in summary VSD patterns where appropriate as a guide to sequence quality for that alignment. Also noted were samples with truncated 5' and 3' UTR ends as these could be cause the loss of key information, such as putative "riboswitch" sites in these regions.

5. Each curated SNV in the protein coding regions (CDS) was then classified by

   a. The CDS SNV type such as C>T, G>A, A>G, T>C, G>C, G>T etc. C/G-sites are implied as APOBEC changes, A/T-sites are implied ADAR mediated changes (Lindley and Steele 2018). These will be further analysed in detail in a follow-up paper (Hall, Mamrot, Steele, Lindley In Preparation). In some cases, G>T SNVs were deduced to be more likely caused by reactive oxygen species (ROS) producing 8oxoG modified guanosines at that site. In these cases the 8oxoG modifications may well be preferred at W<u>G</u> sites as noted previously for cancer genomes viz. the single base substitution (SBS) signature describing this pattern is Signature 18 of Alexandrov *et al.* (2013) and see the COSMIC website for all updated mutational signature information, https://cancer.sanger.ac.uk/cosmic/signatures. We have recently explained the rationale for diagnosis of this ROS signature in Franklin *et al.* (2020).

   b. The likely strand was identified on which the deamination event occurred: the +ve sense strand for mRNA or -ve template strand for replication of COVID-19 sequence copies in the dsRNA Replicating Form (RF) of the virus in the putative membraneous web in the cytosol (Thimme *et al.* 2012, Yang and Leibowitz 2015).

   c. The codon context (Lindley 2013, Lindley *et al.* 2016, Lindley and Steele 2018) of the change viz. whether in the MC1, MC2, MC3 positions or first, second and third positions of the mutated codon (by convention read 5 prime to 3 prime to allow subsequent assignment of specific codon-context deaminase associated mutation signature and motif location assignment (In Preparation).

   d. The nature of the amino acid (AA) change and whether that SNV in the protein is "Conserved", "Benign" or "Radical" in its putative change of protein secondary structure and function. All nonsynonymous changes within an AA functional class are considered, like synonymous changes, as "Conservative" (black in VSD patterns). However, by definition, all observed SNVs are likely to be "benign' in terms of their likely impact on viral protein structure and replicative ability of the RNA viral genome — since the variant virus sequence has already made the "Darwinian Cut". However in this qualitative scheme a "likely benign" nonsynonymous change (green in VSD patterns) would be AA interchanges for Polar<->NonPolar, Basic<->Polar,

Acidic<->Polar. A Radicle change is a full AA charge change "Basic<->Acidic" and Basic<->NonPolar, Acidic<->NonPolar (deep red in VSD patterns). In the various Variable Site Diagrams (VSD) in **RESULTS and DISCUSSION** the following colour codes and qualifications for entries are shown in Figure 1.

6. Throughout the CDS regions, the SNVs were also analysed in terms of likely change to RNA secondary structure based on the SNV's conserved nature at the protein level (as defined, Figure 1) and whether two or more apparent co-ordinated SNV changes are required in presumptive "Haplotype" generation. As explained below we consider this could be a reflection of putative co-ordinately deaminase-targeted "Riboswitch" positions (e.g. as reviewed in Yang and Leibowitz 2015). If they occur frequently, in independent collections from different regions, and are apparently independent sequences, they were noted and the Haplotypes they appear associated with were tabulated and factored into the analysis of sequences and their mutated derivatives (Table 2). The literature on Riboswitches, RNA secondary structure and associated changes in cellular functions has been well documented (Gilbert and Fontane 2006, Tan *et al.* 2015, Widom *et al.* 2018).

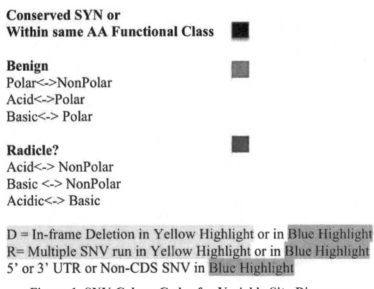

**Conserved SYN or
Within same AA Functional Class**

Benign
Polar<->NonPolar
Acid<->Polar
Basic<-> Polar

Radicle?
Acid<-> NonPolar
Basic <-> NonPolar
Acidic<-> Basic

D = In-frame Deletion in Yellow Highlight or in Blue Highlight
R= Multiple SNV run in Yellow Highlight or in Blue Highlight
5' or 3' UTR or Non-CDS SNV in Blue Highlight

Figure 1. SNV Colour Codes for Variable Site Diagrams

RESULTS AND DISCUSSION

1. A Rationale for Ordering the Data on COVID-19

Table 2 summarises our collected observations for sequences analysed from different regions. It is provisional as it may well be revised with additions, or as qualified deletions as more sequence data and patterns emerge. It shows our current assessment of Haplotypes and coordinated Riboswitch SNVs mainly at the RNA level (not predominantly at the protein level) which we consider useful in our analyses. The colour coding in the table

Table 2 Haplotypes and Sites Defining COVID-19 Common Strain Variants in China, USA, Spain

HAP	AA class-> 5'UTR p.241	P<>NonP Thr<>Ile p.1059	SYN Phe<>Phe p.3037	SYN Ser<>Ser p.8782	NonP<>NonP Phe<>Tyr p.9477	NonP<>NonP Leu<>Phe p.11080/83	P<>NonP Ser<>Leu p.11916	NonP<>NonP Pro<>Leu p.14408	P<>P Tyr<>Tyr p.14805	NonP<>NonP Pro<>Leu p.17747	P<>P Tyr<>Cys p.17858	SYN Leu<>Leu p.18060	NonP<>NonP Ala<>val p.18998	Acid<>NonP Asp<>Gly p.23403	P<>Basic Gln<>His p.25563	NonP<>NonP Gly<>Val p.25979	NP<>NP Gly<>Val p.26144	P<>NonP Leu<>Ser p.28144	SYN Asp<>Asp p.28657	P<>NonP Ser<>Leu p.28863	near 3'UTR non-CDS gap p.29540
L (Hu-1)	C	C	C	C	T	G	C	C	C	C	A	C	C	A	G	G	G	T	C	C	G
Ln	C	C	C	C	T	T	C	C	T	C	A	C	C	A	G	G	T	T	C	C	G
L-241a	T	T	T	C	T	G	C	T	C	C	A	C	C	G	T	G	G	T	C	C	G
L-241a.1	T	T	T	C	T	G	T	T	C	C	A	C	T	G	T	G	G	T	C	C	A
L-241b	T	T	C	C	T	G	C	T	C	C	A	C	C	G	T	G	G	T	C	C	G
L-241c	T	C	T	C	T	G	C	T	C	C	A	C	C	G	T	G	G	T	C	C	G
L-241d/s	T	T	T	C	T	G	C	C	C	C	A	C	C	G	T	G	G	T	C	C	G
L-241e	T	C	C	C	T	G	C	T	C	C	A	C	C	G	T	G	G	T	C	C	G
L-241f	T	C	T	C	T	G	C	T	C	C	A	C	C	G	G	G	G	T	C	C	G
L-241g	T	C	C	C	T	G	C	T	C	C	A	C	C	G	G	G	G	T	C	C	G
S	C	C	C	T	T	G	C	C	C	C	A	C	C	A	G	G	G	C	C	C	G
Sa	C	C	C	T	T	G	C	C	C	T	G	T	C	A	G	G	C	C	C	C	G
Sb	C	C	C	T	A	G	C	C	T	C	A	C	C	A	G	G	C	C	C	C	G
Ss	C	C	C	T	A	G	C	C	T	C	A	C	C	A	G	T	G	C	T	T	G

focuses attention on the distinction between L and L-241 RNA haplotypes as revealed between the Wuhan and New York COVID-19 collections. In other targeted mutagenesis studies numerous RNA secondary structure variant hotspots have been revealed related to efficacy of the replicative phases of the HCV viral life cycle and other translated genes (Pirakitikulr *et al.* 2016; also see Buhr *et al.* 2016, Widom *et al.* 2018), and, as indicated SARS-CoV-1 appears to have also deployed an RNA secondary structure polymorphic adaptation strategy (Yang and Leibwitz 2015). The most notable example is the L *v* S Haplotypes as revealed first in the China data by phylogenetic relationships with SARS-CoV-1 and apparent animal variant relationships (Tang *et al.* 2020). The current simple sequencing methods thus identify the different haplotype-defined RNA strains of L and S and their subtypes. This depends first on detecting a C at p.8782 and T at p.28144 thus identifying the L haplotypes and a T at p.8782 and a C at p.28144 thus identifying the S haplotypes. Another key site is the p.241 C>T in the 5'UTR-other, RNA-only and thus putative Riboswitch sites are presented in Table 2. No other strain RNA haplotypes have been identified using such binary (or even higher number) sequence tests. The L/S test cannot define changes implicating putative RNA secondary structure modifications in currently arising circulating strains. This is the utility of the putative riboswitched haplotypes arrayed in Table 2 — other strains can be haplotyped and much of the current sequence diversity in COVID-19 can be identified and understood in terms of haplotype diversification during global spread of the disease.

Deaminase-Driven Riboswitch Hypothesis: Haplotype Variation in the Initial First Infection?

In support of this interpretation of the data is the fact that the two SNVs defining the S Haplotype are rarely observed by themselves — thus at the canonical S defining site p.8782 the C>T (= p.8785 in the current China alignment Table S1, is MC3, TTT AG**C** CAG) is always paired with the S defining canonical site p.28,144 of a T>C (= p.28,147 in current Table S1 alignment MC2 TGT T**T**A CCT). However, these criteria for defining that haplotype might also apply to the other putative haplotypes identified in Table 2. Thus, it can be inferred that the COVID-19 viral diversification strategy is locked into the productive and coordinate combinations of *RNA Riboswitch modifications* which logically implies RNA secondary structure with downstream affects on function and replication. Thus, the simplest and the most parsimonious interpretation of the data assumes the L-to-S Haplotype variations, and the others listed in Table 2 (L-to-L-241 variants), are largely deamination-driven *in vivo* during the first infection cycle by unmutated source viruses e.g. L Hu-1. That is, the variation is not expected to pre-exist in the initial source virus population prior to first infection — it makes better biological sense that the haploytype switch actually occurs during the innate immune response in the first infection cycle in that subject. Accordingly, in our view, the host-parasite interaction, and the innate immune response to the virus, ultimately determines the observed haplotype that emerges in the complete COVD-19 genome. In our observations the proportion of S Haplotypes to total sequences in any given collection alignment can range from 5–50% (for example in 206 NY samples March 14–22, 6 sequences are S, and 10 are L, below). We have not generally observed haplotype recombinants (on scale) at this stage of our survey — although we expect it to occasionally occur. In a small number of cases a SNV site can be shared between haplotypes (p.14805, C>T site), indicative of deaminase (or reactive oxygen species mutagenesis, ROS, on oxidised guanosines, 8oxoG) activity at that site viz. it could be a hot spot for mutagenesis. If key SNVs defining that haplotype are reverted to Hu-1 reference sequence they are rare (although some undoubtedly occur on inspection of data sets, see below). It is possible that novel conversions can take place on further person-to-person transmissions. However, given that APOBEC deaminations (C>T) can in theory be reverted by ADAR deaminations (T>C) such reversions must be considered as possible, and may often occur during the innate immune response of that infection cycle in that subject. Also, important non-CDS RNA only regions, like the G>A SNV in the non-CDS gap at p.29540 may contribute to additional haplotypes in a wider data set (as that data seems to imply for the L241a.1 subhaplotype, below). The Aspartic Acid to Glycine change at Spike amino acid 614 (D614G) at p.23403 is significant and it has now become the dominant, and thus "haplotype", now detected globally (Korber *et al.* 2020). This has replaced all other detected haplotypes at time of writing (July 17 2020). Of interest is that this change in Spike structure significantly facilitates infection and thus replication of COVID-19 but apparently not disease severity.

Each of the SNV-defined haplotypes identified comprises approximately 0.02% difference from the Hu-1 reference sequence. On average there are approximately 5 SNV differences from Hu-1 defining each haplotype. Thus, there is ≥99.98% identity between any haplotype and the Wuhan reference sequence whether that sequence is collected in China, Spain, the US West Coast or New York City.

So this is our operating hypothesis: the germline encoded innate immune responses in the first day or two after infection with, for example, source Hu-1 virions (L) can generate deaminase-mediated C>U and A>I changes in the replicating viral sequences, and less frequent down-stream miscopied transversions (e.g. opposite inosine template residues). Thus, a range of +ve strand RNA quasi-species are produced in an infected cell with changes at particular deaminase hot spots or riboswitch sites determining compatible RNA secondary structures allowing rapid replication. Host-directed deaminase-mediated riboswitches are expected to create adaptive options for the virus which if then selected allows more rapid replication in that cellular environment. This hypothesis is a great simplification conceptual tool, and it has allowed us to order the complex data sets now emerging in the pandemic in a rational way.

2. Analysis of China COVID-19 complete genomes

All China COVID-19 sequences collected from patients during December 2019 into January 2020 (to Feb 5) were selected into the alignment during a period of explosive exponential increases in COVID-19 cases in Hubei province, particularly its major city Wuhan (Figures S1, S2, S3). These numbers account for ≥90% of all the China COVID-19 cases (and deaths) reported. However, the sequences curated at NCBI Virus do not reflect that case bias, as surrounding regions and provinces are over-represented in the collected sequence-set compared to density of case incidence as shown in Figure S2.

Table 3a. Types of SNVs observed in China outbreak

REF Base	Variant Base				TOTAL	%
	A	T	C	G		
A		1	1	7	9	22.5
T	3		4		7	17.5
C	2	14			16	40
G	4	3	1		8	20
					40	

Transitions - 72.5% Transition: Tranversion ratio 3.4:1
Transversions - 27.5%

Note MT226610 and MT019530 data excluded

Table 3b. Types SNV in California + Cruise Ship Outbreaks Jan 22- Feb 24

REF Base	Variant Base				TOTAL	%
	A	T	C	G		
A		4		2	6	10.7
T			4		4	7.14
C	1	29			30	53.6
G	6	7	3		16	28.6
					56	

Transitions - 73.2% Transition: Tranversion ratio 2.73:1
Transversions - 26.8%

Table 3c. Types SNV in CA outbreaks Feb 27-Mar 4

REF Base	Variant Base				TOTAL	%
	A	T	C	G		
A			1	6	7	23.3
T			4		4	13.3
C	1	11			12	40
G	3	4			7	23.3
					30	

Transitions - 80% Transition: Tranversion ratio 4:1
Transversions - 20%

Table 3d. Types SNV in Spain Outbreaks Mar 6-Mar 10

REF Base	Variant Base				TOTAL	%
	A	T	C	G		
A				4	4	14.8
T	1		2		3	11.1
C		12			12	44.4
G	2	6			8	29.6
					27	

Transitions - 74.1% Transition: Tranversion ratio 2.86:1
Transversions - 25.9%

Table 3e. Types of SNV in NY Outbreaks Mar 5-9

REF Base	Variant Base				TOTAL	%
	A	T	C	G		
A		2		6	8	20
T	1		2		3	7.5
C	1	19			20	50
G	3	6			9	22.5
					40	

Transitions - 75% Transition: Tranversion ratio 3:1
Transversions - 25%

Table 3f. Types of SNV in L and S Haplotypes collected NYC Mar 14-Mar 22.

REF Base	Variant Base				TOTAL	%
	A	T	C	G		
A		2		4	6	34.92
T	2		5		7	17.46
C		16		1	17	17.93
G	4		2		12	29.77
					42	

Transitions - 69% Transition: Tranversion ratio 2.22:1
Transversions - 31%

Table 3g. Types of SNV in collected NYC Mar 14-Mar 19.

REF Base	Variant Base				TOTAL	%
	A	T	C	G		
A		1	2	11	14	34.92
T	3		10		14	17.46
C	1	41		1	43	17.93
G	9	11	3		23	29.77
					94	

Transitions - 75.5% Transition: Tranversion ratio 3.08:1
Transversions - 24.5%
Note: 7 of 11 G>T are potentiall 8oxoG modifications at W G sites

Table 3 Types of SNVs in the different outbreaks analysed. Correction 6 April 2022 of errors in published version in Tables 3f and 3g. The extreme left marginal totals as percent (%) off Ref Base A,T,C,G are: for Table 3f 14.3, 16.7, 40.5 and 28.6 respectively, and for Table 3g 14.8, 14.8, 46.2, 24.5 respectively.

Caveat on all Analyses in this Paper

Apart from this type of bias in sequence selection, there is a major caveat on all other hidden biases present in the aligned data. The clinical decision to seek sequence information on the collected COVID-19 sample assumes that the patient had full blown disease symptoms with respiratory complications (in the main). All other analyses (below) on USA and Spain data lack specific clinical information and the interactive relationships between patients with putative sequences (Sequence IDs or GenBank Accession Numbers), the subject's age, sex, racial origin (Caucasian, Asian, African-American, Latinos etc). Absent here then is the known prior state of health (co-morbidities) or whether the subject survived the acute respiratory infection. In some cases, such as observations on specific outbreaks, we can make inferences because of the location and timing and person-to-person transfers (P-to-P, e.g. hospital outbreaks in Kirkland in Seattle, Washington State) — but that is all they are. In the case of China and Spain we can safely infer dominant Chinese ethnicity and Caucasian/Latino ethnicity of patients (in the main). However we lack key information in a putative P-to-P spreading chain such as "..who actually gave the virus to whom? ..." — that data must exist in some form, somewhere, but we do not have that data. And "community spreads" without a controversial "known link to China" is a background factor in trying to interpret P-to-P spreading. We can only plausibly infer P-to-P transfers from the mutation patterns in the sequence data. But we can say with confidence (see Figure 2, Table 3) as we did earlier for acute HCV, ZIKV infections (Lindley and Steele 2018), that the great bulk of SNVs analysed are at APOBEC (C-site) and ADAR (A-site) deamination motifs viz. APOBEC1 and ADAR1/2 deaminases (Rosenberg *et al.* 2011, Lindley and Steele 2018). They appear to be the responsible drivers of the mutations — including the causative deaminases most likely to drive riboswitching at simultaneous (linked) deamination events by APOBEC/ADAR at functionally-coupled C-site and A-site hotspots. However, motif specificity of other APOBEC RNA C-site editors such as APOBEC3A (Sharma *et al.* 2015, 2016a) and APOBEC3G (2016b) should also be searched for in these sequence data during acute phase COVID-19 infections, and that analysis is underway.

Variable Site Diagram (VSD) of 47 China COVID-19 Sequences (Figure 2)

This is a valuable and informative way to present the SNV data and make logical inferences on the genesis of mutational patterns and relations among sequences. Such patterns, we believe, are far more informative at the molecular and cell biology level than simple construction of phylogenetic trees — the P-to-P issue of "who gave what viral variant to whom" is a far more relevant genetic question in connecting apparently different sequences.

This variable site diagram (VSD) is displayed in Figure 2 for the 47 complete China COVID-19 genomes Dec 20 2019 through January 2020. There were originally 48 selected sequences in the alignment. Sequence LR757997 however had to be removed as there were far too many N runs and other sequence gaps that created real problems not only for a respectable alignment but also in alignment scrolling and analysis. This sequence was thus deleted leaving 47 compete COVID-19 sequences for analysis during the height of the China epidemic.

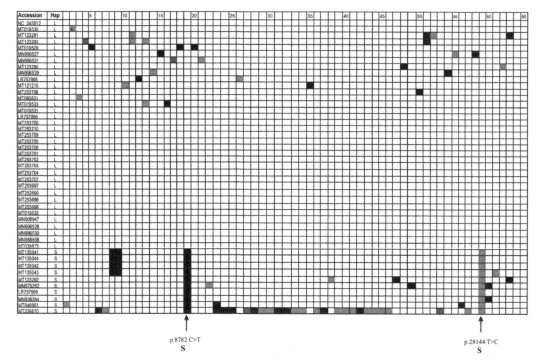

p.8782 C>T
S

p.28144 T>C
S

Figure 2 Variable Site Diagram of SNVs in each aligned sequence in the 47 China sequence alignment, which includes Hu-1 ref NC_045512.2. Variable site number across the top, and Sequence ID down left hand side and Haplotype assignment. Note MT226610 has 27 SNVs and is discussed separately in text. MT019530 may have corrupted sequence in 5' UTR (site 2) but included as identical in rest of sequence to Hu-1 reference. The SNV key with respect to putative impact on protein structure of each SNV is discussed in text and Figure 1. S Hap sites are indicated for sites 19 and 59 and arrowed (and see Table 2). The data in Table S1 should be consulted for further details. The variable site column number followed by SNV position in the alignment are: 1, p.76, C>A; 2, p.107–127, T>A, T>C, T>G, C>G, T>C, G>A; 3, p.189, C>T; 4, p.657, G>A; 5, p.3781, A>G; 6, p.4291, G>T; 7, p.4310, A>C; 8, p.4405, T>C; 9, p.5065, G>T; 10, p.6029, C>T; 11, p.6822, G>T; 12, p.6971, C>A; 13, p.6999, T>C; 14, p.7019, G>A; 15, p.7482, A>G; 16, p.7869, G>T; 17, p.8004, A>C; 18, p.8391, A>G; 19, p.8785, C>T; 20, p.8890, T>A; 21, p.9537, C>T; 22, p.9564, C>T; 23, p.11086, G>T; 24, p.11210, G>C; 25, p.11236, T>G; 26, p.11767, T>A; 27, p.12044, G>C; 28, p.12163, G>C; 29, p.12205, G>C; 30, p.12211, G>T; 31, p.12358, G>C; 32, p.12381, G>A; 33, p.12467, G>T; 34, p.12470, G>T; 35, p.12476, C>T; 36, p.12494, G>T; 37, p.12517, G>C; 38, p.12537, C>T; 39, p.12575, G>T; 40, p.12581, G>A; 41, p.12585, G>T; 42, p.12603, G>A; 43, p.12663, G>C; 44, p.12688, G>C; 45, p.12776, G>T; 46, p.12796, G>T; 47, p.13075, C>T; 48, p.15327, C>T; 49, p.15610, T>C; 50, p.162250, C>T; 51, p.17376, C>T; 52, p.19613, C>T; 53, p.20983, G>C; 54, p.21140, A>G; 55, p.21319, G>A; 56, p.21647, T>A; 57, p.21787, T>A; 58, p.24328, A>G; 59, p.28147, T>C; 60, p.29098, C>T; 61, p.29304, A>T; 62, p.29306, C>T; 63, p.29530, G>A.

Overview of Mutation Pattern of 47 China COVID-19 Sequences

The most striking general patterns displayed by these data (and the California and Cruise Ship SNV data, Figure 3) are their resemblance to the similar variable site patterns seen *in vivo* among the viral quasi-species (Eigen and Schuster 1975, Andino and Domingo 2015) of HCV patients during the acute phase of HCV infection (first week or so) — as seen in the single molecule HCV sequencing of a number of such patients reported by Stoddard *et al.* (2015). Indeed, quasi-species acute phase HCV data were used by us in the *Flavivirus* analysis previously reported (Lindley and Steele 2018). This raises the whole issue of exactly "What a COVID-19 RNA consensus sequence actually is?" Thus, future deep single-molecule sequencing should be conducted on separate COVID-19 swab or bronchial fluid collections from the *same* patient (Li *et al.* 2012) to establish a more realistic assignment of the "consensus" sequence in some patients. The acute phase "quasi-species" like pattern — is distributed in many subjects in the Chinese COVID-19 patient population, rather than as assessed in a single patient *in vivo* by deep sequencing. The same general pattern is evident in the California and Cruise Ship data (Jan 22– Feb 24, below), and for the dominant haplotypes in the explosive New York epidemic (Mar 14–Mar 22).

In Figure 2, there are 63 variable sites. For the CDS region there are 60 variable sites. Of the three sites in the 5'UTR two look legitimate #1 and #3: MT049951 C>A at p.76, MT093631 C>T at p.189. The third #2 is MT019530 and involves a cluster of 6 changes from Hu-1, most are T>C (or T>Y) and could be sequencing artefacts. Our judgement is these sequence sites be ignored, but the CDS region SNVs in MT019530 be kept in the analysis as a legitimate unmutated derivative of the Hu-1 reference sequence. Of the 46 sequences 36 are of L Haplotype and 10 are of the S Haplotype as defined Table 2.

The types of SNVs are displayed in Table 3a. Mutations at C-sites exceeds mutations at A-sites, with an excess of C>T suggesting APOBEC C>U deaminations mainly on the +ve strand either in completed COVID-19 genomic copies or in the single stranded regions of the displaced +ve strand at Transcription Bubbles during replication. ADAR A>I events occur equally on both the +ve and -ve strands suggesting A>I events on dsRNA regions of the RF form as well as in completed stem loops of completed +ve strand copies. The number of transition mutations exceeds the number of transversions more than three to one (an expectation in all deaminase-driven mutagenic systems, see Steele and Lindley (2017).

L Haplotype Analysis of the China data

Among sequences in the major L Hap group there are 26 unique variable sites (MT226610 sites are ignored — as these are all in S Hap).

• 25 L sequences are identical to Hu-1 ref i.e. unmutated
• 11 L sequences were variable from Hu-1 ref.

- 3 sites are shared MT123291, MT123293 and MT019533/MT123293. This implies either *in vivo* deamination hot spots or first generation P-to-P transfers with additional deaminase mediated mutational events laid down on that common sequence structure.
- 24 of the variable sites are thus unique singleton sites — a feature highlighted by Stoddard *et al.* 2015 for the *in vivo* pattern among quasi species for acute phase patterns in individual HCV patients.
- In general, by the criteria for AA impact applied (Figure 1), there is much 'functional sequence conservation' or 'benigness' in these sequences. There is therefore qualified support for the supposition that these are the "Darwinian Cut" survivors of a host innate immune deaminase attack on the acute phase viral sequences (although a small portion are deduced to be the result of ROS 8oxoG modifications — indeed ROS attack is a common innate immune defence against intracellular pathogens).

Putative APOBEC and ADAR Deaminations among L Hap Group

Among the L Hap SNVs in the 11 L sequence set we have: 9 C>T (one shared, presumed APOBEC (+) strand RF); 4 G>A (presumed APOBEC (-) strand RF); 5 A>G (presumed ADAR1/2 (+) strand RF); 1 T>C (shared, presumed ADAR1/2 (-) strand RF); 1 G>T (presumed 8oxoG at WG site (+) strand RF); 1 C>A (presumed APOBEC/8oxoG (-) strand RF); 1 A>C (presumed ADAR1/2 (+) strand RF); 2 T>A (presumed ADAR1/2 (-) strand RF). The identified APOBEC and ADAR putative changes are at typical motifs as observed for HCV, ZIKV (Lindley and Steele 2018). Further specific clarification is a focus of our and ongoing investigations (see also Rosenberg *et al.* 2011, Sharma *et al.* 2015, 2016, Eifler *et al.* 2013).

SNVs per Sequence in L Hap Group

Among the L Hap sequences the number of unique SNV differences per sequence from Hu-1 ref. are: 4, 3, 3, 2, 2, 2, 2, 2, 1, 1, 2; thus a range of about 2–4 differences per sequence for the assumed first infection cycle might be concluded.

So apart from one possible single P-to-P interchange or transfer (MT123291<-> MT123293) all appear to be part of the acute phase deaminase-mediated innate immune host response in the first infection with L Hu-1 viruses. So, the distribution of SNV numbers in order are summarised as:

No. L Seqs.	No. SNV *v* Hu-1
25	0
2	1
5	2
2	3
2	4

There is very little P-to-P spread at the height of the epidemic in Wuhan and surrounding regions. Most COVID-19 positive subjects appear to be infected with the same virus viz. Hu-1 ref. This conclusion is consistent with the same conclusion based on the phylogenetic analysis in January 2020 during the exponential rise in COVID-19 cases in Wuhan (Anderson 2020).

An alternative, and partial, explanation is that many of those L haplotypes showing complete sequence identity to Hu-1 are actually products of P-to-P transfers with no further laying down of deaminase-mediated mutations in the recipient host from which the collection was made. The large number of unmutated COVID-19 L sequences displaying the Hu-1 reference L sequence was also observed a month later in infected patients on board the *Grand Princess* cruise ship off the Californian coast (February 18–24, Figure 3).

S Haplotype Analysis of the China data

The typical sequences in the minor S Hap group, apart from outlier MT226610, are represented by:

MT049951, MT135041, MT135044, MT135042, MT135043, MT123292, MN975262, LR757995, MN938384.

The SNVs are: 1 T>C (shared by MT135041, MT135044, MT135042, MT135043); 1 G>T (8oxoG ? shared by MT135041, MT135044, MT135042, MT135043); 4 C>T (one shared with L Hap, thus hotspot? MN996531, MN975262; another shared MT123262, MN938384); 1 A>T; 1 G>A (shared between MT123292, and MT123 291 a L Hap variant, thus APOBEC hotspot?); 1 G>C; 1 T>A.

After an assumed L Hu-1 primary infection there is a group of four Beijing subjects sharing a S Hap pattern: MT135041, MT135044, MT135042, MT135043. This might be indicative of P-to-P in the second/third infection cycle as one of this group MT135043 has an additional unique SNV. The other five S Hap variants have 3, 3, 3, 1, 0 differences from Hu-1 with an additional possible P-to-P transfer (MN975<->MN938384).

However, as we highlighted in our *Caveats* section, much unknown information limits the scope of this analysis i.e. "Who met who" or "Who most likely gave the COVID-19 variant to whom?" For the limited set of S Hap variants there is evidence of P-to-P, and additional layers of deaminase-driven mutagenesis after transfer on top of the putative L to S switch. It is conceivable that on first infection with Hu-1 the sequences in MT135041, MT135042, MT135043 were shared by P-to-P transfer. It is further conceivable that other S Hap variants were also created in the first infection in the putative quasi-species L pool, namely MT123292, MN195262, LR757995, MN938384, with transfer between MN195262<->MN938384 and other unknown recipients (i.e. those not in our collection). Thus, three of the four S Hap variants appear to be created *in vivo* during a putative L>S deaminase-driven riboswitch then P-to-P transfer creating MN195262<->MN938384 sequences.

Conclusions on SNV Differences from Presumed Source Virus Hu-1

Understanding what happened in the early phase of the COVID-19 pandemic at its agreed epicentre in Wuhan city and regions is important to understand before analysing the further spread of the virus during the pandemic to other countries. Most COVID-19 isolates display the unmutated sequence of the L Hu-1 reference virus. Smaller numbers display 1 to 4 SNV differences from L Hu-1. The SNVs at position "63" look like independent deamination events at a hot spot as they are of different haplotypes (MT123291, MT123292).

These mutagenic patterns in Hu-1 are consistent with host-derived deaminase-mediated mutation signatures at the Wuhan epicentre and wider Hubei region and neighbouring provinces. Among the other unknowns we have no estimate of the *magnitude of the infective dose* from the source COVID-19 virus in Wuhan/Hubei. As suggested, the many unmutated sequences might infer Wuhan patients were older co-morbids who failed to adequately mount defensive deaminase-mediated innate immunity. However, this interpretation is speculative without knowing patient outcomes, and patient-patient relationship for P-to-P inferences (as previously discussed). Thus, it is important to conduct further analysis of this pattern at the explosive epicentre of the COVID-19 outbreak to hopefully inform the analysis of later outbreaks elsewhere in the USA and Europe.

The sequence MT226610 is a clear outlier. It has 27 SNVs compared with the Hu-1 reference and is of the S Hap group.It may represent serial mutagenic episodes (relapsing under clinical treatment) in one patient. The other interpretation is that it is the product of multiple (x8-x9) P-to-P chain transfers of infection with additional layers of mutations laid down during each infection prior to the next transfer. If so, this sequence could be an immune 'escape variant' well on the way to immune evasion and thus higher 'virulence' (?). If the latter is correct, we should note that we have not seen it crop up again in the sample sets we have analysed in Spain and USA. Alternatively, as suggested by a reviewer, the sequence is an artefact of poor assembly and sequencing.

3. Analyses of sporadic early USA outbreaks in California and *Grand Princess* cruise ship Jan 22–Mar 4

The early appearance of COVID-19 in the USA began in California and Washington State, and particularly the sharp outbreak on the *Grand Princess* cruise ship (off the coast of San Francisco which occurred mid to late Feb with swab collections Feb 18–24). This early appearance in the USA West coast, instance California and Washington State prior to any significant infections in the rest of the USA (Figures S1, S3) is reminiscent of the early time course of the pandemic spread to the USA from a similar China-originating pandemic outbreak of influenza H3N2 in 1968 in the USA (Figure S6). For this reason, we have decided to conduct a detailed COVID-19 sequence analysis of isolates of the sporadic and smaller scale USA West coast outbreaks that occurred before significant outbreaks in Europe and New York city.

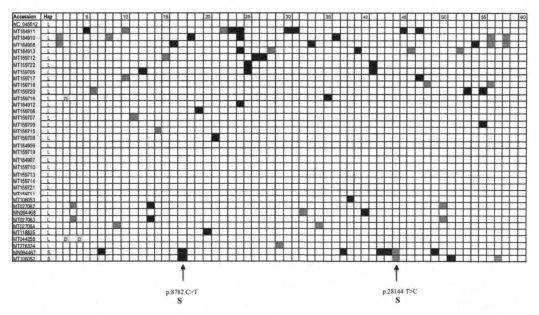

Figure 3 Variable Site Diagram of SNV in each aligned sequence in the 36 CA + Cruise Ship sequence alignment (Jan 22–Feb24) which includes Hu-1 ref NC_045512.2. Variable site number across the top, and Sequence ID down left hand side and Haplotype. The SNV key with respect to putative impact on protein structure of each SNV is discussed in text and Figure 1. S Hap sites are indicated for sites 17 and 44 and arrowed (and see Table 2). Cruise Ship Accession IDs are in orange highlight and grouped. The data in Table S2 should be consulted for further details. The variable site column number followed by SNV position in the alignment are: 1, p.254, C>T, 5'UTR; 2, p.508–522, GHVM in-frame deletion; 3, p.614, G>A; 4, p.686–694, KSF in-frame deletion; 5, p.1063, C>T; 6, p.1385, C>T; 7, p.1548, G>A; 8, p.1911, C>T; 9, p.2091, C>T; 10, p.3099, C>T; 11, p.3259, G>T; 12, p.3738, C>T; 13, p.5084, A>G; 14, p.5845, A>T; 15, p.6636, C>T; 16, p.8312, A>T; 17, p.8782, C>T; 18, p.9157, T>C; 19, p.9474, C>T; 20, p.9924, C>T; 21, p.10036, C>T; 22, p.10083, C>T; 23, p.10507, C>T; 24, p.11083, G>T; 25, p.11410, G>A; 26, p.11750, C>T; 27, p.11956, C>T; 28, p.12513, C>T; 29, p.14718, G>T; 30, p.15193, G>C; 31, p.15810, C>T; 32, p.17000, C>T; 33, p.20988, T>C; 34, p.21710, C>T; 35, p.22033, C>A; 36, p.22104, G>T; 37, p.24034, C>T; 38, p.24325, A>G; 39, p.25587, C>T; 40, p.26144, G>T; 41, p.26326, C>T; 42, p.26729, T>C; 43, p.28077, G>C; 44, p.28147 (= p.28144 "S" site), T>C; 45, p.28253, C>T; 46, p.28367, C>T; 47, p.28381, G>T; 48, p.28409, C>T; 49, p.28792, A>T; 50, p.28854, C>T; 51, p.28878, G>A; 52, p.28916, G>A; 53, p.29230,C>T; 54, p.29596, A>T; 55, p.29635, C>T; 56, p.29736, G>T, 3'UTR; 57, p.29742, G>A, 3'UTR; 58, p.29751, G>C, 3'UTR.

Analysis of the Alignment of 35 Sequences from VSD Figure 3

In this alignment there are 58 variable sites. For the CDS region there are 54 variable sites. Of the 35 sequences, 33 are of L Haplotype — 25 are on the Cruise Ship, 8 on CA mainland and 2 are of the S Haplotype, both on the CA mainland. The break-down of the types of SNV are shown in Table 3b. Again C>T(U) transitions dominate the data set and the strand bias pattern is very similar to the China data (Table 3a) with the same implications as discussed. Far fewer A-site mutations are evident in these data, but appear strand balanced.

L Haplotype Analysis — e.g. Cruise Ship v CA Mainland

Among sequences in the major L Hap group there are 50 unique variable sites. Two are in-frame deletions, one shared between MT159716 and MT044258 suggestive of possible P-to-P transfer between these two subjects. Nine of 25 Cruise L sequences are identical to Hu-1 reference i.e. unmutated. No mainland L Hap sequences are unmutated. For the Cruise Ship the distribution of the number of SNV differences per sequence from Hu-1 for zero difference to 9 per sequence are 9, 6, 3, 2, 0, 1, 1, 1, 0, 9; for the CA mainland the corresponding numbers are 0, 3, 2, 2 1, 0, 0, 1, 0, 0. The two shared sequences on the CA Mainland suggestive of P-to-P are between MT027062<-->MT027063. Similarly, Cruise Ship passengers MT159722 and MT159705 display evidence of sequence sharing and P-to-P transfer of MT159722 to MT159705. The common in-frame deletion p.686–694 suggests some earlier P-to-P transfer connecting MT159716 (Cruise Ship) and MT044258 (CA Mainland). It is also conceivable that Cruise Ship sequences MT184910 and MT184908 are derived (by P-to-P) from a common ancestral sequence as they have identical SNVs in the 5' and 3' UTRs. However, to qualify, in these cases the UTR changes maybe at putative riboswitch hotspots and thus indicative of an emerging new deaminase and ROS driven haplotype seeking to be established? It is observations like this that suggest that sequencers should aim for complete full length genome sequences that include both 5' UTR and 3' UTR regions (as is the case for the Hu-1 reference sequence).

Overall, the "quasi-species" acute phase infection pattern seen *in vivo* in individual subjects infected with a positive strand RNAv iruses (e.g. as shown by Figure 2 in Stoddard *et al.* 2015 for HCV), is now observed in the population of COVID-19 infected individuals (see Figures 2, 3). This is supported by our observation that MT184910<->MT184908 share three putative riboswitch changes in 5' and 3' UTRs (p.254, p.29736, p.29751 with further possible deaminase-mediated and ROS 8oxoG mutagenesis in both subjects during their separate infections with COVID-19.

On the Cruise ship the cases with putative evidence of P-to-P sequence sharing with further layers of deamination mutations in transferred infection appears evident e.g. MT159722<->MT159705, and MT159716 ship<->MT044258 mainland. On the CA Mainland two shared sets of mutations are suggestive of P-to-P between MT027062<--> MT027063. Finally, as noted MT184910<->MT184908 shared putative 5' and 3' UTR riboswitch variants.

Both S Hap variants are CA Mainland-derived carrying 4 and 7 differences from Hu-1 (the differences between the S Hap members, MN994467, MT106052). The other CA Mainland subjects display the sets of apparently random array of differences from Hu-1 per sequence (above). As with the China data (Figure 2) from 2 to 4 differences from Hu-1 in the first infection with L Hu-1 sequence seems to be the norm. The outlier

MT184911 on the Cruise ship suggests that up to 9 differences can accrue in a single sequence, although the precursor sequence for this variant appears to be MT159718, based on P-to-P transfer to MT184911 and then producing the additional 7 SNV variants in that sequence during that subjects innate immune response to the virus.

In the L Hap alignment the distribution of largely deaminase driven SNVs is approximately, 29x C>T (4 are shared), 5x G>A (2 are shared), 11x G>T (8 are shared and putative 8oxoG G>T at W<u>G</u> sites are noted possibles), 3x (G>C (2 are shared), 3x A>T, 2x A>G (shared), 2x T>C plus two in-frame deletions of codons in the two S Hap sequences 1x A>T, 2x T>C (shared), 3x C>T (2 shared), 3x G>A and 1x G>C.

Conclusions on CA + Cruise Ship Data (Jan 22–Feb 24)

Among COVID-19 patients sequenced on the Cruise Ship we observe no mutational evidence of P-to-P spread at the height of this localised epidemic outbreak. From the limited data of confirmed cases this also applies to the surrounding CA Mainland region. Most COVID-19 positive subjects appear to be infected with the same viral strain viz. the putative Hu-1 ref initiated by "community spreads" with no obvious Patient X. This conclusion is again consistent with the phylogenetic analysis by K. Anderson in January 2020 during the exponential rise in COVID-19 cases in Wuhan (Anderson 2020).

So, the conclusions here are strikingly similar to the far larger outbreak in Wuhan, China. Most are unmutated representatives of the L Hu-1 reference virus. Smaller numbers display from 1 to 4 differences from L Hu-1. Although the sample size is small, the proportion of the S Hap variant is just 2 out of 35 sequences (at canonical p.8782 and p.28144 that define L>S as in Tang *et al.* 2020); this compares with an estimated 20% S Haplotype in China (Figure 2).

In Summary again, as in the China data analyses, these mutagenic patterns in Hu-1 are indicative of host-derived deaminase-mediated mutation signatures, particularly striking in the case of the *Grand Princess* cruise ship outbreak (where location at sea at outbreak is defined). Low mutation, low P-to-P spread (although some have likely occurred in 1 or 2 step transfers). The many unmuted sequences on the cruise ship might infer again that patients were older co-morbids who failed to adequately mount defensive deaminase-mediated innate immunity. But we believe that the data show that transfers between a couple can be inferred. That all these patients with unmuted Hu-1 sequences maybe of Chinese ethnicity can also only be inferred.

4. Analyses of sporadic USA outbreaks in California mainland February 27–March 4, 2020

Analysis of the Alignment of 24 CA sequences from VSD Figure 4

The VSD pattern for the California outbreaks Feb 27–Mar 4 are displayed in Figure 4 sorted into the two main haplotypes, L and Sa. Again, quasi-species type variants carrying about 4 SNV randomly distributed variants from either Hu-1 or the Sa haplotype are noted (with limited putative P-to-P sequence sharing e.g.

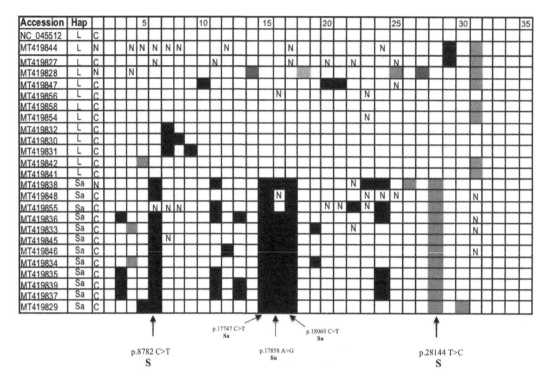

Figure 4 Variable Site Diagram of SNV in each aligned sequence in the 24 CA sequence alignment (Feb 27–Mar 4) which includes Hu-1 ref NC_045512.2. Variable site number across the top, and Sequence ID down left hand side and Haplotype. The SNV key with respect to putative impact on protein structure of each SNV is discussed in text and Figure 1. S Hap sites are indicated for sites 6 and 28, and Sa subsites defined by p.177747, p.17858, p.18060 and arrowed (and see Table 2). A screen shot record of flanking sequences around each SNV in codon-context was made, and this record used to construct the pattern in Figure 4. In some cases an N or N run created uncertainty, and this is recorded here as N to reflect the quality of the sequencing in this batch of complete genomes uploaded to NCBI Virus. This qualification allows assessment of assignment of variable site 16, p.17858, A>G for MT419855 — it should be "G" by Haplotype imputation at this position. However, the generally poor sequence of MT419855 (many N runs) suggest that this assignment is in likely error as well. The variable site column number followed by SNV position in the alignment are: 1, p.241, Hu-1 ref is C, some are N, so most are unlikely of L241 Hap; 2, p.3046, A>G; 3, p.5184, C>T; 4, p.7798, G>T; 5, p.7815, C>T; 6, p.8782, C>T; 7, p.9924, C>T; 8, p.9951, C>T; 9, p.15641, A>C; 10, p.16240, G>A; 11, p.16467, A>G; 12, p.16679, C>T; 13, p.16975, G>T; 14, p.17725, A>G; 15, p.17747, C>T; 16, p.17858, A>G; 17, p.18060, C>T; 18, p.19169, T>C; 19, p.20148, C>T; 20, p.21796, G>A; 21, p.21838, T>C; 22, p.22139, G>T; 23, p.23014, A>G; 24, p.23185, C>T; 25, p.24989, C>A; 26, p.25468, T>C; 27, p.28117, A>G; 28, p.28144, T>C; 29, p.28178, G>T; 30, p.29253, C>T; 31, p.29711, G>T, 3' UTR — possibly 8oxoG ROS product at W<u>G</u> hotspot and thus potential riboswitch?

MT419832◇MT419830◇MT419831; MT419833◇MT419834; MT419836◇MT419835◇ MT419839◇MT419837). The Sa haplotype differs from the S haplotype detected in China (or earlier on the CA Mainland) by coordinated SNV changes seen at p.17747 (C>T), p.17858 (A>G) and p.18060 (C>T) — all these SNVs involve conserved changes (or lack of change) at the amino acid level, and because of their common strain status qualify as riboswitched haplotype changes within the S haplotype (as discussed, Table 2).

The types of SNV are displayed in Table 3c. and are similar to other collections discussed (Table 2), C>T changes dominate, on the +ve RNA strand.

5. Analyses of the outbreak in Washington State, Kirkland, Nursing Home Outbreak near Seattle February 27–March 1, 2020

This is a small alignment (extracted from a larger alignment) relevant to the early spread pattern in the USA (Figure S6) up to and including collections Mar 4. It involved targeted collections and sequencing in the Seattle area. The tabulated data is in Table S3 and a data summary is recounted here.

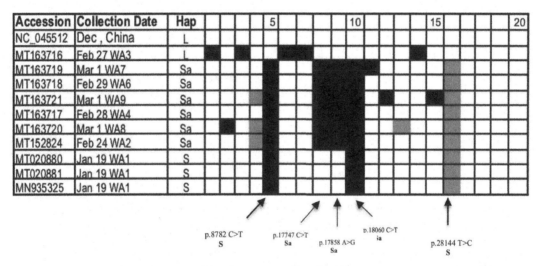

Figure 5 Variable site plot of SNV in each aligned sequence in the 10 sequence alignment for the WA State outbreak Feb 27–Mar 1 2020 versus the Hu-1 ref NC_045512.2. Variable site number across the top, and Sequence ID down left hand side and Haplotype. The SNV key with respect to putative impact on protein structure of each SNV is discussed in text and Figure 1. S, and Sa Hap designations as indicated and arrowed (and see Table 2) and tabulated data in TableS3. This alignment was part of the larger alignment done for Figure 4. Putative (speculated) P-to-P transfers are shown in Figure 6, including the Patient X, MN985325, the first case nCo-2019 in the United States collected Jan 19 2020; the others are the same virus from culture isolates (MT020880, MT020881). The variable site column number followed by SNV position in the alignment are: 1, p.2446, T>C; 2, p.3406, A>C; 3, p.5573, G>T; 4, p.5782, C>T; 5, p.8782, C>T; 6, p.11083,G>T; 7, 14085, C>T; 8, p.17747, C>T; 9, p.17858, A>G; 10, p.18060, C>T; 11, p.20282, T>C; 12, p.20580, G>T; 13, p.23528, C>T; 14, p.26147, G>T; 15, p.26733, G>A; 16, p.28147 (read as .28144), T>C.

The Kirkland nursing home outbreak was widely reported in the media, occurring more or less at the same time in late February as the California outbreaks and involving the at-Sea cruise ship *Grand Princess* just analysed. A Variable Site Analysis diagram is shown in Figure 5.

It is evident that P-to-P transfers have occurred as Patient X (WA1) appears, from all our previous analyses, to be a patient who was infected with the L_{Hu-1} reference virus sequence which underwent a L>S>Sa haplotype switch at the two canonical S-sites, as well as the additional three sites at p.17747, p.17858, p.18060. In this targeted, University of Washington sequencing analysis of COVID-19 patients, we can construct putative patient-to-patient transfers of the virus which lays down a further small number (about 2–3 further mutations in each infection) a pattern typical of quasi-species with mutations away from the L_{Hu-1} reference virus sequence. Thus all the data in Figure 5 can be logically explained in terms of haplotype switching, P-to-P transfers and then largely deaminase-mediated mutagenesis, that together lay down further mutational signatures in each productive infection (there are also some putative ROS 8oxoG or G>T changes that can be identified).

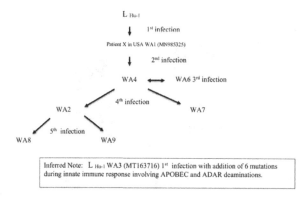

Figure 6. Putative P-to-P Transmissions in Kirkland Outbreak.

Possible P-to-P transfer chains inferred from Figure 5.

6. Analyses of COVID-19 complete genomes collected mainly in Spain Feb 26–Mar 5, Mar 6–10, 2020

The variable site patterns of one of two alignments of sequences largely from Spain collected Mar 6–Mar 10 are shown in Figure 7. The haplotype variations from S as Ss is shown, including the L241c variation observed in Spain but not so much NYC (below). Apart from the small numbers of unique SNV positions there is very little mutation away from the main haplotype group.Presumably, the collections were targeted on known groups suffering disease. However, the Ss haplotype assignment appears solid. It was observed with little further mutations also a week earlier in another set of Spain collections (involving an alignment of MT233519, MT233520, MT233521, MT233522, MT233523, MT198653, MT198651, MT198652). The types of SNVs are summarised in Table 3d, revealing a pattern that is similar to all other collections with a dominance of C-site deaminations on the +ve strand (C>U/G>A) over A-site deaminations, and more or less balanced to both +ve and -ve strands.

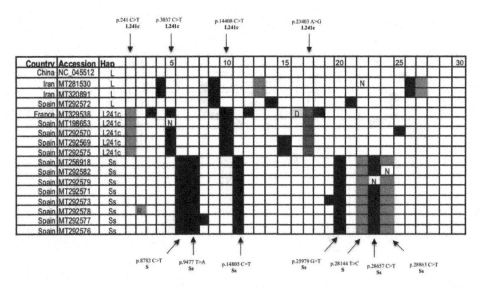

Figure 7 Variable site plot of SNV in each aligned sequence in a 17 sequence alignment for mainly Spain (13 sequences) versus the Hu-1 ref NC_045512.2. Variable site number across the top, and Sequence ID down left hand side and Haplotype assignment. The SNV key with respect to putative impact on protein structure of each SNV is discussed in text and Figure 1. L, L-241, S, and Ss Hap designations as indicated and arrowed (see Table 2). The variable site column number followed by SNV position in the alignment are: 1, p.241, C>T; 2, p.242,244, G>T, C>T; 3, p.618, A>G; 4, 1397, G>A; 5, p.3037, C>T; p.8782, C>T; 7, p.9477, T>A; 8, p.10156, C>T; 9, p.11083, G>T; 10, p.14408, C>T; 11, p.14805, C>T; 12, p.15324, C>T; 13, p.18377, C>T; 14, p.18835, T>C; 15, p.20268, A>G; 16, p.21880, in-frame deletion; 17, p.23403, A>G; 18, p.24025, A>G; 19, p.24928, G>T; 20, p.25979, G>T; 21, p.26144, G>T; 22, p.28144, T>C; 23, p.28657, C>T; 24, p.28863, C>T; 25, p.29144, C>T; 26, p.29374, G>A; 27, p.29742, G>T, 3'UTR.

7. Analyses of COVID-19 complete genomes collected in New York Mar 5–9

The genomes of a small number of collections for COVID-19 sequencing in New York Mar 5–9 just prior to the exponential increase in cases (from about March 14 onwards) were aligned against the Hu-1 reference. The VSD pattern is shown in Figure 8, and the types of SNV recorded in Table 3e. It appears that overt COVID-19 cases were targeted for sequencing and that the sample is clinically biased. The genomes appear harvested from small groups of subjects where putative P-to-P transfers was suspected — several groups share a common COVID-19 sequence with additional unique SNVs added following transfer to suspected recipients. For example, MT143800 may have transferred its COVID-19 sequence to MT434786, with one additional SNV added. In the L Hap group of sequences (MT434807, MT434787, MT434783, MT434784) putative transfers may have been MT434787-> MT434783<>MT434784 with a further additional 2–4 unique SNVs laid down after transfer. The common SNVs in four sequences at sites 17 (p.148805, C>T, synonymous Tyr<>Tyr) and 18 (p.17247, T>C, synonymous Arg<>Arg) could suggest both P-to-P transfers and/or deamination hot spot changes.

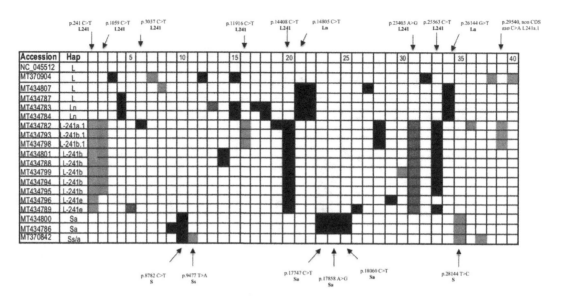

Figure 8 Variable site plot of SNV in each aligned sequence in an 18 sequence alignment for collections New York Mar 5–9 versus the Hu-1 ref NC_045512.2. Variable site number across the top, and Sequence ID down left hand side and Haplotype. The SNV key with respect to putative impact on protein structure of each SNV is discussed in text and Figure 1. L, S, and Sa Hap designations are indicated (see Table 2) and the main S and L haplotype sites are in sites 10 and 35. The other main sites for the L241 haplotypes (Table 2) are also highlighted in bold and arrowed. The variable site column number followed by SNV position in the alignment are: **1, p.241, C>T**; **2, p.1059, C>T**; 3, p.1397, G>A; 4, p. 1625, C>T; 5, p.2592, C>A; **6, p.3037**, C>T; 7, p.3242, G>A; 8, p.5730, C>T; 9, p.6639, A>G; 10, p.8782, C>T; 11, p.9477, T>A; 12, p.9514, A>G; 13, p.10155, A>G; 14, p.10851, C>T; 15, p.11083/11080, G>T; **16, 11916, C>T**; 17, p.12992, C>T; 18, p.13265, A>T; 19, p.13536, C>T; **20, p.14408, C>T**; 21, p.14805, C>T; 22, p.17237, T>C; 23, p.17747, C>T; 24, p.17858, A>G; 25, p.18060, C>T; 26, p.18877, C>T; 27, p.18985, G>T; **28, p.18998, C>T**; 29, p.20268, A>G; 30, p.21846, C>T; **31, p.23403, A>G**; 32, p.25215, C>T; **33, p.25563, G>T**; 34, p.26144, G>T; 35, p.28144, T>C; 36, p.28989, A>T; 37, p.28863, C>T; 38, p.29027, G>T; **39, p.29540, G>A, non-CDS gap**; 40, p.29742, G>T, 3'UTR. Note that sequence MT370842 was collected Mar 4, and sequence MT370904 was collected Feb 29.

Overall the numbers of common and unique SNVs among the L group is similar to that observed in the Wuhan outbreak and the earlier outbreaks on the West coast USA (CA + Cruise ship). Among the L-241 haplotype series there are also examples of P-to-P transfers and further additions of SNVs after transfer. Novel unique mutations per infection are low (but MT370904 has no SNV from the Hu-1 L sequence) as observed earlier for first or second infections (2-6 SNVs per sequence per P-to-P transfer). Again C>T transition SNVs on the +ve strand dominate the sample numbers (Table 3e).

8. Analyses of COVID-19 complete genomes collected in New York Mar 14–22
The genomes of 206 COVID-19 subjects were selected for the period Mar 14–22. A screen shot tabulation was created of alignments against Hu-1 in approximate groups of

10. It was noted, in an initial survey, that most sequences were of the L-241 haplotype with the distinctive C>T at p.241 in the 5' UTR Our analyses of NY sequences during the explosive exponential rise of confirmed COVID-19 cases proceeded in several steps. We separately assess the types of L and S haplotypes in these 206 sequences. We analysed 16 L + S sequences that were clearly not of the L-241 haplotype. We then analysed a sample of the first 58 in sequences in their temporal order of curation/upload to NCB Virus.

8a. Analysis of L and S Haplotype derivatives collected in New York Mar 14–22
The VSD pattern for the set of these 16 sequences, seven S and nine L is displayed in Figure 9. The types of SNV are tabulated in Table 3f. Among L we only see the Ln variant haplotype, defined by SNVs from Hu-1 at p.11080/83, p.14805, p.26144 (Table 2). The Wuhan L variant is not seen in this sample, unlike the week earlier. Thus, Ln is the dominant haplotype and likely sharing of sequences are evident e.g. MT370852, MT370866, MT370903, indicative of P-to-P transfers. However little further mutation is observed on transfer.

Similar P-to-P patterns are evident among MT370971, MT370973, MT370980. In addition, the quasi-species type patterns of apparently random SNVs are also evident in these data — as commented on above for the Wuhan and Cruise Ship patterns (Figures 2, 3).

Among S Haplotype mutational derivatives, the S in Spain (Ss) is found in one case (MT370985). Other examples of sequence sharing (P-to-P) among S are evident in these data.

8b. Analysis of a sample of 58 sequences collected in New York Mar 14–19
The VSD pattern for the set of these 58 sequences, grouped by Haplotype is displayed in Figure 10, and the tabulated data in Table S4. The types of SNV are shown in Table 3g. The striking pattern of apparent mutational diversity compared with the that in Wuhan is apparent. In Wuhan there was a dominant, largely unmutated (or lightly mutated) L haplotype of the Hu-1 sequence (Figure 2). The pattern in New York in the exponential phase is complex and diverse. However, as discussed above, the great bulk of this diversity resides at key sites that determine the main haplotypes (Table 2), particularly for the L-241 series haplotypes, and some L-241a Hap which is dominant (much like the L in Wuhan). As discussed already the L and S haplotypes form a minor component of the NY variable site pattern (Figure 9). The L-241b Hap which was the major one present in the small sample in NY in the week before case numbers began to explode (Figure 8) has been replaced in this sample, by L-241a which was a minor haplotype identified in that earlier period.

Whilst there are some cases of sharing of sequences (putative P-to-P transfers), an important finding is that the L-241a haplotype set (defined by changes from Hu-1, at p.241, p.1059, p.3037, p.14408, p.23403 and p.25563) has a very low number of mutations. If P-to-P transfers are ongoing then the recipients are not laying down a significant deaminase-mutagenic pattern in their own infection prior to transfer as one might expect given the nature of the deaminase driven host-parasite relationship. This

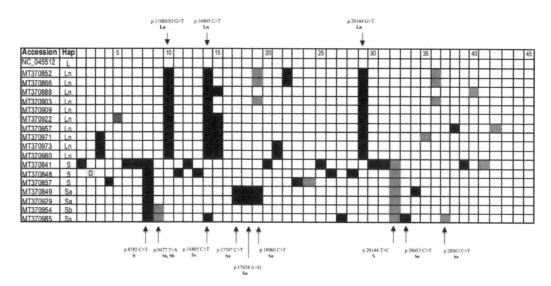

Figure 9 Variable site plot of SNV in each aligned sequence in a 16 sequence alignment for collections New York Mar 5–9 versus the Hu-1 ref NC_045512.2 focusing on L and S haplotype derivatives. Variable site number across the top, and Sequence ID down left hand side and Haplotype. The SNV key with respect to putative impact on protein structure of each SNV is discussed in text and Figure 1. L, S Hap designations as indicated (see Table 2) and the main S and L haplotype sites are indicated (site in bold and arrowed) — for S p.8782 site 8, p.28144 site 32; for Ln sites p.11080/83 site 10, p.14805 site 14, p.26144 site 29. The variable site column number followed by SNV position in the alignment are: 1, p.490, T>A; 2, p.1600–1616, in frame deletion LNDNL; 3, p.1625, C>T; 4, p.2676, C>T; 5, p.2745, A>T; 6, p.3177, C>T; 7, p.6040, C>T; **8, p.8782, C>T; 9, p.9477, T>A; 10, p.11080/83, G>T;** 11, p.12274, G>A; 12, p.12478, G>A; 13, p.13115, C>T; **14, p.14805, C>T;** 15, p.17247, T>C; **16, p.17747, C>T; 17, p.17858, A>G; 18, p.18060, C>T;** 19, p.18086, C>T; 20, p.18735, T>C; 21, p.19166, A>G; 22, p.21137, A>G; 23, p.22606, A>T; 24, p.23525, C>T; **25, p.24034, C>T;** 26, p.25541, T>C; **27, p.25979, G>T;** 28, p.26087, C>T; **29, p.26144, G>T;** 30, p.26729, T>C; 31, p.28077, G>C; **32, p.28144, T>C; 33, p.28657, C>T;** 34, p.28708, C>T; 35, p.28739, G>T; 36, p.28842, G>T; **37, p.28863, C>T;** 38, p.28878, G>A; 39, p.28896, C>G; 40, p.29543, G>C, non-CDS gap; 41, p.29700, A>G, 3'UTR; 42, p.29742, G>A, 3'UTR.

could be the result of dysregulated interferon gene expression (suppression) as has been recently observed in COVID-19 patients (Acharya *et al.* 2020, Blanco-Melo *et al.* 2020, Hadjadj *et al.* 2020). This is an interesting possibility and may explain why there is little or no evidence of a full innate immune response resulting in deaminase mutagenic signatures.

There are a small number of putative ROS mediated 8oxoG modifications found at W<u>G</u> sites that may contribute to the G>T SNVs. Thus, 6 of the L-241a Hap set are unmutated from Hu-1 (MT370845, MT370865, MT370867, MT370872, MT370873, MT370877; 8 within this haplotype set have one SNV difference from Hu-1 viz. MT370834, MT370836, MT370838, MT370843, MT370876, MT370881, MT370884,

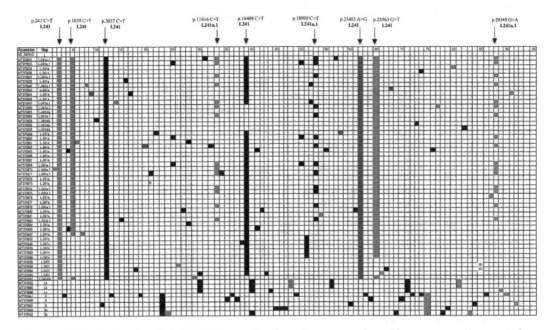

Figure 10 Variable site plot of SNV in each aligned sequence in a 58 sequence alignment for collections New York Mar 14 – 19 versus the Hu-1 ref NC_045512.2. Variable site number across the top, and Sequence ID down left hand side and Haplotype. The source data is in the tabulation in Table S4. The SNV key with respect to putative impact on protein structure of each SNV is discussed in text and Figure 1. L, S Hap and L-241 subset Hap designations as indicated (see Table 2). The variable site column number followed by SNV position in the alignment are in order with the L-241 sites listed in Table 2 in bold and arrowed. Ln, S, Sa, Sb, Ss already summarised for NYC collection as in Figure 9. Other features whether in UTR, non-CDS region or G>T most likely caused by oxidation of G (8oxoG) are added given the complexity of the data set: 1, p.199, G>T, 5'UTR; **2, p.241, C>T, 5' UTR**; 3, p490, T>A; 4, p.619, C>T; **5, p.1059, C>T**; 6, 1820, G>A; 7, p.1917, C>T; 8, 2091, C>T; 9, p.2165, A>G; 10, 2632, G>T, 8oxoG at W<u>G</u>; 11, p.2676, C>T; **12, p.3037, C>T**; 13, 3175, T>A; 14, p.4035, T>C; 15, p.4113, C>T; 16, p.4456, C>T; 17, p.4810, C>T; 18, p.5140, C>T; 19, p.6040, C>T; 20, p.6324, A>G; 21, 7291, A>G; 22, p.7770, A>G; **23, p.8782, C>T**; **24, p.9477, T>A**; 25, p.10015, C>T; 26, p.10265, G>A; 27, p.10369, C>T; 28, p.10851, C>T; 29, p.11003, C>T; **30, p.11083/80, G>T, 8oxoG at W<u>G</u>**; 31, 11101, A>G; 32, 11191, T>A; **33, p.11916, C>T**; 34, p.12153, C>T; 35, p.12274, G>A; 36, 12478, G>A; 37, 13110, C>T; 38, p.14104, T>C; **39, p.14408, C>T**; **40, p.14805, C>T**; 41, p.14912, A>G; 42, p.15324, C>T; 43, p.16293, C>T; 44, 17247, T>C; **45, p.17747, C>T**; **46, p.17858, A>G**; **47, p.18060, C>T**; 48, p.18086, C>T; 49, p.18736, T>C; 50, p.18744, C>T; 51, p.18877, C>T; 52, p.18988, C>T; **53, p.18998, C>T**; 54, p.20755, A>C; 55, p.20844, C>T; 56, p.21137, A>G; 57, p.21830, G>T, 80xoG at W<u>G</u>; 58, p.22455, A>G; 59, p.22468, G>T; 60, p.22606, A>T; 61, p.23284, T>C; **62, p.23403, A>G**; 63, p.24034, C>T; 64, p.25541, T>C; **65, p.25563, G>T, 8oxoG at W<u>G</u>**; 66, 25575, A>C; 67, 25644, G>T, 8oxoG at W<u>G</u>; 68, p.25688, C>A; 69, p.25979, G>T; 70, p.26088, C>T; **71, p.26144, G>T**; 72, p.26729, T>C; 73, p.28061, T>C; 74, p.28077, G>C; **75, p.28144, T>C**; 76, p.28199, T>C; 77, p.28472, C>T; **78, p.28657, C>T**; 79, p.28708, C>T; 80, p.28836, C>T; 81, p.28842, G>T, 8oxoG at W<u>G</u>; 82, p.28849, C>T; 83, p.28863, C>T; 84, p.28878, G>A; 85, p.28881-3, G>A, G>A, G>C; 86, p.28896, C>G; 87, p.29274, C>T; **88, p.29540. G>A, non-CDS gap**; 89, p.29543, G>C, non-CDS gap; 90, p.29700, A>G, 3'UTR; 91, p.29711, G>T, 8oxoG at W<u>G</u>, 3'UTR; 92, p.29742, G>A, 3'UTR.

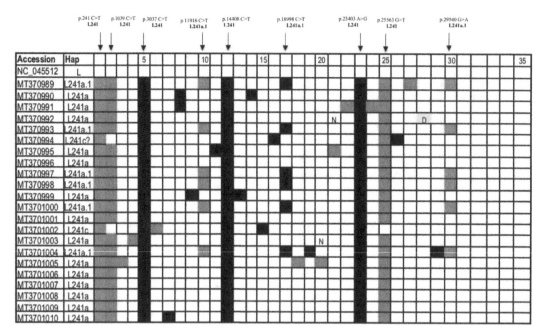

Figure 11 Variable site plot of SNV in each aligned sequence in a 22 sequence alignment for collections New York Mar 19–22 versus the Hu-1 ref NC_045512.2. Variable site number across the top, and Sequence ID down left hand side and Haplotype. The source data are from a screen shot record. The SNV key with respect to putative impact on protein structure of each SNV is discussed in text and Figure 1. L-241 and subset Hap designations as indicated (see Table 2). The variable site column number followed by SNV position in the alignment are in order with the L-241 sites listed in Table 2 in bold and arrowed. Other features whether in UTR, non-CDS region or G>T most likely caused by oxidation of G (8oxoG) are added given the complexity of the data set: **1, p.241, C>T, 5'UTR**; **2, p.1059, C>T**; 3, p.1917, C>T; 4, p.2222, T>C; **5, p.3037, C>T**; 6, p.4575, C>T; 7, p.10831, T>C; 8, p.10851, C>T; 9, p.11781, A>G; **10, p.11916, C>T**; 11, p.13548, C>T; **12, p.14408, C>T**; 13, p.16381, G>A; 14, p.18395, C>T; 15, p.18486, C>T; 16, p.18877, C>T; **17, p.18998, C>T**; 18, p.20005, G>A; 19, p.20553, A>G; 20, p.21458, T>C; 21, p.21485, G>T, 8oxoG at W$\underline{G}$ site?; 22, p.22530, C>T; **23, p.23403, A>G**; 24, p.25305, G>T, 8oxoG at W$\underline{G}$ site?; **25, p.25560/63, G>T, 8oxoG at W$\underline{G}$ site?**; 26, p.26681, C>T; 27, p.28115, T>C; 28, p.29367-29384, in-frame deletion (PTNPKKD); 29, p.28957, C>T; **30, p.29540, G>A, non-CDS gap near 3' UTR**.

MT370887; three have 2 SNV differences from Hu-1 (MT370859, MT370861, MT370885); and MT370880 and MT370863 have 3 and 4 SNV differences respectively.

There are also patterns within the VSD in Figure 10 showing probable P-to-P transfer of a lightly mutated sub-haplotype viz. defined by SNV differences from Hu-1 at p.11916, p.18998, and the change in the RNA only non-CDS gap at site p.29540 near the 3' end of the genome. Other cases of sequence conservation (L-241c) and likely sharing of sequences (indicative of P-to-P) and the addition of one SNV on transfer can be seen in the sequences MT370832, MT370846, MT370879, MT370883, MT370886.

The L-241d Hap set lacks the C>T SNV at p.14408. Even among this set there is very low further mutation, MT370853 is unmutated within the haplotype from Hu-1; and MT370858, MT370856, MT370855 have only one SNV difference from Hu-1 within the haplotype.

These patterns of very low mutation and sequence conservation among individual subjects is reminiscent of that observed in the major Wuhan epidemic, and on a smaller scale, on the *Grand Princess* cruise ship.

To further check on and confirm these observations of very low mutation and haplotype conservation a set of 22 sequences collected in NYC Mar 19–22 were aligned against Hu-1. The VSD plot is show in Figure 11. Once again, the L241a and variant L241a.1 are dominant members of this set. Five L241a sequences have no mutation (MT3701001, MT3701006, MT3701007, MT3701008, MT3701009) and the rest have one (MT3701010, MT3701003) or two to three mutations (MT370990, MT370995, MT3701005, MT370991). A similar haplotype mutation pattern applies to the L241a.1 subset, where four show no mutation (MT370997, MT370998, MT3701000, MT370993) and two one or two mutations (MT370989, MT3701004).

SUMMARY AND CONCLUSIONS

The mutational patterns presented here are for the origin of the COVID-19 virus (Dec–Jan 2020 China, mainly Wuhan), early spread to West Coast USA (mid to late February 2020), the exponential case rises in Spain (Mar 6–10, 2020), and New York just before (Mar 4–9, 2020) and during its key exponential rise in infections (Mar 14–19, 2020). The patterns evident within COVID-19 samples are thus for collections at key informative times and locations during the pandemic.

Our main finding has been the identification of a set of nucleotide sequence sites defining new COVID-19 RNA haplotypes — which have been created during the first infections with the Hu-1 sequence or its close relative. These key riboswitch sites (Table 2), in our view, are driven largely by the APOBEC and ADAR deaminases during the acute phase of infection in each individual: the virus varies largely at the RNA level, presumably to adjust its replicative efficacy to the biochemical and genetic background in which it finds itself. There is a surprising high level of sequence conservation in the functional status of the AA sequences in the mature proteins in the CDS mutations. As explained, the discovery of the generation of these haplotypes during the innate immune response to the virus, allows rational ordering of the data on COVID-19.

A reviewer has asked an important question, to paraphrase: "How likely is it that these apparent mild alterations in strain haplotypes are more adaptive, and could they contribute to conditions of P-to-P transmissions?" We have largely addressed this already — in epicenters during explosive outbreaks the "dominant" haplotype seems to be unmutated (or lightly mutated with largely synonymous changes). We have mentioned this may reflect in part the possible P-to-P sharing amongst vulnerable elderly co-morbids in a localised outbreak situation (nursing facility) of the *same unmutated sequence* (as they are expected to all have compromised or poor innate immune defences). As well as the examples we have seen already in Wuhan/China (Figure 2), the Californian cruise ship (Figure 3) and at the height of the NYC epidemic itself (Figure 10) we have also found a striking example of this phenomenon among a group of COVID-19 sequences collected on the same day, March 13 in Washington State and released as one upload batch on March 31 into NCBI Virus. These 21 sequences are MT262896-MT262916 inclusive. All of the Sa haplotype (Table 2). Nine have a synonymous T>C change at MC3 in a Tyrosine encoding UAU codon at p.11320. This could be a newly identified riboswitch generating a new P-to-P spreading haplotype on the Sa haplotype background? The only other changes are in MT262899 with a synonymous T>Cat p.13845; and in MT262915 a putative "benign" Non-Polar-to-Polar nonsynonymous G>T change at a W$\underline{G}$ site implying an 8oxoG modification. Otherwise, all other sequences are unmutated in relation to the Hu-1 reference. This is the most extreme example of this phenomenon uncovered and supports the implied speculation in the reviewer's question and thus adds to our understanding of how COVID-19 may spread in defined situations.

Our caveats are laid out — we lack clinical and patient data, nor do we have any evidence for dose at time of infections, particularly in the explosive epicentres of Wuhan and New York. We also do not have temporal COVID-19 sequence data for individual patients to identify virus sequence changes in a single host during the acute phase of infection. We can only make inferences about such matters. The striking difference between the diversity of haplotypes, and extent of SNV patterns, between COVID-19 sequence collections from patients in Wuhan/China versus New York is striking. In our view such patterns are consistent with the prediction of the deaminase-driven riboswitch RNA haplotype model that we have used to order the data on COVID-19. i.e. the incoming virus adapts by locking in an RNA haplotype suitable for rapid replication in that host cell under selection. We would expect the ethnic genetic diversity in New York City to far exceed almost pure Chinese genotypes in Wuhan and throughout China.

In our opinion, the implications for vaccine design should incorporate boosting innate immunity, for example by BCG vaccination as for the lung infection tuberculosis. This may involve the use of Interferons to stimulate deaminase expression during the acute stage of infection (Acharya *et al.* 2020), although further work is required. Since BCG is a widely accepted non-specific activator of innate immunity we might expect it to contribute to elevated APOBEC and ADAR expression and thus mutagenic attacks on the virus genome. Such vaccinations logically imply that innate immune responses, and boosting mutagenic APOBEC and ADAR levels could be an important part of vaccine design.

A legitimate question, posed by a reviewer has been whether we can systematically independently test the hypothesis or compare an array of evidence supporting or against the plausibility of the haplotype hypothesis. We therefore ask can we find situations where the "world set" of the main COVID-19 haplotypes in the Northern Hemisphere may be sampled by travellers coming into Australia? This is important as all outbreaks in Australia have been by travellers returning home from the Northern Hemisphere. Over the period of the pandemic Victoria, Australia has been the destination for Australians returning home as "COVID-19 refugees" from Northern Hemisphere locations in Europe,

China, USA. On arrival they have all been quarantined for two weeks to limit spread of the disease to local citizens. We ask: Are the main set of haplotypes as tabulated here (Table 2) evident among these incoming travellers from exposure to the Northern Hemisphere pandemic? First there is no real dominant haplotype among these COVID-19 +ve travellers to Victoria. The distribution of major haplotypes (Table 2) in these incoming travellers for the haplotypes L, Ln, L241a, L241c, L241f, S and Sa were 13, 19, 7, 11, 1, 11 and 15 a reflection of the main haplotypes in circulation in China, USA and Europe in this period (collections January 24–March 16 2020, MT450919-MT450995).

In follow up studies we plan to definitively identify the APOBEC and ADAR variants and isoforms responsible for the mutagenesis of the COVID-19 genome during the innate immune response phase in infected COVID-19 patients as demonstrated for HCV and ZIKV (Lindley and Steele 2018).

ACKNOWLEDGEMENTS

We thank N Chandra Wickramasinghe, Reginald M Gorczynski, Nathan E Hall, Jarod Mamrot and Pat Carnegie for discussions

CONFLICT OF INTEREST

The authors declare that no competing or conflict of interests exist. The funders had no role in study design, writing of the manuscript, or decision to publish.

AUTHORS' CONTRIBUTIONS

Both authors contributed equally to conceptualisation, analysis and writing of manuscript.

REFERENCES

Acharya, D., Liu, G-Q. and Gack, M.U. (2020) Dysregulation of type I interferon responses in COVID-19. *Nat. Rev. Immunol.* DOI https://doi.org/10.1038/s41577-020-0346-x

Alexandrov, L.B., Nik-Zainal, S., Wedge, D.C., Aparicio, S.A., Behjati, S., Biankin, A.V., *et al.* (2013) Signatures of mutational processes in human cancer. *Nature* **500**, 415–421. https://www.ncbi.nlm.nih.gov/pubmed/23945592

Andersen, K. (2020) Clock and TMRCA based on 27 genomes. Novel 2019 coronavirus. http://virological.org/t/clock-and-tmrca-based-on-27-genomes/347

Andino, R. and Domingo, E. (2015) Viral quasispecies. *Virology* 479–480, 46–51. DOI: 10.1016/j.virol.2015.03. 022

Blanco-Melo, D., Nilsson-Payant, B.E., Liu, W-C., Uhl, S., Hoagland, D., Møller, R., *et al.* (2020) Imbalanced Host Response to SARS-CoV-2 Drives Development of COVID-19. *Cell.* **181**, 1036–1045 May 28, 2020 a 2020 Elsevier Inc. https://doi.org/10.1016/j.cell.2020.04.026

Buhr, F., Jha, S., Thommen, M., Mittlestael, J., Kutz, F., Schwalbe, H., Rodina, M.V. and Komar, A.A. (2016) Synonymous codons direct cotranslational folding towards different protein conformations. *Mol. Cell.* **61**, 341–351. http://dx.doi.org/10.1016/j.molcel.2016.01.008

Dorp, L.V., Acman, M., Richard, D., Shaw, L.P., Ford, C.E., Ormond, L., *et al.* (2020a) Emergence of genomic diversity and recurrent mutations in SARS-CoV-2. *Infect. Genet. Evol.* **83**, 104351. https://doi.org/10.1016/j.meegid.2020.104351

Dorp, L.V., Richard, D., Tan, C.C.S., Shaw, L.P., Acman, M. and Balloux, F. (2020b) No evidence for increased transmissibility from recurrent mutations in SARS-CoV-2. BioRxiv reprint. doi: https://doi.org/10.1101/2020.05.21.108506 posted May 21, 2020

Eigen, M. and Schuster, P. (1979) The Hypercycle: A Principle of Natural Self-Organization. Springer, Berlin.

Eifler, T., Pokharel, S. and Beal, P.A. (2013) RNA-Seq analysis identifies a novel set of editing substrates for human ADAR2 present in Saccharomyces cerevisiae. *Biochemistry* **52**, 7857–7869. DOI: 10.1021/bi4006539

Franklin, A., Steele, E.J. and Lindley, R.A. (2020) A proposed reverse transcription mechanism for (CAG)n and similar expandable repeats that cause neurological and other diseases. *Heliyon* **6**, e03258. doi: 10.1016/j.heliyon.2020.e03258

Gilbert, S.D. and Lafontaine, R.T. (2006) Riboswitches: Fold and Function. *Chemistry & Biology* **13**, 857–868. https://doi.org/10.1016/j.chembiol.2006.08.002

Hadjadj, J., Yatim, N., Barnabei, L., Corneau, A., Boussier, J., Péré, H., *et al.* (2020) Impaired type I interferon activity and exacerbated inflammatory responses in severe Covid-19 patients medRxiv preprint. doi: https://doi.org/10.1101/2020.04.19.20068015

Korber, B., Fischer, W., Gnanakaran, S., Yoon, H., Theiler, J., Abfaltere, W., Hengartner, N., *et al.* (2020) Tracking changes in SARS-CoV-2 Spike: evidence that D614G increases infectivity of the COVID-19 virus, Cell In Press. doi: https://doi.org/10.1016/j.cell.2020.06.043

Li, H., Stoddard, M.B., Wang, S., Blair, L.M., Giorgi, E.E., Parrish, E.H., Learn, G.H., Hraber, P., Goepfert, P.A., Saag, M.S., *et al.* (2012) Elucidation of hepatitis C virus transmission and early diversification by single genome sequencing. *PLoS Pathog* **8**(8), e1002880. doi: 10.1371/journal.ppat.1002880

Lindley, R.A. (2013). The importance of codon context for understanding the Ig-like somatic hypermutation strand- biased patterns in TP53 mutations in breast cancer. *Cancer Genetics* **5**, 2619–2640. DOI: 10.1016/j.cancergen. 2013.05.016

Lindley, R.A. and Hall, N.E (2018) APOBEC and ADAR deaminases may cause many single nucleotide polymorphisms curated in the OMIM database. *Mutat. Res. Fund. Mol. Mech. Mutagen* **810**, 33–38. https://doi.org/10.1016/j.mrfmmm.2018.03.008

Lindley, R.A. and Steele, E.J. (2018) ADAR and APOBEC editing signatures in viral RNA during acute- phase Innate Immune responses of the host-parasite relationship to Flaviviruses. Research Reports 2: e1–e22. doi:10.9777/rr.2018.10325

Lindley, R.A., Humbert, P., Larmer, C., Akmeemana, E.H. and Pendlebury, C.R.R. (2016) Association between targeted somatic mutation (TSM) signatures and HGS-OvCa progression. *Cancer Med.* **5**, 2629–2640. DOI: 10.1002/cam4.825

Pirakitikulr, N., Kohlway, A., Lindenbach, B.D. and Pyle, A.M. (2016) The coding region of the HCV genome contains a network of regulatory RNA structures. *Mol. Cell.* **61**, 1–10. http://dx.doi.org/10.1016/j.molcel.2016.01.024

Sharma, S., Patnaik, S.K., Taggart, R.T., Kannisto, E.D., Enriquez, S.M., Gollnick, P. and Baysal, B.E. (2015) APOBEC3A cytidine deaminase induces RNA editing in monocytes and macrophages. *Nat. Commun.* **6**, 6881. doi: 10.1038/ncomms7881

Sharma, S., Santosh, K.. Patnaik, S.K., Kemera, Z. and Baysal, B.E. (2016a). Transient overexpression of exogenous APOBEC3A causes C-to-U RNA editing of thousands of genes. *RNA Biology* **5**, 1–8. doi: 10.1080/15476286.2016.1184387

Sharma, S., Patnaik, S.K., Taggart, R.T. and Basal, B.E. (2016b) The double-domain cytidine deaminase APOBEC3G is a cellular site-specific RNA editing enzyme. *Sci. Rep.* **6**, 39100. doi: 10.1038/srep39100 (2016)

Schneider, W.M., Chevillotte, M.D. and Rice, C.M. (2014) Interferon-stimulated genes: acomplex web of host defenses. *Annu. Rev. Immunol.* **232**, 513–545. doi:10.1146/annurev-immunol-032713-120231

Schoggins, J.W. and Rice, C.M. (2011) Interferon-stimulated genes and their antiviral effector functions. *Curr. Opin. Virol.* **1**, 519–525. doi: 10.1016/j.coviro.2011.10.008

Shi, Y., Wang, Y., Shao, C., Huang, J., Gan, J., Huang, X., *et al.* (2020) COVID-19 Infection: The Perspectives on Immune Responses. *Cell. Death Differ.* **27**, 1451–1454. doi: 10.1038/s41418-020-0530-3

Steele, E.J. and Lindley, R.A. (2017) ADAR deaminase A-to-I editing of DNA and RNA moieties of RNA: DNA Hybrids has implications for the mechanism of Ig somatic hypermutation. *DNA Repair* **55**, 1–6. doi: 10.1016/j.dnarep.2017.04.004

Stoddard, M.B., Li, H., Wang, S., Saeed, M., Andrus, L., Ding, W., Jiang, X., Learn, G.H., von Schaewen, M., Wen, J., Goepfert, P.A., Hahn, B.H., Ploss, A., Rice, C.M. and Shaw G.M. (2015) Identification, molecular cloning, and analysis of full-length hepatitis C virus transmitted/founder genotypes 1, 3, and 4. *mBio* **6**(2), e02518–14. doi: 10.1128/mBio.02518-14

Tan, Z., Zhang, W., Shi, Y. and Wang, F. (2015) RNA Folding: Structure Prediction, Folding Kinetics and Ion Electrostatics. *Adv. Exp. Med. Biol.* **827**: 143–83. doi: 10.1007/978-94-017-9245-5_11. PMID: 25387965

Tang, X., Wu, C., Li, X., Song, Y., *et al.* (2020) On the origin and continuing evolution of SARS-CoV-2. *National Science Review* (2020). nwaa036, https://doi.org/10.1093/nsr/nwaa036

Thimme, R., Binder, M. and Bartenschlager, R. (2012) Failure of innate and adaptive immune responses in controlling hepatitis C virus infection. *FEMS Microbiol. Rev.* **36**, 663–683. DOI: 10.1111/j.1574-6976.2011.00319.x

Widom, J.R. Nedialkov, Y.A., Rai, V., Hayes, R.L., Brooks,C.L., 3rd, Artsimovitch, I. and Walter, N.G. (2018) Ligand modulates cross-coupling between riboswitch folding and transcriptional pausing. *Mol. Cell.* **72**, 541–552.e6. doi: 10.1016/j.molcel.2018.08.046. PMID: 30388413

Yang, D. and Leibowitz, J.L. (2015) The structure and functions of coronavirus genomic 3′ and 5′ ends. *Virus Research* **206**, 120–133. https://doi.org/10.1016/j.virusres.2015.02.025

Implications of Haplotype Switching for the Origin and Global Spread of COVID-19

Edward J. Steele[1,2,3], Reginald M. Gorczynski [4], Herbert Rebhan[1], Patrick Carnegie[5], Robert Temple[6], Gensuke Tokoro[7], Alexander Kondakov[8], Stephen G. Coulson[7], Dayal T. Wickramasinghe[3,9] and N. Chandra Wickramasinghe[3,7,10,11]

[1]CYO'Connor ERADE Village Foundation, 24 Genomics Rise, Piara Waters, 6112

[2]Melville Analytics Pty Ltd, Melbourne, Vic, AUSTRALIA

[3]Centre for Astrobiology, University of Ruhuna, Matara, Sri Lanka

[4]University Toronto Health Network, Toronto General Hospital, University of Toronto, Toronto, ON, Canada

[5]School of Biological Sciences and Biotechnology, Murdoch University, WA, Australia

[6]History of Chinese Science and Culture Foundation Conway Hall, London, UK

[7]Institute for the Study of Panspermia and Astroeconomics, Gifu, Japan

[8]193/ Sinyavinskaya str 16/11, Moscow, Russia

[9]College of Physical and Mathematical Sciences, Australian National University, Canberra

[10]Institute of Fundamental Studies, Kandy, Sri Lanka.

[11]Buckingham Centre for Astrobiology, University of Buckingham, Buckingham, United Kingdom

Abstract

When analysed in patients at epicentres of outbreaks over the first three months of the 2020 pandemic, the virus responsible for COVID-19 cannot be classed as a rapidly mutating virus. It employs a haplotype-switching strategy most likely driven by APOBEC and ADAR cytosine and adenosine deamination events (C>U, A>I) at key selected sites in the ~ 30,000 nt positive sense single-stranded RNA genome (Steele and Lindley 2020). Quite early on (China, through Jan 2020) the main haplotype was L with a minor proportion of the S haplotype. By the time of the explosive outbreaks in New York City (mid-to late-March 2020) the haplotype variants expanded to at least 13. The COVID-19 genomes analysed at the main sites of exponential increases in cases and deaths over a 2 week time period (explosive epicentres) such as Wuhan and New York City showed limited mutation *per se* of the main haplotypes engaged in disease. When mutation was detected it was usually conservative in terms of significant alterations to protein structure. The coronavirus haplotypes whether in Wuhan, West Coast USA, Spain or New York differ by no more than 2-9 coordinated nucleotide changes and all genomes are thus ≥99.98% identical to each other. Further, we show that the most similar SARS-like CoV animal virus sequences (bats, pangolins) could not have caused the assumed zoonotic event setting off this explosive pandemic in Wuhan and regions: zoonotic causation via a Chinese wild bat SL-CoV reservoir jumping to humans by an intermediate amplifier (e.g. pangolins) is clearly not possible on the basis of the available data. We also discuss the evidence for airborne transmission of COVID-19 as the main infection route and highlight outbreaks on certain ships at sea consistent with their hypothesised cosmic origins. We conclude that the virus originated as a pure genetic strain in a life-bearing carbonaceous meteorite which was first deposited in the tropospheric jet stream over Wuhan. Over the next month or so this viral-laden dust cloud not only descended through the troposphere to target Wuhan and its environs, but was also transported in a Westerly direction through the mid-latitude northern jet stream causing explosive in-fall events sequentially over Iran, Italy, Spain and then New York City in the early months of the pandemic to the end of March 2020.

Keywords: Origin COVID-19 Pandemic • COVID-19 Haplotype Switching • Panspermia • Cosmic Adaptation

Introduction

The new coronavirus pandemic of 2019 causing severe acute respiratory syndrome (SARS-CoV-2) has been named COVID-19 by the World Health Organization. This newly emergent virus is related by RNA sequence similarity to the earlier pandemic SARS-CoV-1 (2002-2003). However, the genetic distance between the causative viruses is considerable, with sequence similarity of just 79.45%. This is equivalent to a difference of about 6000 single nucleotide variants accruing over a short evolutionary time period to account for the re-emergence of SARS-CoV-1 leading to the origin of the observed explosive outbreak of COVID-19 in the central China Wuhan region in December 2019.

*Corresponding authors: Dr. Edward J Steele, Melville Analytics Pty Ltd, Level 2, 517 Flinders Lane, Melbourne, VIC 3000, AUSTRALIA, E-mail, e.j.steele@bigpond.com; Professor N Chandra Wickramasinghe , Buckingham Centre for Astrobiology, University of Buckingham MK18 1EG, England, UK, Tel: +44 (0)2920752146/+44 (0)7778389243; E-mail: ncwick@gmail.com,

Received: July, 24 2020; Accepted: August 11, 2020; Published: August 15, 2020

DOI: 10.37421/vcrh.2020.4.135

https://www.hilarispublisher.com/open-access/implications-of-haplotype-switching-for-the-origin-and-global-spread-of-covid19-49285.html

Steele EJ et al.   Virol Curr Res, Volume 4: 2, 2020

Cosmic Origin Hypothesis for COVID-19

We have reviewed the range of evidence [1] consistent with the hypothesis that the virus arrived via a presumed life-bearing cometary bolide possibly, though not necessarily, linked to a fireball event seen over North-Central China on the night of 11 October 2019. A few weeks later a viral-laden dust cloud entered the tropospheric jet stream, thus leading to the explosive disease outbreaks in Wuhan city and surrounds in Hubei province China [1,2]. We can argue that this viral in-fall settling on property, people and animals (domestic and wild) was on a region-wide scale, thus igniting an almost synchronous epidemic epicentre over the ensuing weeks extending well into late January 2020 (Note : A report that COVID-19 emerged in Barcelona in March 2019 was in our view based on false positive evidence, Supplementary File A).

In this paper we review the evidence and critical arguments for and against theories of terrestrial origin (animal-to-human jump and also bioweapon release models) versus the wider array of evidence supporting a cosmic origin. We argue that our proposed model is compatible with all the known facts, genetic and immunological [3], epidemiological, temporal and geophysical [2,4-6]. It is also consistent with all previously documented astrophysical and astrobiological evidence which supports the idea of a spatially interconnected cosmic biology extending to the earliest origins of the known universe [7,8,9,10,11,12,13].

The fact that pathogenic viruses including SARS-CoV-2 are genetically adapted so as to attack particular evolved host species is often cited as evidence against their extraterrestrial origins. This criticism ceases to be valid if we take account of an interconnected cosmic biosphere with genetic exchanges taking place over astronomical distances and timescales. In such a schema the host-parasite adaptation becomes an artefact of a cosmically connected evolutionary process [10,11,13].

We next focus attention on the recently reported genetic data of COVID-19 which shows that the virus does not "rapidly mutate" as is popularly believed but displays a clear haplotype switching genetic strategy in adapting to and spreading between human hosts [3]. We assume the same type of haplotype-switching spread could also occur if the virus were to infect susceptible animal hosts. Thus, initially in Chinese hosts, the numbers of complete genome sequences show the relevant haplotypes are mainly L (Hu-1, dominant) and some developed as S (minor). As the viral-laden cometary dust spread globally in the tropospheric jet streams [4,5,6] it has now become diversified via haplotype switching, displaying infections in populations with diverse genetic backgrounds across the globe. In our view the diverse haplotypes emerge as a consequence of the diversity of the host-parasite interaction via the Innate Immune response of APOBEC and ADAR deaminase-mediated C>U and A>I(G) mutagenesis at key sites in the COVID-19 RNA genome (Table 1).

Thus, haplotypes diversified from 2 (in China) to another 11 emerg-emerging in Europe (Spain, France) and New York City. We confirmed that we had captured most haplotypes emerging during this period by showing they were recovered in the airplane travelers into Victoria, Australia, between January 24 and March 15, and also for all COVID-19 sequences collected in the month of March 2020 in France [3]. This n ≥ 13 haplotype diversity evidently occurred between January – March 2020 culminating in the explosive epidemic in New York City from March 14 – March 22 [3]. However, it should be pointed out that the difference between the original Wuhan L haplotype sequence (Hu-1) and any other haplotype ranges from 2 (S haplotype) to 9 (L-241a.1) apparently coordinated single nucleotide variant (SNV) differences (Figure 1). "Thus, each of the SNV-defined haplotypes identified comprises approximately 0.02% difference from the Hu-1 reference sequence. On average there are approximately 5 SNV differences from Hu-1 defining each haplotype. There is ≥99.98% identity between any haplotype and the Wuhan reference sequence whether that sequence is collected in China, Spain, the US West Coast or New York City" [3]. It needs to be stressed at this point that the same spread of sequence similarity (≥ 99.98%) in geographically dispersed sequences was observed also in the more limited 2002-2003 coronavirus outbreak caused by the SARS-CoV-1 virus [14].

Genomic Structure of COVID-19

Figure 1 is the comparative genomic structure of SARS-CoV-1 (2002-2003) and SARS-CoV-2 (2019-2020) illustrating the SNV site positions of the two main haplotype series (L-241, S) as shown in Table 1 where site combinations defining different haplotypes can be referenced.

The two coronavirus genomes are similar at the nucleotide sequence level at 79.45% (Table 2). The MERS-CoV genome (2012) is strikingly very different again from these two related coronaviruses [15,16]. The key amino acid site in the Spike protein that is clearly altered in the L-241 haplotypes (D614G) now dominates the globe outside China. In China the L-241 haplotypes were not observed in the surveyed cases (Dec 2019-Jan 2020) by Steele and Lindley [3].

The two main global haplotype series are currently L-241 and S, and the provisional range of other haplotypes are listed in Table 1. The Aspartic Acid to Glycine change at Spike (S) amino acid 614 (D614G) at p.23403 is significant as it has now become the dominant genetic change and "haplotype-associated" SNV detected globally [19]. Thus L-241 haplotypes containing D614G appear to have replaced the Wuhan L haplotype and most other detected haplotypes at time of writing (July 2020). But this "replacement" reflects the outcome of the host-parasite relationship as we expect the Hu-1 sequence to be of the L haplotype in endogenous infections via the viral-laden dust in China. Of particular interest is the fact that the D614G change in S protein structure significantly facilitates infection/replication of COVID-19 but not disease severity [19]. This plausibly explains the apparent ease of spread via fomites and person-to-person spreads in contaminated environments (hospital and nursing home clusters, cruise ships, airplane environments etc).

Steele EJ et al.   Virol Curr Res, Volume 4: 2, 2020

HAP	p.241 5'UTR	p.1059 P<>NonP Thr<>Ile	p.3037 SYN Phe<>Phe	p.8782 SYN Ser<>Ser	p.9477 NonP<>NonP Phe<>Tyr	p.11080/83 NonP<>NonP Leu<>Phe	p.11916 P<>NonP Ser<>Leu	p.14408 NonP<>NonP Pro<>Leu	p.14805 P<>P Tyr<>Tyr	p.17747 NonP<>NonP Pro<>Leu	p.17858 P<>P Tyr<>Cys	p.18060 SYN Leu<>Leu	p.18998 NonP<>NonP Ala<>val	p.23403 Acid<>NonP Asp<>Gly	p.25563 P<>Basic Gln<>His	p.25979 NonP<>NonP Gly<>Val	p.26144 NP<>NP Gly<>Val	p.28144 P<>NonP Leu<>Ser	p.28657 SYN Asp<>Asp	p.28863 P<>NonP Ser<>Leu	p.29540 near 3UTR non-CDS gap
L (Hu-1)	C	C	C	C	T	G	C	C	C	C	A	C	C	A	G	G	G	T	C	C	G
Ln	C	C	C	C	T	T	C	C	T	C	A	C	C	A	G	G	T	T	C	C	G
L-241a	T	T	T	C	T	G	C	T	C	C	A	C	C	G	T	G	G	T	C	C	G
L-241a.1	T	T	T	C	T	G	T	T	C	C	A	C	T	G	T	G	G	T	C	C	A
L-241b	T	T	C	C	T	G	C	T	C	C	A	C	C	G	T	G	G	T	C	C	G
L-241c	T	C	C	C	T	G	C	T	C	C	A	C	C	G	T	G	G	T	C	C	G
L-241d/s	T	T	T	C	T	G	C	C	C	C	A	C	C	G	T	G	G	T	C	C	G
L-241e	T	C	C	C	T	G	C	T	C	C	A	C	C	G	T	G	G	T	C	C	G
L-241f	T	C	C	C	T	G	C	T	C	C	A	C	C	G	G	G	G	T	C	C	G
L-241g	T	C	C	C	T	G	C	T	C	C	A	C	C	G	G	G	G	T	C	C	G
S	C	C	C	T	T	G	C	C	C	C	A	C	C	A	G	G	G	C	C	C	G
Sa	C	C	C	T	T	G	C	C	C	T	G	T	C	A	G	G	G	C	C	C	G
Sb	C	C	C	T	A	G	C	C	T	C	A	C	C	A	G	G	G	C	C	C	G
Ss	C	C	C	T	A	G	C	C	T	C	A	C	C	A	G	T	G	C	T	T	G

Table.1 Main COVID-19 haplotypes Jan-Mar 2020. From Steele and Lindley [3].

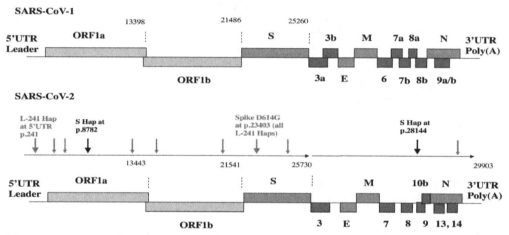

Schematic adapted from Coleman and Frieman 2014, Lu et al 2020 – relative positions , accessary proteins in red. Arrows are approx. relative positions of the key SNV differences from Wuhan Hu-1 ref. sequence associated with L-241 and S COVID-19 haplotypes, see Table 2 in Steele and Lindley 2020. The combinations are shown for L-241 series haplotypes (blue arrows) and for the major positions at p.241, p.23403; and S haplotypes (black arrows) . Also see molecular biology and coronavirus replication strategy in Masters 2006, Yang and Leibowitz 2015.

Figure 1. Schematic comparison of the genomic structure of SARS-CoV-1 (2002-2003) and SARS-CoV-2 (2019-2020). All sources cited are in reference list [15-18,3].

Coronavirus	Percent Identity Matrix Multiple Clustal12.1 Alignment (date 6.7.20)						
	NC_045512.2 Hu-1 (Wuhan)	AY278741.1 SARS-CoV	DQ022305.1 Bat 1	KC881005.1 Bat 2	KC881006.1 Bat 3	MG772933.1 Bat 4	MG772934.1 Bat 5
Hu-1 (Wuhan)	100	79.45	79.32	79.56	79.65	88	87.98
SARS-CoV (Urbani)	79.45	100	87.9	95.32	95.6	80.82	80.94
Bat 1	79.32	87.9	100	88.3	88.26	82.66	82.3
Bat 2	79.56	95.32	88.3	100	98.83	81.11	81.14
Bat 3	79.65	95.6	88.26	98.83	100	81.18	81.18
Bat 4	88	80.82	82.66	81.11	81.18	100	97.46
Bat 5	87.98	80.94	82.3	81.14	81.18	97.46	100

Coronavirus	Accession	Year Published	Ref	Bat Species
Hu-1 (Wuhan)	NC_045512.2	2019		
SARS-CoV	AY278741.1	2003	Masters 2006	
Bat 1	DQ022305.1	2005	Lau et al 2005	*Rhinolophus sinicus* (wild Chinese horseshoe bats)
Bat 2	KC881005.1	2013	Ge et al 2013	*Rhinolophus sinicus* (wild Chinese horseshoe bats)
Bat 3	KC881006.1	2013	Ge et al 2013	*Rhinolophus sinicus* (wild Chinese horseshoe bats)
Bat 4	MG772933.1	2018	Hu et al 2018	*Rhinolophus pusillus* (wild Chinese horseshoe bats)
Bat 5	MG772934.1	2018	Hu et al 2018	*Rhinolophus pusillus* (wild Chinese horseshoe bats)

For 1% difference assume about 300 single nucleotide changes per genome (based on Hu-1 29903 nt in length)
For 10% difference assume about 3000 single nucleotide changes per genome
For 20% difference assume about 6000 single nucleotide changes per genome

Table 2. Percent Identity Matrix between COVID-19 reference sequence (Hu-1), SARS-CoV and various Bat coronavirus sequences.

Steele EJ et al.   Virol Curr Res, Volume 4: 2, 2020

Early COVID-19 Origins and Explosive Epicentres

The COVID-19 pandemic began with the first Chinese cases of severe acute respiratory pneumonia-like diseases in late November to early December 2019 in Wuhan, Hubei province China. Of the first 41 COVID-19 patients 27 were connected and 14 were not connected at all to the Wuhan Meat and Seafood market [20,21]. So even at this early stage the clear evidence showed that one third of all patients had no connections at all to animal wet markets. Yet the common belief is that the pandemic began with a jump from a SARS-like CoV infected animal, probably a bat and/or pangolin [22,23] which then triggered the explosive region-wide epidemic in central China focused on Wuhan city and its regions [1]. The animal jump model, if true, needs to explain this extensive region-wide infection in a remarkably short period of time.

After a number of explosive epidemics, the pandemic then developed further through January 2020 through to end of March 2020: first in Wuhan (first week January increasing exponentially from Jan 21 to Feb 10), next in Tehran/Qom and Italy/Lombardy (from March 1), then Spain (from the end first week March) and then New York City (March 14 – through into April) see Figure 1 [3,5]. This early temporal order of the epicentres is important to keep clearly in mind as most of the rest of the world had little or no evidence of the disease spreading at this point. Indeed, as we noted at the time, all these explosive epicentres fell on a narrow latitude band centred on the Latitude 40o N allowing us to predict that the next major local epidemic after Tehran, Italy and Spain would be New York City [5]. The disease has now spread extensively across the globe from the combination of infall events with person-to-person infection, as well transcontinental transport of virus-laden dust via wind/weather systems. To date some 11 million or more people in both northern and southern hemispheres have come to be infected by the virus [6]. There are also large local explosive outbreaks mainly in certain southern and south west locations in USA (Texas, Florida, Arizona and California) and to a lesser extent in nearby regions (Louisiana, Alabama, New Mexico) suggesting the possibility of a further viral-laden dust cloud in-fall directly from the troposphere or laterally by wind transport across the United States from June-into July 2020 (see charts as 18 July in Supplementary File D). At the time of writing there have been perhaps 500,000 deaths worldwide (a death to confirmed case rate of about 5%).

The vast majority of the deaths are in vulnerable elderly already co-morbid subjects, >65 years of age, [24]. However, based on definitive (and comprehensive) data relating to an outbreak of disease on the cruise ship Diamond Princess a more accurate estimate of the COVID-19 case fatality rate emerges which varies anywhere from 0.05% to 1% [25]. And at the time of writing John Ioannidis estimates that in excess of 300 million globally may have already been infected with COVID-19, a good 10 to 20 times higher than the currently widely publicized estimates [26]. Thus, with the benefit of hindsight the disease itself, while new and striking in the speed of its global spread, should be considered at least in a figurative sense a mild common cold on a par with seasonal Influenza with vulnerabilities manifesting mainly in those with already compromised innate immune defenses.

The widely reported early induced cytokine storm and severe inflammatory sequelae has much support [27] and requires attention (via inflammation suppression) in vulnerable subjects who may also have possibly suppressed innate immunity; dysregulated interferon gene expression (suppression) as has been recently observed in COVID-19 patients [28,29,30]. This may explain why there is little or no evidence of a full innate immune response resulting in deaminase mutagenic signatures [31] in the full-length genomes of many COVID-19 patients [3]. We suspect many of the genomes examined in Steele and Lindley [3] (2020) were in fully developed diseased cases and not "asymptomatics", who may have better developed innate immunity and may thus display a higher level of APOBEC and ADAR mutagenesis in any shed viral genomes. In a Leading Edge Perspective published in Cell Netea and colleagues describe the disease thus " SARS-CoV-2 infection is mild in the majority of individuals but progresses into severe pneumonia in a small proportion of patients. The increased susceptibility to severe disease in the elderly and individuals with co-morbidities argues for an initial defect in anti-viral host defense mechanisms. " and further " Epidemiological data show that the elderly and those with co-morbidities (diabetes, obesity, and cardiovascular, respiratory, renal, and lung diseases) are most susceptible to COVID-19 and more likely to suffer from the most severe disease complications. Interestingly, young children, including infants who are more susceptible to other infections, have milder symptoms and less severe COVID-19" [24]. We would further add that future research on the pathogenesis of COVID-19 in healthy versus susceptible subjects should reveal the important role of the innate immune system - in particular in contributing to a better understanding eventually as the reason for so many asymptomatic infections and for mild symptoms.

Before analyzing the COVID-19 haplotype data further in terms of its putative cosmic origin we need to review the evidence for the two widely believed popular theories of the origin of COVID-19.

The Bat to Human Jump Theory

We will briefly discuss the data on this widely accepted popular theory as it figures prominently not only in the introductory sections of all scientific papers published on the topic, but in many major newspapers around the world including articles by Wildlife Disease Surveillance groups in Science magazine [32].

The process of human infection by animal viruses is termed zoonosis. The first clear point to make is that this theory with respect to the origin of COVID-19 has no direct scientific evidence in its support (unlike the well-documented one step (yet limited) horse -to-human transmission of Hendra virus see CDC [33].

This fact is often overlooked in current public and scientific discussions [32]. Further, the same animal jump model, assumed solely on phylogenetic correlations (then further human-to-human spread) has been applied to all suddenly emergent pandemic diseases over the past 40-50 years : influenza virus epidemics come from migrating birds, domestic chicken flocks or domestic swine [7]; HIV from higher primates (e.g. chimpanzees, "viz. HIV crossed from chimps to humans in the 1920s in what is now the Democratic

Steele EJ et al.   Virol Curr Res, Volume 4: 2, 2020

Republic of Congo. This was probably as a result of chimps carrying the Simian Immunodeficiency Virus (SIV), a virus closely related to HIV, being hunted and eaten by people living in the area. Oct 30 2019" [34].We should stress that there is no direct scientific evidence to support these assumed zoonotic events or animal to human transfers.

Other recent coronavirus diseases associated with acute respiratory diseases such as MERS -CoV (2012) are assumed to have arisen from camels and/or bats in combination [15] and SARS-CoV-1 (2002-2003) from bats [35-38] and/or pangolins in combination [39,40]. In all cases there are suggestive phylogenetic relationships between the putative virus sequence and the human sequence but no direct evidence that any of the major human disease pandemics have actually originated this way. The great genetic hurdles are vividly displayed in Table 2 which shows representative bat SARS-like CoV examples showing the closest sequence similarities with both SARS-CoV-1 and SARS-CoV-2 (COVID-19). These comparisons need to be taken into account when we consider the bat to human jump theory for origin of SARS-CoV-2 (2019-2020) or the more limited SARS-CoV-1 pandemic also originating in China in 2002-2003 [15]. More recently, an intermediate 'amplifying' wild host also eaten in China (pangolins) has been implicated in the explanation [39, 40, 41].

Taking the full length of Hu-1 as a reference (SARS-CoV-2, 29903 nt) the genetic distance from any bat sequence to the human SARS-CoV-1, or SARS-CoV-2 ranges from about 1300 to over 3000 single nucleotide variants (SNVs). We present the sequence similarities this way rather than in the form of a "tree" or percent sequence similarity as the mutational hurdle can be addressed directly and logically by independent observers without trying to interpret what the "tree" means (or be misled by the optimistic estimates of 90% to 96% sequence similarity). This is contrasted with the ≥ 99.98% sequence identity of the known range of COVID-19 haplotypes, despite extensive supposed human passage, during the current pandemic, Table 1 [3] – indeed the same range and stability on human passage was observed for the diversity of SARS-CoV-1 in isolates during 2002-2003 [14].

Generally speaking, many molecular evolutionists who work on these types of phylogenetic data accept our assessment that the bat-to-human genetic hurdle is too big to bridge in the time periods available. Thus, in commenting on putative jumps of this type by bat coronaviruses [35,36,42,22] state "This seriously divides the experts. Australian virologist Edward Holmes has estimated that RaTG13 would take up to 50 years to evolve the extra 4 per cent that would make it a 100 per cent match with the COVID-19 virus". Martin Hibberd, of the London School of Hygiene & Tropical Medicine, believes it might take less than 20 years to morph naturally into the virus driving the current pandemic. Others say such arguments are based on the assumption the virus develops at a constant rate. "That is not a valid assumption" asserts Richard Ebright of Rutgers University's Waksman Institute of Microbiology. "When a virus changes hosts and adapts to a new host, the rate of evolutionary change is much higher. And so it is possible that RaTG13, particularly if it entered humans prior to November 2019, may have undergone adaptation in humans at a rate that would allow it to give rise to Sars-Cov-2. I think that is a distinct possibility".Indeed Ebright believes an even more controversial theory should not be ruled out [22].

"It also, of course, is a distinct possibility that work done in the laboratory on RaTG13 may have resulted in artificial in-laboratory adaptation that erased those three to five decades of evolutionary distance." That latter comment also feeds into the Cold War conspiracy theories that claim that COVID-19 is a Chinese bioweapon that was accidently released from the Wuhan Institute of Virology, a genetically engineered upgraded version of the RaTG13 isolated from an abandoned mine in 2012-2013 below, and [23]. However, what is clear, as reported at the time on January 31 2020 by Jon Cohen of Science magazine [43]. "One of the biggest takeaway messages [from the viral sequences] is that there was a single introduction into humans and then human-to-human spread," this assertion being attributed to Trevor Bedford, a bioinformatics specialist at the University of Washington and Fred Hutchinson Cancer Research Center.

Further support of a bat origin has appeared [42] claiming that the bat SARS-like CoV, RaTG13, has 96.2% whole genome sequence similarity with SARS-CoV-2 (COVID19, the Hu-1 sequence). This virus was originally named RaBtCoV/4991, a name change itself which has fuelled the bioweapon conspiracy theory as well [23]. In any case, this close match would still require approximately 1140 SNV changes to become a COVID-19 exact match (≥ 99.98% sequence identity), a genetic hurdle we believe is too great. This however remains the mainstream view held by most workers at the present time [22].

Our view, given all of what we know on the natural haplotype switching adaptive strategy of COVID-19 coupled to its observed relatively low mutation on human passage [3] is that the genetic jumps as required by the variant distances summarized in Table 2 are impossible to bridge. If coronaviruses infecting bat colonies [35,36,38,42] are the long term "festering" endemic reservoir the sobering facts are that SARS-CoV-1 came and went rapidly in 2002-2003 and never came back [15] which also still currently applies to the more limited outbreak of MERS-CoV in the middle east in 2012.

Why many suddenly emergent epidemic viruses also go quickly and never come back is a key unsolved problem, as well as a major feature of many suddenly emerging pandemics in history [7]. It may well be a combination of natural self-limiting processes such as adaptive T/B lymphocyte "Herd Immunity", heightened and 'trained' non-specific innate immunity [24] as well as degradation of the virus in the physical environment are all involved. If bats are an 'intermediate' host/reservoir and thus a widely available endemic reservoir as suggested [35,36,42] it is a real puzzle why none of the original coronavirus diseases have ever returned if the bat to human (or via animal X?) theory is indeed the explanation for the cause of pandemics such as COVID-19.

Pangolins as an Intermediate Host from Bats then to Human?

The current orthodox theory is that if the bat to human jump is a genetic bridge too far, then perhaps bats are the primary natural reservoirs of zoonotic coronaviruses and that the actual jump occurs by an intermediate host acting as an 'evolutionary amplifier' - presumably some type of evolutionary genetic fine-tuning for the

Steele EJ et al.   Virol Curr Res, Volume 4: 2, 2020

zoonotic leap? [39-41]. However, it seems the genetic distance for such pangolin-nursed SL CoVs maybe just as great as for the bat SL CoVs (Table 2). Thus, in the report by [40] "Pangolin- CoV is 91.02% and 90.55% identical to SARS-CoV-2 and BatCoV RaTG13, respectively, at the whole- genome level. Aside from RaTG13, Pangolin-CoV is the most closely related CoV to SARS-CoV-2." Using the calculator from Table 2 this constitutes a deficit of 2700 SNVs to match the current COVID-19 reference Hu-1 strain, again a genetic difference itself which is insurmountable in our view. Another recent submitted survey of six novel pangolin coronavirus complete genomes [41] gave approximately 85.5% to 92.4% similarity to the Hu-1 sequence – the number of SNV required for a full match to COVID-19 ranging from 2400 to 4350.

Even if we are generous and assume from the data in Table 2 that only about 1% of the relevant nucleotides switched were mandatory for the bat to human transition to occur (i.e. 99% similarity to COVID-19 which has yet to be observed) the probability of this happening by random mutations is 1 in 4^{300}, which is equivalent to a probability of 1 in 10^{180}. The number of protons in the entire observable universe being only 10^{84}, it is amply clear that the probabilistic resources of the entire "Big Bang" universe is already stretched beyond the limit to cope with this presumed event. (We sketch an extreme and complex hypothetical genetic mechanism that might reduce some of these odds in the Supplementary File C).

If pangolin species are indeed an intermediate natural reservoir and amplifier of SARS-CoV-2-like CoVs it seems to us that the probability of a successful bat-to-pangolin-to-human jump (and then successful human-to-human transmission of COVID-19) is the product of two exceedingly improbable events, which makes the integrated jump highly unlikely – a Panglossian just so story. Thus, the actual evidence for real-time and widespread zoonotic events, though suggestive from phylogenetic analyses does not itself add up to the direct evidence for the rampant zoonosis often implied in the overwhelming majority of the papers we have read on the topic [44, 32].

Cosmic Origins?

A plausible scientific explanation (hypothesis) is expected to account for all existing data and observations whilst also making testable predictions of hitherto unexpected observations into the future.

In our view there is a plausible alternative scientific explanation for the observed diversity of all these animal and human SL-CoV sequences. Indeed, under the cosmic dust in-fall theory which entails a connected evolutionary process over vast cosmological dimensions [13], we expect susceptible terrestrial animal hosts including humans to become infected with an appropriate coronavirus variant. Further, flocks of thousands of bats, in their nocturnal scavenging flights, are ideal samplers of in-falling cometary dust clouds, some of which may plausibly harbour viruses. Bats could therefore be ideal sentinels for incoming cosmic coronavirus variants. In some cases, an informative seasonal variation has been observed in longitudinal sampling [35]. "Twenty-seven of the 117 samples (23%) were classed as positive by PCR and subsequently confirmed by sequencing. The species origin of all positive samples was confirmed to be R. sinicus by cytochrome b sequence analysis... A higher prevalence was observed in samples collected in October (30% in 2011 and 48.7% in 2012) than those in

April (7.1% in 2011) or May (7.4% in 2012)... and analysis of the S protein RBD sequences indicated the presence of seven different strains of SL-CoVs". This seasonal variation may perhaps coincide with the crossing times of the Orionid meteorite stream [45] in October-November each year as well as seasonal downdrafts from the troposphere, which we commented on in an earlier paper in this series [4].

These considerations have an important bearing on the genetic similarities and variations observed in coronaviruses isolated from animals as well as human beings. It is entirely conceivable that the primary "large distance" genetic variation in (say) the beta coronavirus family (as instanced by examples in Table 2) pre-exists in the dust in the troposphere at times of in-fall (a genetic scenario which we believe applies to all incoming cosmic viral variants whether they be coronaviruses, influenza viruses or other potential pathogens such as the more sophisticated retroviruses). According to our point of view the primary viral growth and propagation occurs in cellular sources (involving evolved eukaryotic cells) throughout a vast cosmic limitless biosphere over the aeons of cosmic time. The interiors of comets transporting these virions to Earth may well be clonally partitioned with differences thus showing up in the multitude of cometary fragments that enter the Earth [7,46,8,12]. These issues are updated and discussed further in a forth coming *Advances in Genetics* Elsevier volume (No. 106) on "Cosmic Genetic Evolution" which is being finalized and In Press at time of writing (Editors: E.J. Steele, N.C.Wickramasinghe).

The Chinese Bioweapon Release Theory

This theory is much discussed in the popular and serious press [22,23]. Not surprisingly both the bioweapon theory and the animal jump theory (from wet markets), have now been rejected by Chinese scientists reviewing all the data [47]. However Jon Cohen of Science magazine was clear when reporting back on Jan 30 2020 " The role of Huanan Seafood Wholesale Market in Wuhan, China, in spreading 2019-nCoV remains murky, though such sequencing, combined with sampling the market's environment for the presence of the virus, is clarifying that it indeed had an important early role in amplifying the outbreak. The viral sequences, most researchers say, also knock down the idea the pathogen came from a virology institute in Wuhan." [43].

It is therefore difficult to discuss the viability of such an engineered-origins theory in the absence of hard objective scientific evidence. In our view, the way the virus has adapted to different human populations via a host-parasite-dependent haplotype riboswitching strategy has the hallmark of a pure natural biology – a biological adaptation strategy. We believe the only re-joiner is at the cold-war political level itself through rhetorical questioning: "Why design a virus bioweapon which does not lethally target the whole span of age groups in the population? Indeed, why design a weapon that targets only vulnerable elderly co-morbid human beings?" Further, if such a weapon did escape from the Wuhan Virology Institute it would need to have escaped on such a massive scale and at high assumed dose levels to ignite the first synchronous epidemic wave over a wide region of central China centred on Hubei province.

Steele EJ et al.   Virol Curr Res, Volume 4: 2, 2020

Genetic Strategy of COVID-19 is Compatible with its Putative Cosmic Origins

In our view all the animal jump models and the bioweapon idea are flawed and scientifically implausible.

The most plausible explanation, in our view, goes as follow:

• SARS-CoV-2 came as part of the fragmented carbonaceous meteorite as we have advocated earlier, fragmenting and entering the tropospheric jet stream [1-6] and this comes in as a more or less pure 'culture' clonal variant [48,2].

• Further, we strongly suspect SARS-CoV-1 is related to SARS-CoV-2 as they are putative fragments, bearing clonal variants, of the same fragmented cometary source in the Orionid meteor stream [4,45].

• Our genetic analyses have focused on the first 2-3 months of the pandemic, and for informative explosive outbreaks in the main. We focused attention on the main epidemic explosions, and initial spreads, as viral genetic patterns in these collections would be likely to be most revealing about the viral origins and mode of spread. Thus, the putative fall-out times in temporal sequence are Wuhan, China (mainly Dec 20-30 2019, Jan 2020, Feb 2-5 2020) ->West Coast USA and Grand Princess cruise ship (Jan 22- Feb 27 2020, then to Mar 4), Spain (February 26-March 10), then New York City March 5-9, then March 14 -22, 2020 (see details Table 1 in Steele and Lindley 2020 [3] and Supplementary Information in that paper). In addition, so that our findings could be replicated and checked readily by other scientists, we only sourced GenBank curated SARS-CoV-2 sequences at the NCBI Virus site. At the time of writing very few Iranian and Italian complete COVID-19 sequences had been deposited at NCBI Virus Site.

• At the main epicentres (Wuhan, New York) apart from the already reported haplotype diversification in New York (n ≥ 13) relative to Wuhan (n = 2) there was from low to null mutation in COVID-19 isolates from subjects swabbed for the virus and thus complete genome sequencing. This was the strong repetitive pattern that showed up in the data. Person to Person (P-to-P) spreads could be identified and it was concluded that the high numbers of unmutated haplotype sequences in epicentres (and the cruise ship) could also be a reflection of P-to-P sharing of that sequence between susceptible individuals in local environments e.g. hospitals, nursing homes and other closed centres.

• The key major difference (from other low impact zones largely experiencing only P-to-P spreads), we now surmise, accounting for the explosive outbreaks in Wuhan and New York City (as well as those others on the 40° Latitude N band in Tehran, Italy/Lombardy, Spain) would have been the expected large infective viral doses at these times in these locations - large doses indicative of in-fall of viral-laden dust transported first via the tropospheric jet streams and sequentially brought to ground in these locations via local wind patterns and weather conditions : simultaneously infecting large numbers of people over a short time period. However, on each infection cycle the sequence data suggests that the haplotype fate of the virus is determined by the biochemistry and genetics of the host-

parasite relationship. Thus, an APOBEC and ADAR deaminase-driven innate immune mutagenesis response on the part of the host [31] decides the haplotype. This is mainly at the RNA level through riboswitching and thus which COVID-19 haplotype sequence will survive and thrive in a particular host genetic environment [3]. This has been our operating hypothesis. The immediately reactive innate immune response to simultaneous airborne infections in the first 24-48 hours in the expected thousands of Chinese (Dec-Jan) and New Yorkers (March) to the incoming viral laden dust bearing source Hu-1 virions (L haplotype) can assist deaminase-mediated C-to-U and A-to-I (thus G) changes in the replicating viral sequences. A range of mutated positive strand RNA quasi-species are produced in an infected host cell with changes at particular deaminase hot spots or riboswitch sites determining compatible RNA secondary structures. Coordinated changes at two or more of these sites allows rapid replication in that biochemical background. Thus "host-directed" deaminase-mediated riboswitches are expected to create adaptive options for the virus which if then selected allows more rapid replication in that particular cellular environment. This hypothesis is a great simplification conceptual tool, and it has allowed us to order the complex data sets now emerging in the pandemic in a rational way" [3] Table 1. In our view once a haplotype successfully establishes itself by replicating within a particular biochemical-genetic background it would be expected to spread quickly in those hosts sharing that particular biochemical background. This cosmic-derived genetic strategy is part and parcel of the efficient spread of viruses throughout living systems across the cosmos [10,11].

Airborne Transmission COVID-19 Formally Recognized?

It is being more formally recognized that airborne transmission of COVID-19 is the most likely "highly virulent transmission route" in the spread the disease in the explosive outbreaks in Wuhan, Italy, and New York City [49]. The authors of this paper analysed the trends and mitigation measures in Wuhan, China, Italy, and New York City, from January 23 to May 9, 2020, revealing that the differences of outcome with and without mandated face masks was the main determinant in shaping the pandemic trends in the three epicentres. This significantly reduced the number of COVID-19 infections, by over 78,000 in Italy (April 6 to May 9), and by over 66,000 in New York City (April 17 to May 9). The conclusion is that social distancing rules implemented in the United States, were woefully insufficient by themselves in protecting the public. On the other hand, the wearing of face masks in public spaces appears to be is the most effective means to limit human-to human transmission [49]. This conclusion, while agreeable to our position, has been challenged by others (Supplementary File B).

COVID-19 Outbreaks in Ships at Sea

Numerous reports of this type appeared in the media from February 2020 (Supplementary File B). They are consistent with a global airborne transmission of COVID-19 in the air and winds from above. However strong this putative evidence, it is always difficult to separate it from more conventional explanations of infectious

Steele EJ et al.   Virol Curr Res, Volume 4: 2, 2020

communicable disease theory i.e. the simplest explanation being in all cases it is an imported disease to the ships by infected passengers or crew (or fomites such a luggage and supplies), and the subsequent person-to-person spread. Here we discuss two outbreaks which are not easy to explain by conventional communicable infectious disease theory.

Al Kuwait sheep ship

One of us HR (Dr Herbert Rebhan) was the Veterinary surgeon on board the Al Kuwait sheep ship and supplied these details [50]. The ship, without a sheep cargo as it was returning after delivery of a live consignment to Kuwait, docked in Fremantle harbour on May 22, with 21 of its 48 crews testing positive for COVID-19. At sea approaching Fremantle HR, at the request of the ship's Captain (as there was no medical doctor on the ship), provided medical advice and care. What follows now is largely on the public record [51] and are HR recollections and summaries:

" HR found nearly all of the ill crew members displaying symptoms of a bacterial infection (sore throat and sinusitis). No ill crew member complained of any problems with breathing. In regards to coughing, crew members reported no or mild and infrequent coughing. HR did not expect a viral agent to be at work as all ill crew improved 48 hours after starting antibiotic medication and most were deemed fit for duty 96 hours after the start of antibiotics. HR was as surprised as anyone when these crew members tested positive for COVID-19. As the crew had no outside contact since early March, HR was at a loss to explain the source of the infecting agent."

"Although it cannot be ruled out that the virus entered the ship on supplies obtained from shore, the explanation of exposure via sailing through a "viral cloud" dispersed through sea-spray perhaps, is more plausible for several reasons. One is that the sick crew members who tested positive all fell ill within 48 hours of one another, a clear indication of near simultaneous exposure. There was no evidence of person-to-person transmission. The second objection to infection from supplies at ports of call related to the well-attested properties of the virus. Studies have shown that when the virus is exposed to environmental temperatures greater than 30 degrees C, viability is greatly reduced. The supplies taken aboard the Al Kuwait were exposed to environmental temperatures much greater than 30 degrees C for many hours (in Kuwait). It would be hard to imagine that the incoming provisions would have been contaminated with a great enough viral load to infect all the crew at the same time. The crew members who tested positive for COVID were deck workers and would not have had any direct contact with the goods brought on the ship. The chef, cook, and galley helpers who had the closest contact with the goods brought aboard would have had maximum exposure to any and all viral contaminated supplies – but all subsequently tested negative for COVID-19."

HR further reports as follows (after arrival in Fremantle when all crew were placed in quarantine for two weeks in a Perth hotel).

"Of the 48 crew 21 were COVID-19 positive, and were all deck crew (Phillipinos). The officers (Croatian) were unaffected by COVID-19 including HR." ... "The first crew member that fell ill with flu symptoms was one working at the end of the loading ramp. He was in full PPE and the only one that came close to people other than crew. He tested negative on both PCR and serology tests. He was

extensively tested by Western Australian State Health Department looking for something. He took a full seven days to recover"......."The next three crew members who fell ill within 24 hours of one another and 5 days after the first crew member became ill all tested PCR corona positive. They took three days to recover"........."The crew member who was taken to the hospital tested negative. He was hospitalized for the flu"......."The crew members who were the most poorly did not have coronavirus. Some crew members who were ill and tested positive for coronavirus had milder symptoms and a faster recovery. 75% of those that tested positive for coronavirus were asymptomatic."

This testimony is very informative, and is consistent with an airborne and/or associated sea spray exposure to COVID-19 while the ship was isolated in the Indian Ocean. The high asymptomatic rate is similar to the rate reported by [52] on the small cruise ship MV Greg Mortimer (Supplementary Information B).

Argentinian Fishing Boat Echizen Maru (Agence France-Presse (AFP), July 14 2020)

Of all the reports of COVID-19 outbreaks in ships at sea this is perhaps the most compelling and definitive in limiting the types of causal explanations. It clearly supports Dr Rebhan's observations on the Al Kuwait sheep ship and has been recently discussed by us in Howard et al [51].

"The Echizen Maru fishing trawler returned to port in Ushuaia, Argentina after some of its crew began exhibiting symptoms typical of COVID-19. 57 sailors out of 61 were infected with the coronavirus after 35 days at sea, despite the entire crew testing negative before leaving port [53]. Thus, the reports says "57 sailors, out of 61 crew members, were diagnosed with the virus after undergoing a new test…. Yet all of the crew members had previously undergone 14 days of mandatory quarantine at a hotel in the city of Ushuaia. Prior to that, they had negative results, the ministry said in a statement" As the report went further "….it's hard to establish how this crew was infected, considering that for 35 days, they had no contact with dry land and that supplies were only brought in from the port of Ushuaia," said Alejandra Alfaro, the director of primary health care in Tierra del Fuego. "The head of the infectious diseases department at Ushuaia Regional Hospital, Leandro Ballatore, said he believed this is a "case that escapes all description in publications, because an incubation period this long has not been described anywhere."

"We cannot yet explain how the symptoms appeared," said Ballatore. Sceptical comments suggesting possible alternative explanations have been offered at the AFP online site reporting the story. Of course, there may be ways of escaping this uncomfortable conclusion but the odds are beginning to stack up against this. One might for instance assert that a Pandora's box containing the virus was opened in mid-ocean and that a surviving virus population suddenly emerged to simultaneously infect 57 individuals.

In summary we note that all "ships-at-sea" data and observations (Supplementary File B) are consistent with the airborne arrival of coronavirus-laden dust contaminating the ships and inhabitants directly or by the undoubted sea spray of already heavily contaminated ocean surface waters from earlier in-falls prior to the ship's crossing that particular patch of ocean.

Steele EJ et al.

Virol Curr Res, Volume 4: 2, 2020

Summary: Haplotype Switching as a Cosmic Viral Adaptation Strategy

In summary the COVID-19 genetic haplotype patterns are consistent with an "adaptive genetic" strategy of a new virus from space trying to fit into, and replicate within, the genetic-background and thus biochemistry of the host cells, for example, the cells in the respiratory tracts of human beings. We expect similar processes to be occurring in those species of animals that have been successfully infected by coronaviruses.

The deaminase-driven riboswitch haplotype mechanism thus allows the virus to find the best RNA haplotype for optimum replication in that host cell [3]. This is governed by a small set of approximately 2-9 coordinated changes in RNA sequence – the weighted average is 4-5 coordinated differences from the Hu-1 reference sequence per haplotype sequence. In other words, all the haplotypes are ≥ 99.98% identical in sequence to the Wuhan reference sequence (Hu-1).

In our view this is one example of a universal cosmic genetic strategy for single stranded RNA viruses seeking to find a congenial cellular niche after landing, and within which to grow and replicate. Thus, the COVID-19 genome may give the semblance of "rapidly mutating"- but that is not the case, it is actually switching haplotypes. It may also appear to have an "ethnic or genetic" preference, but only in so far as successfully replicating the haplotype it settles on. Thus, APOBEC and ADAR C-to-U /G-to-A and A-to-I(G)/U-to-C deaminase-mutagenesis generates the coordinated changes and the cell then "selects" that sequence from among the variant quasi-species to replicate in that host cell. It is a "selection" mechanism from the variant set of quasi-species of RNA genomes that appears shortly after successful initial infection. This is a general biological strategy – for example the immune system uses a similar strategy to select the best-fitting antibodies. Thus, with COVID-19 haplotype riboswitching we are witnessing a universal biological adaptation strategy, one that we think has evolved and operates on a truly cosmic scale.

The challenge for mankind is to now systematically introduce near-Earth early warning surveillance (and mitigation) for incoming cosmic in-falls of micro-organisms and viruses from the cometary dust and meteorite streams that our planet routinely encounters as it orbits the Sun.

Acknowledgement

"We thank Max Wallis, Predrag Slijepcevic and Brig Klyce for helpful discussions."

Note in Proof

The role of air pollution in facilitating the global spread and severity of the COVID-19 epidemic has been reported in Coccia, M (2020) Factors determining the diffusion of COVID-19 and suggested strategy to prevent future accelerated viral infectivity similar to COVID. Science of the Total Environment 729 (2020) 138474.

Further, due to the rapid developments of the pandemic many key references are either online or will remain online at time of submission. All references with active URL internet links are listed in Supplementary File E."

References

1. Steele, EJ, Qu J, Gorczynski RM and Lindley RA, et al. Origin of new emergent Coronavirus and Candida fungal diseases — Terrestrial or cosmic? "Cosmic Genetic Evolution" Adv. Genet. (2020)Volume 106. In press

2. Wickramasinghe, NC, Steele EJ, Gorczynski RM and Temple R, et al. "Comments on the origin and spread of the 2019 Coronavirus." Virol Curr Res(2020)4:1.

3. Steele, EJ, Lindley RA. "Analysis of APOBEC and ADAR deaminase-driven riboswitch haplotypes in COVID-19 RNA strain variants and the implications for vaccine design." Research Reports. In press.

4. Wickramasinghe, NC, Steele EJ, Gorczynski RM and Temple R, et al. "Growing evidence against global infection-driven by person-to-person transfer of COVID-19." Virol Curr Res (2020)4:1.

5. Wickramasinghe, NC, Steele EJ, Gorczynski RM and Temple R, et al. "Predicting the future trajectory of COVID-19." Virol Curr Res (2020)4:1.

6. Wickramasinghe, NC, Wallis MK, Coulson SG and Kondakov A, et al. "Intercontinental spread of COVID-19 on global wind systems." Virol Curr Res (2020)4:1.

7. Hoyle, F, Wickramasinghe NC. "Diseases from Space." J.M. Dent Ltd, London (1979).

8. Hoyle, F, Wickramasinghe NC. "Astronomical Origins of Life: Steps Towards Panspermia." Kluwer Academic Publishers (2000).

9. Steele, EJ, Al-Mufti S, Augustyn KK and Chandrajith R, et al. "Cause of Cambrian Explosion: Terrestrial or Cosmic?" Prog. Biophys. Mol. Biol. (2018)136:3–23.

10. Steele, EJ, Gorczynski RM, Lindley RA and Liu Y, et al. "Lamarck and Panspermia - On the efficient spread of living systems throughout the cosmos." Prog. Biophys. Mol. Biol. (2019)149: 10 -32.

11. Steele, EJ, Gorczynski RM, Lindley RA and Liu Y, et al. "The efficient Lamarckian spread of life in the cosmos."Adv. Genet (2020)Volume 106

12. Wickramasinghe, CH. "Proofs that Life Is Cosmic: Acceptance of a new paradigm. " World Scientific Publishing Co, Singapore, ISBN (2018)978-981-3233-10-2.

13. Wickramasinghe, NC, Wickramasinghe DT, and Tout CA, et al. "Cosmic biology in perspective." Astrophys Space Sci (2019)364:205.

14. Holmes, KV, Enjuanes L. "The SARS Coronavirus: A Postgenomic Era Science." (2003)300:1377-1378.

15. Coleman, CM, Frieman MB. "Coronaviruses: Important Emerging Human Pathogens." J.Virol (2014)88:5209–5212.

16. Lu, R, Zhao X, Li J and Niu P, et al. "Genomic characterisation and epidemiology of 2019 novel coronavirus: implications for virus origins and receptor binding." Lancet (2020)395:565–74.

17. Masters, PS. "The molecular biology of coronaviruses." Adv. Virus Res (2006)6:193–292.

18. Yang, D, Leibowitz JL. "The structure and functions of coronavirus genomic 3' and 5' ends." Virus Research (2015)206:120–133.

19. Korber, B, Fischer W, Gnanakaran S and Yoon H, et al. "Tracking changes in SARS-CoV-2 Spike: evidence that D614G increases infectivity of the COVID-19 virus." Cell (2020).

20. Cohen, J. "Wuhan seafood market may not be source of novel virus spreading ." globally Science, January 26 (2020).

21. Huang, C, Wang Y, Li X and Ren L, et al. "Clinical features of patients infected with 2019 novel coronavirus in Wuhan, China." The Lancet (2020)395:497–506.

22. Arbuthnott, G, Calvert J, Sherwell P. "Out of the bat cave: China's deadly maze." The Times London, 6 July (2020).

Steele EJ et al.   Virol Curr Res, Volume 4: 2, 2020

23. Conradi, P. "World health inquiry into Covid will not visit Wuhan laboratory." The Sunday Times (London) July 12 (2020).

24. Netea, MG, Giamarellos-Bourboulis EJ, Domı́nguez-Andrés J and Nigel Curtis N, et al. "Trained Immunity: a tool for reducing susceptibility to and the severity of SARS-CoV-2 infection." Cell (2020)181:969- 977.

25. Ioannidis, JPA. "A fiasco in the making? As the coronavirus pandemic takes hold, we are making decisions without reliable data." STAT News March 17 (2020) In John Miltimore Interview in FEE.

26. Claus, P. "Interview with John PA Ioannidis Up to 300 Million People May Be Infected by Covid-19, Stanford Guru John Ioannidis Says." Greek USA Reporter June 27 (2020).

27. Lee, JS, Park S, Jeong HW and Ahn JY et al. "Immunophenotyping of COVID-19 and influenza highlights the role of type I interferons in development of severe COVID-19 Sci. Immunol. In Press (2020).

28. Acharya, D, Liu GQ, Gack MU. "Dysregulation of type I interferon responses in COVID-19." Nat. Rev. Immunol (2020)20:397-398.

29. Blanco, Melo D, Nilsson Payant BE, Liu WC and Uhl S, et al. "Imbalanced Host Response to SARS-CoV-2 Drives Development of COVID-19." Cell (2020)181:1036–1045.

30. Hadjadj, J, Yatim N, Barnabei L and Corneau, A, et al. "Impaired type I interferon activity and exacerbated inflammatory responses in severe Covid-19 patients." medRxiv (2020).

31. Lindley, RA, Steele EJ. "ADAR and APOBEC editing signatures in viral RNA during acute- phase Innate Immune responses of the host-parasite relationship to Flaviviruses." Research Reports (2018)2:e1- e22.

32. Watsa, M. "Wildlife Disease Surveillance Focus Group." Rigorous wildlife disease surveillance Science (2020)369:145-147.

33. "Transmission of Hendra virus to humans can occur after exposure to body fluids and tissues or excretions of horses infected with Hendra virus". Centers for disease control and prevention.

34. "The link between HIV and SIV". Global information and education on HIV and AIDS, Avert.

35. Ge, XY, Li JL, Yang XL and Chmura AA, et al. "Isolation and characterization of a bat SARS-like coronavirus that uses the ACE2 receptor . Nature (2013)503:535- 540.

36. Ge, XY, Wang N, Zhang W and Hu B, et al. "Coexistence of multiple coronaviruses in several bat colonies in an abandoned mineshaft." VIROLOGICA SINICA (2016)31:1.

37. Hu, D, Zhu C, Ai L and He T, et al. "Genomic Characterization and Infectivity of a Novel SARS-like Coronavirus in Chinese Bats." Emerg Microbes Infect (2018)7:1.

38. Lau, SKP, Woo PCY, Li KSM and T soi, et al. "Severe Acute Respiratory Syndrome Coronavirus- Like Virus in Chinese Horseshoe Bats." Proc Natl Acad Sci USA (2005)102:39.

39. Tang, X, Wu C, Li X and Song Y, et al. "On the origin and continuing evolution of SARS-CoV-2." National Science Review (2020).

40. Zhang, T, Wu Q ,Zhang Z. "Probable Pangolin origin of SARS-CoV-2 associated with the COVID-19 outbreak." Current Biology (2020)30:1346–1351.

41. Lam, TTY, Shum MHH, Zhu HC and Tong YG, et al. "Identification of 2019-nCoV related coronaviruses in Malayan pangolins in southern China." bioRxiv preprint (2020).

42. Zhou, P, Yang XL, Wang XG and Hu B, et al. "A pneumonia outbreak associated with a new coronavirus of probable." bat origin Nature (2020)579:270-274.

43. Cohen, J. "Mining coronavirus genomes for clues to the outbreak's origins." Science (2020)

44. Xu, J, Zhao S, Teng T and Abdalla AE, et al. "Systematic comparison of two animal-to-human transmitted human coronaviruses: SARS-CoV-2 and SARS-CoV." Viruses (2020)12:244.

45. Wickramasinghe, NC, Wainwright M, Narlikar, J. "SARS a clue to its origins?" The Lancet (2003)361:1832.

46. Hoyle, F, Wickramasinghe NC. "Evolution from Space." J.M. Dent Ltd, London (1981).

47. Areddy, JT. "Coronavirus: Wuhan lab theory 'pure' fabrication' says Chinese scientist." The Wall Street Journal May (2020).

48. Andersen, K. "Clock and TMRCA based on 27 genomes." Novel 2019 coronavirus (2020). Cited in [20]

49. Zhang, R, Li Y, Zhang AL and Wang Y, et al. "Identifying airborne transmission as the dominant route for the spread of COVID-19." Proc. Natl Acad. Sci (2020).

50. Garvey, P. "Coronavirus: Vet slams Premier's 'scare tactics' over WA sheep vessel outbreak." The Australian May (2020).

51. Howard, GA, Wickramasinghe NC, Rebhan, H and Steele EJ, et al. "Mid-ocean outbreaks of COVID-19 with tell-tale signs of aerial incidence." Virol Curr Res (2020)4:2.

52. Ing, A, Cocks C, Green JP. "COVID-19: in the footsteps of Ernest Shackleton." Thorax Epub ahead of print (2020)1–2

53. "Mystery as Argentine sailors infected with virus after 35 days at sea." Agence France-Presse (AFP), July 14 (2020).

How to cite this article: Edward J. Steele, Reginald M. Gorczynski, Herbert Rebhan and Patrick Carnegie, et al. "Implications of Haplotype Switching for the Origin and Global Spread of COVID-19". Virol Curr Res 4 (2020) doi:DOI: 10.37421/Virol Curr Res.2020.4.116

Supplementary Information

Implications of haplotype switching for the origin and global spread of COVID-19

Edward J. Steele, Reginald M. Gorczynski, Herbert Rebhan, Patrick Carnegie, Robert Temple, Gensuke Tokoro,Alexander Kondakov, Stephen G. Coulson,Dayal T. Wickramasinghe, and N. Chandra Wickramasinghe

We address here issues that have emerged through the pandemic, some consistent with our explanations offered and others apparently in contradiction.

A.COVID-19 in Barcelona Sewer System March 2019?

This claim was made in a paper on a pre-print server and has been widely reported in both the popular press and social media (Chavarria-Miró et al 2020). There is no discussion anywhere on PCR precautions for COVID-19 genome contamination given that Spain has been saturated with viral genomes for many months. One positive 2019 date suggests contamination. Also, there was no mention of the technical precautions against contamination and sensitivities they have taken. In such a heavily contaminated environment PCR is notorious for finding contaminants. The issue is not discussed. The authors say " Technical details are included in the Appendix" yet those relating to controls, contamination etc. could not be found. The key text is: "This possibility prompted us to analyse some archival WWTP samples from January 2018 to December 2019 (Figure 2). All samples came out to be negative for the presence of SARS-CoV-2 genomes with the exception of March 12, 2019, in which both IP2 and IP4 target assays were positive. This striking finding indicates circulation of the virus in Barcelona long before the report of any COVID-19 case worldwide." This is a classic PCR contaminant pattern, a false positive in a heavily contaminated environment - a false positive outlier with another explanation. Our assessment is replicated by others who have read the paper, see comments at the site https://www.medrxiv.org/content/10.1101/2020.06.13.20129627v1

B. COVID-19 Outbreaks in Ships at Sea

A key task we have with outbreaks in ships at sea lies in separating infections brought to the ship by passengers or supplies prior to departure *versus* unexpected and hitherto unexplained, outbreaks at sea. That is the challenge, and we included in the main text only the strong data and observations (*Al Kuwait, Echizen Maru*)*.* However there is in addition an overall pattern that needs to be addressed, as many other types of ships became engaged with COVID-19 outbreaks while at sea. All these observations are, we believe, consistent with, and best explained by, the in-fall of COVID-19 dust clouds from the tropospheric jet streams. We document the numerous other reports of this type that appeared in the media from February 2020, particularly the *Princess* cruise ships. These ships would be expected to have a high proportion of elderly retirees and thus many who may have co-morbidities and thus would be quite vulnerable to common cold and flu-type respiratory diseases. As indicated some of these outbreaks may be accounted for by already infected travellers boarding the ships and infecting others by P-to-P spreads and fomite contamination (e.g. luggage from contaminated airplanes and airports). Some outbreaks such as the *Al Kuwait* animal transportation ship (empty and approaching Fremantle, Western Australia at time of outbreak) are not so easy to understand by conventional P-to-P infectious disease theory.

• *MV Greg Mortimer*- In the case of the outbreak on the *MV Greg Mortimer* a small cruise ship to Antartica (Ing et al 2020) there is a suggestion of a possible at-sea viral dust exposure in the South Atlantic at a time we have previously argued that viral dust clouds were known to be spreading into the Southern Hemisphere over South America, particularly Brazil (Wickramasinghe et al 2020b). However, the alternative view that

2

the coronavirus was introduced, either on their person or luggage, by passengers who travelled to Argentina by airplanes from already infected zones cannot be excluded. This introduction of virus would have had to occur despite pre-screening of passengers which took place- thus " all 128 passengers and 95 crew were screened for COVID-19 symptoms, and body temperatures were taken before boarding. No passengers or crew that had transited through China, Macau, Hong Kong, Taiwan, Japan, South Korea or Iran in the previous 3 weeks were permitted to board, given that these countries were where COVID-19 infection was most prevalent at the time. Multiple hand hygiene stations were positioned throughout the ship and especially in the dining area."

Almost all passengers on board were infected, and the great majority had mild infections. All the relevant data are highly detailed as the medical practitioners among the passengers actively organised the sampling, surveillance and testing of passengers, in real time. " Of the 217 passengers and crew on board, 128 tested positive for COVID-19. Of the COVID- 19 -positive patients, 19% (24) were symptomatic; 6.2% (8) required medical evacuation; 3.1% (4) were intubated and ventilated; and the mortality was 0.8% (1). The majority of COVID-19-positive patients were asymptomatic (81%, 104 patients). We conclude that the prevalence of COVID-19 on affected cruise ships is likely to be significantly underestimated, and strategies are needed to assess and monitor all passengers to prevent community transmission after disembarkation." This description can also apply to the infection experience on the *Diamond Princess* (Ioannidis 2020).

Events on the *MV Greg Mortimer* unfolded thus – "The first recorded fever on board the ship was a febrile passenger on day 8. Isolation protocols were immediately commenced, with all passengers confined to cabins and surgical masks issued to all. Full personal protective equipment was used for any contact with any febrile patients, and N95 masks were worn for any contact with passengers in their cabins. The crew still performed duties, including meal services to the cabin doors three times a day, but rooms were not serviced. Expedition staff helped with crew duties at meal service. …Further fevers were detected in three crew on day 10, two passengers and one crew on day 11, and three passengers on day 12". …" As Argentina had closed its borders, and permission to disembark at Stanley, Falkland Islands, was refused, the ship sailed to Montevideo, Uruguay, arriving the evening of day 13…The majority of febrile patients had improved with symptomatic treatment and were afebrile on arriving at Montevideo."…." Of the 217 passengers and crew on board, 128 tested positive for COVID-19 (59%). These included all passengers who tested negative" by an antibody test… and " there were 10 instances where two passengers sharing a cabin recorded positive and negative results".

While 128 (59%) of the population tested positive, " fever and mild symptoms were present in only 16 of 128 COVID-19- positive patients (12.5%), with another 8 medically evacuated (6.2%) and 4 requiring intubation and ventilation (3.1%). There has was one death (0.8%)… with a total of 24 COVID-19-positive patients who were symptomatic (19%), with the majority being asymptomatic (104 patients or 81%)."

This is a valuable study and is consistent with the observations by Herbert Rebhan on the *Al Kuwait* sheep ship.

• *Outbreak on "American Triumph" an Alaskan factory fishing vessel*
As this paper was being finalised another report of outbreaks of COVID-19 among many crew from a fishing boat was reported. viz. "Alaska fishing boat has 85 crew members infected with virus"
The Associated Press via The Charlotte Observer, July 20
https://www.charlotteobserver.com/news/article244351137.html

• *Aircraft Carriers* - Both US ships in North West Pacific (*USS Theodore Roosevelt* and *USS Ronald Reagan*) and the French aircraft carrier *Charles de Gaulle* (operating we assume in the North Atlantic) reported many thousands of cases, but details of these at-sea outbreaks are hard to examine and verify properly as the information release has been limited.

3

In late March the two U.S. aircraft carriers were in the western Pacific and both reported cases of the new coronavirus among their crews. After eight sailors on the U.S. aircraft carrier *Theodore Roosevelt* tested positive for COVID- 19 the ship went to Guam, where the rest of the crew would be tested (Stashwick 2020, Evans 2020). The *Theodore Roosevelt* was out of action for 10 weeks, docked in Guam while the crew was tested. More than 1150 of its 4800 crew tested positive and one sailor died.

The French aircraft carrier *Charles de Gaulle* arrived at its base in the bay of Toulon, southern France, Sunday April 12, 2020. The French Defence Ministry said in a statement that around 40 sailors initially showed symptoms compatible with COVID-19. However the coronavirus was shown to have infected more than 1,000 sailors aboard the *Charles de Gaulle.* (Schaeffer and Ganley 2020).

Apart from these basic details little else was shared with the US or French public.

• *Princess cruise ships-* In the case of the *Diamond Princess* operating in the South China Sea/Sea of Japan in February the timing and location of the outbreaks at sea are certainly consistent with a fragment of the Wuhan viral dust cloud drifting into the South China Sea. The report of the level of COVID-19 antibody positive subjects on the ship suggests widespread exposure on the ship, by P-to-P or fomites or both (Ioannides 2020).

The sudden outbreak on the *Grand Princess* off California mid to late February (Snowden 2020) involved exclusively the Wuhan L haplotype, both non-mutated, and lightly mutated with some P-to-P spreads (Steele and Lindley 2020). The news reports suggest many infected persons were crew The timing is consistent with a presumptive viral dust cloud affecting the USA West Coast at this time, much like the 1968 H3N2 influenza virus, also originating in China, which affected the USA from the West to East coasts in such a similar directional manner in 1968 (Wickramasinghe et al 2020a).

NOTE: The study discussed in the main text on airborne transmission that was published in PNAS by Zhang, Li et al has been challenged in a Letter transmitted to the PNAS editorial board

(https://metrics.stanford.edu/sites/g/files/sbiybj13936/f/files/pnas_loe_061820_v3.pdf)

C. Hyper and Non-Random Recombination Mechanisms in Coronavirus Adaptation?
Supplied by EJS : Can these odds be reduced by a special type of hypermutation-recombination mechanism deployed by coronaviruses? That is to say, a non-random complex mechanism involving a recombination process via multiple variant strain infections of the same cell – a type of replicase -linked strand jumping (copy choice) known to happen in part in experimental selection situations (Masters 2006) or as for influenza virus the recently described process of host-virus hybrid gene formation involving cleaved and 5'-m7G-capped host transcripts to prime viral mRNA synthesis (Ho et al 2020). To put simply: recombination of pre-existing variant SNV sequence templates which are all stitched together in a single host cell to arrive at a perfect COVID-19 sequence match – a form of natural genetic engineering? Each new sequence then would be a mosaic of blocks of sequence coped from other variant templates, a mosaic pattern much like the PCR recombinant pattern that can be generated by Taq or Pfu polymerases PCR runs from multiple different templates in vitro (Zylstra et al 1998). What are the odds given current known data on the sequence similarity of the closest bat strain RaTG13 which is 96.2% similar to, or 1140 SNV differences from, SARS-CoV-2? These considerations are reminiscent of the earlier discussions (1960s through 1980s) over targeted recombinational 'gene conversion' mechanisms of somatic hypermutation (SHM) in rearranged antibody variable genes (reviewed in Steele 1991). SHM is now known to be achieved by a combination of both locus-targeted APOBEC and ADAR deaminase mutagenesis and an error-prone reverse transcription process involving the Y family DNA repair polymerase, DNA Polymerase – eta (η) (Lindley and Steele 2013, Steele

3

4

2016, Franklin , Steele and Lindley 2020). Given that a reverse transcription step is not known to be involved at any stage of the coronavirus replication cycle – unlike HIV or Hepatitis B Virus - COVID-19 recombination would be driven by replicase 'strand jumping' coupled to deaminase hypermutagenesis. The SNV differences between the closest match strains to COVID-19 are formidable and it has to remain doubtful that such a mechanistic process in the cytosolic membraneous webs harbouring the "replication and transcription factories" actually can be assembled for the availability of variant templates in close proximity. In the case of HIV a strong case can be put that even this retrovirus may have co-opted the B lymphocyte somatic hypermutation mechanism to its own adaptive variation strategy (Steele and Dawkins 2016) but hypermutation is not a feature of COVID-19 in the human passages examined (Steele and Lindley 2020). Finally, however, COVID-19 recombination variation patterns were not an easily recognizable feature over the first three months of human disease episodes and passage at explosive epicentres as assessed in Steele and Lindley (2020).

D. Recent Epidemics in USA June -July 2020

Apparent "2nd Wave" epidemics with rising numbers of cases showed up in a number of southern and western states of the USA. This appears to be part of a general pattern - the first wave being followed by large epidemics in the north-eastern regions states New York, New Jersey, Maryland, Washington DC in March-April 2020. So the infective explosions occurred in a patchy manner across different regions. Some examples are shown, from Google Searches viz " <Type in State> covid-19 cases by county". These patterns suggest the descent of viral-laden dust clouds of varying size and viral load are now striking (as July 18 2020) the southern and western states in the USA, to varying degrees.

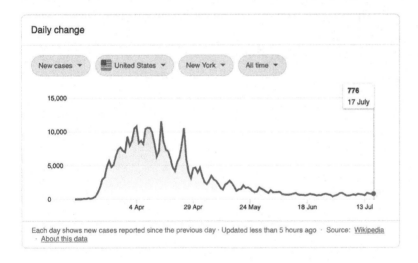

5

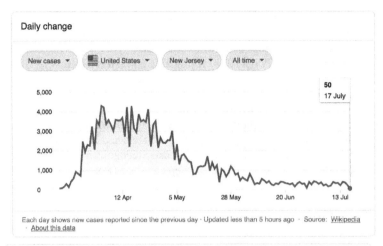

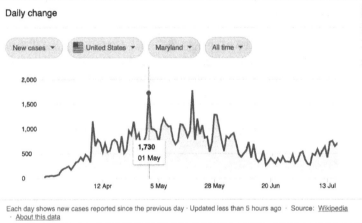

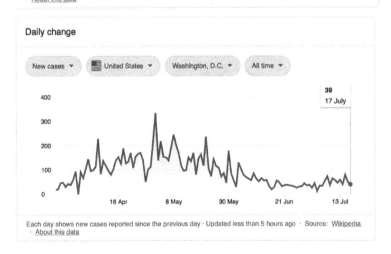

6

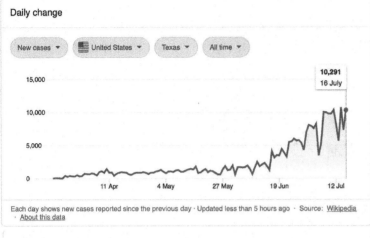

Each day shows new cases reported since the previous day · Updated less than 5 hours ago · Source: Wikipedia · About this data

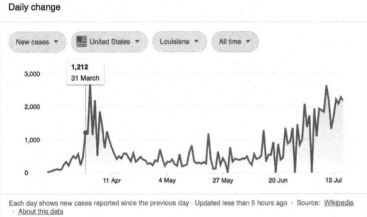

Each day shows new cases reported since the previous day · Updated less than 5 hours ago · Source: Wikipedia · About this data

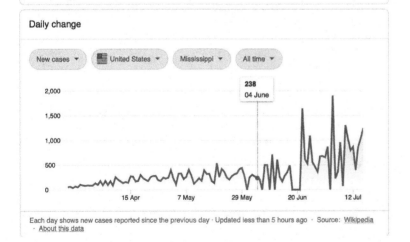

Each day shows new cases reported since the previous day · Updated less than 5 hours ago · Source: Wikipedia · About this data

7

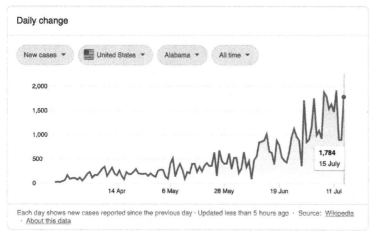

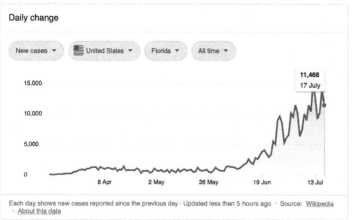

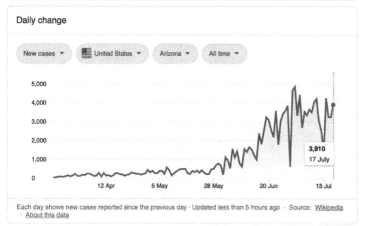

8

References cited

Chavarria-Miró, G., Anfruns-Estrada, E., Guix, S.,Paraira, M., Galofré, B., Sánchez, G., et al. (2020) Sentinel surveillance of SARS-CoV-2 in wastewater anticipates the occurrence of COVID-19 cases medRxiv preprint doi: https://doi.org/10.1101/2020.06.13.20129627.this version posted June 13, 2020.

Evans, M (2020) " Uncle Sam doubles down in naval display" *The Times (London)* June 23 2020 reprinted in *The Australian*
https://www.theaustralian.com.au/world/the-times/uncle-sam-doubl...own-in-naval-display/news-story/142048bc6afcc2aa159ce4c9f3c05d0a

Franklin, A., Steele, E.J., Lindley, R.A. (2020) A proposed reverse transcription mechanism for (CAG)n and similar expandable repeats that cause neurological and other diseases. Heliyon 6, e03258
doi: 10.1016/j.heliyon.2020.e03258

Ho,J.S.Y., Angel, M.,Ma, Y., Sloan, E., Wang, G., Martinez-Romero, C., et al.,
(2020) Hybrid Gene origination creates human-virus chimeric proteins during Infection
Cell 181, 1–16 https://doi.org/10.1016/j.cell.2020.05.035

Ing, A.., Cocks, C., Green, J.P. (2020) COVID-19: in the footsteps of Ernest Shackleton Thorax Epub ahead of print 2020;0:1–2. doi:10.1136/thoraxjnl-2020-215091

Lindley, R.A., Steele, E.J. (2013). Critical analysis of strand-biased somatic mutation signatures in TP53 versus Ig genes, in genome-wide data and the etiology of cancer ISRN Genomics, 2013 Article ID 921418, 18 pages. https://www.hindawi. com/journals/isrn/2013/921418/.

Schaeffer, J., Ganley, E. (202) France finds more than 1,000 virus cases on aircraft carrier. Associated Press Apr 17, 2020 / 11:06 AM EDT / Updated: Apr 17, 2020 / 03:07 PM https://www.news10.com/news/french-seek-clue-to-900-plus-virus-cases-on-aircraft-carrier/

Snowden, A. 2020. "Four Australians stuck on new coronavirus cruise ship *Grand Princess*" *The Australian*, March 5 , 2020.

Stashwick, S. Mar 30 2020 COVID-19 Cases Reported on Both US Aircraft Carriers in Western Pacific in https://thediplomat.com
https://thediplomat.com/2020/03/covid-19-cases-reported-on-both-us-aircraft-carriers-in-western-pacific/

Steele, E. J. (1991) Somatic Hypermutation in V-Regions . CRC Press, Boca Raton, Florida , USA. 1991.

Steele, E.J. (2016). Somatic hypermutation in immunity and cancer: critical analysis
of strand-biased and codon-context mutation signatures. DNA Repair 45, 1-24.
https://doi.org/10.1016/j.dnarep.2016.07.001.

Steele, E.J., Dawkins, R.L. (2016) . New Theory of HIV Diversification : Why it May Never Be Possible to Make a Protective Vaccine viXra.org 1612.0346.
https://vixra.org/abs/1612.0346?ref=9160630

9

Steele, E.J., Lindley, R.A. (2020) Analysis of APOBEC and ADAR deaminase-driven riboswitch haplotypes in COVID-19 RNA strain variants and the implications for vaccine design. Accepted Research Reports https://vixra.org/abs/2006.0011 replaced on 2020-06-29 20:33:02.

Zylstra, P., Rothenfluh, H.S., Weiller, G.F., Blanden, R.V., Steele, E.J. (1998). PCR amplification of murine germline V genes: strategies for minimization of recombinant artefacts. Immunol. Cell Biol. 76, 395–405. DOI: 10.1046/j.1440-1711.1998.00772.x

Wickramasinghe, N. C., Steele, E. J., Gorczynski, R. M., Temple, R., Tokoro, G., Wallis, D. H., et al. (2020a). Growing evidence against global infection-driven by person-to-person transfer of COVID-19. Virology: Current Research, 4(1). https://doi. org/10.37421/Virol Curr Res.2020.4.110

Wickramasinghe, N.C., Wallis, M.K. Coulson, S.G., Kondakov, A., Steele, E.J., Gorczynski, R.M., et al. (2020b) Intercontinental spread of COVID-19 on global wind systems Virology :Current Research 4(1) doi: 10.37421/Virol Curr Res.2020.4.113 https://www.hilarispublisher.com/open-access/intercontinental-spread-of-covid19-on-global-wind-systems.pdf

Zhang, R., Li, Y., Zhang, A.L.,Wang, Y., Molina, M.J. (2020) Identifying airborne transmission as the dominant route for the spread of COVID-19. Proc. Natl Acad. Sci. In Press https://www.pnas.org/cgi/doi/10.1073/pnas.2009637117

E. Full details with URL Links of references cited in main text of paper

Acharya, D., Liu, G-Q., Gack, M.U. (2020) Dysregulation of type I interferon responses in COVID-19 Nat. Rev. Immunol. 20, 397-398 DOI https://doi.org/10.1038/s41577-020-0346-x

Agence France-Presse (AFP), July 14 (2020) "Mystery as Argentine sailors infected with virus after 35 days at sea" reported Yahoo News https://news.yahoo.com/mystery-argentine-sailors-infected-virus-35-days-sea-035702418.html

Arbuthnott, G., Calvert, J., Sherwell, P. (2020) Out of the bat cave: China's deadly maze . *The Times (London)* 6 July 2020 re-printed in *The Australian* July 6 2020 p.12

Areddy, J.T. (2020) Coronavirus: Wuhan lab theory 'pure' fabrication' says Chinese scientist *The Wall Street Journal* May 2020, Reprinted in *The Australian* May 27 2020.

Andersen, K. (2020). Clock and TMRCA based on 27 genomes . Novel 2019 coronavirus http://virological.org/t/clock-and-tmrca-based-on-27-genomes/347

Blanco-Melo, D., Nilsson-Payant, B.E., Liu, W-C., Uhl, S., Hoagland, D., Møller, R., et al. (2020) Imbalanced Host Response to SARS-CoV-2 Drives Development of COVID-19 Cell 181, 1036–1045 May 28, 2020 a 2020 Elsevier Inc. https://doi.org/10.1016/j.cell.2020.04.026

Claus, P. (2020) Interview with John P.A. Ioannidis "Up to 300 Million People May Be Infected by Covid-19, Stanford Guru John Ioannidis Says*."* *Greek USA Reporter* June 27 , 2020

10

https://usa.greekreporter.com/2020/06/27/up-to-300-million-people-may-be-infected-by-covid-19-stanford-guru-john-ioannidis-says/

Cohen, J. (2020). Wuhan seafood market may not be source of novel virus spreading globally. Science, January 26. https://doi.org/10.1126/science.abb0611.

Cohen, J. (2020). Mining coronavirus genomes for clues to the outbreak's origins. *Science* Jan 31, 2020 https://www.sciencemag.org/news/2020/01/mining-coronavirus-genomes-clues-outbreak-s-origins

Coleman, C.M., Frieman, M.B. (2014). Coronaviruses: Important Emerging Human Pathogens J.Virol. 88, 5209–5212 doi:10.1128/JVI.03488-13

Conradi, P. 2020 World health inquiry into Covid will not visit Wuhan laboratory. *The Sunday Times (London).* July 12 2020, reprinted *The Australian* July 13 2020, p.9.

Garvey, P. (2020) "Coronavirus: Vet slams Premier's 'scare tactics' over WA sheep vessel outbreak" *The Australian* May 28, 2020

Ge, X-Y., Li, J-L., Yang, X-L., Chmura, A.A., Zhu, G., Jonathan H. Epstein, J.H., et al. (2013). Isolation and characterization of a bat SARS-like coronavirus that uses the ACE2 receptor . Nature 503, 535- 540 doi:10.1038/nature12711

Ge, X-Y., Wang, N., Zhang, W., Hu, B., Li, B., Zhang, Y-Z., et al. (2016)Coexistence of multiple coronaviruses in several bat colonies in an abandoned mineshaft VIROLOGICA SINICA 2016, 31 (1): 31–40 DOI: 10.1007/s12250-016-3713-9

Hadjadj, J., Yatim, N., Barnabei, L., Corneau, A., Boussier, J., Péré, H. et. al. (2020) Impaired type I interferon activity and exacerbated inflammatory responses in severe Covid-19 patients   medRxiv preprint doi: https://doi.org/10.1101/2020.04.19.20068015

Holmes, K.V., Enjuanes, L. 2003. The SARS Coronavirus: A Postgenomic Era Science 300, 1377-1378. doi: 10.1126/science.1086418

Howard, G.A., N.Chandra Wickramasinghe,Rebhan,H., Steele, E.J., Gorczynski, R.M., Temple, R., Tokoro, G., Klyce, B., Slijepcevic, P. (2020) Mid-ocean outbreaks of COVID-19 with tell-tale signs of aerial incidence Virology :Current Research Submitted July 18 2020. In Press.

Hoyle, F., Wickramasinghe, N.C. 1979. *Diseases from Space*. J.M. Dent Ltd, London.

Hoyle, F., Wickramasinghe, N.C., 1981. *Evolution from Space*. J.M. Dent Ltd, London.

Hoyle, F., Wickramasinghe, N.C. 2000. *Astronomical Origins of Life: Steps Towards Panspermia*. Kluwer Academic Publishers. Dordrecht/Boston/London.

Hu, D., Zhu, C., Ai, L., He, T., Wang, Y, Ye, F., et al (2018). Genomic Characterization and Infectivity of a Novel SARS-like Coronavirus in Chinese Bats Emerg Microbes Infect 7(1),154. doi: 10.1038/s41426-018-0155 https://pubmed.ncbi.nlm.nih.gov/30209269/

Huang, C., Wang, Y., Li, X., Ren, L., Zhao, J., Hu, Y., et al. (2020). Clinical features of patients infected

11

with 2019 novel coronavirus in Wuhan, China. The Lancet, 395, 497–506. Published online January 24,2020. https://doi.org/10.1016/S0140-6736(20) 30183-5.

Ing, A.., Cocks, C., Green, J.P. (2020) COVID-19: in the footsteps of Ernest Shackleton Thorax Epub ahead of print 2020;0:1–2. doi:10.1136/thoraxjnl-2020-215091

Ioannidis, J.P.A. (2020) A fiasco in the making? As the coronavirus pandemic takes hold, we are making decisions without reliable data STAT News March 17 2020 In John Miltimore Interview in FEE https://fee.org/articles/modelers-were-astronomically-wrong-in-covid-19-predictions-says-leading-epidemiologist-and-the-world-is-paying-the-price/?fbclid=IwAR2qLXB6PZevlxmVAHJP9B2rfzpYYKGZVguDWxPXn4BH0uDqEEgEiq-kpA4

Korber, B., Fischer, W., Gnanakaran, S., Yoon., H, Theiler, J., Abfalterer, W., Hengartner, N., et al. (2020). Tracking changes in SARS-CoV-2 Spike: evidence that D614G increases infectivity of the COVID-19 virus, Cell (2020) In Press , doi: https://doi.org/10.1016/j.cell.2020.06.043

Lam, T.T-Y., Shum, M. H-H. , Zhu, H-C., Tong, Y-G., Ni, X-B., Lao, Y-S., et al. (2020) Identification of 2019-nCoV related coronaviruses in Malayan pangolins in southern China bioRxiv preprint doi: https://doi.org/10.1101/2020.02.13.945485. this version posted February 18, 2020.

Lau, S.K.P., Woo, P.C.Y., Li, K.S.M., Tsoi, H-W., Wong, B.H.L., Wong, S.S.Y., et al (2005) Severe Acute Respiratory Syndrome Coronavirus- Like Virus in Chinese Horseshoe Bats Proc Natl Acad Sci U S A. 2005 Sep 27;102(39):14040-5. doi: 10.1073/pnas.0506735102 https://www.ncbi.nlm.nih.gov/pmc/articles/PMC1236580/

Lee, J.S., Park, S., Jeong, H.W., Ahn, J.Y., Choi, S.J., Lee, H., et al. (2020). Immunophenotyping of COVID-19 and influenza highlights the role of type I interferons in development of severe COVID-19 Sci. Immunol. In Press 10.1126/sciimmunol.abd1554 (2020). https://immunology.sciencemag.org/content/5/49/eabd1554

Lindley, R.A., Steele, E.J. (2018) ADAR and APOBEC editing signatures in viral RNA during acute- phase Innate Immune responses of the host-parasite relationship to Flaviviruses. Research Reports 2:e1- e22. doi:10.9777/rr.2018.10325.

Lu, R., Zhao, X., Li, J., Niu, P, Yang, B., Wu, H., et al. (2020). Genomic characterisation and epidemiology of 2019 novel coronavirus: implications for virus origins and receptor binding Lancet 2020; 395: 565–74 https://doi.org/10.1016/ S0140-6736(20)30251-8

Masters, P.S. (2006). The molecular biology of coronaviruses. Adv. Virus Res. 6 , 193–292. doi: 10.1016/S0065-3527(06)66005-3

Netea, M.G., Giamarellos-Bourboulis, E.J., Domı́nguez-André s, J., Nigel Curtis, N., van Crevel, R., van de Veerdonk, F.L., Marc Bonten, M. (2020). Trained Immunity: a tool for reducing susceptibility to and the severity of SARS-CoV-2 infection Cell 181, 969- 977, May 28, 2020 https://doi.org/10.1016/j.cell.2020.04.042

Steele, E.J., Al-Mufti, S., Augustyn, K.K., Chandrajith, R., Coghlan, J.P., Coulson, S,G., Ghosh, S., Gillman, M., et al (2018) Cause of Cambrian Explosion: Terrestrial or Cosmic? Prog. Biophys. Mol. Biol. 136, 3 – 23. https://doi.org/10.1016/j.pbiomolbio.2018.03.004

12

Steele, E.J., Lindley, R.A. (2020) Analysis of APOBEC and ADAR deaminase-driven riboswitch haplotypes in COVID-19 RNA strain variants and the implications for vaccine design. Accepted Research Reports https://vixra.org/abs/2006.0011 replaced on 2020-06-29 20:33:02.

Steele, E.J., Gorczynski, R.M., Lindley, R.A., Liu, Y., Temple, R., Tokoro, G., Wickramasinghe, D.T., Wickramasinghe, N.C. (2019) Lamarck and Panspermia - On the efficient spread of living systems throughout the cosmos. Prog. Biophys. Mol. Biol. 2019 149, 10-32 https://doi.org/10.1016/j.pbiomolbio.2019.08.010

Steele, E.J., Gorczynski, R.M., Lindley, R.A., Liu, Y., Temple, R., Tokoro, G.,. Wickramasinghe, D.T., Wickramasinghe, N.C. (2020). The efficient Lamarckian spread of life in the cosmos. In Steele, E.J., Wickramasinghe, N.C (Eds) "Cosmic Genetic Evolution" Adv. Genet. (Elsevier) Volume 106, In Press

Steele E.J., Qu, J., Gorczynski, R.M., Lindley, R.M.,Tokoro, G.,Temple, R., Wickramasinghe, N.C. (2020) Origin of new emergent Coronavirus and Candida fungal diseases—Terrestrial or cosmic? In Steele, E.J., Wickramasinghe, N.C (Eds) "Cosmic Genetic Evolution" Adv. Genet. (Elsevier) Volume 106. doi: 10.1016/bs.adgen.2020.04.002 [Epub ahead of print]

Tang, X., Wu, C., Li, X., Song, Y., et al. (2020) On the origin and continuing evolution of SARS-CoV-2. National Science Review (2020). nwaa036, https://doi.org/10.1093/nsr/nwaa036

Xu, J., Zhao, S., Teng, T., Abdalla, A.E., Zhu, W., Xie, L., Wang, Y., Guo , X. (2020) Systematic comparison of two animal-to-human transmitted human coronaviruses: SARS-CoV-2 and SARS-CoV Viruses 2020, 12, 244; doi:10.3390/v12020244

Watsa, M., and Wildlife Disease Surveillance Focus Group (2020). Rigorous wildlife disease surveillance Science 369 , 145-147. DOI: 10.1126/science.abc0017

Wickramasinghe, Chandra, (2018). *Proofs that Life Is Cosmic: Acceptance of a new paradigm* . World Scientific Publishing Co, Singapore, ISBN 978-981-3233-10-2.

Wickramasinghe, N. C., Steele, E. J., Gorczynski, R. M., Temple, R., Tokoro, G., Qu, J., et al. (2020a). Comments on the origin and spread of the 2019 Coronavirus. Virology: Current Research, 4(1). https://doi.org/10.37421/Virol Curr Res.2020.4.109.

Wickramasinghe, N. C., Steele, E. J., Gorczynski, R. M., Temple, R., Tokoro, G., Wallis, D. H., et al. (2020b). Growing evidence against global infection-driven by person-to-person transfer of COVID-19. Virology: Current Research, 4(1). https://doi. org/10.37421/Virol Curr Res.2020.4.110.

Wickramasinghe, N. C., Steele, E. J., Gorczynski, R. M., Temple, R., Tokoro, G., Kondakov, A., et al. (2020c). Predicting the future trajectory of COVID-19. Virology: Current Research, 4(1). https://doi.org/10.37421/Virol Curr Res.2020.4.111.

Wickramasinghe, C, Wainwright, M., Narlikar, J.(2003) SARS a clue to its origins? The Lancet 361, 1832. Doi: https://doi.org/10.1016/S0140-6736(03)13440-X

Wickramasinghe, N.C., Wallis, M.K. Coulson, S.G., Kondakov, A., Steele, E.J., Gorczynski, R.M., et al. (2020d) Intercontinental spread of COVID-19 on global wind systems Virology :Current Research 4(1) doi: 10.37421/Virol Curr Res.2020.4.113

13

https://www.hilarispublisher.com/open-access/intercontinental-spread-of-covid19-on-global-wind-systems.pdf

Wickramasinghe, N.C., Wickramasinghe , D.T.,   Christopher A. Tout, C.A., Lattanzio, J.C., Steele, E.J. (2019) Cosmic biology in perspective. Astrophys Space Sci 364:205 https://doi.org/10.1007/s10509-019-3698-6

Yang, D., Leibowitz, J.L. (2015) The structure and functions of coronavirus genomic 3′ and 5′ ends Virus Research 206 :120–133. https://doi.org/10.1016/j.virusres.2015.02.025

Zhang, R., Li, Y., Zhang, A.L.,Wang, Y., Molina, M.J. (2020) Identifying airborne transmission as the dominant route for the spread of COVID-19.Proc. Natl Acad. Sci. In Press https://www.pnas.org/cgi/doi/10.1073/pnas.2009637117

Zhang, T., Wu, Q.,Zhang, Z. (2020) Probable Pangolin origin of SARS-CoV-2 associated with the COVID-19 outbreak Current Biology 30, 1346–1351, April 6, 2020 https://doi.org/10.1016/j.cub.2020.03.022

Zhou, P., Yang, X-L., Wang, X-G., Hu, B., Zhang, L., Zhang, W., et al. (2020) A pneumonia outbreak associated with a new coronavirus of probable bat origin Nature 579 , 270-274 , 12 March 2020 https://doi.org/10.1038/s41586-020-2012-7

Received: 3 May 2021 | Revised: 28 August 2021 | Accepted: 29 August 2021

DOI: 10.1111/sji.13100

REGULAR ARTICLE

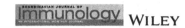

Analysis of SARS-CoV-2 haplotypes and genomic sequences during 2020 in Victoria, Australia, in the context of putative deficits in innate immune deaminase anti-viral responses

Robyn A. Lindley[1,2,3] | Edward J. Steele[3,4]

[1]GMDxgen Pty Ltd, Melbourne, Victoria, Australia

[2]Department of Clinical Pathology, The Victorian Comprehensive Cancer Centre, Faculty of Medicine, Dentistry & Health Sciences, University of Melbourne, Melbourne, Victoria, Australia

[3]Melville Analytics Pty Ltd, Melbourne, Victoria, Australia

[4]CYO'Connor ERADE Village Foundation, 24 Genomics Rise, Piara Waters, Australia

Correspondence
Edward J. Steele, Melville Analytics Pty Ltd, Level 2, 517 Flinders Lane, Melbourne, VIC 3000 Australia.
Email: e.j.steele@bigpond.com

Funding information
Supported entirely by in-house company funding (GMDxgen Pty Ltd and Melville Analytics PTY Ltd)

Abstract

The SARS-CoV-2 epidemic infections in Australia during 2020 were small in number in epidemiological terms and are well described. The SARS-CoV-2 genomic sequence data of many infected patients have been largely curated in a number of publicly available databases, including the corresponding epidemiological data made available by the Victorian Department of Health and Human Services. We have critically analysed the available SARS-CoV-2 haplotypes and genomic sequences in the context of putative deficits in innate immune APOBEC and ADAR deaminase anti-viral responses. It is now known that immune impaired elderly co-morbid patients display clear deficits in interferon type 1 (α/β) and III (λ) stimulated innate immune gene cascades, of which APOBEC and ADAR induced expression are part. These deficiencies may help explain some of the clear genetic patterns in SARS-CoV-2 genomes isolated in Victoria, Australia, during the 2nd Wave (June–September, 2020). We tested the hypothesis that predicted lowered innate immune APOBEC and ADAR anti-viral deaminase responses in a significant proportion of elderly patients would be consistent with/reflected in a low level of observed mutagenesis in many isolated SARS-CoV-2 genomes. Our findings are consistent with this expectation. The analysis also supports the conclusions of the Victorian government's Department of Health that essentially one variant or haplotype infected Victorian aged care facilities where the great majority (79%) of all 820 SARS-CoV-2 associated deaths occurred. The implications of our data analysis for other localized epidemics and efficient coronavirus vaccine design and delivery are discussed.

1 | INTRODUCTION

The coronavirus pandemic due to SARS-CoV-2 has engulfed the world and has exacted enormous health and economic tolls. Since it first emerged in Wuhan, China, in late November and early December 2019,[1-3] the health impact has been mainly on our elderly co-morbid citizens. In designing an effective vaccine, it is important, in our view, to understand how this pandemic coronavirus genetically diversifies at the RNA and protein levels as it infects different human populations. This is particularly the case for the elderly co-morbid subgroup where the deficits in innate immunity are clearly evident[4-8] as well as compromised adaptive immunity.[9,10] Type I and type III interferon (IFN) inducible anti-viral immunity is particularly effected.[11] Longitudinal studies show that patients in this subgroup appear 'immune defenceless' to coronavirus respiratory tract infections and are at a very high risk for severe outcomes including death.[11] Important reviews on the special susceptibility of this aged co-morbid group have appeared.[10,12] An integrated schematic of the innate immune deficits in relation to adaptive immune responses and severity of viral replication in healthy and susceptible human subjects has been published by Sette and Crotty[10] which clearly shows the barrier of induced innate immunity which normally quells viral replication in infected healthy subjects in the first few days of infection. Such a picture is completely consistent with a very large population-level observational study in Denmark (4 million PCR-tested individuals) showing that the elderly are more often immunologically vulnerable to reinfection with SARS-CoV-2.[13]

We have started the process of investigating exactly how SARS-CoV-2 varies genetically to gain insight into more effective vaccine design. In a previous study, we analysed the full-length genomic sequences generated over the first three months of the pandemic from late December 2019 through January 2020 in China (mainly Wuhan), then via the hot spot zones in Spain, some early sporadic outbreaks in California and Washington State (through February 2020) and then to the large-scale explosive outbreak in New York City in mid to late March 2020.[14] In that study, we used a haplotype rather than the more mainstream phylogenetic tree approach to the temporally emerging SARS-CoV-2 sequence data[15-17] The haplotype approach directly compares the full-length test sequence aligned against the Hu-1 reference. This type of comparison provides insights into the putative APOBEC and ADAR deaminase-driven cystosine to uracil (C > U) and adenosine-to-inosine (A > I/G) variation mechanisms per se which are not necessarily obvious or available with the phylogenetic approach of the Pangolin classification system[15-17] (which generates putative person-to-person or P-to-P lineages, clusters and clades). Indeed, RNA-sequence haplotypes, in our view, are functional strings implying stable RNA secondary structures required for maximal replicative efficiency in that host's genetic/biochemical background.[14] The other implication is that new vaccine designs and therapies may need to specifically target functionally important secondary structures with the presumptive replicative stability of the viral RNA genome (eg reviewed in Robson et al[18]).

Our detailed haplotype and sequence analyses reported here further extend the main findings from the previous

work[14] but now within a small well defined geographical urban setting. The main findings show how a single viral clone or haplotype of SARS-CoV-2, either unmutated or lightly mutated, can dominate a local epidemic and cause considerable health impacts on elderly citizens who are putatively immune defenceless. The person-to-person (P-to-P) spread of the same haplotype clone in closed institutions and between institutions was most likely affected by more healthy asymptomatic carriers of the disease. We are thus testing the hypothesis that due to *expected deficits* in type I and type III IFN inducible innate anti-viral immunity[11] involving activated APOBEC and ADAR deaminase expression[19-21] there will be a lowered level of observed mutagenesis in isolated SARS-CoV-2 genomes isolated from such patients. As we discussed earlier[14] the anti-viral properties of the induced innate immune APOBEC and ADAR deaminases are well documented in the literature. They are powerful viral genome mutators causing predominantly transition mutations such as C > T /G > A and A > G/T > C single nucleotide variations (SNV) in single-stranded and double-stranded viral RNA and DNA genomes.[21-25] Such mutations at some deaminase sites can be pro-viral.[21] On occasion, such mutators can also go off target affecting host genomes and thus contributing to cancer mutagenesis as recently reviewed by Lindley.[26]

Here, we report on an exhaustive analysis of the levels of mutagenesis in full-length SARS-CoV-2 genomes that have been, due to the mass testing coverage in Victoria, isolated mainly from putative elderly infected patients (and their carers and tending health professionals according to media and government reports) in order to assess a fit with the hypothesis that a predicted lowered innate immune APOBEC and ADAR anti-viral deaminase responses in a significant proportion of elderly patients would be consistent with/reflected in a low level of observed mutagenesis in many isolated SARS-CoV-2 genomes. The data, in an epidemiologically somewhat unique cohort (isolated island community, excellent biomedical research environment, first class public health response system), are consistent with our stated hypothesis.

2 | MATERIALS AND METHODS

2.1 | Publicly available data resources

Supporting Information Files A, B, C, D, E, F, G summarize much of this publicly available data and information and are cited below.

a. *Victorian Government Website* : Summary statistics of COVID-19 new cases and whether they were acquired in Australia (ie in Melbourne or Victorian regions) from a known source or from an unknown source have been recorded by the Government of Victoria at the Department of Health website https://www.dhhs.vic.gov.au/victorian-coronavirus-covid-19-data and in the *Herald Sun* newspaper, Figures 1, 2, 3, 4 and 5 and Table 1, and Supporting Information File A and F summarizes these infection data. Clearly as Table 1 shows most elderly people who died in Victoria (97.8%) on contracting SARS-CoV-2 were over 60 years, of median age 80-89 years, and these were concentrated in aged care facilities (Supporting Information File F). However, not all infected resident cases in aged care died; yet it was a significant yet variable fraction across a range of institutions, approximately 30%–40% of resident cases (Supporting Information File F).

b. *Herald Sun newspaper*: A full page of SARS-CoV-2 infection statistical data and detailed Victorian State map of case incident summaries (from mid-July to October 28) appeared each day in this Melbourne daily tabloid newspaper. Many of these pages were preserved and a scanned (pdf) digital record created. Examples for late July and early August—just before hard Stage 4 lock downs began on August 2—are shown in Supporting Information File A. Data in this newspaper record were used to construct the summary in Figure 2 from data in Supporting Information File C. This page of the newspaper also had a story of the day discussing the main challenges which the health authorities confronted. In our considered view, the most important reports, and there were many, were those on the very high incidence of 'Community Transmissions'. These cases, which are defined by rigorous epsidemiological contact tracing and genomic sequencing linked to a known cluster, are defined as SARS-CoV-2 infections

acquired from an unknown source (Figures 2, 3, 4 and 5, and Supporting Information file A, and see 'COVID-19 Hotel Quarantine Inquiry, Final Report and Recommendations'[27]). These cases were largely absent or rare in the Victorian 1st Wave where all secondary cases acquired in Australia came largely from infected overseas travellers into Melbourne. The numerous 'Community Transmission' cases in the 2nd Wave largely drove the Victorian Government's social distancing lock down policies. During the period from August 1 to September 6, these numbers went from highs of 94-174 per day (recorded across the City and the State) to 55-8 per day by September 6. (Supporting Information File C). They eventually declined as a significant driving source of infections as the epidemic petered out. The numbers per day are listed here to indicate they are small enough in daily aggregates for the teams of contract tracing units across the state to manage. However, the phrase 'Community Transmissions' quickly evolved over many detailed news reports of joint press conferences (Supporting Information File A) by the Chief Victorian Health Officer (Professor Brett Sutton) and the Premier of Victoria (Hon. Daniel Andrews) to become genuine 'Mystery Cases'—as they could not be traced to an acquisition from a known contact case, that is no patient zero, or linked to a known genomic sequence cluster.

a. *GenBank/NCBI Virus*. This publicly accessible site is hosted at The National Center for Biotechnology Information (NCBI) at the National Institutes of Health (NIH), Bethesda, Maryland, USA, which curates SARS-CoV-2 sequences at https://www.ncbi.nlm.nih.gov/sars-cov-2/#nucleotide-sequences. This was also used

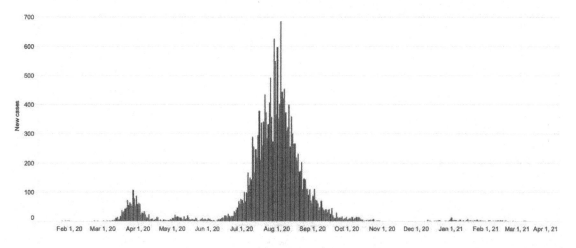

FIGURE 1   New SARS-CoV-2 cases per day recorded in Victoria, Australia, during 2020. These data can be accessed at https://www.dhhs.vic.gov.au/victorian-coronavirus-covid-19-data

for all sequences haplotyped and analysed in Steele and Lindley.[14] As before, the simple and straight forward NCBI Virus alignment tool at the site was used for all sample alignments against the original Wuhan Hu-1 reference sequence (NC_045512.2). The data for the haplotyping screens of 96 alignments of variable size can be found in the Supporting Information File B. It has sheets showing

TABLE 1   People who have passed away with coronavirus (COVID-19) in Victoria throughout 2020

Age Group	Male	Female	Total
00-09	0	0	0
10-19	0	0	0
20-29	1	0	1
30-39	2	0	2
40-49	1	0	1
50-59	10	4	14
60-69	20	9	29
70-79	83	46	129
80-89	166	182	348
90+	107	189	296
Total	390	430	820

Notes: Data from Victorian Department Health and Humans Services website as 13 March 2021. https://www.dhhs.vic.gov.au/victorian-coron avirus-covid-19-data

Numbers of deaths of all SARS-CoV-2 cases in Victoria 2020. This is from the Victorian Government Department of Health website as 17 March 2021. The median age at death assumed by COVID-19 is 80-89 years, and 97.8% of all deaths were in patients >60 years; and 94.3% are aged >70 years.

https://www.dhhs.vic.gov.au/victorian-coronavirus-covid-19-data

the alignment number and sequence IDs; the alignments grouped by collection period from patients; a summary of numbers of various haplotypes versus collection dates; tables showing accumulated haplotype numbers over different collection times. An excel table and histogram plots (see Figures 6 and 7) showing the emergence of the almost clonal L241f.1vic haplotype over time versus the related L241f.1 haplotype in collections from early March 2020 to early September 2020 is assembled from data in Supporting Information File B and D and also presented in Supporting Information File E.

An important caveat is there is no metadata available in the public domain linking a particular patient's clinical/epidemiological data to a given GenBank Accession number for a full-length SARS-CoV-2 genomic sequence. All associations are thus inferred from the sheer dominance of all main SARS-CoV-2 case data (and deaths) amongst the elderly and within aged or nursing care facilities (Supporting Information F). Inquiries in writing were made to The Victorian Department of Health and The Peter Doherty Institute, and these were unsuccessful in securing metadata information.

2.2 | Analysis of SARS-CoV-2 sequences at NCBI virus

a. Main Haplotype Screen. The haplotype analyses using the NCBI Virus 'Align' tool screened 12,798 SARS-CoV-2 genomes collected in Victoria from first travellers into Melbourne from Wuhan and other world cities from January through to October 2 (Supporting Information

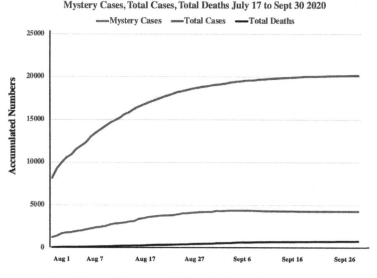

Mystery Cases, Total Cases, Total Deaths July 17 to Sept 30 2020

From Melbourne *Herald Sun* newspaper July 27, July 30, July 31, Aug 1 through Sept 30

FIGURE 2   Total accumulated mystery cases, total cases and total accumulated deaths from July 27 through September 30—as published daily in the *Herald Sun* newspaper (Supporting Information File C)

SCANDINAVIAN JOURNAL OF Immunology AN INTERNATIONAL MONTHLY JOURNAL -WILEY | 5 of 20

FIGURE 3 Numbers of confirmed cases acquired versus cases acquired from unknown cause sin Victoria 1st wave March through May 2020. Primary data in NCOV_COVID_Cases_by_Source_20210131.csv at: https://www.dhhs.vic.gov.au/victorian-coronavirus-covid-19-data

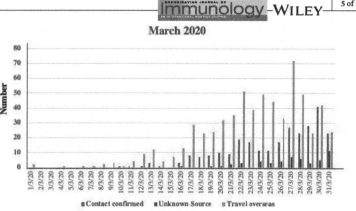

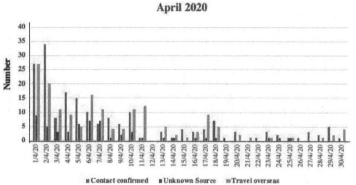

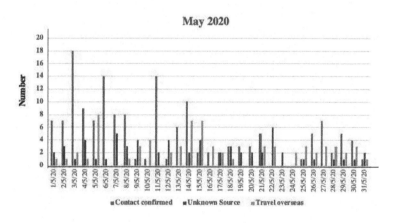

File B). The haplotype markers across the Hu-1 SARS-CoV-2 genome are those shown in Table 2 which includes the L241f.1vic haplotype which was defined more clearly in the detailed later Sequence Alignment analyses of all L241f.1 haplotypes from March, April, May and June and sample collection times in July, August and September (Supporting Information File D). Table 2 is thus a refinement and revised update of the original provisional haplotyping table.[14] The main addition is the L241f.1 haplotype with the distinctive SNV tandem

changes GGG>AAC at p.28881-3. This was in international circulation as it was observed at low frequency in New York City (late March 2020)[14] and also in many collections in Florida through April, May, June and July 2020 (data not shown).

Summaries of all the data on the haplotype screen are in the Supporting Information File B, Excel Book Sheets S1-S5. This large haplotype screen employed SNV markers at p.241, p.1059, p.3037, p.8782, p.11083, 14 408, p.25563, p.28144, p.28881-3.

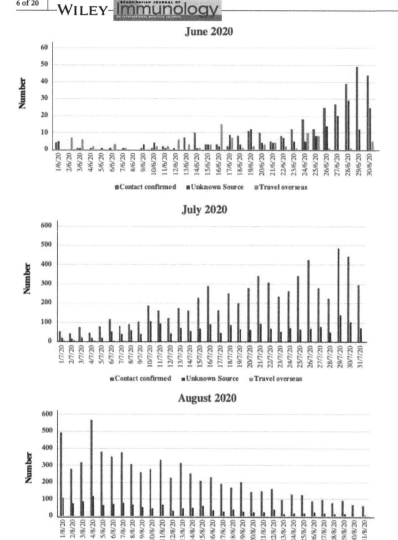

FIGURE 4 Numbers of confirmed cases acquired versus cases acquired from unknown cause in Victoria 2nd wave June through August 2020. Primary data in NCOV_COVID_Cases_by_Source_20210131.csv at: https://www.dhhs.vic.gov.au/victorian-coronavirus-covid-19-data

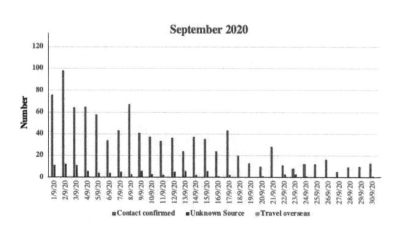

FIGURE 5 Numbers of confirmed cases acquired versus cases acquired from unknown cause in Victoria 2nd wave tail September 2020. Primary data in NCOV_COVID_Cases_by_Source_20210131.csv at: https://www.dhhs.vic.gov.au/victorian-coronavirus-covid-19-data

FIGURE 6   Haplotype numbers by collection period in first screen from data at NCBI virus. The primary summarized data are in Supporting Information File B, and these plots are from Sheet S4

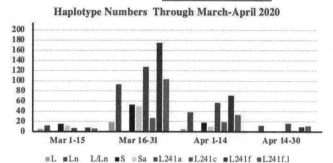

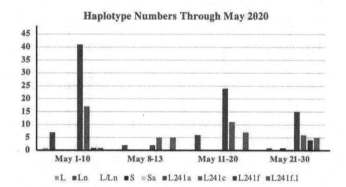

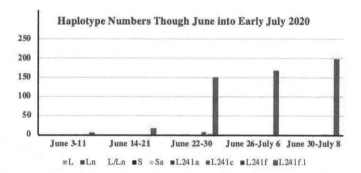

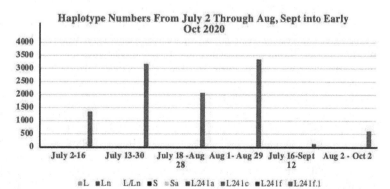

b. Genomic Sequence Alignments of L241f.1 haplotypes March, April, May, June and for Selected Collection Times July, August and September. Full-length genomic sequence analyses of L241f.1 haplotypes with collection times were conducted (Supporting Information File D) where the full patterns of SNV variability across many

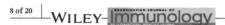

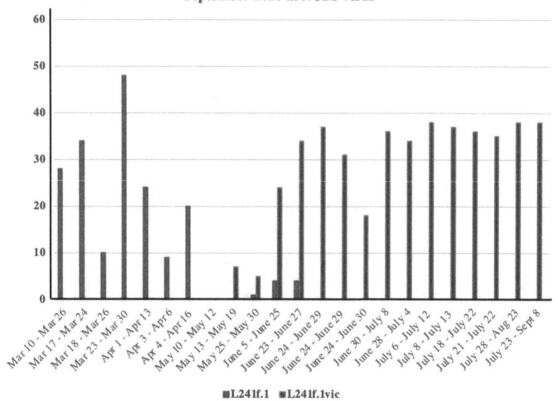

Numbers L241f.1 and L241f.1vic Sequences Sampled March through September 2020 at NCBI Virus

■L241f.1   ■L241f.1vic

FIGURE 7   Emergence of L241f.1vic haplotypic sequence and disappearance of the L241f.1 haplotypic sequence from the uploads at GenBank/NCBI Virus. From Supporting Information Files D and E

collection time points can be inspected in that wider data set. The alignments discussed here were preserved as screen shot records of each NCBI Virus alignment for later construction of Variable Site Diagrams, or VSDs which clarify haplotype analysis as discussed[14] (Supporting Information File D). The putative impact of SNV changes on protein structure and function was qualitatively assessed as in Steele and Lindley[14] using the colour code for amino acid conservation or change in Supporting Information File D.

The VSDs were sorted by sub-variants of the L241f.1 haplotype and also by sequences that were clearly unmutated, usually grouped at the bottom of each VSD figure. In this way, lightly mutated haplotypes can also be easily identified and P-to-P transfers and P-to-P groups can also be readily identified. The SNV patterns from VSDs for the L241f.1vic haplotype are summarized in Table 3.

2.3 | Independent haplotype analysis of 'Vic' tagged SARS-CoV-2 sequences uploaded to GISAID database

An independent check was kindly conducted by Dr Jared Mamrot on the above haplotype screen and sequence alignment analyses on Victoria, Australia SARS-CoV-2 sequence data at NCBI Virus. The catalogue of Victorian SARS-CoV-2 sequences at the GISAID db (with GenBank ID links) was downloaded and screened for haplotype numbers using the haplotype markers defined in Table 2 at given collection dates spanning the 2nd wave, June 1 to September 30. Specifically, all SARS-CoV-2 viral genomes were obtained from GISAID (https://www.gisaid.org/) on 15 March 2021 and from GenBank (https://www.ncbi.nlm.nih.gov/sars-cov-2/) on 23 March 2021. FASTA sequences with 'Vic' in the identifier (case-insensitive search) were extracted from both databases, combined, and duplicates were removed.

Sequences collected between 01/06/2020 and 30/09/2020 were extracted (n = 12,009) and aligned to the NC_045512.2 SARS-CoV-2 reference genome using MAFFT (v7.475; https://mafft.cbrc.jp/alignment/software/) with options '--6merpair --keeplength --addfragments'. Haplotypes were defined according to 19 genomic positions, relative to the reference genome as listed in Table 2: p.241, p.1059, p.3037, p.1163, p.7540, p.8782, p.11083, p.14408, p.16647, p.17747, p.17858, p.18060, p.18555, p.22992, p.23401, p.23403, p.25563, p.28144, p.28881-3. Nucleotides at these positions were identified for each sample, collated and summarized. These data are in Supporting Information File G and for further ease of principle haplotype identification and analysis were sorted first by column T (p.28881-3), then by column F (p.7540), then by column C (p.1059) and then by column D (p.3037).

2.4 | Correspondence between Pangolin classification and main haplotypes in Table 2

At time of writing, we are in the process of forming a translation table for the main Steele-Lindley (S/L) 'replicative' haplotypes (Table 2) with the PANGO classification system'. At this stage it is evident that.

PANGO 'B' = L Hap of S/L = Wuhan ref seq December 2019 (Hu-1).

PANGO 'P.1 and B.1.1.7 and B.1.1.348' = L241f.1 haplotype variants of S/L. This would cover the 'UK Mutant' and the different 'Vic Mutant' (L241f.1vic) that infected many Melbourne aged care and nursing home and presumed secondary asymptomatic contacts.

PANGO 'B.1 and B.1.526 and B.1.429 and B.1.526.1' = L241a of S/L. A common and frequent haplotype seen in overseas air travellers in the Vic 1st Wave March-April 2020.

PANGO 'B.1.525' = L241f of S/L. A common and frequent haplotype seen in overseas air travellers in the Vic 1st Wave March–April 2020.

Therefore, a number of PANGO lineages in this first small sample tested can be understood in terms of the sequence architecture of the main coordinated positional changes in the 29 903 nt Hu-1 RNA sequence (which is 'B' or 'L'). Evidently, PANGO is tracking human passaged variants in local global regions and they appear as Sub-Haplotype variants of the main Haplotypes we have recorded in the first three months of the pandemic.[14] In other NCBI Virus, multiple alignment analyses of pairs or groups of the same PANGO variants collected at different times in different geographical regions it is apparent to us these PANGO variants are the end products of multiple P-to-P transfers accumulating largely deaminase-mediated[14] mutations at each transfer. Estimates of the number of putative

mutagenic P-to-P transfers away from the primary haplotypes reported in Steele and Lindley[14] range from 4 P-to-P transfers for B.1.1.7 to 6 or 7 transfers to generate B.1.525 and 3 or 4 transfers to generate B.1.526 lineages (data not shown, Steele EJ, Gorczynski RM et al in preparation).

3 | RESULTS

The opportunity to gain a deeper insight into the SARS-CoV-2 genetic variation mechanisms and viral adaptation strategies during the pandemic was offered by the definitive sets of observations on SARS-CoV-2 case numbers in Victoria, (mainly in Melbourne) Australia. The Victorian epidemics are scientifically definitive for several reasons:

1. The genesis of the two epidemics were clearly different, the 1st Wave due solely to overseas travellers entering Australia from Northern Hemisphere infected zones, the 2nd Wave to infections clearly acquired in Australia (Figures 1, 3, 4, 5). This is a very important demarcation in the case data.
2. The health authorities implemented strict lock downs and social distancing protocols, including mandatory mask wearing and mass PCR testing as well as quarantining of overseas travellers on arrival.
3. The health authorities identified hot zones all over the state and convinced tens of thousands of citizens to get PCR-tested on a mass scale whether showing symptoms or not (upwards of 30,000 PCR tests on oro-nasal swabs per day through May, June, July, August and September 2020).
4. Teams of contact tracers were actively coordinated throughout Melbourne and regions and were largely comprehensive despite some failures and much public political criticism of the regimentation of public behaviour involved.

As a consequence, a large amount of epidemiological data, PCR testing data and full-length genomic sequences were generated and largely placed in the public domain. This allows the comprehensive analysis and conclusions we record here. These observations and genomic sequence data are represented in 2020 by the main 1st and 2nd Wave SARS-CoV-2 epidemics: the 1st Wave in March-April (with a May blip in new cases and secondary transmissions) and the 2nd Wave beginning mid-June through July, August and September (Figure 1). Thus, many of the full-length genomic sequences for these epidemics (≥12,000) are publicly available for direct analysis using the alignment tools at the NCBI GenBank/NCBI Virus website. Moreover, whilst these two epidemics in Australia have been very controversial and caused much political dysfunction in

TABLE 2 Haplotypes and main sites defining SARS-CoV-2 common strain variants updated and revised for Victoria -Corrected 30.6.21

	AA class->	P<>NonP	SYN	P<>NonP	SYN	SYN	NonP<>NonP	NonP<>NonP	SYN
	5'UTR	Thr<>Ile	Phe<>Phe	Ile<>Phe	Thr<>Thr	Ser<>Ser	Leu<>Phe	Pro<>Leu	Thr<>Thr
HAP	p.241	p.1059	p.3037	p.1163	p.7540	p.8782	p.11080/83	p.14408	p.16647
L (Hu-1)	C	C	C	A	T	C	G	C	G
Ln	C	C	C	A	T	C	T	C	G
L-241a	T	T	T	A	T	C	G	T	G
L-241b	T	T	C	A	T	C	G	T	G
L-241c	T	C	T	A	T	C	G	T	G
L-241d/s	T	T	T	A	T	C	G	C	G
L-241e	T	C	C	A	T	C	G	T	G
L-241f	T	C	T	A	T	C	G	T	G
L-241f.1	T	C	T	A	T	C	G	T	G
L-241f.1vic	T	C	T	*T*	*C*	C	G	T	*T*
L-241g	T	C	C	A	T	C	G	T	G
S	C	C	C	A	T	T	G	C	G
Sa	C	C	C	A	T	T	G	C	G
Sb	C	C	C	A	T	T	G	C	G
Ss	C	C	C	A	T	T	G	C	G

Notes: p.11080/83 is a pan-Haplotype marker (G/T) of putative 8oxoG non-deaminase modification at a WG site that can occur across haplotypes.

Key changes in *italic* to focus on for Victorian 2nd wave analyses.

The table shows haplotypes and main sites defining SARS-CoV-2 common strain variants documented in China, USA, Spain (January-March) Florida (May, June, July), California (March), with Update and Revision for Victoria as 16.3.21 Post Publication Steele and Lindley.[14]

p.7540 site annotation corrected as 30.6.21 from P<>P Ser<>Thr tp SYN Thr<>Thr.

Victoria,[27] the epidemics nevertheless have features that allow succint scientific analysis not necessarily available to Northern Hemisphere infected zones (where the great bulk of global infections have occurred and continue to occur at the time of writing).

The Results section thus highlights the statistics of the SARS-CoV-2 cases through 2020, the complete haplotyping of all publicly available SARS-CoV-2 genomes, and a detailed comparative full-length sequence analysis of all L241f.1genomes collected in March, April, May, June and sample sets selected at different times through early, mid and late July, and though August and September (all these alignments are summarized as VSD in Supporting Information File D, with SNV summary in Table 3).

3.1 | Overview SARS-CoV-2 case statistics of the 1st and 2nd waves in Victoria in 2020

The pandemic in Australia began with travellers into Australia from overseas infected zones, beginning in late January 2020 and continuing through to the end of April and also later times into May 2020.[28] The numbers of New Cases per Day are shown in Figure 1.

The main 1st and 2nd Waves are shown—March–April, then from June through September and early October. There is a slight blip in May which can be considered for operational purposes the tail of the 1st Wave. The 1st wave was generated solely by infected travellers into Melbourne, and the 2nd Wave from mid-June through to the end of October generated almost exclusively by new cases acquired in Australia. About 79% of all cases acquired in Australia (ie Victoria) in the 2nd wave were by contact with an identifiable SARS-CoV-2 'case' or by assignment to a known SARS-CoV-2 genomic sequence cluster. Many however were acquired from an unknown source and could not be assigned by contact tracing or linked to a known cluster by genomic sequencing (Figures 2-5).

Further insight into these case categories is provided at the Victorian Department of Health website in the data displayed in Figures 3-5 for March, April, May, June, July, August and September. This is a very informative set of plots based on recorded daily Acquired Cases in

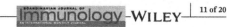
NonP<>NonP	P<>P	SYN	SYN	P<>P	SYN	Acid<>NonP	P<>Basic	P<>NonP	RADICLE
Pro<>Leu	Tyr<>Cys	Leu<>Leu	Asp<>Asp	Ser<>Asn	Gln<>Gln	Asp<>Gly	Gln<>His	Leu<>Ser	Arg, Gly>Lys, Arg
p.17747	p.17858	p.18060	p.18555	p.22992	p.23401	p.23403	p.25563	p.28144	p.28881-3
C	A	C	C	G	G	A	G	T	GGG
C	A	C	C	G	G	A	G	T	GGG
C	A	C	C	G	G	G	T	T	GGG
C	A	C	C	G	G	G	T	T	GGG
C	A	C	C	G	G	G	T	T	GGG
C	A	C	C	G	G	G	T	T	GGG
C	A	C	C	G	G	G	T	T	GGG
C	A	C	C	G	G	G	G	T	GGG
C	A	C	C	G	G	G	G	T	AAC
C	A	C	T	A	A	G	G	T	AAC
C	A	C	C	G	G	G	G	T	GGG
C	A	C	C	G	G	A	G	C	GGG
T	G	T	C	G	G	A	G	C	GGG
C	A	C	C	G	G	A	G	C	GGG
C	A	C	C	G	G	A	G	C	GGG

Victoria confirmed by contact with an infected source, against those Acquired from an Unknown Source, and Infected Travellers from Overseas. It clearly shows that 'Community Transmissions' or 'Mystery Cases' (acquired in Victoria from an unknown source) were low in the 1st Wave March, April (from putative secondary transmissions from infected travellers from overseas), were low in May into the middle of June at which point they began to rise significantly rising from about 10 per day (June 17) to 20-30 per day by the end of June, and then maintained, apart from occasional spikes, at about 50-60 per day right through to about August 10. They were spread all over widely separate suburbs and regions near Melbourne (see case incident data by local government area at https://www.dhhs.vic.gov.au/victorian-coronavirus-covid-19-data). In contrast acquired cases with a confirmed contact displayed, a more explosive rise each day through late June and rose sharply each day staying high throughout July into mid-August when clear declines were setting in (see the flaring New Cases Per Day spikes in Figure 1 during this period). All of the confirmed contact cases were associated with known putative cases in aged care and nursing facilities, which dominated the 2nd Wave. These case and death data, for residents, health workers and carers can be viewed in Supporting Information File F. These foci of explosive hotspots, on the data available at GenBank/NCBI Virus, putatively fuelled the spread of the main infective clones of the dominant L241f.1vic haplotype variant (Table 2).

The data in Figures 3-5 are significant because they attest to the robustness of the contact tracing and genomic sequence assignment system in place in Victoria. The numbers per day were small enough for the contact tracing teams coupled to SARS-CoV-2 genomic sequencing at The Peter Doherty Institute to establish or eliminate links of the patient to known clusters. We can deduce this because as the clones of L241f.1vic infecting aged care facilities were being amplified their sheer spiking numbers (see Figure 1, particularly during July) reduced the apparent proportion of cases with an unknown source, which, as discussed, remained remarkably constant with an array of haphazard spikes. It can be seen in the 'Mystery Case' data for August 2020 as recorded in the media by the *Herald Sun* newspaper (Supporting Information File C).

TABLE 3 SNV frequency and P-to-P spread among L241f.1vic haplotype sequences 5 June through 8 September 2020

| Collection Date 2020 | No. of L241f.1vic | No. L241f.1vic Sequences with SNV Differences | | | | | No. P-to-P Clusters with Shared SNV Differences | | | |
L241f.1 Alignment	Sequences	0	1	2	3	≥4	1	2	3	≥4
June 7-June 25 (L241f.1 Align#1)	25	4	6	1	2	0	4	0	0	0
June 23-June 27 (L241f.1 Align#2)	34	9	1	5	0	0	3	0	0	0
June 24-June 29 (L241f.1 Align#3)	37	14	13	4	2	0	3	2	9	0
June 24-June 29 (L241f.1 Align#4)	31	7	3	6	0	0	3	0	0	0
June 24-June 30 (L241f.1 Align#5)	18	6	3	2	1	0	3	0	0	0
June 30-July 8 (L241f.1 Align#16)	36	4	1	8	3	0	4	0	0	0
June 28-July 4 (L241f.1 Align#13)	34	7	10	10	0	1	6	0	0	0
July 6-July 12 (L241f.1 Align#17)	38	13	13	5	4	3	6	0	0	0
July 8-July 13 (L241f.1 Align#18)	37	8	16	9	1	2	5	2	0	2
July 18-July 22 (L241f.1 Align#19)	36	12	12	7	4	1	5	0	2	0
July 21-July 22 (L241f.1 Align#20)	35	4	7	10	7	8	2	3	1	1
July 28-Aug 23 (L241f.1 Align#15)	38	4	9	10	10	5	6	2	0	0
July 23-Sept 8 (L241f.1 Align#14)	38	4	10	9	10	5	4	2	2	0

Note: Sequence collections times, alignment number from variable site diagrams in Supporting Information File D.

3.2 | Haplotype analyses of NCBI virus publicly available genomic sequencing data

The positional SNV markers for the first haplotype screen of 12,798 genomic sequences at NCBI Virus (versus the Hu-1 reference) were (Table 2) at p.241, p.1059, p.3037, p.8782, p.11083, p.14408, p.23403, p.25563, p.28144 and p.28881-3. Variants of the S haplotype (p.8782/p.28144) were further subtyped by markers at p.17747, p.18858 and p.18060. The marker p.11083 G/T we have noted as a pan-haplotype SNV but does distinguish L (Wuhan) from Ln (New York). In some cases in the aligned sequence data (Supporting Information File B), an N run across the

p.11083 site meant the haplotype was either L or Ln. L, Ln or L/Ln were common in the 1st Wave of travellers to Melbourne. A summary of all the haplotypes available at GenBank/NCBI Virus March 1 through October 2 is shown in Figure 6.

It is clear that there is considerable haplotype diversity through March and April. These haplotype patterns are consistent with the lineage and cluster patterns reported in Seemann et al[28] and in the sample we reported in Steele and Lindley.[14] For our immediate purposes here, note that the L241f.1 haplotype was prominent, but not dominant, in March 2020 and was at low frequency in late April and into first week of May. These markers, defining the

L241f.1 sequence, then picked up sequence signals at low frequency from May 8 to 13 and maintained at low numbers right through to mid-June. Notice that by mid-June, most of the other haplotypes typical of the travellers entering Australia had dropped to low or undetectable numbers as numbers of international flights arriving in Australia were reduced.

Then from the third week of June, right through to the end of the collection period, (Oct 8) the L241f.1 haplotype (as defined Table 2) dominated all uploaded sequences at the NCBI Virus website.

It later became apparent when the actual full-length sequences of these L241f.1 haplotypes were examined in greater detail, that a clear new variant of L241f.1 had emerged from about May 10 with additional six coordinated changes (at largely riboswitch sites as defined earlier) at p.1163, p.7540, p.16647, p.18555, p.22992 and p.23401 now defining the L241f.1vic haplotype (as named by us here). This haplotype was the L241f.1vic variant that dominated all sequences uploaded to GenBank/NCBI Virus through to the end of the 2nd Wave (Figure 7). We have no clear sequence-linked metadata, but a plausible assumption is these were causally associated with the daily reported flareups of case numbers (see spikes in Figure 1, particularly through July) in the many Victorian SARS-CoV-2 case hotspots at aged care facilities across the inner and outer Western (and some Eastern) suburbs of Melbourne (Supporting Information File F). The flare ups in late June-early July are consistent with the well-publicized outbreaks in Melbourne in the nine tower blocks in the north west of the city in Kensington. All these high population density towers, with many three generation families from migrant communities, were '.. put into "hard" lockdown on 4 July, with 3000 residents told not to leave their homes for five days. State police was brought in to ensure compliance, and as community transmission continued to grow, lockdown measures were applied across Melbourne'.[29]

3.3 | Full-length genomic sequence alignments of L241f.1 haplotypes of NCBI virus uploaded sequence data

We then set out to establish whether or not the set of SARS-CoV-2 full-length sequences of the L241f.1 haplotype, as defined by the markers in Table 2, is the same basic genomic sequence throughout the 1st and 2nd Waves. All the L241f.1 haplotypes available from March, April, May, June and at later sample collection times in July, August, September (we sampled groups across representative collection times as the numbers there were very large) were aligned against Hu-1 and the sequence

alignments presented as VSD as shown in Supporting Information File D, and SNVs analysed as summarized in Table 3 for these collection times. The full set of sample times is in Supplementary Information File D which shows a more detailed trend in the VSD patterns over time, particularly in the L241f.1vic haplotype that went on to dominate sequence uploads exclusively from mid-June. The type of SNV change at a given VSD position relative to the Hu-1 reference sequence (C > T, A > G, T > C, G > A, G > T etc) can be deduced from the entries in the body of the table against the Hu-1 line at the top of each VSD figure (NC_045512). Note that a detailed compilation of the main types of SNV changes at APOBEC deamination C-sites and ADAR deamination A-sites for isolates Jan-Mar 2020 from Northern Hemisphere hotspot zones (Wuhan, New York City, West Coast USA, Spain) can be found in Steele and Lindley (2020).[14]

3.3.1 | March

The VSD in Supporting Information File D show the sequence patterns of SNVs across the SARS-CoV-2 full-length L241f.1 genomes collected in March 2020. Note the striking sequence conservation at the RNA and at the amino acid level. In this sample, 12/33 [36%] are unmutated and many are lightly mutated (15/33 [46%]) with 1-2 SNV per sequence. The sharing of sequences in the lightly mutated category can be seen. P-to-P transfers may well be evident in the unmutated set, but patient metadata would be required to establish that. These sequence data suggest that patients from SARS-CoV-2-infected Northern Hemisphere zones brought the unmutated L241f.1 sequence into Melbourne, and if they did transfer the sequence on by secondary P-to-P the recipient subject on average introduced one or two new SNVs into the sequence. This was also observed repeatedly in our first report.[14] The smaller numbers of more heavily mutated sequences (eg MT451254 with 8 SNVs) may indicate the endpoint of possibly two P-to-P transfers, and we assume in healthy subjects with active APOBEC and ADAR deaminase mutator responses. In the same vein, some of the unmutated sequences could be primary or secondary P-to-P infections circulating in subjects with deficits in Innate Immune deaminase mutagenesis.

3.3.2 | April through May

These sample VSD alignments (Supporting Information D) capture the VSD patterns from March, April though to May 19, and reveal the emergence of the L241f.1vic sequence in collections on May 13 (unmuted or lightly mutated). There are other interesting features in these data including sharing of sequences indicative of a number of P-to-P secondary transfers to at least 1 or 4 other recipient patients (close interacting groups such as a family?). Notice clear additional mutagenesis on secondary transfer in these groups, suggesting these recipients could be healthy subjects with functioning Innate Immune deaminase mutagenesis. The L241f.1vicm sequence identified did not flourish much further during June and early July (Supporting Information File D).

3.3.3 | June 5–June 25

This sample alignment (Supporting Information File D) illustrates features already discussed and shows that the L241f.1vic sequence begins to dominate the sequences uploaded to NCBI Virus through June. Note that a residue of L241f.1 sequences, initiated as secondary transfers and thus derivatives from incoming overseas travellers (?) display sequences that are heavily mutated, in contrast to many other sets (both L241f.1vicm and L241f.1vic sequences). What is notable about the L241f.1vicm and L241f.1vic sequences is largely the absence of mutation, or evidence of lightly mutated sequences on P-to-P transfer (Table 3).

3.3.4 | June 23–June 30

These sample alignments (Supporting Information D) show a continuation of the trend discussed (Table 3). Thus, largely unmutated representatives of the L241f.1vic haplotype clearly dominate all uploaded sequence collections from infected subjects. Again, on secondary transfer of the unmutated sequence, one or two SNVs may be introduced but most are not further mutated or lightly mutated (Table 3).

3.3.5 | June 28–July 22

The alignments over these collection periods (Supporting Information File D) were for samples collected when the explosive epidemic was reaching its peak (Figure 1). Whilst there are still many unmutated and lightly mutated l241f.1vic sequences (1-2 SNVs per sequence), there is also evidence of multiple P-to-P secondary transfers with a higher number of SNVs per sequence (Table 3)—this could plausibly suggest transfers in closed aged care facilities to healthier medical and carer staff (or other visitors) in such institutions. This latter group dominate sets

of cases, outnumbering infected residents by about fifty per cent (Supporting Information File F).

3.3.6 | July 28 to August 23

These alignments (Supporting Information File D) cover sequence collections as the epidemic was declining though August into September (right hand side of Figure 1). The increased SNV density pattern per sequence has now become far more pronounced. Whilst there are clearly some unmutated Ll241f.1vic sequences, the great majority are now mutated and evidence of secondary transfer of group sizes 2-4 are now evident in the data (Table 3). The dominance of clearly multiply mutated sequences is plausible evidence of P-to-P transmission into and from healthy subjects introducing Innate Immune deaminase-mediated mutations into the viral genome (which could also be introductions, or infections, into elderly co-morbid patients as well, but patient metadata would be required to identify such P-to-P transfers).

3.3.7 | July 23 to September 8

These alignments (Supporting Information File D) cover sequence collections as the epidemic was in evident decline though August into September (right-hand side of Figure 1). The patterns of SNV and P-to-P transfers are very similar to that discussed above in Section 3.3.6 July 28 to August 23 (Table 3).

The data just presented is either comprehensive or were selected to be representative and illustrative of the SARS-CoV-2 sequence changes in Victoria in the 1st and 2nd Waves (as made public at the NCBI Virus website). The wider set of SNV patterns showing this clear quantitative and qualitative trend in the VSD plots can be found in Supporting Information File D. The clear trend from mid-June to end of July is the amplification of the L241f.1vic haplotype clone virtually unmutated (or very lightly mutated) as summarized also in Table 3.

3.4 | Biases in uploaded sequence data

The uploaded sequence data at NCBI Virus for collections in Victoria, Australia, whilst substantial are clearly biased and do not report the complete numbers of known full-length genomes, estimated to be approximately 3500-4000 'Community Transmissions' or 'Mystery Cases' described above. For the period covering the entire 2nd Wave June 1-September 30, the numbers of these acquired cases from an unknown source totalled 3571 (from data in Figures 3-5). That is, we do not know the extent of the types of haplotype diversity (see Table 2) or mutational loads in such haplotypes of such subjects, nor do we have information on such 'Mystery Cases' amongst residents and other cases in aged care facilities (see Supporting Information F). The clear biased deficit in numbers of putative mystery case SARS-CoV-2 genomic sequences, which would have differed significantly in haplotype sequence from the main amplified L241f.1vic haplotype (unmutated or lightly mutated), requires further comment.

Either these collections were not sequenced: that is, contact tracing established by conventional means failed to identify a confirmed case contact X was considered sufficient evidence. Alternatively, they were routinely sequenced given the scale of the sequencing operation at The Peter Doherty Institute. This seems more plausible as all public commentary through June, July and August including testimony by lead epidemiologist at the Victorian Department of Health (Dr Charles Alpren) to the formal government inquiry into aged care outbreaks[27] directly implied that mystery cases were full-length genomes sequenced to formally exclude them from the main known hot spot clusters in aged care. They were not made publicly available to GenBank/ NCBI Virus. We can only speculate that they were not made available as they were considered 'uninteresting sequences' in explaining the wild-fire spread of the main SARS-CoV-2 'clone' (L241f.1vic) through Victorian aged care and nursing facilities. This is a possible yet speculative explanation given the medical emergency at the time. Indeed as reported in the *British Medical Journal,* Professor Ben Howden, director of the Microbiological Diagnostic Unit Public Health Laboratory at The Peter Doherty Institute, told the government inquiry[29] in mid-August 2020.. '..that, of the 1837 cases of local transmission that have been sequenced since 8 May, 99.8% came from three clusters, one from the Rydges Hotel and two from the five star Stamford Plaza Hotel'.[29] We can plausibly associate the major L241f.1vic haplotype with the Rydges Hotel cluster, and the other minor haplotypes through May and June with the L241f.1vicm, L241a, L241c and L241f.1 haplotypic variants (Figure 6, Supporting Information Files B, D and section e. below, analysis of GISAID db available sequencing data). Yet everyday throughout July and August official public references were made (by the Premier of Victoria Hon. Daniel Andrews and Chief Health Officer Professor Brett Sutton) to the continuing high numbers of mystery cases as it was feared they were contributing also by allowing transmissions to aged care facilities causing infection cluster flare ups (the spikes in daily case numbers as seen in Figure 1).

TABLE 4   Total statistics in Victorian aged care in 2nd wave 2020

Confirmed cases	Staff cases	Resident cases	Other cases	Deaths
5078	2009	1947	1122	647
-	(39.6%)	(38.3%)	(22.1%)	(12.7%)

Note: Summary of totals from Supporting Information F.

3.5 | Haplotype analyses of GISAID publicly available genomic sequencing data

An independent check at the GISAID db (and GenBank db) on total Victorian sequences and their haplotypes (Table 2) was conducted by Dr Jared Mamrot on the sequences uploaded by The Peter Doherty Institute for collections in the period June 1 through September 30. The magnitude of sequence numbers established in the analysis at NCBI Virus and the dominance of the L241f.1vic sequences in June, July, August and September were confirmed. In addition, the sporadic occurrences of other minor haplotypes are consistent with our above analyses, in June 2020. We have concluded that genomic sequences from the cases from an unknown cause, that is the expected large numbers of sequences quite different from the dominant L241f.1vic sequence, were not present in the GISAID repository at the time of submission of this paper. The haplotyping analysis is in Supporting Information File G. In this separate analysis, all Victorian GISAID and associated GenBank ID sequences (at both low and high coverage) allow estimates of the extreme haplotype dominance of the L241f.1vic haplotype (>99% of all sequences collected) and the occurrence of other minor variants and haplotypes: the 18 nt in-frame deletion variant of L241f.1vic, from p.288879 removing the p.28881-3 marker (Supplementary Information File B); the minor L241f.1vicm variant ($n \sim 214$) detected in May and June in GenBank/NCBI Virus uploaded data, which did not further appear in high numbers through July and August in sequence data uploaded to both GenBank/NCBI Virus and GISAID databases; and lower numbers of L241f $n \sim 5$, L241fc $n \sim 41$, L/Ln $n \sim 6$ and S with $n \sim 1$.

4 | DISCUSSION

In our considered view, as listed above, there are a number of scientific advantages in analysing the data on what exactly happened at the SARS-CoV-2 genomic sequence level during the 1st and 2nd Waves in Victoria, Australia. Thus, despite the extreme personal hardships, the SARS-CoV-2 epidemics in Australia enabled many types of observations based on a set of almost 'controlled conditions' or 'biomedical experiments of nature' (despite the biases in the data highlighted). For example, as we discuss below, it allows a considered reflection on how the 'UK Mutant' first arose to dominance and why this publicized highly putatively contagious SARS-CoV-2 mutant did not spread when it appeared in Australia in January 2021 brought in by multiple travellers from the UK into many different major Australian cities (Adelaide, Perth, Brisbane, Melbourne, Sydney).

Using publicly available data and observations, we have recorded here some key genomic features of the 1st and 2nd Wave SARS-CoV-2 epidemics in Victoria that can be discerned which involves mainly the city of Melbourne and some nearby regional towns and cities to the north west (Macedon, Mitchell, Bendigo, Ballarat) and south-west of the city along Port Phillip Bay (Geelong, Colac) comprising upwards of 5 million people in a small area of land mass (as the greater eastern part of the state was basically virus free). The large numbers of publicly available SARS-CoV-2 genomes at the NCBI Virus database could be systematically analysed by the simple accessible alignment tools provided at that site. This has allowed us considerable insight into the mode of SARS-CoV-2 haplotype variation strategies and the major infection transmission mode of the virus in the Victorian aged care and elderly community.

To summarize our main findings.

a. The severity and quantitative patient dominance of the Victorian 2nd Wave epidemic in 2020 was focussed almost exclusively on elderly citizens (Tables 1 and 4), presumed vulnerable and immune defenceless as discussed already due to clear deficits in first-line IFN -driven innate immunity.[4-11] Many of these 'immune defenceless' elderly co-morbid citizens were concentrated in closed aged care communities (Supporting Information F and Table 4). Given that APOBEC and ADAR innate immune 'mutators' are activated by the same IFN type I and type III stimulated gene pathways[19-26] it is a logical priority to consider the level of their mutagenic impact on the SARS-CoV-2 clones being transferred within and between aged vulnerable groups (eg VSD analysis in the Supporting Information D).

b. It is clear that the L241f.1vic clone dominated the effective 'fire storm' of infections in the Victorian elderly. The spread of *largely unmutated clones* of this haplotype, particularly in second half June 2020 into late July 2020, is striking and suggests little or no APOBEC and ADAR mutagenesis on P-to-P transfers, and this plausibly implies the infections were rampant in patients with clear deficits in IFN type I and type III stimulated gene pathways (see in particular the VSD patterns in

Supplementary Information Files D and F, and Table 3 summary).

The data reported herein are thus consistent with the following P-to-P infection model which is also the operational hypothesis under test: clusters of immune defenceless elderly co-morbid citizens in many aged care and nursing facilities were all systematically struck with devastating force (high infection rates and death rates), with a single unmutated (or lightly mutated) SARS-CoV-2 haplotype variant (L241f.1vic). Through late June, July, August and September in 2020, this putatively cloned variant must have been spread unimpeded by carriers who were asymptomatic or lightly symptomatic infected healthcare professionals and carers working across multiple age care institutions.[30-33] The large-scale amplifications of the L241.1vic variant—instanced by the size of the multiple 'New case' spikes (shown in Figure 1), particularly through July 2020—could have produced many trillions of L241f.1vic virions in each location thus contaminating numerous surfaces (fomites, personal effects of all types) and could have contaminated or infected human carriers in each institution. This then fuelled the further putative quantitative dominant rapid spread of this apparently capricious L241f.1vic variant into the local community and particularly to other aged care facilities leading to further putative viral amplifications in elderly co-morbid subjects. If anything, the Victorian experience underlines why elderly co-morbid citizens require very special care, protection and therapies during cold and flu seasons.[31,32] Such an approach now seems obvious to handle the viral-induced respiratory crises in vulnerable aged care patients. There is a need for much further research on how to boost innate and specific adaptive immunity defences in such vulnerable patients—so as to achieve a survival infection outcomes in such vulnerable patients (see Sette and Crotty[10] integrated summary, and Lucas et al[11]).

The fact that the L241f.1vic variant remained largely unmutated or very lightly mutated on secondary transfer (1-2 SNVs, Table 3) implies that the main amplifying source of viral replication in each aged care facility were patients with extreme deficits in first-line innate immune IFN type 1 and III dependent anti-viral immunity, see Figure 2C in Lucas et al[11]. The levels of both APOBEC and ADAR host deaminase anti-viral mutators are normally induced by invading pathogens in a healthy cellular innate immune response.[19-25] The lack of apparent mutation in the main transmitted L241f.1vic clone through June and July is consistent with the hypothesis that the virus was replicating almost unimpeded in immune defenceless elderly co-morbids. Indeed many travellers into Australia carrying the L241f.1 haplotype variant in March-April 2020, and their presumed putative secondary transfer recipients also display unmutated or lightly mutated sequences (Supporting Information File D). This suggests those incoming overseas travellers were probably also elderly immune defenceless patients. There is further support for this interpretation. Through August and into September, the incidence and frequency of mutations in mutated derivatives of the L241f.1vic haplotype increased, significantly, a pattern consistent with P-to-P transfer and passage of the L241f.1vic clone through healthy asymptomatic carriers with intact innate immune system and functioning APOBEC/ADAR mutators (Table 3, Supporting Information File D).

Our further hypothesis is that the L241f.1vic variant, which emerged as an escape haplotype variant from a hotel quarantine site on May 8 (Rydges Hotel)[27] gained a low level P-to-P foothold in the community for a month through late May and into mid-June where upon it was fortuitously and explosively amplified and spread on scale when introduced into closed groups of immune defenceless elderly co-morbid patients living in the Kensington Towers in north west Melbourne and aged care facilities.[29] Through late June and into July, its large amplification factors and numerous cross-institutional spreading 'vectors' (asymptomatic family members, aged carers and health workers, and their presumed fomites) ensured it took over and spread quickly through all of Melbourne's and nearby regional aged care facilities. The sequencing effort by the Victorian Department of Health in association with The Peter Doherty Institute and epidemiological interpretation was thus focussed on the L2411f.1vic haplotype to try and prevent its further spread.

Our further related hypothesis is that the much publicized 'UK Mutant' (B.1.1.7) that emerged in the United Kingdom in the latter months of 2020 spread and came to dominance in much the same way as L241f.1vic in Victoria, Australia—a capriciously amplified SARS-CoV-2 variant in closed communities of immune defenceless elderly co-morbid patients.

The UK Mutant is of the L241f.1 haplotype (L241f.1uk)—but different from L241f.1vic which has a smaller number (n = 7) of 'riboswitch' type key distinctive SNV markers that distinguish it from L241f.1 (Table 2)—with about 17-19 additional sequence changes from L241f.1, four being deletions and one a STOP codon (Rambaut et al[16]). Apart from distinctive radicle changes, all the other SNV changes in L241f.1uk appear conserved or benign, a picture consistent with all our sequence analysis here and in Steele and Lindley.[14] The advance news media notice on the 'UK Mutant' as it arrived with travellers into Australia in early 2021 described the variant as a 'highly contagious rapidly spreading mutant'. On arrival with travellers from overseas, it inevitably escaped quarantine into the community

and in public airport domestic departure lounges in Adelaide, Brisbane, Perth and then Melbourne exposing potentially many hundreds of Australian residents and other travellers. These escapes each caused severe hard Stage 4 lock downs (2-5 days) of the entire city populations, and in Victoria and Western Australia almost the entire State populations for 5 days. Given all the advance publicity and the hundreds of putative reported P-to-P contacts and opportunities for further P-to-P spreading (and further interstate by aeroplanes by many more hundreds of putative contacts), the UK Mutant *was not contagious* and did not spread into the wider Australian community.[34,35] These very clear negative transmission data led the noted Australian epidemiologist at The Australian National University, Professor Peter Collignon, to release his considered opinion to *The Australian* newspaper[34]:

> ' ..In retrospect, the Melbourne lockdown was unnecessary... From my perspective, if you've got very little community transmission, I'm not sure that a short lockdown achieves much extra, if you've got good contact tracing and good testing', he said. ... 'If I look at the lockdowns done in Adelaide, Brisbane, Perth, and now Melbourne, it didn't turn up one more case than contact tracing did. ... 'The UK strain has not spread uncontrollably and wildly'.

Clearly, further research is required to understand exactly why the 'UK Mutant' did not spread when multiply introduced via multiple entry points into Australia in the first few months of 2021. One possibility is that it really was not that contagious in normal healthy people, it had been attenuated but behaved as a putative capriciously amplified variant in elderly co-morbids. That is clearly dangerous for that vulnerable group (which by chance were not in large numbers in the public places the infected travellers were supposed to have visited).

In our view, what has unfolded with the L241f.1vic, as documented here, is a clear putative exemplar. Our hypothesis is that the 'UK Mutant' (B.1.1.7) or L241f.1uk haplotype was a capricious P-to-P generated SARS-CoV-2 variant haplotype that was fortuitously amplified on scale to quantitative clonal dominance in and between aged care facilities in southern England from September 2020, much like the L241f.1vic haplotype in Victoria, Australia. The main difference between the otherwise similar countries (both economically, culturally and multi-ethic diverse composition) is one of population scale given the population differential between UK and Victoria is about ten-fold, and given similar land areas the population density in the UK would be far higher than Victoria.

Given all these findings what then of appropriate vaccine design? Apart from any safety or adverse reaction issues with the current set of spike protein mRNA expression vector vaccines, there are, in our opinion, three main issues to be addressed, two arise from our analysis. These relate in general to the vulnerable *target group* to be protected—the immune defenceless elderly co-morbids—and *the type* of protective acquired immunity to be induced by any vaccine (the relevant vaccine data is under detailed review elsewhere Gorczynski RM, Lindley RA, Steele EJ, Wickramasinghe NC. 2021 'Nature of acquired immune responses, epitope specificity and resultant protection from SARS-CoV-2', under submission).

First, boosting innate immunity would seem a priority medical strategy in the vulnerable elderly, as for example BCG vaccination is expected to do for the lung infection tuberculosis. This could involve the use of IFNs to stimulate deaminase expression during the acute stage of infection. BCG is a safe and widely accepted non-specific activator of innate immunity, and it could contribute to elevated APOBEC and ADAR expression and thus mutagenesis of the coronavirus genome. This logically implies that strategies for boosting or elevation, by 'training' the innate immune responses[7,12] may boost mutagenic APOBEC and ADAR expression levels and other anti-viral gene products.[19,20]

Second, it is still unclear whether the current crop of SARS-CoV-2 vaccines is inducing *the appropriate class of acquired immunity*, namely mucosal responses involving specific secretory IgA responses in nose, saliva and respiratory tract (A. Hapel, discussion and person comm. February 2021). This is also confirmed by the April 20 2021 update report on vaccine efficacy from the US Centers for Disease Control.[36] A careful reading of that report suggests that none of the current 'jab in the arm' vaccines protect against catching SARS-CoV-2, yet may moderate severity. This is consistent with prior historical immunology discoveries. It has been known for over 45 years that the best form of protective immunity for pathogens invading by the nasal or oral route are local secretory IgA responses.[37,38] Therefore, at this juncture, it is not clear whether currently deployed intramuscular (im) parenteral immunization is the best approach for highly effective mucosal immunity against SARS-CoV-2, and the oral-nasal routes of vaccination should be considered. Indeed, recent informed analysis and commentary supports this conclusion.[39,40] Natural infections with SARS-CoV-2 (in recovered patients) would therefore be expected to induce protective dimeric sIgA mucosal immunity. Certainly, the recent longitudinal population scale study in Denmark implies that prior infection with SARS-CoV-2 affords upwards of 80% protection in the population under 65 years against reinfection between the first and second

major surges of SARS-CoV-2 in Denmark in 2020; with the protective rate in the re-infected elderly vulnerable group a half lower again at 47%.[13] These are encouraging findings suggesting, at the time of writing, that natural 'herd immunity' could be well underway in Denmark and similar Northern hemisphere infected zones in 2020 and into likely surges and waves of SARS-CoV-2 in 2021.

Finally, a striking feature of the adaptation strategy of the SARS-CoV-2 coronavirus is the signature of 'haplotype ribo-switching', focussed mainly on C-site and A-site centred motifs targeted by APOBEC and ADAR deamination events.[14] We expect this strategy to be general for coronavirus infections (it is evident in the additional SNVs over the L241f.1 haplotype in the L241f.1vic variant). Thus, whilst some variation can occur at the amino acid level, it is largely conserved as discussed[14] and as illustrated in the haplotyping data of the VSD presented here (Supporting Information File D). The predominant conclusion is the large amount of viral variation that goes on at the RNA level with presumptive links to functional RNA secondary structures, that is downstream consequences for appropriate RNA secondary structures compatible with viral replicative fitness. The striking sequence conservation at the amino acid level after human passage[14] implies that there are key conserved variations mainly at the RNA genomic level. Thus, most recorded SNVs were either synonymous or, if non-synonymous, the SNVs in coding regions lead often to likely functionally benign amino acid outcomes and thus result in likely conservation of viral function at the protein level. This was a striking fact across all data sets examined[14] and in the data reported here (Supporting Information File D). Clearly, all these observed viral sequences survived Darwinian negative selection within each infected subject against malfunctioning and poorly replicating variants in the quasi-species pool as discussed.[14] Targeted mutagenesis studies[41,42] on viral genomes affirm this conclusion. That data demonstrate how sensitive and tightly tuned information-rich single-stranded viral genomes really are to *any* non-synonymous substitutions of many types. In Hepatitis C Virus (HCV) studies, another similar approach has demonstrated how targeted substitutions in the coding regions of the HCV genome reveals a functional network of RNA regulatory structures important in efficacy of viral replication and infectivity OK.[43]

Therefore, new vaccine designs and therapies may need to target these new and putative stable secondary structures thrown up by haplotype ribo-switching for the presumptive replicative stability of the viral RNA genome. This type of RNA secondary structure research and analysis is underway (Lindley RA and associates). This will obviously involve an entirely different approach to vaccine RNA target site design and curative therapies, which will necessitate further research on RNA structure rather than the protein components of the virus (aspects reviewed in Robson et al[18]).

ACKNOWLEDGMENT
We thank Dr Jared Mamrot of GMDxgen Pty Ltd for the independent analysis of the haplotype sequences of Victoria Australia genomes made publicly available at the GISAID database. We thank Dr Andrew Hapel and Professor Patrick Carnegie for discussions and references on secretory IgA mucosal immunity.

CONFLICT OF INTEREST
There is no conflict of interest with the scientific objectivity of this paper.

AUTHOR CONTRIBUTIONS
RAL and EJS conceived the plan, aim and organization of the paper, and EJS wrote the first draft of the paper. EJS did the primary analysis of GenBank/NCBI Virus accessed COVID-19 genomic sequences. Both authors read and worked on the final version of the paper before submission by EJS.

ORCID
Robyn A. Lindley (iD) https://orcid.org/0000-0002-8952-1536
Edward J. Steele (iD) https://orcid.org/0000-0003-4700-3156

REFERENCES
1. Huang C, Wang Y, Li X, et al. Clinical features of patients infected with 2019 novel coronavirus in Wuhan. *Lancet*. 2020;395:497-506.
2. Cohen J. Wuhan seafood market may not be source of novel virus spreading globally. *Science*. 2020;367. https://www.sciencemag.org/news/2020/01/wuhan-seafood-market-may-not-be-source-novel-virus-spreading-globally
3. Pekar J, Worobey M, Moshiri N, Scheffler K, Wertheim JO. Timing the SARS-CoV-2 index case in Hubei province. *Science*. 2021;372:412-417. doi:10.1126/science.abf8003
4. Acharya D, Liu G-Q, Gack MU. Dysregulation of type I interferon responses in COVID-19 Nat. *Rev Immunol*. 2020;20:397-398. doi:10.1038/s41577-020-0346-x
5. Blanco-Melo D, Nilsson-Payant BE, Liu W-C, et al. Imbalanced Host Response to SARS-CoV-2 Drives Development of COVID-19. *Cell*. 2020;181:1036-1045. doi:10.1016/j.cell.2020.04.026
6. Hadjadj J, Yatim N, Barnabei L, et al. (2020) Impaired type I interferon activity and exacerbated inflammatory responses in severe Covid-19 patients medRxiv preprint doi:10.1101/2020.04.19.20068015
7. Netea MG, Giamarellos-Bourboulis EJ, Domınguez-Andreʹs J, et al. Trained Immunity: A tool for reducing susceptibility to and the severity of SARS-CoV-2 infection. *Cell*. 2020;181:969-977.
8. Zhang Q, Bastard P, Liu Z, et al. Inborn errors of type I IFN immunity in patients with life-threatening COVID-19. *Science*. 2020;370:eabd4570.
9. Moderbacher CR, Ramirez SI, Dan JM, et al. Antigen-specific adaptive immunity to SARS-CoV-2 in acute COVID-19 and associations with age and disease severity. *Cell*. 2020;183:996-1012.
10. Sette A, Crotty S. Adaptive immunity to SARS-CoV-2 and COVID-19. *Cell*. 2021;184:1-20.
11. Lucas C, Wong P, Klein J, et al. Longitudinal analyses reveal immunological misfiring in severe COVID-19. *Nature*. 2020;584:463-469.
12. Netea MG, Domınguez-Andres J, Barreiro LB, et al. Defining trained immunity and its role in health and disease. *Nat Rev Immunol*. 2020;20:375-388.
13. Hansen CH, Michlmayr D, Gubbels SM, Mølbak K, Ethelberg S Assessment of protection against reinfection with SARS-CoV-2 among 4 million PCR-tested individuals in Denmark in 2020: A population-level observational study. *The Lancet*. 2021;397 doi:10.1016/S0140-6736(21)00575-4
14. Steele EJ, Lindley RA. Analysis of APOBEC and ADAR deaminase-driven Riboswitch Haplotypes in COVID-19 RNA strain variants and the implications for vaccine design. *Res Rep*. doi:10.9777/rr.2020.10001   https://companyofscientists.com/index.php/rr
15. Rambaut A, Holmes EC, Hill V, et al. A dynamic nomenclature proposal for SARS- CoV-2 to assist genomic epidemiology. *Nat. Microbiol*. 2020;5:1403-1407.
16. Rambaut A, Loman N, Pybus O, et al. Preliminary genomic characterisation of an emergent SARS-CoV-2 lineage in the UK defined by a novel set of spike mutations. Virologic.org In Press Feb 4 2021 https://virological.org/t/preliminary-genomic-characterisation-of-an-emergent-sars-cov-2-lineage-in-the-uk-defined-by-a-novel-set-of-spike-mutations/563
17. Forster P, Forster L, Renfrew C. Forster MJ 2020 Phylogenetic network analysis of SARS-CoV-2 genomes. *Proc Natl Acad Sci USA*. 2020;117:9241-9243.
18. Robson F, Khan KS, Le TK, et al. Coronavirus RNA proofreading: Molecular basis and therapeutic targeting. *Mol Cell*. 2020;79:710-727.
19. Schoggins JW, Rice CM. Interferon-stimulated genes and their antiviral effector functions. *Curr Opin Virol*. 2011;1:519-525.
20. Schneider WM, Chevillotte MD, Rice CM. Interferon-stimulated genes: A complex web of host defenses. *Annu Rev Immunol*. 2014;232:513-545.
21. Samuel CE. Adenosine deaminases acting on RNA (ADARs) are both antiviral and proviral. *Virology*. 2011;411:180-193. doi:10.1016/j.virol.2010.12.004
22. Conticello SG. The AID/APOBEC family of nucleic acid mutators. *Genome Biol*. 2008;9:229. doi:10.1186/gb-2008-9-6-229
23. Harris RS, Bishop KN, Sheehy AM, et al. DNA deamination mediates innate immunity to retroviral infection. *Cell*. 2003;113:803-809.
24. Refsland EW, Harris RS. The APOBEC3 family of retroelement restriction factors. *Curr Top Microbiol Immunol*. 2013;371:1-27. doi:10.1007/978-3-642-37765-5_1
25. Vartanian J-P, Henry M, Marchio A, et al. Massive APOBEC3 editing of hepatitis B viral DNA in cirrhosis. *PLoS Pathog*. 2010;6(5):e1000928. doi:10.1371/journal.ppat.1000928

26. Lindley RA. Review of the mutational role of deaminases and the generation of a cognate molecular model to explain cancer mutation spectra. *Med Res Arch*. 2020;8(8):2177.

27. COVID-19 Hotel Quarantine Inquiry, Final Report and Recommendations, Volume I Parl paper no. 191 (2018–2020) ISBN 978-0-6450016-1-7 (Victorian Government Inquiry).

28. Seemann T, Lane CR, Sherry NL, et al. Tracking the COVID-19 pandemic in Australia using genomics. *Nat Com*. 2020;11(1):4376. doi:10.1038/s41467-020-18314-x

29. Smith P. Covid-19 in Australia: most infected health workers in Victoria's second wave acquired virus at work. *BMJ*. 2020;370:m3350. doi:10.1136/bmj.m3350

30. ABC News. "Workplace coronavirus transmission driving Victorian case numbers, including in aged care" Sunday 19 July 2020 at 2:27pm, updated Monday 20 July 2020 at 12:30 am. https://www.abc.net.au/news/2020-07-19/workplace-coron avirus-transmission-in-victoria-in-aged-care/12470704

31. Cousins S. Experts criticise Australia's aged care failings over COVID-19. *The Lancet*. 2020;396:1322-1323.

32. Hashan MR, Smoll N, King C, et al. Epidemiology and clinical features of COVID-19 outbreaks in aged care facilities: A systematic review and meta-analysis. *EClinicalMedicine*. 2021;33:100771. doi: 10.1016/j.eclinm.2021.100771

33. Rose T Carer tracking lacking. Herald-Sun, Melbourne 31 August 2020 p.12

34. Baxendale R, Robinson N. Spread of UK coronavirus variant limited to close contacts. *The Australian*. February 20, 2021

35. Robinson N. Why didn't others get the hotel virus. The Australian February 9, 2021.

36. CDC Update: Science Brief: Background Rationale and Evidence for Public Health Recommendations for Fully Vaccinated People Centers for Disease Control and Prevention, COVID-19 Updated Apr. 2, 2021 https://www.cdc.gov/coronavirus/2019-ncov/science/science-briefs/fully-vaccinated-people.html

37. Steele EJ, Chaicumpa W, Rowley D. Isolation and biological properties of three classes of rabbit antibody to Vibrio Cholerae. *J Infect Dis*. 1974;130:93-103.

38. Steele EJ. 1975. Efficiency of antibody classes in cholera immunity. PhD diss. University of Adelaide.

39. Bleier BS, Ramanathan M, Lane AP. COVID-19 vaccines may not prevent nasal SARS-CoV-2 infection and asymptomatic transmission. *Otolaryngol Head Neck Surg*. 2021;164:305-307. doi:10.1177/0194599820982633

40. Schiavone M, Gasperetti A, Mitacchione G, Viecca M, Forleo GB. Response to: COVID-19 re-infection vaccinated individuals as a potential source of transmission. *Eur J Clin Invest*. 2021;00:e13544. doi:10.1111/eci.13544

41. Sanjuan R, Moya A, Elena SF. The distribution of fitness effects caused by single- nucleotide substitutions in an RNA virus. *Proc Natl Acad Sci USA*. 2004;2004(101):8396-8401.

42. Sanjuan R, Nebot MR, Chirico N, et al. Viral mutation rates. *Virology*. 2010;84:9733-9748.

43. Pirakitikulr N, Kohlway A, Lindenbach BD, Pyle AM. The coding region of the HCV genome contains a network of regulatory RNA structures. *Mol Cell*. 2016;61:1-10. doi:10.1016/j.molcel.2016.01.024

SUPPORTING INFORMATION

Additional supporting information may be found online in the Supporting Information section.

How to cite this article: Lindley RA, Steele EJ. Analysis of SARS-CoV-2 haplotypes and genomic sequences during 2020 in Victoria, Australia, in the context of putative deficits in innate immune deaminase anti-viral responses. *Scand J Immunol*. 2021;94:e13100. https://doi.org/10.1111/sji.13100

SECTION 6

The Second Year and Role of Human Passaged Plumes in Viral Spread and Vaccine Efficacy

Commentary

Cometary Origin of COVID-19

Edward J. Steele[1,2,3]*, Reginald M. Gorczynski[4], Robyn A. Lindley[5,6], GensukeTokoro[7], Daryl H. Wallis[7], Robert Temple[8] and N. Chandra Wickramasinghe [3,7,9,10]

[1]C.Y.O' Connor ERADE Village Foundation, Piara Waters, Perth, WA, Australia

[2]Melville Analytics Pty Ltd, Melbourne, VIC, Australia

[3]Centre for Astrobiology, University of Ruhuna, Matara, Sri Lanka

[4]University Toronto Health Network, Toronto General Hospital, University of Toronto, Toronto, ON, Canada

[5]Department of Clinical Pathology, Faculty of Medicine, Dentistry & Health Sciences, University of Melbourne, Melbourne, VIC, Australia

[6]GMDx Group Ltd, Melbourne, VIC, Australia

[7]Institute for the Study of Panspermia and Astroeconomics, Gifu, Japan

[8]The History of Chinese Science and Culture Foundation, Conway Hall, London, United Kingdom

[9]University of Buckingham, Buckingham, United Kingdom

[10]National Institute of Fundamental Studies, Kandy, Sri Lanka

*Corresponding author: Edward J. Steele, C.Y.O' Connor ERADE Village Foundation, Piara Waters, Perth, WA, Australia; E-mail: e.j.steele@bigpond.com

Received: May 06, 2021; Accepted: May 11, 2021; Published: May 18, 2021

Abstract

The evidence for the cometary origin then rapid global spread of COVID-19 through 2020 is critically reviewed. We outline why it is an alternative plausible scientific explanation to the current bat/pangolin animal jump theories. In our view this explanation is consistent with all the available temporal unfolding scientific data (genomic, immunologic, epidemiologic, geophysical, astrophysical and astrobiological). Thus COVID-19 arrived as infective cryopreserved virions in cometary meteoritic dust clouds from space in a bolide strike in the stratosphere over China on October 11 2019. Prevailing high-level and low-level wind systems then globally distributed the infective viral dust clouds, striking different regions at different times. Given this possibility, a new space challenge for mankind is to develop near-Earth early warning biological surveillance (and mitigation) systems for incoming cosmic in-falls of micro-organisms and viruses from the cometary dust and meteorite streams that our planet routinely encounters as it orbits the Sun.

Since it first emerged in Wuhan, China in late November into December 2019 the coronavirus pandemic due to COVID-19 (SARS-CoV-2) has been engulfing the world with considerable economic and health impact targeting mainly our elderly co-morbid citizens with clear deficits mainly in type I and type III interferon inducible anti-viral immunity [1-5].

How credible then is our conclusion, embodied in our title, that the COVID-19 pandemic could have arrived from space? The journal has invited us to outline this evidence for an extra-terrestrial origin, which we began publishing from early 2020 [6-10] and then in a mid-year review which appeared in November 2020 [11]. Our initial focus has been to explain the key events of the first months of the pandemic so as to understand its origin and rapid global spread. We marshalled not only the geophysical and temporal global epidemiological evidence [6-8,12], the prior knowledge from astrophysical and astrobiological evidence [13-16] but also gained insight into the genetic adaptation strategy of the virus, based on APOBEC and ADAR deaminase driven responses in infected subjects. These host innate immune responses designed to mutate and thus cripple the viral RNA genome actually helps steer viral haplotype diversification for optimal replicative efficacy. We view this as a ribo-switching host-parasite selection process for the fittest transmissible RNA haplotypic genome in a subject host [12,17].

Our short narrative summary of one possible scenario not considered as mainstream thinking goes like this: A life-bearing loosely held carbonaceous cometary bolide arrived in the stratosphere over Jilin in North East China on the night of Oct 11 2019. This well-documented and widely observed event is recorded at the Space.com website. The viral-laden cometary dust particles and clumps (typically micron size) were released prior to the fireball in a fragmentation process, and they began their expected slow descent from the stratosphere in the 40° N Latitude band (30-50°). Over the next month some of this cometary-meteorite dust cloud was brought down to ground by local weather precipitation (rain) targeting the central Chinese city of Wuhan in Hubei province. This event, within another month, ignited by mass simultaneous infective exposure caused the explosive rise of COVID-19 cases through January in Wuhan and its wider contaminated regions. About 30% of all such infections were demonstrably not connected to any food or wet market [18,19]. However much of the upper troposphere/stratosphere viral laden dust remained there in the East to West (E-W) jet streams and was distributed around the globe at great speed (jet-streams circle the globe in ~ 3 days at speeds 150-200 km/hr). We speculate that explosive outbreaks on the ground of human person-to-person (P-to-P) passaged COVID-19 viruses could have created a secondary rising plume of viral-laden pollution and dust [20,21] over Wuhan and

DOI: 10.31038/IDT.2021212

https://researchopenworld.com/cometary-origin-of-covid-19/

Infect Dis Ther, Volume 2(1): 1–1, 2021

Hubei province containing trillions of dust-associated COVID-19 virions. We think that this plume was then carried by the lower level West to East (W-E) prevailing wind systems across the Pacific (Max Wallis, pers comm) engaging cruise ships through February in the South China Sea and Sea of Japan (*Diamond Princess, Westerdam*). This mode of transfer, including early first wave in-falls in South Korea and Japan and, by mid-February, to the US West Coast [7], could explain the virus outbreak on the *Grand Princess* cruise ship sailing out of San Francisco. This scenario for the *Grand Princess* outbreak has supportive genetic evidence as the main COVID-19 haplotype in infected passengers was identical to the unmutated (and lightly mutated) L haplotype that dominated the Wuhan outbreak [12,22]. The deposits in the higher E-W jet streams could have been brought down by capricious local weather conditions during early-mid March 2020 in Tehran/Qom, Lombardy/Italy and Spain, and then on the 40° N Latitude band to engage New York City as our earlier analysis had predicted [7,8].

The explosive outbreaks at widely dispersed global sites are consistent with this scenario. Further, they happened at great speed, with exponential growth rates of case numbers per day, that defied initial expectations of P-to-P spreading with the expected 1-2 week infection incubation periods. Aerial infective in-fall by viral laden dust over large population centres seems the most logical explanation for the simultaneous infections with little evidence of delay due to incubation time. The same explosive apparent simultaneous large-scale outbreaks occurred in clearly documented cases of deck crew members on ships at sea [17,23] and in the remote Chilean Bernardo O'Higgins Army Station in Antarctica in late December 2020 [24]. In a similar vein, the island of Sri Lanka flat lined in case numbers for many months with hardly any cases, and became suddenly engaged in a mass outbreak of over a 1000 COVID-19 cases in the period Oct 4-6 [10] and see also Sri Lanka at the Google URL search link below [25].

By March into April part of the E-W 40° N stream transporting the dust clouds was diverted into South America, particularly Brazil by prevailing Atlantic ocean wind systems [9]. From there on the prevailing wind systems of the Southern Hemisphere became engaged as the principal carriers of the infalling viral laden dust clouds. The high profile infective outbreaks were those in June through September occurring predominantly in South Africa and Victoria Australia, which coincidently are on the same prevailing W-E 40° S Latitude band (the French Polynesian Islands became engaged several months later from September). The latter interpretation for Victoria, Australia, is at odds with the prevailing local belief that the 2nd Wave outbreak was caused by hotel quarantine "escapees into the community". This claim infers that infected travellers to Melbourne in March-April from Northern Hemisphere zones inadvertently spread the virus into the community where after several months these "escapee" variants then ignited the 2nd Wave in late June 2020. However, our evaluation of the publicly available Victorian case incidence data and the publicly available COVID-19 genomic sequence data leads to a qualified and quite different explanation which is also consistent with the viral laden dust cloud in-fall interpretation.

Interested readers can perform their own survey of the global COVID-19 cases per day patterns since early 2020 to the present at the Google URL site listed below to verify our claims [25]. It is evident that the disease has now spread all over the globe to all major continents and regions. At the time of writing (April-May 2021) a major in-fall has occurred over India and regions which we speculate is a down draft off the 40° N latitude band on the southern side of the Himalayan Mountains. But it is an exceedingly patchy pattern worldwide as discussed extensively in Hoyle and Wickramasinghe [13] again recently in Wickramasinghe et al [10] and as is evident in the Figures and Supplementary data to be found in Steele and Lindley [12] and Steele et al. [11,17]. Thus epidemics begin and end at different times in different regions and reach different intensities. In our view this behaviour reflects globally dispersed fragmented viral laden dust clouds brought haphazardly and capriciously to ground by local meteorological conditions. Certain regions may not experience a real in-fall event, and this is borne out in islands like Taiwan despite its closeness to China. The vagaries of local weather, prevailing winds, and chance in-fall of viral-laden dust clouds combine to present a capricious pattern of attack.

So in the ongoing pandemic, outbreaks around the globe have their own sudden beginnings and endings, yet major regions on the N 40° Latitude band (North America, Europe Asia Minor and the Indian subcontinent) have experienced several "Waves" already, or by the scenario considered here, separate "wash down" events from the troposphere. An interesting feature across all regions where a clear single mode of in-fall can be discerned is an unmistakable symmetrical bell-shaped curve, such as happened for the 2nd Wave in Victoria Australia, 1st Wave in South Africa, and the 1st Wave in Pakistan. There are many instances of this type if one cares to Google survey the case incident patterns per day across the globe [25]. Despite the height of the peak or intensity of the epidemic in individual instances, it is remarkable that the base of the symmetrical curve stretches typically over 2-3 months. The simplest interpretation is that this reflects the decay time of the virions in the physical environment, which remains remarkably the same across the globe.

With respect to the symmetrical nature of the bell-shaped curves describing the distributions of cases per day seen in such well documented epidemics such as the Victorian 2nd Wave an important deduction can be drawn about the impact of extreme 'lockdown' social distancing measures aimed at reducing viral reproduction rate R_o to less than 1. We have statistically analysed the Gaussian features of the Victorian 2nd Wave (which peaked on August 1-2, 2020). The best Gaussian fit with R^2 gives 0.8999 which implies an almost perfect statistical fit to a symmetrical bell-shaped curve. Such a result would be consistent with the epidemic curve being overwhelmingly dominated by the growth and decay of a localised atmospheric in-fall event. The hard Stage 4 lockdown in Victoria came into effect on August 2, 2020. Given this perfect symmetry we conclude that the hard lock down measures had little impact, if any, on the course of the 2nd Wave COVID-19 epidemic in Victoria, Australia. This conclusion is consistent with the independent analyses of the impact of extreme lockdown measures on the course of the COVID-19 lockdowns introduced in a number of States in the USA during 2020 [26].

Edward J. Steele (2021) Cometary Origin of COVID-19

The patterns we have discussed apply generally to the manner in which suddenly emergent pandemics run their course throughout history [13]. It seems plausible to us that many might be a combination of wash down from the troposphere, leading to population wide exposures, eventually inducing herd immunity and a natural decay of the virions in the environment. However, we admit that there are many unknowns and that there are alternative explanations for these effects. Yet, on some specific details presented to us, the scenario presented here is a possible new reality that will need much future research.

Thus, from our viewpoint, the bulk of the key global evidence is consistent with an extra-terrestrial origin of COVID-19. Are there alternative explanations for the sudden origin and rapid global spread of the pandemic? We have dealt with this issue at some length [17], and there is one possible yet highly unlikely scientific explanation, and a bio weapon conspiracy theory explanation. Both are discussed in detail in Steele et al [17], but it is the zoonotic theory that can be dealt with rationally and scientifically, namely that COVID-19 arose in a jump from an animal reservoir, either in one or two steps or in combination, with SARS CoV related variants growing in bats and/or pangolins. In reviewing all the known related bat and pangolin SARS-CoV-like sequences the closest possible precursors are 96.2 % similar to the COVID-19 Hu-1 reference sequence (29903 nt). To get an exact match, in the normal haplotype range for globally dispersed COVID-19 of 99.98% sequence similarity [12,17] this involves>1100 specific nucleotide changes in the precursor to get such an exact COVID-19 match. These numbers imply super astronomical odds against a successful jump. Indeed, even if we are generous and assume only a 1% difference (which has not been seen in the wild) this gives odds of one successful mutational jump in 10^{180} trials, which also is a super astronomical number, far exceeding the molecular, and statistical, resources of the known universe. In our view a zoonotic explanation for the origin of COVID-19, although a valid scientific concept, is implausible on the current evidence [17].

This leaves us then with an alternative plausible scientific explanation that is consistent with the available data: the arrival of COVID-19 as infective cryopreserved virions in cometary meteoritic dust clouds from space. Given this possibility, a new space challenge for mankind is to develop near-Earth early warning biological surveillance (and mitigation) systems for incoming cosmic in-falls of micro-organisms and viruses from the cometary dust and meteorite streams that our planet routinely encounters as it orbits the Sun.

Acknowledgement

We acknowledge for discussion and contributions in development of ideas in this and earlier articles, Stephen G Coulson, Max K Wallis, Brig Klyce, Predrag Slijepcevic, Alexander Kondakov, Dayal T Wickramasinghe, George Howard, Herbert Rebhan, Pat Carnegie, Ananda Nimalasuriya and Milton Wainwright

References

1. Acharya D, Liu G-Q, Gack MU (2020) Dysregulation of type I interferon responses in COVID-19. *Nat Rev Immunol* 20: 397-398. [crossref]

2. Blanco-Melo D, Nilsson-Payant BE, Liu WC, Uhl S, Hoagland D, et al. (2020) Imbalanced Host Response to SARS-CoV-2 Drives Development of COVID-19. *Cell* 181: 1036-1045. [crossref]

3. Hadjadj J, Yatim N, Barnabei L, Corneau A, Boussier J, et al. (2020) Impaired type I interferon activity and exacerbated inflammatory responses in severe Covid-19 patients. *Science* 369: 718-724. [crossref]

4. Netea MG, Giamarellos-Bourboulis EJ, Domínguez-Andrés J, Curtis N, van Crevel R, et al. (2020) Trained Immunity: a tool for reducing susceptibility to and the severity of SARS-CoV-2 infection *Cell* 181: 969- 977. [crossref]

5. Lucas C, Wong P, Klein J, Castro TBR, Silva J, et al. (2020) Longitudinal analyses reveal immunological misfiring in severe COVID-19. *Nature.* 584: 463-469.

6. Wickramasinghe NC, Steele EJ, Gorczynski RM, Temple R, Tokoro G, et al. (2020) Comments on the Origin and Spread of the 2019 Coronavirus. *Virology : Current Research* 4:1.

7. Wickramasinghe NC, Steele EJ, Gorczynski RM, Temple R, Tokoro G, et al. (2020) Growing Evidence against Global Infection-Driven by Person-to-Person Transfer of COVID-19. *Virology : Current Research* 4:1.

8. Wickramasinghe NC, Steele EJ, Gorczynski RM, Temple R, Tokoro G, et al. (2020) Predicting the Future Trajectory of COVID-19. *Virology : Current Research* 4:1.

9. Wickramasinghe NC, Wallis MK, Coulson SG, Kondakov A, Steele EJ, et al. (2020) Intercontinental Spread of COVID-19 on Global Wind Systems. *Virology: Current Research* 4:1.

10. Wickramasinghe NC, Steele EJ, Nimalasuriya A, Gorczynki RM, Tokoro G, et al. (2020) Seasonality of Respiratory Viruses Including SARS-CoV-2. *Virology: Current Research* 4:2.

11. Steele EJ, Gorczynski RM, Lindley RA, Tokoro G, Temple R, et al. (2020) Origin of new emergent Coronavirus and Candida fungal diseases- Terrestrial or Cosmic? *Advances in Genetics* 106: 75-100. [crossref]

12. Steele EJ, Lindley RA (2020) Analysis of APOBEC and ADAR deaminase-driven Riboswitch Haplotypes in COVID-19 RNA strain variants and the implications for vaccine design. *Research Reports* Vol 4.

13. Hoyle F, Wickramasinghe NC (1979) Diseases from Space. JM Dent Ltd, London.

14. Hoyle F, Wickramasinghe NC (2000) Astronomical Origins of Life: Steps Towards Panspermia. Klower Academic Publishers, Dordrechl, Netherlands.

15. Steele EJ, Al-Mufti S, Augustyn KA, Chandrajith R, Coghlan JP, et al. (2018) Cause of Cambrian Explosion: Terrestrial or Cosmic? *Prog Biophys Mol Biol* 136: 3-23. [crossref]

16. Steele EJ, Gorczynski RM, Lindley RA, Liu Y, Temple R, (2019) et al. Lamarck and Panspermia - On the Efficient Spread of Living Systems Throughout the Cosmos. *Prog Biophys Mol Biol* 149 : 10 -32.

17. Steele EJ, Gorczynski RM, Rebhan H, Carnegie P, Temple R, et al. (2020) Implications of haplotype switching for the origin and global spread of COVID-19. *Virology: Current Research* 4:2. Supplementary data at: https://www.hilarispublisher.com/open-access/implications-of-haplotype-switching-for-the-origin-and-global-spread-of-covid19.pdf

18. Huang C, Wang Y, Li X, Zhao J, Ren L, et al. (2020) Clinical Features of Patients Infected with 2019 Novel Coronavirus in Wuhan. *Lancet* 395: 497 - 506.

19. Cohen J (2020) Wuhan seafood market may not be source of novel virus spreading globally. *Science* Vol 367.

20. Coccia M (2020) Factors determining the diffusion of COVID-19 and suggested strategy to prevent future accelerated viral infectivity similar to COVID. *Science of the Total Environment* 729: 138474. [crossref]

21. Martelletti L, Martelletti P (2020) Air Pollution and the Novel Covid-19 Disease: a Putative Disease Risk Factor. *SN Compr Clin Med* 2: 383-387.

22. Andersen K (2020) Clock and TMRCA based on 27 genomes. *Novel 2019 coronavirus.* http://virological.org/t/clock-and- tmrca-based-on-27-genomes/347

23. Howard GA, Wickramasinghe NC, Rebhan H, Steele EJ, Reginald M, et al. (2020) Mid-Ocean Outbreaks of COVID-19 with Tell-Tale Signs of Aerial Incidence *Virology: Current Research* 4:2.

24. Antartica Base: The remote Chilean Army Base in Antartica suddenly became engaged in late December 2020 by multiple simultaneous COVID-19 cases https://www.bbc.com/news/world-latin-america-55410065; https://www.abc.net.au/news/2020-12-23/more-covid-cases-linked-to-chilean-antarctic-base/13009706

Edward J. Steele (2021) Cometary Origin of COVID-19

25. Google: **"Coronavirus disease statistics"** URL is https://www.google.com.au/search?hl=en&ei=vWxyX7ipM4-m9QP18If4CQ&q=Coronavirus+disease+statistics&oq=Coronavirus+disease+statistics&gs_lcp=CgZwc3ktYWIQAzICCAAyAggAOgQIABBHOgcIABCxAxBDOgQIABBDULZUWPh1YJF7aABwAXgAgAH2AYgBvA6SAQYwLjEwLjGYAQCgAQGqAQdnd3Mtd2l6yAEGwAEB&sclient=psy-ab&ved=0ahUKEwj4-47e-4zsAhUPU30KHXX4AZ8Q4dUDCAw&uact=5 This gives you the "Australia" dashboard (from there you can choose your country in the menu bar scroll)

26. Luskin DL (2020) The failed experiment of COVID-19 lockdowns. *The Wall Street Journal.*

Citation:

Steele EJ, Gorczynski RM, Lindley RA, Tokoro G, Wallis DH, et al. (2021) Cometary Origin of COVID-19. *Infect Dis Ther* Volume 2(1): 1-4.

Infect Dis Ther, Volume 2(1): 4-4, 2021

Research Article

COVID-19 Sudden Outbreak of Mystery Case Transmissions in Victoria, Australia, May-June 2021: Strong Evidence of Tropospheric Transport of Human Passaged Infective Virions from the Indian Epidemic

Edward J. Steele[1,2,3*], **Reginald M. Gorczynski**[4], **Patrick Carnegie**[5], **Gensuke Tokoro**[6], **Daryl H. Wallis**[6], **Robert Temple**[7], **Milton Wainwright**[3] and **N. Chandra Wickramasinghe**[3,6,8,9]

[1]C.Y.O' Connor ERADE Village Foundation, Piara Waters, Perth, WA, Australia

[2]Melville Analytics Pty Ltd, Melbourne, VIC, Australia

[3]Centre for Astrobiology, University of Ruhuna, Matara, Sri Lanka

[4]University Toronto Health Network, Toronto General Hospital, University of Toronto, Toronto, ON, Canada

[5]School of Biological Sciences and Biotechnology, Murdoch University, WA, Australia

[6]Institute for the Study of Panspermia and Astroeconomics, Gifu, Japan

[7]The History of Chinese Science and Culture Foundation, Conway Hall, London, United Kingdom

[8]University of Buckingham, Buckingham, United Kingdom

[9]National Institute of Fundamental Studies, Kandy, Sri Lanka

Corresponding author: Edward J. Steele, C.Y.O' Connor ERADE Village Foundation, Piara Waters, Perth, WA, Australia; **E-mail:** e.j.steele@bigpond.com

Received: June 20, 2021; **Accepted:** July 05, 2021; **Published:** July 12, 2021

Abstract

A sudden yet very small outbreak of COVID-19 mystery community transmissions occurred in a defined arc across the inner Western and outer Northern suburbs of Melbourne in May-June 2021. An infection zone that could be 1000 km² in size. These sudden outbreaks of genuine mystery cases could not be traced to any direct infected contacts nor could they be directly genomically linked to any known infection clusters (e.g. among infected international travellers in hotel quarantine). In response the Government of Victoria on the recommendation of the Chief Medical Officer and the Victorian Department of Health locked down the entire State of Victoria in an extreme Stage 4 emergency. As a consequence, large numbers of PCR COVID-19 tests on oro-nasal swabs were conducted (> 30, 000 per day at peak) and all positives quarantined at home, a directive enforced by police and in some cases the Australian Army. Citizens were neither allowed to leave Melbourne nor from Victoria to any other State of Australia. Contact tracing was conducted on a very large scale by teams of experienced tracers. Several sudden mystery outbreaks continued to occur despite the lock-down on people movements. This included restriction of numbers of visitors at homes, crowd-size limitations, curtailment of sporting events, school closures, mandatory mask wearing, and personal tracking of all individuals in shops and supermarkets (via a personal "QR" digital tracking system linked to mobile phones or via written personal contact statements at store or shop entry). Many of the COVID-19 variants of concern (PANGO classification) were clearly mature human-passaged virions, many of which have been identified in the current and very large 2nd Wave Indian epidemic. We show here there is plausible strong evidence that a heterogeneous set of these "Indian" variants may have been transported by prevailing tropospheric global wind systems via the Indian Ocean and Southern Ocean (Roaring Forties West to East on the 40° S Latitude line) to Victoria, Australia. There is much precedent for such global wind transportations in the history of past Influenza virus pandemics in the last 100 years and the present observations relating to COVID-19 events in Australia are discussed in that context.

Introduction

A cool and objective scientific understanding the origins and global spread of the COVID-19 virus is the most pressing issue of our time. The multifactorial evidence that we have assembled through 2020 is fully consistent with COVID-19 arriving first via a loosely-held life-bearing carbonaceous cometary bolide that dispersed its viral cargo in the stratosphere on the 40° N Latitude line over Jilin in North East China on the night of October 11 2019 [1-3]. A long series of air-sampling experiments carried out in the stratosphere over the past 20 years have revealed unequivocal evidence of biological entities ranging in size from tens of nanometres, identifiable as virions, to several microns corresponding to bacteria at heights of up to 41 km [4,5]. More recently, Grebennikova et al. have identified by PCR techniques several bacterial species on the outside of the International Space Station (orbiting at a height of 400km) which are most plausibly of cometary origin [6]. A variable population of bacteria and viruses in the stratosphere thus appears to have a firm empirical basis, and is moreover consistent with the theory of cometary panspermia for which there is now a formidable body of evidence [7,8].

DOI: 10.31038/IDT.2021214

https://researchopenworld.com/covid-19-sudden-outbreak-of-mystery-case-transmissions-in-victoria-australia-may-june-2021-strong-evidence-of-tropospheric-transport-of-human-passaged-infective-virions-from-the-indian-epidemic/

Edward J. Steele (2021) COVID-19 Sudden Outbreak of Mystery Case Transmissions in Victoria, Australia, May-June 2021: Strong Evidence of Tropospheric Transport of Human Passaged Infective Virions from the Indian Epidemic

A critical evaluation of all the relevant evidence suggests the causative virus of the COVID-19 pandemic could not have come from an infected bat or pangolin to infect all of the central region of China around Wuhan city and Hubei province on the scale that was witnessed in Nov 2019-Jan 2020 [2,9]. In our opinion, guided by the relevant evidence and observations of many similar instances of suddenly emergent pandemics throughout history [10], this pandemic is entirely natural which is by no means unique. It represents a natural phenomenon consistent with the emerging paradigm that life is an all pervasive cosmic phenomenon [10-12]. It is unrelated to putative explanations based on non-scientific *ad hoc* human-induced conspiracy theories - such as those currently in vogue in the popular press e.g. "Wuhan Virus Lab Leak" theories. It cannot be emphasised too strongly that all such explanations are non-scientific. They require too many *ad hoc* assumptions, many incoherent and contradictory, when rationally examined in the light of *all* the unfolding *temporal key* evidence. The appropriate scientific domains in which the relevant data *must* be addressed and analysed for this pandemic must of necessity include immunology, genetics, epidemiology, astrobiology and atmospheric physics. The group of scientists that we represent has been tracking, analysing, explaining as well as predicting with accuracy the course of this suddenly emergent virus disease from its origin and early spread in Wuhan in late November 2019 through January 2020, following in our view the arrival at the Earth of a putative life-bearing cometary bolide [1,3]. We then analysed the early evidence *against* the standard explanation of global infection-driven solely by person-to-person (P-to-P) transfer of the COVID-19 virus [13]. The long-distance transfer of infection after the initial Wuhan strike to other far-flung global regions occurred primarily not by P-to-P transfer but via upper level tropospheric/stratospheric jet streams on a $40° - 60°$ N latitude band from East to West [14]. This process combined with more localised lower-level tropospheric wind systems (West-to-East) explains much of the unfolding data in the early weeks of the pandemic. This includes the otherwise mysterious transport across the Pacific Ocean of the L haplotype of the Wuhan-plumed P-to-P virus to infect the *Grand Princess* cruise ship off San Francisco [3].

The pandemic next appeared to move into lower - level Atlantic Ocean prevailing wind systems and thence into the Southern Hemisphere [15]. During this early period, up to May 2020, many ships at sea became engaged with sudden and seemingly mysterious COVID-19 outbreaks: cruise ships (*Diamond Princess, Westerdam Grand Princess*), aircraft carriers (*USS Theodore Roosevelt*, the French Navy's *Charles de Gaulle*), various fishing trawlers and live animal transportation ships [9,16]. Wherever these 'ship at sea' strikes could be cleanly analysed it became evident that all such outbreaks are best understood as mid-ocean depositions of COVID-19 virions with all the tell-tale signs of aerial pathogenic attack [9,16]. Moreover, sudden strikes on isolated islands such as Sri Lanka that had flat-lined in COVID-19 case incidence all year (2020) and then suddenly became engaged in a few days (Oct 4-6, 2020) with over a thousand active cases are difficult to understand in terms of traditional P-to-P spreads considering the associated minimum incubation time between transfers of infections of about one week [3,17]. Another remarkable incident of a similar kind is the isolated Chilean military base in

Antartica, thousands of kilometres from civilisation that became suddenly engaged late December 2020 [3]. A cool objective assessment of all these types of striking sudden COVID-19 outbreaks are inconsistent with traditional P-to-P infectious disease epidemiology, but entirely consistent with transportation via tropospheric winds and precipitation (rain) bringing the viral-laden clouds to ground. In this way we can explain the sudden and simultaneous appearance of sporadic mass infections in widely separated geographical locations that are mutually isolated, and thus cannot be cross-infecting one another by a P-to-P spread process. The intensity of each outbreak in any given geographical zone depends only upon viral density at in-fall, and the exposed susceptible human population density in that area. The viral density detected at ground level is predicted to be quite patchy, on scales determined by the turbulence patterns caused by thermal fluctuations determined by local heat sources.

The modern tendency to invoke the *ad hoc* concepts of super spreaders, asymptomatic carriers or "stranger-to-stranger" spread to explain any baffling aspects of the pandemic is a desperate attempt to maintain the *status quo* of the terrestrial origin of the virus and its P-to-P spread. It is interesting to recall that this is strikingly reminiscent of the Ptolemaic epicycles that were invoked in the last days of the Copernican revolution (Supplementary Information). It was the multiplication of such epicycles that finally led to the rejection of the Ptolemaic Earth-centred universe. Whether we have now come anywhere near this critical point in the story of COVID-19 epidemiology is left to be seen. Through 2020 we analysed the genetics of adaption of the COVID-19 virus in the first few months of the pandemic in 2020 at clear explosive hotspot locations (Wuhan, New York City, US West Coast) and defined the initial (*ab initio*) haplotype sorting process used by all respiratory epithelial lining cells in the innate -immune driven host -parasite relationship in the first 24-48 hrs of infection - APOBEC and ADAR deaminase-driven ribo-switching of a common set of COVID-19 haplotypes. These are best understood as co-ordinated single nucleotide variant (SNV) changes consistent with successful effective replicative RNA secondary structures [9,18]. This is discussed further in 'Haplotype Analysis' in Materials and Methods.

In a review of all the relevant key evidence the most parsimonious explanation seems to be that COVID-19 came from space [2,3], just as have many other similar suddenly emergent pandemics past and recent: such as the Spanish Flu 1918-1919 and the other pandemics that punctuate history over millennia, and in particular over the best documented period over the past 100 years spanning the 20th and 21st centuries [10-12]. In this report we now critically evaluate the publicly available infection and COVID-19 genomic data for the sudden, yet small, outbreak of COVID-19 cases in Victoria, Australia in May - June 2021. Many of the initiating cases prior to P-to-P spreading within a local cluster are genuine mystery/community transmissions that have still not been resolved as this paper was submitted (as June 19 2021) – either by contact tracing or by genomic sequencing matching with already known clusters in the epidemic target zone. Given the global isolation of Australia as an island continent, and the further isolation of the State of Victoria, taken together with the stringent quarantine and isolation regulations combined with diligent contact tracing that have been in place, we have here a remarkable setting for a controlled experiment for

Edward J. Steele (2021) COVID-19 Sudden Outbreak of Mystery Case Transmissions in Victoria, Australia, May-June 2021: Strong Evidence of Tropospheric Transport of Human Passaged Infective Virions from the Indian Epidemic

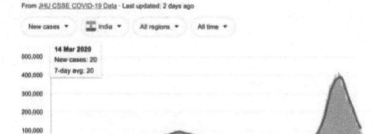

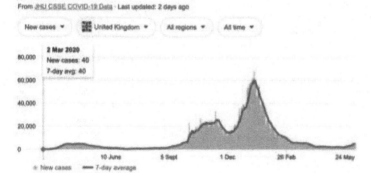

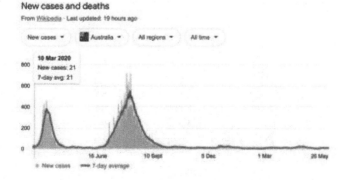

Figure 1: Magnitude and timing of the COVID-19 epidemics in Inda, United Kingdom amd Australia during 2020 and 2021.

Google: "**Coronavirus disease statistics**"URL is https://www.google.com.au/search?hl=en&ei=vWxyX7ipM4-m9QP18If4CQ&q=Coronavirus+disease+statistics&oq=Coronavirus+disease+s tatistics&gs_lcp=CgZwc3ktYWIQAzICCAAyAggAOgQIABBHOgcIABCxAxBDOgQIABBDULZUWPh1YJF7aABwAXgAgAgAH2AYgBvA6SAQYwLjEwLjYAQCgAQGgAQGqAQdnd3Mtd2l6yAEGwAEB&sclient=psy-ab&ved=0ahUKEwj4-47e-4zsAhUPU30KHXX4AZ8Q4dUDCAw&uact=5

This gives you the "Australia" dashboard (from there you can choose your country in the menu bar scroll).

Edward J. Steele (2021) COVID-19 Sudden Outbreak of Mystery Case Transmissions in Victoria, Australia, May-June 2021: Strong Evidence of Tropospheric Transport of Human Passaged Infective Virions from the Indian Epidemic

testing transmission models of the COVID-19 pandemic. As seen in Figure 1 all the case numbers in Australia are minuscule in comparison with the Northern Hemisphere infected zones (and see Supplementary Information). Further advantages in the situation in Victoria include the scale of mass PCR COVID-19 testing (≥30,000 per day, Figure 2); and a strictly policed social distancing/mask covering with Stage 3 and Stage 4 lock down regulations enforced in Victoria with the deployment of police and sometimes the army. The available data in the public domain allows scientific conclusions not as easily derived for the Northern Hemisphere infected zones, where the disease is of far greater intensity and wider geographic extent (two to four orders of magnitude greater than the greater metropolitan area of Melbourne, Victoria - this has, however, had well over 90% of all COVID-19 cases in Australia in 2020 and 2021 c.f. Figure 1 and URL link).

There are two general tropospheric viral-laden in-fall hypotheses that could serve to explain the patterns in these mystery infection data. They could operate together, or one or other may prevail in quantitative terms.

The two possibilities are:

A. The sudden outbreaks are due to precipitation bringing down virus-laden cometary dust in an arc around inner-outer Melbourne (West-North, approximately 1000 Km²) thus contaminating the environment and causing spot mystery infections of SARS-CoV-2 respiratory disease (generating simple haplotype variants *ab initio*, as Steele and Lindley [18]).

B. The sudden outbreaks are caused by the same precipitation (rain) bringing down human passaged virions transported in global wind circulation from Northern Hemisphere infected zones, in particular from the Indian outbreaks.

The most likely source, in our view, would be the putative and massive viral plume over India of virions which have already "gone through" human passage (P-to-P), and thus showing substantially modified genomic sequences as multiple P-to-P products from the early *ab initio* haplotype sequences These were discussed, using data from the first three months of 2020, for haplotype diversification between Wuhan and New York City [9,18].

Here we assemble the evidence that strongly supports hypothesis B, that all the community transmission 'mystery cases' in the Victorian epidemic in May - June 2020 may have been caused by a range of Indian human-passaged viruses delivered to Victoria, Australia, from elsewhere, most likely via the Indian subcontinent viral plume via tropospheric wind systems. This conclusion is not inconsistent with low level tropospheric prevailing wind systems spreading viral pandemics in the recent past via non P-to-P processes on scale [10]. Many striking non P-to-P spreading events like this were reviewed over 30 years ago by Hammond et al. [19].

Materials and Methods

Publicly Available Data Resources

a. *GenBank/NCBI Virus db*

For full length COVID-19 genomic sequences and their haplotype analysis against the Wuhan Hu-1 29903 nt long RNA reference sequence (NC_045512.2) all Genbank Accession sequence data were obtained and aligned (multiple sequence alignments) using the *NCBI Virus* database and alignment tools. This publicly accessible site is hosted at The National Center for Biotechnology Information (NCBI) at the National Institutes of Health (NIH), Bethesda, Maryland, USA, which curates SARS-CoV-2 sequences at https://www.ncbi.nlm.nih.gov/sars-cov-2/#nucleotide-sequences

b. *Epidemiological Information*

This is from that published daily by the national newspaper *The Australian* and other information from Melbourne's *Herald-Sun* newspaper. All specific details are referenced or expanded on in the Supplementary Information. Other data for background long term cross checking can be access at The Victorian Department of Health website https://www.dhhs.vic.gov.au/victorian-coronavirus-covid-19-data

c. *Weather Information*

This was from The Australian Bureau of Meteorology (BOM) and also news reports through April and May 2021

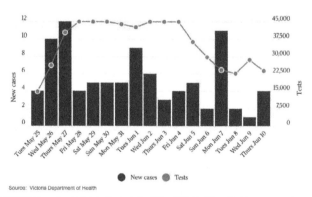

Figure 2: New Cases per Day and Total PCR Tests per Day in Victoria. *The Australian* 10 June 2021. Hard Stage 4 lockdown across entire state of Victoria introduced on May 27.

Edward J. Steele (2021) COVID-19 Sudden Outbreak of Mystery Case Transmissions in Victoria, Australia, May-June 2021: Strong Evidence of Tropospheric Transport of Human Passaged Infective Virions from the Indian Epidemic

http://www.bom.gov.au/climate/dwo/202105/html/IDCJDW3050.202105.shtml

Haplotype Analysis

The haplotype approach to COVID-19 sequence diversification [18] differs from the PANGO classification system which uses a phylogenetic approach which generates putative person-to-person (P-to-P) lineages, clusters and clades [20,21]. The *ab initio* haplotype-sort/selection explanation, during first infection of respiratory epithelial cells in the first Host-Parasite encounter - by viral-laden meteorite tropospheric dust - is a better primary explanation of the APOBEC/ADAR-driven deaminase ribo-switching process and informs classification of sequences through molecular understanding based on variant RNA secondary structures. In the first three months of the pandemic this ribo-switching haplotype sorting and quasi-species selection process operates in the first subject infected host [22,23]. This generates, in our view, a range of quasi-species and then host-parasite selection allows successful emergence of a replicative 29903 nt long RNA *secondary structure haplotype* in that subject host (Steele and Lindley 2020 [18] Table 1). The PANGO variants published in *The Australian* newspaper (Saturday 5 June 2021) which are of concern

to the Victorian Department of Health (Figure 3) have been assigned haplotypes using these markers (Table 2).

Criteria for a SNV in the Coding Regions (CDS) Classed as Conserved, Benign, Radical (Table 2) - as defined in Steele and Lindley (2020) [18]

Conserved: These are synonymous SNVs or a SNV change leading to the same amino acid (AA) functional class. *Benign:* These are AA changes which are Polar<-> NonPolar, Acid <-> Polar, or Basic<-> Polar. *Radicle:* These are AA changes Acid<-> NonPolar, Basic<-> NonPolar, Acidic<-> Basic.

Multiple PANGO Sequences Used to Determine Haplotypes as Shown in Table 2

Shown in Table 3 are the GenBank accession numbers of many of the PANGO variants of concern in Victoria from the *NCBI Virus* website for the haplotype analysis in the Melbourne, Victoria outbreak of mystery cases in May-June 2021- all haplotyped in multiple alignments v Hu-1 (NC_045512).

Among a Set of the Same "PANGO Designated Variants"

Table 1: Putative *Ab Initio* Haplotypes and Main Sites Defining COVID-19 Common Strain Variants in first 3 months of the pandemic (Jan-Mar 2020).

HAP	AA class-> 5'UTR p.241	P<>NonP Thr<>Ile p.1059	SYN Phe<>Phe p.3037	P<>NonP Ile<>Phe p.1163	SYN Thr<>Thr p.7540	SYN Ser<>Ser p.8782	NonP<>NonP Leu<>Phe p.11080/83	NonP<>NonP Pro<>Leu p.14408	SYN Thr<>Thr p.16647	NonP<>NonP Pro<>Leu p.17747	P<>P Tyr<>Cys p.17858	SYN Leu<>Leu p.18060	SYN Asp<>Asp p.18555	P<>P Ser<>Asn p.22992	SYN Gln<>Gln p.23401	Acid<>NonP Asp<>Gly p.23403	P<>Basic Gln<>His p.25563	P<>NonP Leu<>Ser p.28144	RADICLE Arg/Gly/Lys/Arg p.28881-3
L (Hu-1)	C	C	C	A	T	C	G	C	G	C	A	C	C	G	G	A	G	T	GGG
Ln	C	C	C	A	T	C	T	C	G	C	A	C	C	G	G	A	G	T	GGG
L-241a	T	T	T	A	T	C	G	T	G	C	A	C	C	G	G	G	T	T	GGG
L-241b	T	T	C	A	T	C	G	T	G	C	A	C	C	G	G	G	T	T	GGG
L-241c	T	C	T	A	T	C	G	T	G	C	A	C	C	G	G	G	T	T	GGG
L-241d/s	T	T	T	A	T	C	G	C	G	C	A	C	C	G	G	G	T	T	GGG
L-241e	T	C	C	A	T	C	G	T	G	C	A	C	C	G	G	G	T	T	GGG
L-241f	T	C	T	A	T	C	G	T	G	C	A	C	C	G	G	G	T	T	GGG
L-241f.1	T	C	T	A	T	C	G	T	G	C	A	C	C	G	G	G	T	T	AAC
L-241g	T	C	C	A	T	C	G	T	G	C	A	C	C	G	G	G	T	T	GGG
S	C	C	C	A	T	T	G	C	G	C	A	C	C	G	G	A	G	C	GGG
Sa	C	C	C	A	T	T	G	C	G	T	G	T	C	G	G	A	G	C	GGG
Sb	C	C	C	A	T	T	G	C	G	C	A	C	C	G	G	A	G	C	GGG
Ss	C	C	C	A	T	T	G	C	G	C	A	C	C	G	G	A	G	C	GGG

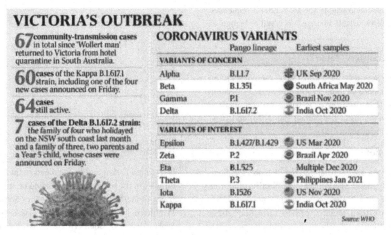

Figure 3: *The Australian* Saturday 5 June 2021.

Edward J. Steele (2021) COVID-19 Sudden Outbreak of Mystery Case Transmissions in Victoria, Australia, May-June 2021: Strong Evidence of Tropospheric Transport of Human Passaged Infective Virions from the Indian Epidemic

Table 2: PANGO variants of COVID-19 of interest and concern in Melbourne, Victoria outbreak of mystery cases in May-June 2021.

PANGO Variant	Steele and Lindley *Ab Initio* HAP seq	Numbers of additional variations accrued on top of S&L HAP sequence when aligned against Hu-1										Total	From *Ab Initio* number putative P-to-P transfers?
		5' UTR	5' UTR	3' UTR	3' UTR	Non-CDS	Non-CDS	SNV CDS variants recorded as :					
		SNV	Indel	SNV	Indel	SNV	Indel	Conserved	Benign	Radical	In-frame Indel		
B.1.1.7	L241f.1	0	0	0	0	0	0	7	3	6	1 to 3	17-19	4
B.1.351	L241a	1	0	0	0	0	0	5	3	3	2	14	3 or 4
P.1	L241f.1	0	0	2	0	0	1	11	9	2	1	26	5 or 6
B.1.617.2	L241f	1	0	1	0	0	1	6	8	4	1	22	4 or 5
B.1.427/B.1.429	L241a	0	0	0	0	1	0	3	3	1	0	8	2
P.2	Nd	Nd	Nd	Nd	Nd	Nd	Nd	Nd	Nd	Nd	Nd	Nd	Nd
B.1.525	L241f	0	0	0	1	1	0	18	5	1	4	30	6 or 7
P.3	Nd	Nd	Nd	Nd	Nd	Nd	Nd	Nd	Nd	Nd	Nd	Nd	Nd
B.1.526	L241a	0	0	0	0	0	1	7	5	1	1	15	3 to 4
B.1.617.1	L241f	1	0	1	0	0	1	5	7	5	0	17	3 or 4

The PANGO variants from *The Weekend Australian* June 5-6 2021.

There Will be Variable Sites – that is *"Not All PANGOS are Identical"*

It is important to understand that when newly isolated COVID-19 genomic sequences are assigned a PANGO variant/lineage label, all PANGO variants with that label are not necessarily identical. Human passaged (P-to-P) will introduce further new variable sites within that haplotypic framework. For example in a multiple alignment against the Hu-1 reference of six B.1.617.2 variants (MZ318750, MZ318917, MZ320553, MZ317762, MZ318262, MZ318150) the number of non-haplotypic shared sites above the 22 listed in Table 2 for B.1.617.2, there are 49 other sites that can vary. A similar pattern like this applies to sets of the other PANGO haplotypes in Table 2 aligned against Hu-1. Thus the statement that a freshly isolated sequence "has a particular PANGO variant sequence (i.e. haplotype) *should **not** be taken to mean all members of that variant are identical* as APOBEC/ADAR-driven variation at P-to-P transfers ensures most **will be not** identical. Most of these differences (>95%) result in conserved or benign AA changes i.e. there is considerable sequence conservation at the protein level due to Darwinian purifying selection (e.g. in the six B.1.617.2 sequences discussed above 48 of the 49 variable sites are conserved or benign as defined).

Estimates of P-to-P Transfers (Table 2)

It should be noted here that the estimates of the numbers of putative P-to-P transfers since *ab initio* creation in the first infection from raw meteorite dust-derived virus, is based on conservative estimates from the observations in the Wuhan (Jan 2020) and New York City (Mar 2020) hotspot zones [18].

Results and Discussion

To focus on the relevant geographical infected Melbourne region, Figures 4A and 4B show Google Maps of the West-North Melbourne arc where the great majority of waste water catchment COVID-19 fragment detections have been found (April to early May 2021, Supplementary Information) and where the suddenly emergent mystery case-generated clusters of COVID-19 infections have *later*

Table 3: Gen Bank accession numbers of all PANGO sequences multiply aligned for haplotype assignment.

Accession	Collect 2021	Geo Location	PANGO
MZ310552	04-12	India	B.1.1.7
MZ310908	05-05	USA.SC. Lancaster	B.1.1.7
MZ317817	05-10	USA, Rhode Island	B.1.351
MZ317890	02-02	India	B.1.351
MZ317892	02-02	India	B.1.351
MZ318331	04-15	USA, North Carolina	B.1.351
MZ311471	05-14	USA. Mass	P.1
MZ311478	05-19	USA. New Hampshire	P.1
MZ317762	05-04	USA Mass	B.1.617.2
MZ318159	04-10	India	B.1.617.2
MZ318262	04-30	USA	B.1.617.2
MZ318750	05-11	USA Texas	B.1.617.2
MZ318817	05-09	USA Arkansas	B.1.517.2
MZ318917	05-09	USA New Jersey	B.1.617.2
MZ310942	05-20	USA. Mass	B.1.617.2
MZ304709	05-08	USA. California	B.1.617.2
MZ317766	05-03	USA, Mass	B.1.427
MZ317895	04-01	Germany, Frankfurt	B.1.427
MZ317896	01-14	Germany, Frankfurt	B.1.429
MZ318827	05-10	USA, California	B.1.429
MZ318829	05-11	USA, Texas	B.1.427
P.2 -Nd			
MZ317699	2021-05	USA Virginia	B.1.525
MZ321539	05-12	USA Mass	B.1.525
P.3-Nd			
MZ311490	05-14	USA. New Hampshire	B.1.526
MZ311497	05-20	Rhode Island	B.1.526
MZ310590	03-17	India	B.1.617.1
MZ310588	02-12	India	B.1.617.1

been found (below and Supplementary Information). A conservative estimate of the size of the region could be at least 1000Km², stretching from Altona/Maidstone in Melbourne's South West to the northern Whittlesea local government area (LGA) in which the suburb of Wollert is on the southern edge. The distance from Altona to the northern edge of Whittlesea LGA is at least 30 Km.

Edward J. Steele (2021) COVID-19 Sudden Outbreak of Mystery Case Transmissions in Victoria, Australia, May-June 2021: Strong Evidence of Tropospheric Transport of Human Passaged Infective Virions from the Indian Epidemic

Weather in Melbourne and Environs through April into May 2021

There was significant April rain in greater Melbourne, usually at night and cold, on 9th (6.2mm), 10th (0.2 mm), 11th (3.4 mm), 12th (10 mm), 13th (0.6mm), 16th (1mm), 21st (10.4 mm), 23rd (0.4 mm), 25th (2.6 mm), 26th (1.2 mm), 27th (0.6mm), 28th (0.4mm) ; then again further rains well into May and June including severe flooding in the same regions covered in the Google Maps above. Precipitation coming up from the Southern Ocean in a SW to E direction (the typical prevailing way the winter weather visits Victoria) would be a necessary pre-condition for any tropospheric clouds of COVID-19 virion dust-associated particles to be brought to ground.

PCR COVID-19 Fragments Detected in Waste-Water Catchments Prior to Sudden Outbreak

The West-North arc and range of these detections is specifically covered in the Supplementary Information. They occurred during a period *when no COVID-19 cases had been detected for many weeks* (prior to May 11). These significant PCR detection signals occurred in late April early May *before* 'Wollert Man' the putative infective P-to-P trigger for the entire outbreak (see below and Supplementary Information) left the Adelaide quarantine hotel (May 4) and cover the *same environment footprint* where all the key putative mystery cases have been reported or deduced to have emerged. Thus, significant environmental contamination with COVID-19 genomes appears to

have occurred and are manifest in waste-water catchment reservoirs in the W-N arc under discussion and analysis - it stretches incredulity that all the PCR fragments signals, in the face of massive dilution factors, are due to undetected high-rate urine shedders of COVID-19 virions by undetected asymptomatic infected subjects. The maps in Figures 4A and 4B can assist in visualising this COVID-19 fragment footprint in association with Supplementary Information.

Analysis of Key Mystery Cases and Clusters

The caveats to this analysis are the absence of meta-data (ethnicity, clinical status, exact likely locations at infection) and the non-availability of exact COVID-19 genomic sequence(s) apart from muted PANGO variant of the infected subjects as well as considerable mis-information about each case in the mass media. There is only limited knowledge of the genomic sequence (shown in Figure 3) - some are either Indian variant kappa (B.1.617.1) or delta (B.1.617.2) as assigned below. When it was neither variant that was acknowledged in the press release we can only deduce that in that particular mystery case the sequence was "one of concern" as summarised in Figure 3 and Table 2. All the key public information around the origin of each mystery cluster is provided in the Supplementary Information for the reader to independently weigh up the evidence *pro* and *con*. In our considered view every case in the list below is a real mystery community transmission- *no definitive genomic links nor P-to-P contact links with any other cluster*. There has been considerable speculation in the mass media with state-wide (and even nation-wide)

Figure 4(A): Map West-North Melbourne Infected zones centred on "Reservoir".

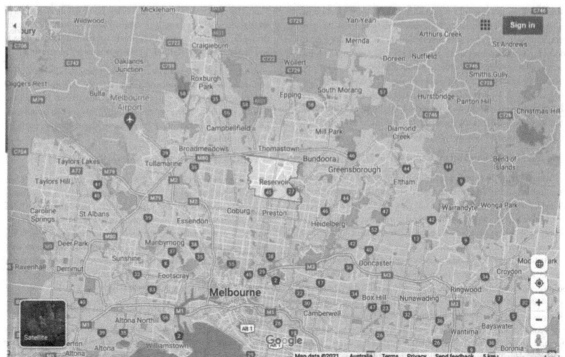

Edward J. Steele (2021) COVID-19 Sudden Outbreak of Mystery Case Transmissions in Victoria, Australia, May-June 2021: Strong Evidence of Tropospheric Transport of Human Passaged Infective Virions from the Indian Epidemic

Figure 4(B): Map West-North Melbourne Infected zones centred on "North Melbourne Primary School".

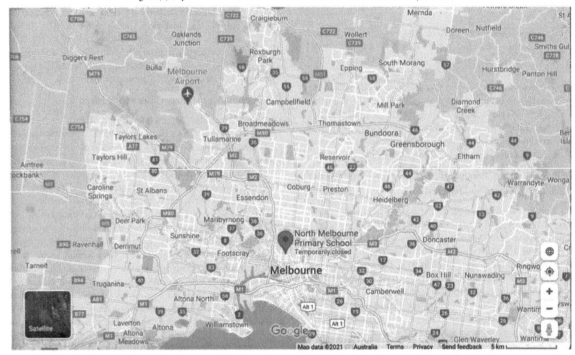

searches for the 'missing links' between clusters. They have not been found. To claim, as indicated in **Materials & Methods**, that Wollert Man or those in the larger Whittlesea LGA cluster are of the kappa Indian variant does not constitute evidence of a direct genomic link-in a situation as in Wollert v Whittlesea where no direct physical P-to-P links can be established. The article by *The Australian's* Stephen Lunn on the origins of 'Wollert Man' catching a kappa variant by a putative fleeting 18 second contact in a corridor at the Playford quarantine hotel in Adelaide CBD cannot be taken seriously in the light of all the other epidemiological evidence (discussed below)

• **Wollert Man (Indian Variant Kappa B.1.617.1)**

Wollert Man, a 30 yr male returned home to Australia on April 20 from India via Adelaide airport and went into hotel quarantine. Over the next 2 weeks he had 3 negative PCR tests. On May 4 he travelled to Adelaide airport, caught a plane to Melbourne, travelled from the airport by Sky bus to Melbourne's Southern Cross Station in the CBD, then caught the train north to Wollert, where he lived. According to reports he had some symptoms on May 8 and was PCR positive on May 11. His close contacts in the household have not become PCR positive. He had limited movement while in Wollert (in the Whittlesea LGA) but all subsequent tests on all those putatively contacted by him on his May 4 travel to Wollert and since (several hundred contacts) have scored PCR negative. In addition there was no transmission of the Playford hotel kappa Indian variant in Adelaide or anywhere in South Australia. The later kappa Indian cluster in Whittlesea LGA (on

May 24) some 5 to 10 km from his Wollert home has no direct link to Wollert man- only the loose 'kappa variant' associations highlighted by the media and the Victorian Department of Health discussed already and in **Materials and Methods** (and Supplementary Information).

The most parsimonious interpretation of these data is that Wollert Man became infected when he returned to the already COVID-19 contaminated environment in Wollert on his return. He did not overtly transfer the infection after that date. This is a real genuine in-fall infection from the troposphere with an already human passaged common Indian variant (Table 2).

• **Whittlesea Cluster (Indian Variant Kappa B.1.617.1)**

This is a much larger cluster that emerged suddenly on May 24 and grew to about 20 cases in a few days (Figure 2), then to even greater numbers > 60 cases (Figure 3 and Supplementary Information). We have established there is no link with Wollert Man. We have no idea if there is more than one kappa mystery infection that initiated the P-to-P expansion. It is conceivable there may have been more than one pro-band. The situation remains confused and that point is not resolved. This cluster is not linked genomically or by any P-to-P contact with the other mystery clusters (below).

• **Arcare Outbreak (Variant Non-Indian Kappa or Delta)**

This case appeared suddenly on May 30 2021 in a 55 yr female carer at the Arcare aged care facility in Maidstone, West Melbourne (see Supplementary Information). It was passed to several elderly residents (>

Edward J. Steele (2021) COVID-19 Sudden Outbreak of Mystery Case Transmissions in Victoria, Australia, May-June 2021: Strong Evidence of Tropospheric Transport of Human Passaged Infective Virions from the Indian Epidemic

80 yr) and also to another female carer who was also working in another local aged care facility (Sunshine). Of interest the 55 yr female carer had already had one COVID-19 vaccination, and the resident she passed it to (90 yr male) had a full course of two vaccinations. The elderly infected residents were transferred to hospital and seem to have recovered at time of writing. The Arcare facility is in lockdown at time of writing.

• Delta Cluster, Nth Melbourne (Indian Delta B.1.617.2)

This cluster emerged around June 4. It involved two families from North Melbourne who travelled together on holiday to the South Coast of NSW in the same large people moving van. Most members of that travelling group have become PCR positive. There are no physical or genomic links to any other cluster. But a supposed link with a 'delta' Indian variant brought from overseas by a Sri Lankan traveller to Melbourne has been hypothesized (see Supplementary Information). The most parsimonious explanation is this is a genuine mystery cluster as recognized by authorities. Whether one or several mystery infected probands in that van is responsible for initiating P-to-P spreads is not known.

• Reservoir Cluster (Variant Non-Indian Kappa or Delta)

This appeared suddenly on June 10 2021 and "includes a man in his 80s, a woman in her 70s, a man in his 50s and a man in his 20s who all live in the same household in Reservoir in Melbourne's northern suburbs" (see Supplementary Information). There is no genomic or physical P-to-P link with any other cluster. It is clear the coronavirus variants driving the mystery clusters in the Victoria outbreak are diverse and typical of prior P-to-P passaged virus variants (Table 2). Where did they suddenly and mysteriously come from? This, we would argue, is a classic signature of spot "infections from the sky" over a regional arc known to have been previously contaminated with COVID-19 genomes on a regional scale. So all these cases are fully consistent with an aerial pathogenic attack from the troposphere, contaminating the environment and capriciously infecting unsuspecting victims as we have discussed in other recent papers.

Possible Explanations

Ab Initio haplotype sorting of meteorite dust raw virus seems highly unlikely given the clear evidence of complex human-passaged variants, many of which appear to have come from the Indian subcontinent epidemic (Table 2). The variant diversity in India is remarkably wide, and not confined to the main "Indian variants" kappa and delta. It includes even the 'UK Mutant' (B.1.1.7) which has become engaged in the Indian epidemic (Figures 1, 3 and Table 2). Indeed, in a sample of recent Indian PANGO variants that were uploaded to *NCBI Virus* we find at least 5 that are of concern in Victoria (Figure 3 and Table 2) have also been found in India. Thus PANGO variants and numbers uploaded in this small sample, as determined over the first two hundred upload web pages – each page can accommodate 200 entries- on June 6 and 7 (in brackets) are : B.1.1.7 (11), B.1.617.1 (4), B.1.617.2 (33), B.1.36.8(10), B.1.36 (14), B.36.10 (1), B.1 (2), B.1.1.216 (3), B.1.367 (2), B.1.1 (4), B.1.1.306 (1), B.1.36.17 (1), B.1.351, (5), B.1.427/B.1.429 (2) (see Supplementary Information). So just how did these mature human-passaged Indian variants appear mysteriously in Victoria from a tropospheric in-fall?

The recent outbreak in India is massive and cataclysmic. It has engaged almost all Indian provinces suddenly across the entire sub-continent (not shown, use URL in Figure 1 to check this fact out). We have speculated in the past that it has been triggered on scale by a viral laden dust comet dust in-fall off the 40° N Latitude band on the southern side of the Himalayan Mountains [3]. However, we can plausibly include, at a slightly later time, the Sri Lankan and Maldives outbreaks as also coming from India (Supplementary Information). Indeed, as we continue to marshal the relevant evidence, there is in fact a temporal sequential order of outbreaks further south on that same longitude line down the East African coast. New COVID-19 outbreaks of variable magnitude, temporally following India, appear evident in Kenya, Madagascar and South Africa. It is thus conceivable that the putative virus-laden plume (heterogeneous collection of human passaged COVID-19 viral variants) over India has been transported by tropospheric Indian Ocean and Southern Ocean prevailing winds to also cause the comparatively minor outbreak in Victoria, Australia in May-June 2021.

The prevailing winds in the Indian and Southern Ocean (Figure 5) make this global tropospheric transport route entirely credible. And indeed, the recent "upticks" in the rolling waves of Chilean epidemics suggest that the entire Roaring Forties 40° S line may now be entrapped by the tropospheric viral clouds from the plume of the Indian epidemic (Supplementary Information). Other independent evidence supporting this interpretation has been documented in the past for the global transport and spread of previous Influenza pandemics by global weather and wind systems [10,19]. Further, in the case COVID-19 in the first few months of the pandemic, the Wuhan plume carrying the dominant human passaged haplotype (L) appeared to have crossed the North Pacific by mid-February 2020 to infect passengers on the *Grand Princess* cruise ship who displayed genomic sequences of unmutated or lightly mutated L haplotype as discussed [3,18].

Conclusions

It is plausible in the light of this analysis of a defined small COVID-19 outbreak that other global transfers of viral plumes are conceivable. The "UK Mutant" B.1.1.7 is now widespread and very common in the USA (inspection of the *very large numbers* of uploads of B.1.1.7 variants to *NCBI Virus* confirms this impression) and including many parts of Europe. These global transportations again via lower-level E-to-W and W-to-E tropospheric winds seem plausible given the expected size of the viral plume over the UK epidemic Dec-Feb (Figure 1). There are many unknowns on the size and potential rising-height of the putative viral plumes, so plausible speculation is required. From available epidemiological data (e.g. Figure 1) which suggest an estimated 10 million active Indian cases at any given time over several weeks (20 days of say 500,000 cases per day), we would have ~ 10^7 virus exhalers who undoubtedly contribute virions into the lower atmosphere. If we assume that each infected "exhaler" conservatively contributes 10^{12} aerosol virions we would have a total of 10^{19} virions potentially arising from the surface of the Indian subcontinent. Such virions which pass through regions of high humidity would be expected to acquire outer mantles of water ice that could help to retain viability to some degree. Fukuta et al. have recently

Edward J. Steele (2021) COVID-19 Sudden Outbreak of Mystery Case Transmissions in Victoria, Australia, May-June 2021: Strong Evidence of Tropospheric Transport of Human Passaged Infective Virions from the Indian Epidemic

Figure 5: Prevailing winds in Indian and Southern Oceans
Google link to Indian Ocean winds at: https://www.google.com.au/search?source=univ&tbm=isch&q=indian+ocean+prevailing+winds&hl=en&sa=X&ved=2ahUKEwiKpNCLqoTxAhUmzT
gGHQEfBHkQjJkEegQIChAB&biw=1018&bih=602&dpr=2

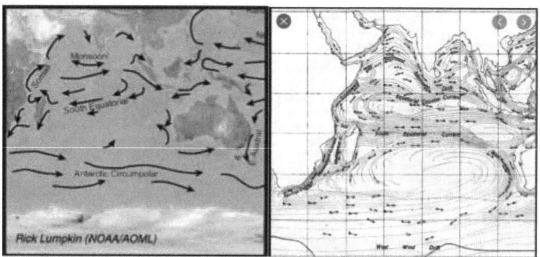

Indian Ocean- a Cruising Guide
cruiserswiki.org

Indian Ocean Gyre - Wikipedia

shown that COVID-19 remains highly infectious for prolonged periods in cold and wet conditions [24]. In addition, Kwon et al. [25] have determined the stability of the virus in a variety of biological fluids (nasal mucus, sputum, saliva, tear, urine, blood, and semen) and "it remained infectious significantly longer under winter and spring/fall conditions than under summer conditions". This suggests that dispersed viruses in aerosol biological fluid protective wraps may add to putative stability. If say 10% of these aerosol-protected virions survive lofting into the troposphere and subsequent wind transport, we have some 10^{18} virions (all amplified by victims in India) that are in circulation and which could contribute to the outbreaks of the so-called mystery clusters in Victoria, Australia. Indeed as this paper was being submitted it seems that the southern Chinese city of Guangzhou may be engaged in a sudden tropospheric strike of variants from India. Further, many other Northern Hemisphere countries (Russia, UK, USA) are also reporting the sudden spread of the Indian delta variant on real population wide scale (for news links see Supplementary Information File)

Given these developments, and on reflection, the sudden large outbreak in Sri Lanka October 4 – 6 2020 may well have been due to the 1st Wave Indian human-passaged viral plume (see Figure 1 and Supplementary Information). In contradistinction, the recent In Press report of Althoff et al. [26] of early spot detections and spreads of COVID-19 (late 2019-early 2020) suggest early fragmented in-fall of small clouds of raw (non P-to-P passaged) meteorite dust COVID-19 from the stratosphere on the 40° N latitude line as discussed viz [14]. "7 individuals had detectable SARS-CoV-2 immunoglobulin G prior to the first confirmed case in the states of Illinois, Massachusetts, Wisconsin, Pennsylvania, and Mississippi, suggesting that SARS-CoV-2 infections were occurring weeks prior to recognized cases in at least 5 US states [26]."

What lessons can we learn? Certainly, near-Earth surveillance of incoming pathogens from space, such as the suggested "Hoyle" shield needs to be an international imperative [27], as often reiterated by us [3,28], including for monitoring for tropospheric global transport of viral plumes as discussed here. But it seems also that once a viral pandemic is already underway, rising viral-plumes from major infected zones can potentially be transported to infect other global regions on a mass scale. Indeed pathogenic re-circulation via the troposphere during a pandemic is a major factor to consider for societies whose thinking seems restricted to "hard lockdowns and social distancing" to prevent or alleviate the spread of airborne viruses. If it is considered feasible a procedure by which the lower atmosphere and environments of infected areas could be sprayed with suitable disinfectants from the air must surely deserve serious attention. Face masks may be useful during an actual tropospheric in-fall event but may not work in the way the health authorities have advocated during a real mass outbreak on the scale of trillions of infective virions falling from the sky. All the evidence from the 2nd Wave in the Victorian 2020 epidemic suggests the Stage 4 lockdown had no impact whatsoever on the course of the epidemic [3], a conclusion supported by critical analysis of similar lock downs in the USA [29].

What of the immediate future? Has all the raw cometary dust-protected virus or the P-to-P plumed-virus (almost certainly assisted and protected by pollution particles) [30,31], washed down from the troposphere? The Spanish Flu took two years to run its full course. COVID-19 is nowhere as lethal but its global reach is similar, implying a similar magnitude of initiating viral inoculation. If that is a valid comparison then full viral wash down could perhaps take another 6 months. This time frame is not incompatible with other micron-sized particle falling-rates as estimated for wash down of radioactive

Edward J. Steele (2021) COVID-19 Sudden Outbreak of Mystery Case Transmissions in Victoria, Australia, May-June 2021: Strong Evidence of Tropospheric Transport of Human Passaged Infective Virions from the Indian Epidemic

tracers following upper-atmosphere nuclear tests in the late 1950s [2]. In conclusion we stress that as scientists we have a responsibility to accept whatever facts that the universe presents us without fear or favour. Distorting or even simply tweaking emerging facts in order to fit a long-established paradigm should be avoided at all cost.

Acknowledgement

We thank Max K. Wallis for critical discussions on the pandemic contributions of rising plumes of P-to-P virus, particularly the Wuhan COVID-19 plume of January 2020. George Howard is thanked for bringing to our attention the recent study by Althoff KN, Schlueter DJ, Anton-Culver H, Cherry J, Denny JC, et al. (2020). We thank John A Schuster for a critical reading of the manuscript first draft.

References

1. Wickramasinghe NC, Steele EJ, Gorczynski RM, Temple R, Tokoro G, et al. (2020) Comments on the Origin and Spread of the 2019 Coronavirus. *Virology: Current Research* 4:1. DOI: 10.37421/Virol Curr Res.2020.4.109

2. Steele EJ, Gorczynski RM, Lindley RA, Tokoro G, Temple R, et al. (2020) Origin of new emergent Coronavirus and Candida fungal diseases- Terrestrial or Cosmic? *Advances in Genetics* 106: 75-100. [crossref] https://doi.org/10.1016/bs.adgen.2020.04.002

3. Steele EJ, Gorczynski RM, Lindley RA, Tokoro G, Wallis DH, et al. (2021) Cometary Origin COVID-19 *Infect Dis & Therapeutics* 2: 1-4. DOI: 10.31038/IDT.2021212

4. Wainwright M, Wickramasinghe NC, Narlikar JV, Rajaratnam P, Perkins Joy (2004). Confirmation of the presence of viable but non-culturable bacteria in the stratosphere. *Int. J. Astrobiology* 3: 13-15. DOI: https://doi.org/10.1017/S1473550404001739

5. Wainwright M, Wickramasinghe NC, Tokoro G (2021) Neopanspermia - evidence that life continuously arrives at the Earth from space. *Advances in Astrophysics*. In Press

6. Grebennikova TV, Syroeshkin AV, Shubralova EV, Eliseeva OV, Kostina LV, et al. (2018) The DNA of bacteria of the world ocean and the Earth in cosmic dust at the international space station. *Sci. World J.* https://doi.org/10.1155/2018/7360147

7. Steele EJ, Al-Mufti S, Augustyn KA, Chandrajith R, Coghlan JP, et al. (2018) Cause of Cambrian Explosion: Terrestrial or Cosmic? *Prog. Biophys. Mol. Biol* 136: 3-23. [crossref] https://doi.org/10.1016/j.pbiomolbio.2018.03.004

8. Steele EJ, Gorczynski RM, Lindley RA, Liu Y, Temple R, et al. (2019) Lamarck and Panspermia - On the Efficient Spread of Living Systems Throughout the Cosmos. *Prog. Biophys. Mol. Biol* 149: 10-32. https://doi.org/10.1016/j.pbiomolbio.2019.08.010

9. Steele EJ, Gorczynski RM, Rebhan H, Carnegie P, Temple R, et al. (2020) Implications of haplotype switching for the origin and global spread of COVID-19 *Virology: Current Research* DOI: 10.37421/Virol Curr Res.2020.4.115

10. Hoyle F, Wickramasinghe NC (1979) *Diseases from Space* JM Dent Ltd, London.

11. Hoyle, F and Wickramasinghe, NC. (2000) *Astronomical Origins of Life: Steps Towards Panspermia*. Klower Academic Publishers, Dordrechl, The Netherlands.

12. Steele EJ, Wickramasinghe NC (Editors) (2020) Cosmic Genetic Evolution. *Advances in Genetics*. 106: 2-143.

13. Wickramasinghe NC, Steele EJ, Gorczynski RM, Temple R, Tokoro G, et al. (2020) Growing Evidence against Global Infection-Driven by Person-to-Person Transfer of COVID-19 *Virology: Current Research* 4:1. DOI: 10.37421/Virol Curr Res.2020.4.110

14. Wickramasinghe NC, Steele EJ, Gorczynski RM, Temple R, Tokoro G, et al. (2020) Predicting the Future Trajectory of COVID-19. *Virology: Current Research* 4:1. DOI: 10.37421/Virol Curr Res.2020.4.111

15. Wickramasinghe NC, Wallis MK, Coulson SG, Kondakov A, Steele EJ, et al.(2020) Intercontinental Spread of COVID-19 on Global Wind Systems *Virology: Current Research* 4:1.DOI: 10.37421/Virol Curr Res.2020.4.113

16. Howard GA, Wickramasinghe NC, Rebhan H, Steele EJ, Gorczynski RM, et al. (2020) Mid-Ocean Outbreaks of COVID-19 with Tell-Tale Signs of Aerial Incidence *Virology: Current Research* 4:2. DOI: 10.37421/Virol Curr Res.2020.4.114

17. Wickramasinghe NC, Steele EJ, Nimalasuriya A, Gorczynki RM, Tokoro G, et al. (2020) Seasonality of Respiratory Viruses Including SARS-CoV-2 *Virology: Current Research* 4:2. DOI: 10.37421/VCRH.2020.4.117

18. Steele EJ, Lindley RA (2020) Analysis of APOBEC and ADAR deaminase-driven Riboswitch Haplotypes in COVID-19 RNA strain variants and the implications for vaccine design. *Research Reports*. https://companyofscientists.com/index.php/rr

19. Hammond GW, Raddatz RL, Gelskey DE (1989) Impact of atmospheric dispersion and transport of viral aerosols on the epidemiology of Influenza. *Reviews of Infectious Disease* 11: 494- 497. [crossref] https://doi.org/10.1093/clinids/11.3.494

20. Rambaut A, Holmes EC, O'Toole Á, Hill V, McCrone JT, et al. (2020) A dynamic nomenclature proposal for SARS- CoV-2 to assist genomic epidemiology. *Nat. Microbiol* 5: 1403-1407. [crossref] https://doi.org/10.1038/s41564-020-0770-5

21. Forster P, Forster L, Renfrew C, Forster M (2020) Phylogenetic network analysis of SARS-CoV-2 genomes. *Proc. Natl. Acad. Sci USA* 117: 9241-9243. https://doi.org/10.1073/pnas.2004999117

22. Eigen M, Schuster P (1979) *The Hypercycle: A Principle of Natural Self-Organization*. Springer, Berlin.

23. Andino R, Domingo E (2015) Viral quasispecies. *Virology* 479-480: 46-51. [crossref] https://doi.org/10.1016/j.virol.2015.03.022

24. Fukuta M, Mao ZQ, Morita K, Moi ML (2021) Stability and Infectivity of SARS-CoV-2 and viral RNA in Water, Commercial Beverages, and Bodily Fluids. *Front. Microbiol* 12: 667956. [crossref] https://doi.org/10.3389/fmicb.2021.667956

25. KwonT, Gaudreault NN, Richt JA (2021) Seasonal Stability of SARS-CoV-2 in Biological Fluids. *Pathogens* 10: 540. https://doi.org/10.3390/pathogens10050540

26. Althoff KN, Schlueter DJ, Anton-Culver H, Cherry J, Denny JC, et al. (2020) Antibodies to SARS-CoV-2 in *All of Us* Research Program Participants, January 2-March 18, 2020. *Clinical Infectious Diseases*. https://academic.oup.com/cid/advance-article/doi/10.1093/cid/ciab519/6294073

27. Smith WE (2013) 2013; Life is a cosmic phenomenon: the Search for Water evolves into the Search for Life. Hoover RB, Levin GV, Rozanov AY, Wickramasinghe NC (Eds.). Proc. SPIE 8865, Instruments, Methods, and Missions for Astrobiology XVI. San Diego, California, United States. https://doi.org/10.1117/12.2046862.

28. Qu J, Wickramasinghe NC (2020) The world should establish an early warning system for new viral infectious diseases by space-weather monitoring. *MedComm* 1: 423-426. DOI: 10.1002/mco2.20

29. Luskin DL (2020) The failed experiment of COVID-19 lockdowns. *The Wall Street Journal*. Sept 2.

30. Coccia M (2020) Factors determining the diffusion of COVID-19 and suggested strategy to prevent future accelerated viral infectivity similar to COVID. *Science of the Total Environment* 729: 138474. https://doi.org/10.1016/j.scitotenv.2020.138474

31. Martelletti L, Martelletti P (2020) Air Pollution and the Novel Covid-19 Disease: a Putative Disease Risk Factor. *SN Compr. Clin. Med* 2: 383-387. https://doi.org/10.1007/s42399-020-00274-4

Citation:

Steele EJ, Gorczynski RM, Carnegie P, Tokoro G, Wallis DH, et al. (2021) COVID-19 Sudden Outbreak of Mystery Case Transmissions in Victoria, Australia, May-June 2021: Strong Evidence of Tropospheric Transport of Human Passaged Infective Virions from the Indian Epidemic. *Infect Dis Ther* Volume 2(1): 1-28.

Edward J. Steele (2021) COVID-19 Sudden Outbreak of Mystery Case Transmissions in Victoria, Australia, May-June 2021: Strong Evidence of Tropospheric Transport of Human Passaged Infective Virions from the Indian Epidemic

Supplementary Information

COVID-19 sudden outbreak of mystery case transmissions in Victoria Australia, May-June 2021 : Strong evidence of tropospheric transport of human passaged infective virions from the Indian epidemic

Edward J. Steele, Reginald M. Gorczynski, Patrick Carnegie, Gensuke Tokoro, Daryl H. Wallis, Robert Temple, Milton Wainwright and N. Chandra Wickramasinghe

We address here issues as Supplementary Information to assist understanding of the main text. For some computer systems the entire URL link may need to be copied and pasted into Search bar to obtain link.

- A. **Fragility of paradigms- Ptolemaic epicycles just prior to the first Copernican revolution from the 16th Century**
- B. **COVID-19 Cases per Day in Australia (Victoria), India, Sri Lanka, Maldives, Kenya, Madagascar, South Africa, Chile**
- C. **Distribution of Cases and Clusters in Greater Melbourne Victoria from May – June 2021**
- D. **Recent Indian PANGO variants** *NCBI Virus* **Page 2/ 2855 pages- Screen Shots as 6 June 2021**
- E. **Newspaper and Media Reports – all significant relevant coverage**
- F. **Indian 'delta' variant (B.1.617.2) now going global as June 19 2021**

A. Figure shows Ptolemaic epicycles just prior to the first Copernican revolution from the 16th Century

See also Wickramasinghe, Steele, Gorczynski et al (2020) *Virology Current Research*
On the Fragility of Empires and Paradigms Virology Current Research Volume 4:1,2020
DOI: 10.37421/Virol Curr Res.2020.4.112
https://www.hilarispublisher.com/open-access/on-the-fragility-of-empires-and-paradigms.pdf

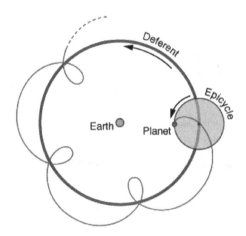

B. COVID-19 Cases per Day in Australia (Victoria), India, Sri Lanka, Maldives, Kenya, Madagascar, South Africa, Chile Google: "Coronavirus disease statistics" URL is
https://www.google.com.au/search?hl=en&ei=vWxyX7ipM4-
m9QP18If4CQ&q=Coronavirus+disease+statistics&oq=Coronavirus+disease+statistics&gs_lcp=CgZwc3ktYWIQAzICCAAyAggA
OgQIABBHOgcIABCxAxBDOgQIABBDULZUWPh1YJF7aABwAXgAgAH2AYgBvA6SAQYwLjEwLjGYAQCgAQGqAQdnd3
Mtd2l6yAEGwAEB&sclient=psy-ab&ved=0ahUKEwj4-47e-4zsAhUPU30KHXX4AZ8Q4dUDCAw&uact=5
 This gives you the "Australia" Victoria dashboard (from there you can choose your country in the menu bar scroll)

Edward J. Steele (2021) COVID-19 Sudden Outbreak of Mystery Case Transmissions in Victoria, Australia, May-June 2021: Strong Evidence of Tropospheric Transport of Human Passaged Infective Virions from the Indian Epidemic

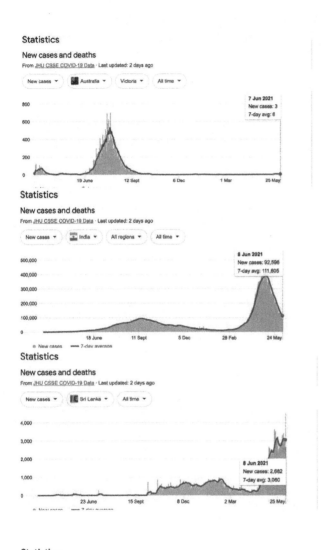

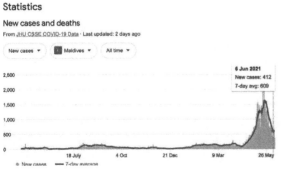

Edward J. Steele (2021) COVID-19 Sudden Outbreak of Mystery Case Transmissions in Victoria, Australia, May-June 2021: Strong Evidence of Tropospheric Transport of Human Passaged Infective Virions from the Indian Epidemic

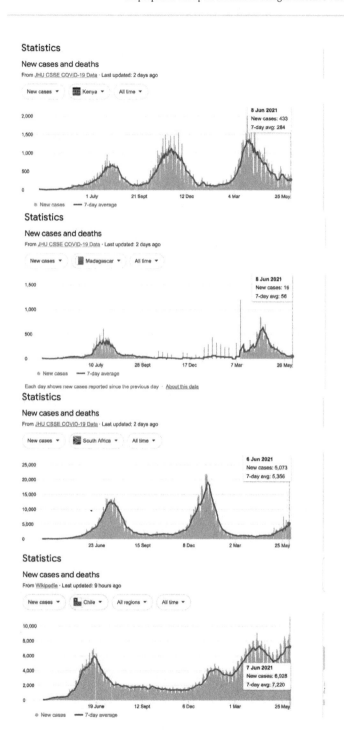

Edward J. Steele (2021) COVID-19 Sudden Outbreak of Mystery Case Transmissions in Victoria, Australia, May-June 2021: Strong Evidence of Tropospheric Transport of Human Passaged Infective Virions from the Indian Epidemic

C. Distribution of Cases and Clusters in Greater Melbourne Victoria from May – June 2021

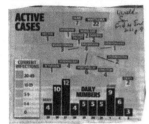

Source : *The Herald-Sun* 4 June 2021

D. Recent Indian PANGO variants *NCBI Virus* Page 2/ 2855 pages- Screen Shots as 6 June 2021

	Accession	Submitters	Release Date	Pangolin	Species	Molecule type	Length	Geo Location
☐	MZ317887	Lemieux,J.,...	2021-06-01	B.1.1.7	Severe acute respiratory s...	ssRNA(+)	29680	USA: Rhode Islan
☐	MZ317890	Sharma,S., ...	2021-06-01	B.1.351	Severe acute respiratory s...	ssRNA(+)	29784	India
☐	MZ317891	Saiyed,Z., e...	2021-06-01	B.1.351	Severe acute respiratory s...	ssRNA(+)	29784	India
☐	MZ317892	Raval,J., et al.	2021-06-01	B.1.351	Severe acute respiratory s...	ssRNA(+)	29784	India
☐	MZ317893	Pandit,R., e...	2021-06-01	B.1.351	Severe acute respiratory s...	ssRNA(+)	29784	India
☐	MZ317894	Savaliya,N.,...	2021-06-01	B.1.36	Severe acute respiratory s...	ssRNA(+)	29802	India
☐	MZ317895	Widera,M.	2021-06-01	B.1.427	Severe acute respiratory s	ssRNA(+)	29782	Germany: Frankf

	Accession	Submitters	Release Date	Pangolin	Species	Molecule type	Length	Geo Location
☐	MZ317896	Widera,M., ...	2021-06-01	B.1.429	Severe acute respiratory s...	ssRNA(+)	29782	Germany: Frankf
☐	MZ317905	Saiyed,Z., e...	2021-06-01	B.1.1.7	Severe acute respiratory s...	ssRNA(+)	29783	India
☐	MZ317906	Soni,T., et al.	2021-06-01	B.1.36.10	Severe acute respiratory s...	ssRNA(+)	29802	India
☐	MZ317907	Sharma,S., ...	2021-06-01	B.1	Severe acute respiratory s...	ssRNA(+)	29802	India
☐	MZ317908	Kumar,D., e...	2021-06-01	B.1.351	Severe acute respiratory s...	ssRNA(+)	29784	India
☐	MZ317915	Pandit,R., e...	2021-06-01	B.1.1.7	Severe acute respiratory s...	ssRNA(+)	29783	India
☐	MZ317916	Raval,J., et al.	2021-06-01	B.1.1.7	Severe acute respiratory s...	ssRNA(+)	29783	India
☐	MZ317917	Kumar,D., e...	2021-06-01	B.1.36	Severe acute respiratory s...	ssRNA(+)	29793	India
☐	MZ317918	Savaliya,N.,...	2021-06-01	B.1.1.7	Severe acute respiratory s...	ssRNA(+)	29783	India
☐	MZ317919	Patel,Z., et al.	2021-06-01	B.1.1.7	Severe acute respiratory s...	ssRNA(+)	29783	India

	Accession	Submitters	Release Date	Pangolin	Species	Molecule type	Length	Geo Location
☐	MZ317919	Patel,Z., et al.	2021-06-01	B.1.1.7	Severe acute respiratory s...	ssRNA(+)	29783	India
☐	MZ317920	Saiyed,Z., e...	2021-06-01	B.1.1.7	Severe acute respiratory s...	ssRNA(+)	29783	India
☐	MZ317921	Sharma,S., ...	2021-06-01	B.1.1.7	Severe acute respiratory s...	ssRNA(+)	29783	India
☐	MZ317922	Soni,T., et al.	2021-06-01	B.1.36	Severe acute respiratory s...	ssRNA(+)	29793	India
☐	MZ318037	Pandit,R., e...	2021-06-01	B.1.1.7	Severe acute respiratory s...	ssRNA(+)	29783	India
☐	MZ318038	Kumar,D., e...	2021-06-01	B.1.1.7	Severe acute respiratory s...	ssRNA(+)	29783	India
☐	MZ318159	Kanani,A., ...	2021-06-01	B.1.617.2	Severe acute respiratory s...	ssRNA(+)	29796	India
☐	MZ318160	Saiyed,Z., e...	2021-06-01	B.1.617.2	Severe acute respiratory s...	ssRNA(+)	29775	India
☐	MZ318161	Kanani,A., ...	2021-06-01	B.1.617.2	Severe acute respiratory s...	ssRNA(+)	29796	India
☐	MZ318201	Patel,Z., et al.	2021-06-01	B.1.617.2	Severe acute respiratory s...	ssRNA(+)	29792	In

4

Edward J. Steele (2021) COVID-19 Sudden Outbreak of Mystery Case Transmissions in Victoria, Australia, May-June 2021: Strong Evidence of Tropospheric Transport of Human Passaged Infective Virions from the Indian Epidemic

	Accession ⇕	Submitters ⇕	Release Date ⇕	Pangolin ⇕	Species ⇕	Molecule type ⇕	Length ⇕	Geo Location ⇕
☐	MZ318161	Kanani,A., …	2021-06-01	B.1.617.2	Severe acute respiratory s…	ssRNA(+)	29796	India
☐	MZ318201	Patel,Z., et al.	2021-06-01	B.1.617.2	Severe acute respiratory s…	ssRNA(+)	29792	India
☐	MZ318202	Raval,J., et al.	2021-06-01	B.1.617.2	Severe acute respiratory s…	ssRNA(+)	29796	India
☐	MZ318243	Pandit,R., e…	2021-06-01	B.1.617.2	Severe acute respiratory s…	ssRNA(+)	29796	India
☐	MZ318244	Savaliya,N.,…	2021-06-01	B.1.617.2	Severe acute respiratory s…	ssRNA(+)	29792	India
☐	MZ318245	Kumar,D., e…	2021-06-01	B.1.617.2	Severe acute respiratory s…	ssRNA(+)	29796	India
☐	MZ318246	Soni,T., et al.	2021-06-01	B.1.617.2	Severe acute respiratory s…	ssRNA(+)	29796	India
☐	MZ318253	Pandit,R., e…	2021-06-01	B.1.617.2	Severe acute respiratory s…	ssRNA(+)	29794	India
☐	MZ318254	Waghela,B.…	2021-06-01	B.1.617.2	Severe acute respiratory s…	ssRNA(+)	29796	India
☐	MZ318255	Waghela,B.…	2021-06-01	B.1.617.2	Severe acute respiratory s…	ssRNA(+)	29796	India

	Accession ⇕	Submitters ⇕	Release Date ⇕	Pangolin ⇕	Species ⇕	Molecule type ⇕	Length ⇕	Geo Location ⇕
☐	MZ318267	Patel,Z., et al.	2021-06-01	B.1.617.2	Severe acute respiratory s…	ssRNA(+)	29796	India
☐	MZ318268	Raval,J., et al.	2021-06-01	B.1.617.2	Severe acute respiratory s…	ssRNA(+)	29802	India
☐	MZ318270	Prajapati,B.…	2021-06-01	B.1.617.2	Severe acute respiratory s…	ssRNA(+)	29797	India
☐	MZ318271	Savaliya,N.,…	2021-06-01	B.1.617.2	Severe acute respiratory s…	ssRNA(+)	29802	India
☐	MZ318277	Prajapati,B.…	2021-06-01	B.1.617.2	Severe acute respiratory s…	ssRNA(+)	29797	India
☐	MZ318279	Purohit,T., …	2021-06-01	B.1.617.2	Severe acu…	ssRNA(+)	29796	India
☐	MZ318282	Purohit,T., …	2021-06-01	B.1.617.2	Severe acute respiratory s…	ssRNA(+)	29796	India
☐	MZ318283	Raval,J., et al.	2021-06-01	B.1.617.2	Severe acute respiratory s…	ssRNA(+)	29802	India
☐	MZ318284	Patel,Z., et al.	2021-06-01	B.1.617.2	Severe acute respiratory s…	ssRNA(+)	29791	India

	Accession ⇕	Submitters ⇕	Release Date ⇕	Pangolin ⇕	Species ⇕	Molecule type ⇕	Length ⇕	Geo Location ⇕
☐	MZ318357	Soni,T., et al.	2021-06-01	B.1.617.2	Severe acute respiratory s…	ssRNA(+)	29796	India
☐	MZ318358	Savaliya,N.,…	2021-06-01	B.1.617.2	Severe acute respiratory s…	ssRNA(+)	29796	India
☐	MZ318359	Kumar,D., e…	2021-06-01	B.1.617.2	Severe acute respiratory s…	ssRNA(+)	29796	India
☐	MZ318364	Goswami,K.…	2021-06-01	B.1.617.2	Severe acute respiratory s…	ssRNA(+)	29792	India
☐	MZ318365	Patel,N., et al.	2021-06-01	B.1.617.2	Severe acute respiratory s…	ssRNA(+)	29797	India
☐	MZ318366	Patel,N., et al.	2021-06-01	B.1.617.2	Severe acute respiratory s…	ssRNA(+)	29797	India
☐	MZ318377	Patel,A., et al.	2021-06-01	B.1.617.2	Severe acute respiratory s…	ssRNA(+)	29796	India
☐	MZ318378	Goswami,K.…	2021-06-01	B.1.617.2	Severe acute respiratory s…	ssRNA(+)	29792	India
☐	MZ318383	Patel,A., et al.	2021-06-01	B.1.617.2	Severe acute respiratory s…	ssRNA(+)	29796	India
☐	MZ318426	Sharma,S., …	2021-06-01	B.1.617.2	Severe acute respiratory s…	ssRNA(+)	29799	India

Edward J. Steele (2021) COVID-19 Sudden Outbreak of Mystery Case Transmissions in Victoria, Australia, May-June 2021: Strong Evidence of Tropospheric Transport of Human Passaged Infective Virions from the Indian Epidemic

PANGO variants in India screen shots *NCBI Virus* page.201of 2855 pages as 7 June 2021

p.201/2855

	Accession ⇕	Submitters ⇕	Release Date ⇕	Pangolin ⇕	Species ⇕	Molecule type ⇕	Length ⇕	Geo Location
☐	MZ310507	Sharma,S., et al.	2021-05-28	B.1	Severe acute respiratory s…	ssRNA(+)	29802	India
☐	MZ310508	Saiyed,Z., et al.	2021-05-28	B.1.1.216	Severe acute respiratory s…	ssRNA(+)	29802	India
☐	MZ310509	Raval,J., et al.	2021-05-28	B.1.36	Severe acute respiratory s…	ssRNA(+)	29802	India
☐	MZ310510	Soni,T., et al.	2021-05-28	B.1.36	Severe acute respiratory s…	ssRNA(+)	29799	India
☐	MZ310511	Sharma,S., et al.	2021-05-28	B.1.36	Severe acute respiratory s…	ssRNA(+)	29799	India
☐	MZ310512	Saiyed,Z., et al.	2021-05-28	B.1.36.8	Severe acute respiratory s…	ssRNA(+)	29802	India
☐	MZ310579	Pandit,R., et al.	2021-05-28	B.1.36.8	Severe acute respiratory s…	ssRNA(+)	29802	India
☐	MZ310580	Raval,J., et al.	2021-05-28	B.1.617.1	Severe acute respiratory s…	ssRNA(+)	29801	India
☐	Accession ⇕	Submitters ⇕	Release Date ⇕	Pangolin ⇕	Species ⇕	Molecule type ⇕	Length ⇕	Geo Location
☐	MZ310587	Kumar,D., et al.	2021-05-28	B.1.617.1	Severe acute respiratory s…	ssRNA(+)	29801	India
☐	MZ310588	Savaliya,N., et al.	2021-05-28	B.1.617.1	Severe acute respiratory s…	ssRNA(+)	29801	India
☐	MZ310589	Patel,Z., et al.	2021-05-28	B.1.367	Severe acute respiratory s…	ssRNA(+)	29801	India
☐	MZ310590	Soni,T., et al.	2021-05-28	B.1.617.1	Severe acute respiratory s…	ssRNA(+)	29801	India
☐	MZ310591	Sharma,S., et al.	2021-05-28	B.1.367	Severe acute respiratory s…	ssRNA(+)	29801	India

	Accession	Submitters	Release Date	Pangolin	Species	Molecule type	Length	Geo Location
	MZ292126	Sharma,S., et al.	2021-05-26	B.1.36	Severe acute respiratory s…	ssRNA(+)	29801	India
	MZ292127	Soni,T., et al.	2021-05-26	B.1.36	Severe acute respiratory s…	ssRNA(+)	29801	India
	MZ292128	Pandit,R., et al.	2021-05-26	B.1.36.8	Severe acute respiratory s…	ssRNA(+)	29801	India
	MZ292129	Raval,J., et al.	2021-05-26	B.1.36.8	Severe acute respiratory s…	ssRNA(+)	29801	India
	MZ292130	Kumar,D., et al.	2021-05-26	B.1.1.216	Severe acute respiratory s…	ssRNA(+)	29801	India
	MZ292131	Soni,T., et al.	2021-05-26	B.1.1.216	Severe acute respiratory s…	ssRNA(+)	29801	India
	MZ292132	Saiyed,Z., et al.	2021-05-26	B.1.36.8	Severe acute respiratory s…	ssRNA(+)	29801	India
	MZ292133	Pandit,R., et al.	2021-05-26	B.1.36.8	Severe acute respiratory s…	ssRNA(+)	29801	India
	MZ292134	Raval,J., et al.	2021-05-26	B.1.36.8	Severe acute respiratory s…	ssRNA(+)	29801	India
	MZ292135	Savaliya,N., et al.	2021-05-26	B.1.36.8	Severe acute respiratory s…	ssRNA(+)	29801	India
	MZ292136	Patel,Z., et al.	2021-05-26	B.1.36.8	Severe acute respiratory s…	ssRNA(+)	29801	India
☐	Accession ⇕	Submitters ⇕	Release Date ⇕	Pangolin ⇕	Species ⇕	Molecule type ⇕	Length ⇕	Geo Location ⇕
☐	MZ292137	Sharma,S., et al.	2021-05-26	B.1.36	Severe acute respiratory s…	ssRNA(+)	29801	India
☐	MZ292138	Soni,T., et al.	2021-05-26	B.1.1.7	Severe acute respiratory s…	ssRNA(+)	29790	India
☐	MZ292145	Saiyed,Z., et al.	2021-05-26	B.1.36	Severe acute respiratory s…	ssRNA(+)	29801	India
☐	MZ292146	Pandit,R., et al.	2021-05-26	B.1.1	Severe acute respiratory s…	ssRNA(+)	29801	India
☐	MZ292147	Patel,Z., et al.	2021-05-26	B.1.1	Severe acute respiratory s…	ssRNA(+)	29801	India
☐	MZ292148	Savaliya,N., et al.	2021-05-26	B.1.1.306	Severe acute respiratory s…	ssRNA(+)	29801	India
☐	MZ292150	Soni,T., et al.	2021-05-26	B.1.36	Severe acute respiratory s…	ssRNA(+)	29801	India
☐	MZ292151	Kumar,D., et al.	2021-05-26	B.1.36	Severe acute respiratory s…	ssRNA(+)	29801	India
☐	MZ292152	Pandit,R., et al.	2021-05-26	B.1.36	Severe acute respiratory s…	ssRNA(+)	29788	India
☐	MZ292153	Saiyed,Z., et al.	2021-05-26	B.1.36	Severe acute respiratory s…	ssRNA(+)	29801	India

6

Edward J. Steele (2021) COVID-19 Sudden Outbreak of Mystery Case Transmissions in Victoria, Australia, May-June 2021: Strong Evidence of Tropospheric Transport of Human Passaged Infective Virions from the Indian Epidemic

	Accession ⇕	Submitters ⇕	Release Date ⇕	Pangolin ⇕	Species ⇕	Molecule type ⇕	Length ⇕	Geo Location ⇕
☐	MZ292154	Sharma,S., et al.	2021-05-26	B.1.36.8	Severe acute respiratory s...	ssRNA(+)	29801	India
☐	MZ292155	Raval,J., et al.	2021-05-26	B.1.36.17	Severe acute respiratory s...	ssRNA(+)	29788	India
☐	MZ292157	Savaliya,N., et al.	2021-05-26	B.1.1	Severe acute respiratory s...	ssRNA(+)	29801	India
☐	MZ292158	Patel,Z., et al.	2021-05-26	B.1.1	Severe acute respiratory s...	ssRNA(+)	29801	India

E. Newspaper and Media Reports – all significant relevant coverage

Use Google Maps if need be to locate the suburbs and regions identified in Melbourne, Victoria , Australia. The main suburbs and areas are Wollert, Whittlesea, Altona North, North Melbourne and Reservoir. Other specific details are in the media reports, although text of key articles is included here.

a. COVID-19 PCR fragments in waste-water catchments during April 2021

• "Two new wastewater COVID-19 viral fragment detections in Daylesford and Benalla " Government advice from early April 2021
https://www.dhhs.vic.gov.au/wastewater-testing-covid-19
Advice:
"Viral fragments of COVID-19 have been detected in wastewater samples recently taken from the inlet to wastewater treatment plants at Daylesford and Benalla.

This follows the detection of viral fragments in Moonee Ponds Main and Ringwood South Branch sewer catchments announced earlier this week.

Given the prolonged period of no community transmission in Victoria and absence of local cases in these areas, these are most likely due to a person or people who are not infectious but are shedding the virus.

Victoria's wastewater testing program is designed to provide early warning of COVID-19, and the possibility that someone is in the early phase of the virus cannot be ruled out.

People who live in or have visited the Daylesford area from 10 to 12 April, or the Benalla area from 10 to 15 April, should monitor for symptoms of COVID-19 and get tested if any develop. "

• *The Australian online* 29.4.21 at 9.45PM by Remy Varga 3 hours ago posted at 6.30 PM

Hundreds told to isolate in Melbourne
Brief:
Hundreds of people in Melbourne's west and northwest have been asked to isolate after "strong" coronavirus fragments were detected in waste water.

A total of 246 people had been contacted as a precaution after a positive case travelled from Western Australia, A Victorian Health Department spokesperson said on Thursday.

"This additional action is being taken due to the strength of the wastewater detection and because a known positive COVID-19 case, from flight QF778, has been in Victoria in the past 14 days," the spokesperson said. "The 246 people who have been contacted today include four primary close contacts of that case and 242 recently returned red and orange zone travel permit holders.

"All of these primary close contacts have recently been tested and have returned negative results. All of the 246 people are being asked to test again out of an abundance of caution."

7

Edward J. Steele (2021) COVID-19 Sudden Outbreak of Mystery Case Transmissions in Victoria, Australia, May-June 2021: Strong Evidence of Tropospheric Transport of Human Passaged Infective Virions from the Indian Epidemic

And it is region wide in arc from West to North and some in east. The official waste water detection methods at: https://www.dhhs.vic.gov.au/wastewater-testing-covid-19

" New Detections:
Northwestern suburbs
April 20-27: Glenroy, Hadfield, Oak Park, Pascoe Vale
April 10-15 and 20-26 (repeat detections): Benalla
Western suburbs
April 20-27: Altona, Altona North, Brooklyn, Newport, South Kingsville, Williamstown, Williamstown North
Northern suburbs
April 20-27: Briar Hill, Bundoora, Diamond Creek, Greensborough, Lower Plenty, Macleod, Mill Park, Montmorency, Plenty, South Morang, St Helena, Viewbank, Watsonia, Watsonia North, Yallambie, Yarrambat
Outer eastern suburbs
April 20-26: Chirnside Park, Coldstream, Kalorama, Lilydale, Montrose, Mooroolbark, Mount Dandenong, Mount Evelyn, Olinda, Yarra Glen, Yering

Active detections
Western suburbs catchment
April 18-26: Persons visiting or residing in Albanvale, Burnside, Burnside Heights, Cairnlea, Caroline Springs, Deer Park, Delahey, Hillside (Melton), Keilor Downs, Kings Park, Plumpton, Ravenhall, Sydenham, Taylors Hill or Taylors Lakes.

Northwestern suburbs catchment
April 18-26: Persons visiting or residing in Avondale Heights, Calder Park, Hillside (Melton), Kealba, Keilor, Keilor Downs, Keilor East, Keilor Lodge, Keilor North, Keilor Park, Sydenham or Taylors Lakes.

Eastern suburbs catchment
April 20-24: Persons visiting or residing in Balwyn, Balwyn North, Blackburn, Blackburn North, Box Hill, Box Hill North, Bulleen, Doncaster, Doncaster East, Donvale, Mitcham, Mont Albert, Mont Albert North, Nunawading or Templestowe Lower.

Outer northern suburbs catchment
April 17-22: Persons visiting or residing in Epping, South Morang or Wollert.

Comment:
Given the wide spread Melbourne and regions "waste water" detections (which would be open to the air, that there have been in-falls with all that pre-winter rain recently early April. Officials are trying to locate source to to infected travellers. But the wide spread nature, the large dilution factors and the "strong positive PCR " detections suggest a region wide in-fall of at least 1000Km^2. But no reported community transmissions or mystery cases at this stage , first is "Wollert Man" on May 11.

• *Herald-Sun* Sunday 6 June 2021 by Laura Placella p.9 " Covid found in suburbs' sewage'.

b. Wollert Man

• In *The Australian* online 25.5.21

Melbourne's May Cluster as 25.5.21

May 4: Man in his 30s returns to his Wollert home, on Melbourne's northern outskirts, having contracted coronavirus in an Adelaide quarantine hotel.

May 6-9: The man is believed to have been infectious during this period, having developed symptoms on May 8, and got tested on May 10. His exposure sites during his infectious period were listed as the Epping

8

Woolworths, a CBD restaurant, Friday night trains between Craigieburn and the city which were packed with footy crowds, an Indian spice shop in Epping, and a warehouse in Altona North.

May 11: The Wollert man's case becomes public. No further cases are identified among his three household contacts and more than 100 other close contacts.

May 21: Victoria's Health Department reveals it incorrectly listed Epping Woolworths as an exposure site for the Wollert man, due to electronic banking records and the supermarket's proximity to the Indian spice shop the man also visited. In fact the man visited Woolworths Epping North. The department also confirms it has detected strong positive results for coronavirus in sewage from the Wollert and Epping areas. All staff at the Epping North Woolworths have since tested negative.

May 24: Four family members spread across three households test positive for coronavirus. All live in the Whittlesea local government area, which takes in Wollert and Epping. Case One of the four is a man in his 30s, with a man and a woman in their 70s and a preschool aged child also infected. A list of exposure sites for the four, for dates spanning May 19 to 23, includes the Epping North Woolworths, a swim school Bundoora, Victoria's third-largest shopping centre Highpoint in the western suburb of Maribyrnong, a stadium in Brunswick, a service station and soccer field in Reservoir, and several other shops and food outlets in Epping and Epping North.

May 25: A fifth case is confirmed in a man in his 60s, who had a business appointment with Case One on May 18. Health authorities say the fifth case developed symptoms earlier than the other four cases, who are believed to have caught the virus via him. Genomic sequencing confirms the five latest cases are closely linked to that of the Wollert man, but no direct links have yet been established.

• How Wollert Man may have caught B.1.617.1 at Adelaide Quarantine hotel

The Australian May 28 2021 9.33AM by Stephen Lunn " The 18-second Adelaide hotel Covid-19 breach that brought misery and despair to seven million Victorians". Full text is

"It was the sliding doors moment that left nearly seven million Victorians facing another soul-crushing lockdown.

Just 18 seconds in duration. On May 3 in the Playford Hotel in Adelaide's CBD, the door to the room of a man known as Case A was opened for a couple of seconds. Just enough time for the 30-something to collect a meal placed outside.

Case A, as SA Health has dubbed him in its investigation into how the virus spread inside the hotel, was near the end of his 14-day quarantine after returning from India. He was tested for Covid-19 on day one, five and 13, returning a negative result each time.

But unfortunately for Case A, and now for Victoria, he was in a room adjacent to Case B.

In what should have been a red flag given previous incidents of hotel quarantine infections, their rooms were at the end of a corridor.

SA Health's report released late Wednesday revealed that twice on May 3 Case A opened his door to collect a meal, but so too did Case B. He hadn't been diagnosed with Covid at the time, only starting to show symptoms

"On one occasion, Case B opened his room door to collect his meal, then 18 seconds later Case A opened his door to collect his meal," the report says. "This was during the time Case B was infectious but prior to staff knowing his positive Covid-19 status. A similar situation was observed again on the same day with a time lapse of less than 12 minutes.

Edward J. Steele (2021) COVID-19 Sudden Outbreak of Mystery Case Transmissions in Victoria, Australia, May-June 2021: Strong Evidence of Tropospheric Transport of Human Passaged Infective Virions from the Indian Epidemic

"Case B opening their door could have resulted in potentially contaminated corridor air either directly exposing Case A or forcing contaminated air into his room, particularly given Case B's room was situated at the end of a corridor and the intervening time period may not have allowed exchange of fresh air to have occurred despite adequate ventilation levels in the corridor."

It was potentially the 18-second window that saw Covid-19 pass from one hotel room to another, then, as we now know from genomic testing, to a northern Melbourne suburb, then across the city into workplaces, nightclubs and football stadiums.

Spreading far and wide

Since then, infected people have spent time in Bendigo and in Cohuna near the NSW border. A netball match in Cohuna against a team from the Riverina in NSW has led to people across the border being urged to get tested. More than 100 people linked to exposure sites who have since returned to South Australia and a number in Western Australia are being urged to isolate and test.

What's it all mean? Small businesses smashed. Again. Melbourne's CBD ghostly quiet. Again. Families denied access to loved ones in hospitals and nursing homes. Again. Parents dealing with children's remote learning. Again. Anxiety and stress. Again.

Part of the anxiety is the unknown. Though Victorian Acting Premier James Merlino and Health Minister Martin Foley say they take some comfort in that the 26 Covid cases identified so far are genomically linked, two concerns stand out.

Filling in the gaps

First is a gap in the chain of transmission. Case A was released from hotel quarantine on May 4 and returned to the north Melbourne suburb of Wollert. He felt unwell and tested for the virus on May 8, receiving confirmation of his positive status on May 11.

While there has been a genomic link established between Case A and the new Covid cases in Melbourne, no direct connection has been identified. Only the most general geographic link — that Case A and the so-called "index case" in the new Melbourne cluster live nearby in the Whittlesea area — has been established.

Second is the pace of the spread. Consider this. The index case, labelled by Victorian health authorities as Case 5 (the fifth positive case identified in this outbreak), is a man in his 60s. He tested positive on Tuesday, but was believed to be infectious since May 15 and had symptoms on May 17.

He had a business meeting with Case 1, a man in his 30s, on May 18. Case 1 tested positive on Monday, as did three of his relatives, including a preschool-aged child.

Four of Case 5's relatives have also tested positive, one of whom works in Stratton Finance, a large financial firm in Port Melbourne. Five work colleagues have tested positive.

It is understood one of those five spent much of last Saturday evening hopping between nightclubs in the Melbourne party zone of Prahran and South Yarra.

Others among the cases identified so far had been to two AFL games. The area of the MCG named as an exposure site following Sunday's Collingwood-Port Adelaide game included the Port cheer squad.

In short, since Case 1 was identified as Covid-positive on Monday, 14,000 primary and secondary contacts have been identified by contact tracers. And more than 150 potential exposure sites, public and private, have been found.

Question of quarantine

10

Edward J. Steele (2021) COVID-19 Sudden Outbreak of Mystery Case Transmissions in Victoria, Australia, May-June 2021: Strong Evidence of Tropospheric Transport of Human Passaged Infective Virions from the Indian Epidemic

Amid the blizzard of numbers is a bleak reminder of Covid's considerable dangers. Of the 26 cases in this cluster, one elderly person is in intensive care. Merlino said the person was "not in a very good way".

Victorians, again the pariahs of the nation, are now wondering if this fourth lockdown could have been avoided.

Certainly the state's chief health officer, Brett Sutton, was blunt when asked on Thursday about the genesis of the outbreak, another case of airborne transmission inside hotel quarantine.

"We have seen it too many times. It happens when doors open in quick succession," he said. "That is something we have tried to mitigate in Victoria as much as possible with filtered air purifiers in corridors. That said, hotels are not the ideal structural environment to keep people (in quarantine)."

c. Whittlesea Cluster

Above timeline and

• *The Australian* online 29.5.21 by Rhiannon Down 6 hours ago 4.35 PM
"Complex web of connections behind Covid outbreak"

d. Arcare Facility Cluster, Maidstone

• Reported on ABC news online
https://www.abc.net.au/news/2021-05-30/victoria-records-five-new-local-covid-cases/100176658

• *The Australian* online May 30 2021 post ed 11.20 PM "Coronavirus: mystery case hits lockdown plan" by Rebecca Urban, Remy Varga, (also reported *Herald-Sun* June 1 2021 p.4-5).

The mystery case of a Melbourne aged care employee who worked for two days while potentially infectious with Covid-19 has emerged as a priority for contact tracers and a risk to Victoria ending its seven-day lockdown.

The healthcare worker, a woman aged in her 50s who tested positive on Saturday, has no known link to other cases in the state's latest outbreak, which has spread to 40 after five new infections emerged on Sunday.

Victoria's Covid-19 response commander Jeroen Weimar said the aged care case was an "extreme concern" due to both the work setting and unknown acquisition source.

Contact tracers were working hard to identify potential exposures within the facility but also the wider community, he said.

"This is the first mystery case we have seen in this particular outbreak," Mr Weimar said.

"I am concerned that at this point in time we don't have an original acquisition source.

"It is our most vulnerable and sensitive setting … and that is why we have put such an important response into this since late last night."

Acting Premier James Merlino described the case as a "very, very serious matter" and declined to be drawn on whether lockdown restrictions would be eased on Friday as initially scheduled.

It was a day-by-day proposition, he warned.

"We are three days into a seven-day lockdown," Mr Merlino said.

Edward J. Steele (2021) COVID-19 Sudden Outbreak of Mystery Case Transmissions in Victoria, Australia, May-June 2021: Strong Evidence of Tropospheric Transport of Human Passaged Infective Virions from the Indian Epidemic

"Today we're talking about a mystery case. Today we're talking about aged care.

"There's a lot of work to do."

Mr Merlino said health officials were working at an "unbelievable rate" and a majority of more than 4000 primary close contacts across all exposure sites had been tested, with about 70 per cent returning negative tests so far.

More than 45,000 Victorians were tested on Saturday. A testing blitz was under way on Sunday at Arcare Aged Care Maidstone, which bills itself as a "five-star" private facility in Melbourne's west, where residents have now been subjected to hard lockdown and confined to their rooms.

Staff were provided with upgraded "tier three" personal protection equipment and additional cleaners were also deployed to the centre, which has recorded seven positive cases throughout the pandemic – all of which were employees – but no deaths

• *The Australian* online by Angelica Snowden 6 June 2021 posted 12.30PM " Two more cases confirmed in Melbourne aged care"

• *The Australian* online May 31 2021 posted 9.52 AM by Rachel Baxendale "Second Melbourne aged care worker test positive"

Brief:

" A second staff member at a second Victorian aged care facility has tested positive for coronavirus.

BlueCross Western Gardens in the western Melbourne suburb of Sunshine have confirmed a staff member tested negative on their last day of work, before returning a positive result on Sunday night.

The news comes after a staff member at the Arcare facility in Maidstone, also in Melbourne's west, tested positive on Saturday, with at least one Arcare resident since infected.

Contact tracers are yet to link the Maidstone case to the Whittlesea cluster of at least 40 coronavirus cases.

At least two other aged care facilities have gone into lockdown after staff worked across multiple centres."

e. Delta Cluster variant, North Melbourne

• *The Australian* online 4 June 2021 at 9.30PM by Rachel Baxendale posted at 8.45 PM "Breakdown cluster sparks hunt for source"

Health authorities in multiple states are checking genomic sequencing data for all known Delta variant cases of coronavirus in Australia, as mystery surrounds the origins of a cluster of seven cases linked to a West Melbourne family who spent six days in NSW.

The revelation that the seven cases are unrelated to Melbourne's other community-acquired cases came amid confusion over the Andrews government's handling of two false positive cases revealed late on Thursday, which contributed to Wednesday's decision to extend Melbourne's lockdown.

Business groups and the state opposition called for the lockdown to end as soon as possible, as Victoria recorded four new cases, all of which were in quarantine and close contacts of existing cases.

Of 67 community-acquired cases diagnosed in Victoria since a man in his 30s caught the virus in an Adelaide quarantine hotel and returned to the outer northern Melbourne suburb of Wollert on May 4, 54 are linked to the

12

Edward J. Steele (2021) COVID-19 Sudden Outbreak of Mystery Case Transmissions in Victoria, Australia, May-June 2021: Strong Evidence of Tropospheric Transport of Human Passaged Infective Virions from the Indian Epidemic

main Whittlesea cluster across Melbourne's northern suburbs and an associated workplace in Port Melbourne, while five are associated with a cluster linked to the Arcare aged-care facility in Maidstone in Melbourne's west.

• *The Australian* online as 4 June 2021 posted 2.39PM PM by Rachel Baxendale "Timeline: what we know about west Melbourne outbreak"

May 19-24:

- Family of four from West Melbourne begin the first day of their holiday, driving from Melbourne to the Green Patch Campground at Booderee National Park near Jervis Bay on the NSW South Coast.
- It's not known where they stopped in Victoria, but their NSW stops include a cafe, craft centre and antique shop in Gundagai and the Shell Coles Express Big Merino service station in Goulburn.
- On Friday May 21 they visited a cafe and bric-a-brac store in Huskisson, and a Coles in Vincentia, and on Sunday May 23 they visited a cafe in Hyams Beach and revisited the Vincentia Coles.
- On Monday May 24 they travelled back to Melbourne, via a bakery and the Big Merino service station in Goulburn, as well as BP truck stops in Glenrowan, Euroa and Wallan in the Victorian side of the border.

May 25:

- Adult male family member develops symptoms.
- He works at GTA Consultants, on Levels 24 & 25 of 55 Collins St in Melbourne on this day.
- Authorities in NSW and Victoria initially consider the man and his family to have likely been infectious from May 23, two days before the onset of symptoms, but extend the period back to May 19 when other family members later test positive.

May 26-31:

- Family members visit a range of sites in Melbourne's CBD and inner north and west while likely infectious, including North Melbourne Primary School, Joeys Scouts Carlton, Flagstaff Gardens, Officeworks QV, Coles Spencer St, male public toilets at 225 Bourke St, and Costco Docklands.

Tuesday, June 1:

- Authorities in NSW and Victoria confirm the adult male family member has tested positive for coronavirus. Initially he is assumed to be part of the wider Melbourne cluster linked to Adelaide hotel quarantine, pending confirmation from genomic sequencing.

Wednesday, June 2:

Three more family members test positive, including an adult female and two children.

Friday, June 4:

- Positive results are received for two adults and a child, understood to be a Grade Five student at North Melbourne Primary School. It's believed the Grade Five caught the virus from a classmate, who is a member of the West Melbourne family.
- An inconclusive result is received for a second child.
- There are now seven confirmed positive cases linked to the West Melbourne cluster.

Edward J. Steele (2021) COVID-19 Sudden Outbreak of Mystery Case Transmissions in Victoria, Australia, May-June 2021: Strong Evidence of Tropospheric Transport of Human Passaged Infective Virions from the Indian Epidemic

- Chief health officer Brett Sutton reveals genomic sequencing has found the family have the Indian B.1.617.2 or Delta strain of the virus, as opposed to the Indian B.1.617.1 Kappa strain found in members of Melbourne's other current clusters.
- While the Delta strain has been detected in hotel quarantine cases up and down Australia's eastern seaboard, none of these cases is a genetic match for the virus found in the West Melbourne family.
- Sutton says it is possible, given the timing of the onset of symptoms, that the family caught the virus in NSW.

• *The Australian* online 5 June 2021 posted 12.40PM by Rhiannon Down "Delta variant cluster now at nine cases"

Victorian testing commander Jeroen Weimar has confirmed that two of today's five new Covid-19 cases are part of a cluster of the Delta variant.

Mr Weimar confirmed the cluster, which was first detected in one family from West Melbourne who spent six days in NSW last month, had grown to nine cases.

"Then of course, our new cluster, the Delta variant cluster that we are most concerned about," he said.

"Nine active cases, that is an increase of two from yesterday.

Mr Weimar said one of the cases was in a child belonging to the second family in the cluster, who have already had one child test positive.

"One of those is a second child of the second family," he said.

"So we have two families of four, both active with Covid, and then one where the primary close contact, a workplace colleague of the first case that was identified a few days ago.

"We have identified some exposure size for that individual."

• *The Australian* online 8 June 2021 by Rachel Baxendale posted 9.30 PM
"Delta dawned from yet another hotel breach"

Link to such a breach is tenuous and unclear see
https://www.abc.net.au/news/2021-06-10/victoria-new-covid-cases-melbourne-lockdown-restrictions/100203632

f. Reservoir Cluster, in northern suburbs

• Outline on ABC news at
https://www.abc.net.au/news/2021-06-10/victoria-new-covid-cases-melbourne-lockdown-restrictions/100203632

• *The Australian* online 10 June 2021 by Rachel Baxendale posted at 6.12PM "Household cluster sounds new alarm"

14

Edward J. Steele (2021) COVID-19 Sudden Outbreak of Mystery Case Transmissions in Victoria, Australia, May-June 2021: Strong Evidence of Tropospheric Transport of Human Passaged Infective Virions from the Indian Epidemic

A new mystery cluster of four cases in a household in Melbourne's north has spooked Victorian health authorities, prompting a backflip on plans to ease rules governing the wearing of masks outdoors.

The about-face came despite an admission from Victoria's Covid logistics chief, Jeroen Weimar, that there has been no evidence of outdoor transmission of the virus this year.

Victoria's health department is also investigating a possible link between a coronavirus-positive couple who left the outer northwestern suburb of Melton on June 1 and travelled through NSW to Queensland, and a shopping centre in Melbourne's outer north visited by nine other cases.

Victoria's latest cases include a man in his 80s, a woman in her 70s, a man in his 50s and a man in his 20s who all live in the same household in Reservoir in Melbourne's northern suburbs.

How they caught the virus remained a mystery on Thursday, with the man in his 80s the first to return a positive test result on Wednesday, followed by the others. Victoria's health department said authorities had also tested "a number of high-risk primary close contacts of the cases outside of the household" and all had returned negative results, although no detail was provided on the nature of the "high-risk".

Exposure sites visited by household members included a shopping centre in Bundoora and a service station in Thomastown on Monday, and a grocery store in Reservoir and Bunnings in Thomastown on Tuesday.

Ahead of an easing of Melbourne's lockdown on Thursday night, Acting Premier James Merlino warned Victoria remained on "high alert" for undetected community transmission.

"I can confirm the easing of restrictions that we announced yesterday will proceed as planned from 11.59pm tonight with one small exception for Melbourne: masks will continue to be required to be worn outdoors in all circumstances," he said.

Mr Weimar was asked if there had been any recent examples of coronavirus being transmitted outdoors in Victoria. "No. We have no evidence that we have seen in this ... outbreak or the most recent ones, of outdoor transmission," he conceded.

Acting deputy chief health officer Allen Cheng said instances of outdoor transmission had been confirmed during Victoria's second wave of coronavirus last year.

"They're not very common but they do occur. When there are active cases in the community, I think it's a small thing to ask for people to continue to wear masks at all times when outside of home," Professor Cheng said.

He said Victoria's public health team estimated "perhaps 5 per cent" of cases in the second wave had been transmitted outdoors "but, again, it can be very difficult to tell".

More than 24 hours after Queensland broke news of a positive test from a traveller from Victoria, and NSW issued a list of sites visited in that state, Victoria was yet to release details of any exposure sites.

The state's health department said a contact tracing interview was ongoing late on Thursday.

The first member of the couple to test positive, a 44-year-old woman, is believed to have been infectious when they left home on June 1 and developed symptoms on June 3.

Contact tracers are investigating a potential link to the Craigieburn Central shopping centre, where one of the couple checked in on May 23, given nine other cases have visited the site during the current outbreak.

Edward J. Steele (2021) COVID-19 Sudden Outbreak of Mystery Case Transmissions in Victoria, Australia, May-June 2021: Strong Evidence of Tropospheric Transport of Human Passaged Infective Virions from the Indian Epidemic

g. Summary of all Mysteries in *The Australian* 13 June 2021

The Australian Online 13.6.21 Rachel Baxendale posted at 4.30PM

The six missing links in Victoria's Covid clusters

There have now been six coronavirus cases among Victoria's two current outbreaks where authorities have been unable to identify a source of infection, including three this week:

1. The first mystery case emerged on May 24. While the initial May 24 case was linked back to at least one prior case, the path of transmission has not been established between what has become known as the Whittlesea cluster and the genomically linked Kappa strain case of a man who returned to the northern suburb of Wollert on May 4 after contracting coronavirus in an Adelaide quarantine hotel. The Port Melbourne cluster is a directly linked offshoot of the Whittlesea cluster, sparked by a close contact who worked at Stratton Finance in Port Melbourne. The Whittlesea cluster and the Port Melbourne cluster each comprise 32 cases, with an overlap of one case which fits into both clusters.

2. The Arcare cluster of 11 cases, the first of which emerged on May 31, is genomically linked to the Kappa strain outbreak. The direct source of acquisition has not been identified.

3. The West Melbourne outbreak of 15 cases are linked to a genomically distinct Delta cluster sparked by a man in his 40s who arrived in Melbourne from Sri Lanka on May 8. The direct link has not been established between the man and the cluster - which comprises two families and their close contacts and first emerged on June 1.

4. Two cases identified on Wednesday and Thursday in a couple from Melton, in Melbourne's outer northwest who tested positive in Queensland. While the cases have been genomically linked to the Kappa outbreak, the direct source has not been identified.

5. Thursday's new case in four members of a Reservoir household in Melbourne's north. While this case has been genomically linked to the Kappa outbreak, the direct source has not been identified. Exposure sites include locations is Reservoir, Thomastown, Epping and Bundoora, all in the northern suburbs.

6. Saturday's single new case in a City of Melbourne resident. Victorian Covid-19 logistics chief Jeroen Weimar said on Sunday authorities were expecting to receive genomic sequencing of the case late on Sunday night or on Monday. The genomic sequencing is expected to confirm whether or not the case is linked to either current Melbourne cluster. "We're seeing a number of close linkages we're exploring between that particular case and other parts of the Kappa outbreak," Mr Weimar said. Exposure sites for the case include locations in Docklands, Southbank, Thornbury, Reservoir and North Geelong.

Note : Through to June 19 2021 number increased a little in each cluster by P-to-P spreads but all clusters were unlinked to each other – missing links not definitively found as documented in this paper.

16

F. Indian 'delta' variant (B.1.617.2) now going global as June 19 2021

As this paper was being submitted it seems that the southern Chinese city of Guangzhou may be engaged in a sudden tropospheric strike of variants from India.

https://www.news.com.au/world/coronavirus/global/china-hit-by-devastating-covid-outbreak-in-the-city-of-guangzhou/news-story/42a8ac41bd27d3a24620e1888671e08e

Further many other Northern Hemisphere countries (Russia, UK, USA) are also reporting the sudden spread of the Indian delta variant on real population wide scale.

https://www.news.com.au/world/coronavirus/global/highly-infectious-delta-variant-quickly-taking-over-the-world/news-story/5325efa0d41c14856a728d92ee597a91

Commentary

An End of the COVID-19 Pandemic in Sight?

Edward J. Steele[1,2,3*], Reginald M. Gorczynski[4], Robyn A. Lindley[5,6], Gensuke Tokoro[7], Daryl H. Wallis[7], Robert Temple[8] and N. Chandra Wickramasinghe[3,7,9,10]

[1]C.Y.O' Connor ERADE Village Foundation, Piara Waters, Perth, WA, Australia
[2]Melville Analytics Pty Ltd, Melbourne, VIC, Australia
[3]Centre for Astrobiology, University of Ruhuna, Matara, Sri Lanka
[4]University Toronto Health Network, Toronto General Hospital, University of Toronto, Toronto, ON, Canada
[5]Department of Clinical Pathology, Faculty of Medicine, Dentistry & Health Sciences, University of Melbourne, Melbourne, VIC, Australia
[6]GMDx Group Ltd, Melbourne, VIC, Australia
[7]Institute for the Study of Panspermia and Astroeconomics, Gifu, Japan
[8]The History of Chinese Science and Culture Foundation, Conway Hall, London, UK
[9]University of Buckingham, Buckingham, UK
[10]National Institute of Fundamental Studies, Kandy, Sri Lanka

Corresponding author: Edward J. Steele, C.Y.O' Connor ERADE Village Foundation, Piara Waters, Perth, WA, Australia; E-mail: e.j.steele@bigpond.com

Received: August 23, 2021; Accepted: August 28, 2021; Published: September 03, 2021

Abstract

We have set out to assess the data on the intensity of the COVID-19 pandemic with a view to making plausible predictions of its decline. A plot of "% COVID-19 Associated Death per Day" versus the timing and extent of the roll out of national vaccination campaigns in Sweden, Denmark, Netherlands, United Kingdom, France, Germany, Italy and USA shows that the decline in the severity of the COVID-19 pandemic was well advanced noticeably before vaccinations began or could have become a significant contributory factor. Israel is an outlier in its manifest decline pattern, yet the data also demonstrate that vaccination has had no discernible impact at all on % Deaths per Day in Israel.

Human societies throughout recorded history have been ravaged by suddenly appearing regional epidemics and in more recent centuries by epidemics that have been observed to spread globally [1,2]. The COVID-19 pandemic caused by coronavirus SARS-CoV-2 has caused serious global health emergencies and associated social and economic destruction on the citizens of many countries on a hitherto unprecedented scale. The disease emerged suddenly in Oct-Nov 2019 in Hubei region of Central China [3].

Pandemics as always emerge without any warning, cause their toll havoc and then predictably subside. They usually last in a severe form no more than a few years – as the data relating to the "Spanish Flu" of 1918-1919 clearly attests. The termination process of pandemics is not clearly understood, but it is generally assumed to be a combination of herd immunity, attenuation of the pathogen (leading to ill-defined mechanisms of endemicity) and its degradation in the physical environment. Thus, there are likely to be a wide range of factors in varying from country to country that contributes to the decline in disease severity and eventual its disappearance. We have attempted in this note to quantitatively measure the progress of the COVID-19 pandemic in a number of Northern Hemisphere countries from available public data from the time of its onset to the present day (August, 2021). We chose "% COVID-19 Associated Death per Day" as an objective end-point of the measure of severity of SARS-Co-V-2 induced disease. Such an index may reasonably allow a comparison across countries over and above country specific variable factors such

as country-and region-specific technical and demographic variations in the application of the diagnostic PCR genomic test as a primary indicator of infection.

We report here a simple observation on the current status of the COVID-19 pandemic (as 15 Aug 2021) that could have a bearing on the timing of the likely end of the pandemic. We chose two straightforward metrics from data that are publicly available at Coronavirus websites (see Source Data URL links below). We selected those countries where much new Cases per Day data are available and where the Vaccination Campaign is ostensibly substantially advanced. The Cases (and Deaths) per Day by Country are at Google: Search "Coronavirus disease statistics". Vaccination Rates by Country are Google Search "COVID-19 vaccination rates by country". We largely chose key time points associated with the clear successive rolling epidemic peaks of new Cases per Day in each country. We then assumed a 14-day lag at that time point before the severe COVID-19 outcome of "Death" as an objective response rate (ORR) metric. These key time-point data were entered into an Excel spread sheet and primary graphic plots were developed for each country, and resulting figure of % Death per day *versus* % Population Vaccinated generated by standard Excel software. These primary plots were then adjusted for scale (mainly on the Y-axis for % Vaccination rate in that country) to allow a visual comparison with the % COVID-19 associated Death rate per Day at that time point.

DOI: 10.31038/IDT.2021222

https://researchopenworld.com/an-end-of-the-covid-19-pandemic-in-sight/

Infect Dis Ther, Volume 2(2): 1–5, 2021

Edward J. Steele (2021) 'An End of the COVID-19 Pandemic in Sight?"

Figure 1: %COVID-19 Deaths per Day versus % Full Vaccination by Country at key times during the epidemic waves.

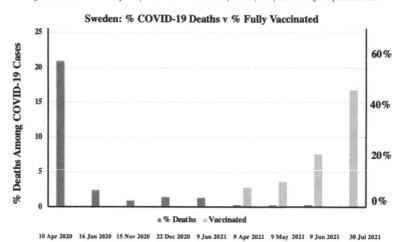

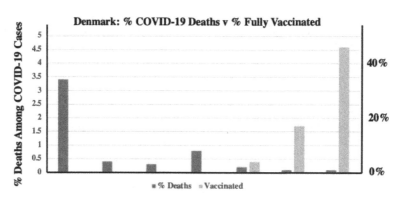

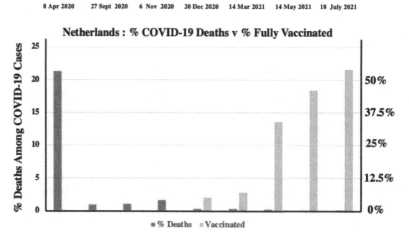

Edward J. Steele (2021) 'An End of the COVID-19 Pandemic in Sight?"

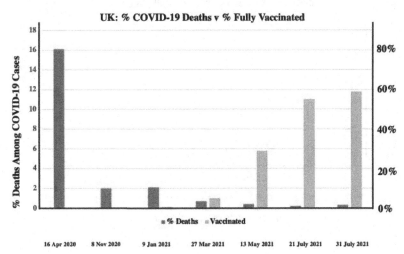

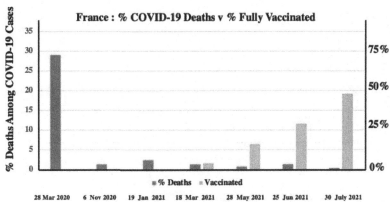

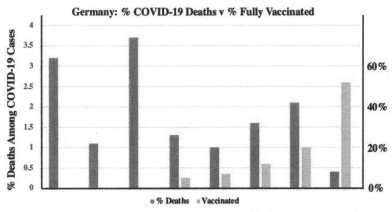

Edward J. Steele (2021) 'An End of the COVID-19 Pandemic in Sight?"

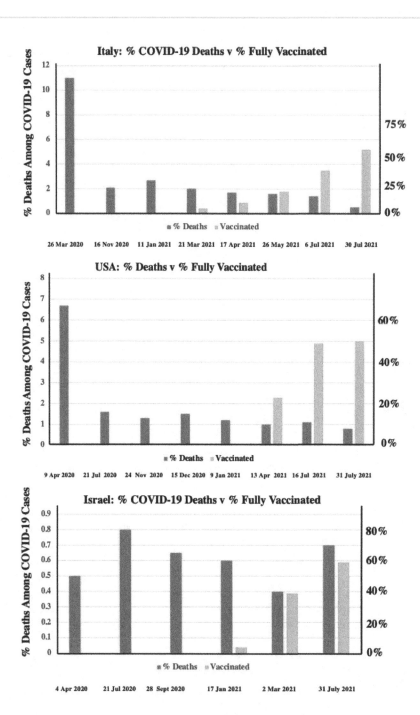

Thus, the reference date along the X-axis in the summary country plots in Figure 1 (above) refers to the time point for new Cases per Day. The reader can draw their own conclusions but a clear trend is evident in all the data – the decline in % COVID-19 associated reported deaths was manifestly well advanced *before* the roll out of the intra-muscular mRNA expression vector vaccine program was begun or had become substantially advanced (e.g. significant in impact, say >20% population vaccinated). The USA is a vast country and its data may need

Edward J. Steele (2021) 'An End of the COVID-19 Pandemic in Sight?"

to be analyzed State-by-State for granular trends in localized regions to become better apparent-like the countries of Europe chosen here. Israel is also a clear outlier in the basic trend - as that country did not suffer the same levels of % COVID-19 associated deaths as the others, even in the first wave in March-April 2020. However, the vaccination program on the basis of this data appears to have had no discernible impact at all on % Deaths in Israel. In many cases the waning of the death rates are seen to have progressed *before* the vaccination rates rose to substantial levels, probably pointing to the development of natural herd immunity as the most reasonable principal cause.

We refrain from further discussion of the many likely factors and variables that would need to be considered in a more exhaustive analysis. To conclude we leave the reader with two crucially important questions that urgently need to be dispassionately addressed. What do these plots mean for possibly heralding the termination of the pandemic? Is the long-awaited end really in sight across the world in mid-August 2021? And does a new world order beckon?

Source Data

COVID-19 Cases per Day, Deaths, Vaccination Rates 15 August 2021

Cases and Deaths per Day site

Google: "**Coronavirus disease statistics**" URL is

https://www.google.com.au/search?hl=en&ei=vWxyX7ipM4-m9QP1 8If4CQ&q=Coronavirus+disease+statistics&oq=Coronavirus+diseas e+statistics&gs_lcp=CgZwc3ktYWIQAzICCAAyAggAOgQIABBHO gcIABCxAxBDOgQIABBDULZUWPh1YJF7aABwAXgAgAH2AYgB vA6SAQYwLjEwLjGYAQCgAQGqAQdnd3Mtd2l6yAEGwAEB&scli ent=psy-ab&ved=0ahUKEwj4-47e-4zsAhUPU30KHXX4AZ8Q4dU DCAw&uact=5

This gives you the "Australia" dashboard (from there you can choose your country in the menu bar scroll)

Vaccination Rates by Country Google " **covid-19 vaccination rates by country**"

https://www.google.com.au/search?q=covid-19+vaccina-tion+rates+by+country&hl=en&source=hp&ei=A80XYfHzKsHY-1sQPlJKyoAY&iflsig=AINFCbYAAAAAYRfbE8FsfFtTOks_fGuW-cDJpb1k5VYyd&oq=COVID-19+vaccination+rates&gs_lcp=Cgd-nd3Mtd2l6EAEYATIFCAAQgAQyBQgAEIAEMgUIABCABDIF-CAAQgAQyBQgAEIAEMgUIABCABDIFCAAQgAQyCAgAEI-AEEMkDMgUIABCABDIFCAAQgAQ6CwgAEIAEELEDEIM-BOggIABCABBCxAzoRCC4QgAQQsQMQgwEQxwEQowI6Dg-guEIAEELEDEMcBEKMCOg4IABCABBCxAxCDARCLAzoOC-C4QgAQQxwEQowIQiwM6CwgAEIAEELEDEIsDOhEILhCABB-CxAxDHARCjAhCLAzoLCAAQsQMQgwEQiwM6DggAEI-AEELEDEIMBEMkDOgUIABCSAzoICAAQgAQQiwM6CA-gAELEDEIMBUJxLWOSJAWDHoQFoAHAAeACAAcUBiAGO-H5IBBDAuMjaYAQCgAQG4AQI&sclient=gws-wiz

This gives you the "Australia" dashboard (from there you can choose your country in the menu bar scroll)

References

1. Creighton C (1891) *History of Epidemics in Great Britain.* Cambridge University Press.

2. Beveridge WIB (1977) *The Last Great Plague.* W. Heinemann, London.

3. Pekar J, Worobey M, Moshiri N, Scheffler K, Wertheim JO (2021) Timing the SARS-CoV-2 index case in Hubei province. *Science* 372: 412-417.

Citation:

Steele EJ, Gorczynski RM, Lindley RA, Tokoro G, Wallis DH, et al. (2021) An End of the COVID-19 Pandemic in Sight? *Infect Dis Ther* Volume 2(2): 1-5.

Review

Nature of Acquired Immune Responses, Epitope Specificity and Resultant Protection from SARS-CoV-2

Reginald M. Gorczynski [1,*], Robyn A. Lindley [2,3], Edward J. Steele [4,5] and Nalin Chandra Wickramasinghe [6,7,8]

1   Institute of Medical Science & Departments of Immunology and Surgery, University of Toronto, Toronto, ON M5S 3G3, Canada
2   Department of Clinical Pathology, Faculty of Medicine, Dentistry & Health Sciences, University of Melbourne, Melbourne, VIC 3000, Australia; robyn.lindley@unimelb.edu.au
3   GMDx Group Ltd., Melbourne, VIC 3000, Australia
4   C.Y.O'Connor ERADE Village Foundation, Piara Waters, Perth, WA 6207, Australia; e.j.steele@bigpond.com
5   Melville Analytics Pty Ltd., Melbourne, VIC 3000, Australia
6   Buckingham Centre for Astrobiology, University of Buckingham, Buckingham MK18 1EG, UK; NCWick@gmail.com
7   Centre for Astrobiology, University of Ruhuna, Matara 81000, Sri Lanka
8   National Institute of Fundamental Studies, Kandy 20000, Sri Lanka
*   Correspondence: reg.gorczynski@utoronto.ca

Abstract: The primary global response to the SARS-CoV-2 pandemic has been to bring to the clinic as rapidly as possible a number of vaccines that are predicted to enhance immunity to this viral infection. While the rapidity with which these vaccines have been developed and tested (at least for short-term efficacy and safety) is commendable, it should be acknowledged that this has occurred despite the lack of research into, and understanding of, the immune elements important for natural host protection against the virus, making this endeavor a somewhat unique one in medical history. In contrast, as pointed out in the review below, there were already important past observations that suggested that respiratory infections at mucosal surfaces were susceptible to immune clearance by mechanisms not typical of infections caused by systemic (blood-borne) pathogens. Accordingly, it was likely to be important to understand the role for both innate and acquired immunity in response to viral infection, as well as the optimum acquired immune resistance mechanisms for viral clearance (B cell or antibody-mediated, versus T cell mediated). This information was needed both to guide vaccine development and to monitor its success. We have known that many pathogens enter into a quasi-symbiotic relationship with the host, with each undergoing sequential change in response to alterations the other makes to its presence. The subsequent evolution of viral variants which has caused such widespread concern over the last 3–6 months as host immunity develops was an entirely predictable response. What is still not known is whether there will be other unexpected side-effects of the deployment of novel vaccines in humans which have yet to be characterized, and, if so, how and if these can be avoided. We conclude by remarking that to ignore a substantial body of well-attested immunological research in favour of expediency is a poor way to proceed.

Keywords: SARS-CoV-2; host resistance; innate immunity; acquired immunity; mucosal immunity; vaccination

Citation: Gorczynski, R.M.; Lindley, R.A.; Steele, E.J.; Wickramasinghe, N.C. Nature of Acquired Immune Responses, Epitope Specificity and Resultant Protection from SARS-CoV-2. *J. Pers. Med.* **2021**, *11*, 1253. https://doi.org/10.3390/jpm11121253

Academic Editor: Roger E. Thomas

Received: 16 October 2021
Accepted: 20 November 2021
Published: 25 November 2021

Publisher's Note: MDPI stays neutral with regard to jurisdictional claims in published maps and institutional affiliations.

1. Introduction

For the past 18 months, the world has been ravaged by a pandemic caused by a coronavirus infection originating in late 2019 in Wuhan, China. By mid-2020 it became apparent that there had arisen global consensus that the way forward from the socioeconomic and medical morass which had occurred was through rapid development and implementation of a universal vaccination program. However, unlike past precedents, this was to take place in the relative absence of detailed knowledge and investigation into the nature of natural host resistance to the pathogen concerned, and by "speed-tracking" novel vaccine

HTML Version: https://www.mdpi.com/2075-4426/11/12/1253/htm
PDF Version: https://www.mdpi.com/2075-4426/11/12/1253/pdf

J. Pers. Med. **2021**, *11*, 1253

designs to clinical use, again in the absence of detailed knowledge of possible short-term and longer-term implications of this vaccine's administration. In a recent review the (then) current status of understanding of immunity to SARS-CoV-2, and how this might affect future approaches to protective vaccination, was discussed [1]. The concern was raised in that review that far too little effort had been focused on understanding the nature of the immune response which might provide optimal immune protection. What follows is an analysis of those advances that have taken place to improve that understanding, and how and if this has affected, and may further affect, the global response to the SARS-CoV-2 pandemic.

Mammalian immunity has both an innate and adaptive arm. Protection mediated by innate immunity, the sole immune mechanism for 95% of the species on earth, develops quickly (1–2 days), with some evidence also implying an immune memory, "training", affording an enhanced protection from reinfection (with the same pathogen) and even enhanced immunity to novel pathogens [2]. This novel idea suggests a much closer parallel with adaptive immunity that has been long thought to be the only immune system to show memory.

Figure 1 shows the causal links between deaminase mutagenic activity, SARs-Cov-2 infection, the role of interferon stimulated gene (ISG) pathways, the host innate and adaptive immune response, and the subsequent possible accumulation of collateral cell damage. Innate immunity involving the deaminases is designed to inhibit pathogens through multiple, mostly non-genetic, pathways. Genetic targeting of the SARs-Cov-2 RNA genome by deaminases, namely innate immunity-induced mutagenesis of the pathogen genome cripples its replicative efficacy. The deaminases are the main ISG induced proteins that attack the DNA or RNA of invading viruses by extensively mutating their genomes with C-to-U (T) and A-to-I(G) mutations [3,4]. The deaminases APOBEC3B and APOBEC3G, in particular, have been studied for two decades, and they are now colloquially known as 'virus smashers' due to their well characterised mechanism of actions that impact viral potency and function [4]. This is the first line of innate immune defence that acts to suppress or eliminate the SARS-CoV-2 virus. During ISG induced attacks on foreign pathogens by deaminases, some *de novo* mutations that remain uncorrected may also accumulate in the DNA of transcribed non-Ig genes, and possibly lead to further cell damage in infected tissue [5].

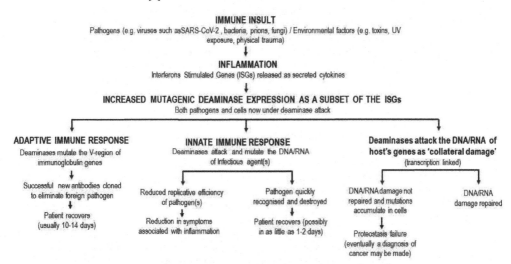

Figure 1. Model linking downstream innate and adaptive immune changes following pathogen insult.

The mechanism(s) involved in training innate immunity likely involve epigenetic changes (altered DNA methylation; histone deacetylase activity) which results in more

J. Pers. Med. **2021**, *11*, 1253

rapid activation of the genes implicated in response to pathogens [6]. Epigenetic chemical alterations on sections of the gene make up a part, or all, of the genetic regions that can potentially be targets for deamination during transcription. Conversely, it makes sense that those regions that are chemically protected from deamination are conserved where DNA fidelity needs to be maintained for survival and the proper functioning of an organism. In a landmark study by Guo et al. [7], it was found that the TET1 gene and the oncogenic adenosine deaminase APOBEC1 are actively involved in region-specific neuronal activity-induced DNA methylation changes [7,8]. This concept of training of innate immune responses may in part help explain why infant mortality, and even adult mortality, is less in Bacillus Calmette-Guerin (BCG) vaccinated cohorts (BCG admixed with adjuvants is an excellent inducer of innate immune responses) than in non-vaccinated cohorts from the same population [9]. BCG-mediated training of innate immunity in vaccine development is the founding principle behind the ACTIVATE trial in elderly volunteers to assess the contribution of BCG vaccine in decreasing susceptibility to bacterial disease [10,11] and, more recently, SARS-CoV-2 infection [12].

Defects in innate immunity, as well as acquired immunity, are particularly evident in the elderly [13–18]. Innate immunity acts rapidly to control viral replication in infected healthy subjects [19], through type I and type III interferon inducible anti-viral immunity [20]. Elderly patients lacking this rapid innate response are at very high risk for severe outcomes following SARS-CoV-2 infection, including increased morbidity and mortality [21]. Type1 and III interferon inducible genes include APOBEC and ADAR induced expression, which as described in Figure 1 and elsewhere can, in turn, play a role in "haplotype switching" of SARS-CoV-2-expressed genes, leading in turn to the diversification of the virus genetic pattern seen in some subjects, but notably not in those with impaired innate immunity (see below and [22]).

Adaptive (acquired) T and B lymphocyte mediated immunity, while certainly primarily responsible for immunologic memory, takes some 10–14 days post pathogen exposure to become active, but in general shows much greater diversity for pathogen recognition than does innate immunity. Given the experience in understanding how acquired immune mechanisms can be brought to play to enhance pathogen resistance by deliberate vaccination, and the numerous successes evident in global disease control reported as a result, it is not surprising that over the last 12–18 months effort has been directed to making this the key strategy employed against the current pandemic. The discussion below reviews what we have learned about the importance of antibody (B cell mediated) and T effector immunity in providing protection following natural infection, or following vaccination, and how the pathogen has, in turn, responded to naturally acquired or vaccine-induced heightened host resistance. In addition, a brief synopsis of some unexpected adverse effects already noted with vaccines currently "in play", and how this might affect the future direction of vaccinology will be mentioned.

1.1. Heterogeneity in SARS-CoV-2 Antibody Responses and SARS-CoV-2 Protection

Entry of virus into the cells of infected individuals was shown early on to depend on the receptor-binding domain (RBD) of the spike (S) protein of SARS-CoV-2 [23]. Accordingly, much of the research on naturally infected and even vaccinated individuals has focused attention on the epitopes (different unique antigenic configurations) of the RBD recognized by antibodies [24] (and see below, T cells [25]). Even though viral neutralizing titers were low following natural infection and convalescence, a commonality was seen amongst recovered individuals for Ig responses to various RBD domains in the S protein [23]. It is important to note that an independent analysis of naturally infected COVID subjects reported only a very weak correlation between antibody titers and neutralizing activity in sera using commercial clinical laboratory assays [26]. This is perhaps not surprising given an independent study looking at the various B cell subsets giving rise to antigen specific Ig responses following SARS-CoV-2 infection [27]. This group reported that B cells could be segregated into discrete functional subsets specific for the spike (S), nucleocapsid

J. Pers. Med. **2021**, *11*, 1253

protein (NP), and open reading frame (ORF) proteins (nomenclature accorded, 7a and 8), but only S-specific B cells were enriched in memory B cell clusters, with monoclonal antibodies (mAbs) from these cells being potently neutralizing. In contrast, B cells specific to ORF8 and NP were enriched in naïve and innate-like clusters, and mAbs against these targets were non-neutralizing. Again, studying serum Ig binding across platforms of viral antigens and antibodies with 15 positive and 30 negative SARS-CoV-2 controls followed by viral neutralization assessment S-IgG3 was reported to provide the highest accuracy for predicting serologically positive individuals with virus neutralization activity [28].

The sophistication of dissecting Ig response to the RBD to assess efficacy in protection is highlighted by more recent analysis of epitope binding. Thirty-eight RBD-binding neutralizing Abs with known structures, mostly isolated from virus-infected patients, were grouped into five general clusters, which were, in turn, able to document distinct non-neutralizing faces on the RBD. A maximum of up to 4 of these neutralizing Abs could bind to the RBD simultaneously, with significant implications for vaccine design [29,30]. These clinical analyses highlighting the importance of responses to the RBD in S protein in protection are in turn supported by independent data from animal model studies. Passive transfer of potent neutralizing antibodies (nAbs) to two epitopes on the receptor binding domain RBD of S protein provided protection against disease, as monitored by the maintenance of body weight and low lung viral titers following high-dose SARS-CoV-2 challenge in Syrian hamsters [31]. In addition, mice immunized with a recombinant vaccinia virus expressing a modified SARS-CoV-2-S protein (which was recognized on virally infected cells by anti-RBD Ig and soluble human ACE2 receptor) produced neutralizing Ig which passively protected humanACE2 transgenic mice from lethal SARS-CoV-2 infection [32]. Transgenic mice immunized with vaccinia vector before SARS-CoV-2 infection had no morbidity and weight loss upon intranasal infection with SARS-CoV-2 either 3 wk or 7 weeks later. In addition, there was no detectable infectious SARS-CoV-2 or subgenomic viral mRNAs in the lungs. Further, a greatly reduced induction of cytokine and chemokine mRNAs was reported, with scant levels of virus found in the nasal turbinates of 1/8 rMVA-vaccinated mice on day 2 (and none later) [32].

Despite these data, it should be acknowledged that clinical manifestations of SARS-CoV-2 infection are not the same in children, and nor is the immune response engendered following infection. Children are largely spared from severe respiratory disease but may develop a multisystem inflammatory syndrome similar to Kawasaki's disease [33]. SARS-CoV-2-specific Igs were less diverse and specific in children compared with adults, with both children and adults producing IgG, IgM and IgA Abs specific for S protein but only adults making significant responses to nucleocapsid (N) protein [33]. Children produced markedly lower neutralizing activity compared to SARS-CoV-2 infected adult cohorts [33]. There is no data yet available on the relative responses of the two cohorts to vaccination.

1.2. The Role of Mucosal Immunity in Protection against SARS-CoV-2

It has been known for many years, that the best form of protective immunity for pathogens invading by the nasal or oral route are local secretory IgA responses [34]. Recent analyses on SARS-CoV-2 reinfections and transmissions in vaccinated individuals [35,36] and studies assessing immunization against influenza and SARS-CoV-2 are consistent with this concept [37,38]. Froberg et al. reported that mucosal IgA responses were detected in naturally infected cases in the absence of serum antibody responses, and in this scenario, mucosal antibody levels correlated strongly with virus neutralization. Given the current focus on SARS-CoV-2 vaccination as the primary path forward to resolve the clinical sequelae of the current pandemic, it is concerning that there has been so little attention paid to vaccine-induced mucosal immunity. This may in part at least help explain observations reported in the 20 April 2021 update report from the US Centers for Disease Control on vaccine efficacy [39] which suggested little vaccine protection from infection, though a clear moderation of disease severity in infected vaccinated individuals. An important dichotomy between systemic and mucosal immunity following SARS-CoV-2 infection

J. Pers. Med. **2021**, *11*, 1253

has been reported by Smithy et al. [40] with important ramifications for treatment, and interpretation of pathology. Independent recent studies by Lopez et al. [41], and Cheemarla et al. [42] show that that the supply of antiviral interferon enables epithelial cells of the nasopharyngeal mucosa to inhibit SARS-CoV-2 growth, with interferon-induced mucosal genes thus serving as biomarkers of infection (see above and below in sections on innate immunity).

A separate study measured humoral responses to SARS-CoV-2, including analysis of the presence of specific neutralizing antibodies in the serum, saliva, and bronchoalveolar fluid of 159 patients following natural infection with SARS-CoV-2. Again, early viral specific humoral responses were dominated by IgA antibodies with peaks during the third week post-infection, with IgA contributing to virus neutralization to a greater extent than IgG or IgM antibodies. While anti-viral IgA serum concentrations decreased after 1 month neutralizing IgA remained detectable in saliva for up to 10 weeks [43]. The same conclusion was reached independently by Butler et al. [44] who acknowledged that while serum neutralization and effector functions correlated with systemic SARS-CoV-2-specific IgG response magnitude, mucosal neutralization was associated with nasal SARS-CoV-2-IgA, along with less severe disease. A recent study has examined the nature of mucosal immunity induced by two independent mRNA vaccines in the USA, BNT162b2 from Pfizer/BioNTech and mRNA-1273 from Moderna [45]. Both vaccines induce antibodies to SARS-CoV-2 S-protein, including neutralizing antibodies (nAbs) to the RBD, with marked increased titers observed following a second dose of vaccine. Again, antibodies to the S-protein and the RBD were reported in saliva samples from mRNA-vaccinated healthcare workers, with 100% of subjects given either vaccine showing IgG in the saliva, and >50% with IgA.

Limited research studies have been reported on vaccine induced mucosal immunity in animals. A chimpanzee adenovirus-vectored vaccine encoding a prefusion stabilized spike protein (ChAd-SARS-CoV-2-S) was studied following intramuscular (im) injection for protection against SARS-CoV-2 infection in mice expressing the human angiotensin-converting enzyme 2 receptor [46]. A single dose induced systemic humoral and cell-mediated immune responses and protected mice against lung infection, inflammation, and pathology, without inducing sterilizing immunity, as confirmed by viral RNA detection after SARS-CoV-2 challenge. In contrast, a single intranasal dose of the same vaccine induced high levels of neutralizing antibodies, enhanced both systemic and mucosal IgA and T cell responses, and prevented SARS-CoV-2 infection in both the upper and lower respiratory tracts [46]. In a study in macaques, a comparison was made between animals receiving both intramuscularly priming and boosting with vaccine and those receiving intramuscularly priming but intranasal boosting with a vaccine. The vaccine used was an adjuvant vaccine with SARS-CoV-2 S protein. While the im only vaccine induced both binding and neutralizing antibody with persistent cellular immunity systemically and mucosal, using a strategy of intranasal boosting resulted in weaker T cell and IgG responses but higher dimeric IgA and IFNα. Following SARS-CoV-2 challenge both groups of animals had no detectable subgenomic RNA in either the upper or lower respiratory tracts compared with naive controls, again supporting the validity of a mucosal immunization strategy [47].

Further insight into the importance of mucosal immunity (and its induction) in effective immunity to SARS-CoV-2 infection comes from studies with children. Unlike other respiratory viruses where disease manifestations are often more severe in children, infection of children with SARS-CoV-2 generally follows a more benign course. Pierce et al. [48] found that SARS-CoV-2 copy numbers, ACE 2, and TMPRSS2 gene expression were similar in children and adults, but infected children had increased expression of molecules indicative of innate immune pathway stimulation (expression of genes associated with IFN signaling, NLRP3 inflammasome, and other innate pathways). Higher levels of IFN-α2, IFN-γ, IP-10, IL-8, and IL-1β proteins were detected in the nasal fluid of children compared with adults, with similar levels of SARS-CoV-2 specific IgA and IgG in

J. Pers. Med. **2021**, *11*, 1253

nasal fluid of both groups. All children had a far more benign course following infection than the adult cohort. Given the importance of secretory dimeric IgA (sIgA) in protecting mucosal surfaces from pathogens, and evidence (see above) implying the importance of mucosal sIgA in immunity to SARS-CoV-2, of further interest is a report by Quinti et al. on the increased susceptibility and more fulminant course of disease in subjects lacking (genetically) in SARS-CoV-2-specific IgA and secretory IgA [49]. As they note, unlike other primary antibody deficiency entities, selective IgA deficiency is often a "silent" unrecognized condition but may be an (unexplored) important cause of variability in response to SARS-CoV-2 infection. Confirmation of increased susceptibility to SARS-CoV-2 in IgA deficiency has also been reported by Colkesen and colleagues [50].

1.3. T Cell Immunity to SARS-CoV-2

It has been known for some time that activated T lymphocytes are crucial for protective immunity to viral infections. This is consistent with what we understand about the quite different antigen recognition by B versus T cells. The latter recognize cell surface MHC-presented epitopes altered following viral infection and thus can act to destroy potential "viral factories" before living viral replication is completed within the infected cell. While monitoring of (serum) Ig may make for easier assessment of the development of an immune response to a pathogen, it may, as inferred above, provide little information about the development of protective immunity in the infected host. The issue is further discussed in some detail in a recent review [51]. Antibody response correlates poorly with disease particularly in mild infections, with a more robust response generally reflective of more severe clinical disease. In contrast, virus-reactive T-cell immunity lasts longer, and natural SARS-CoV-2 infection induces broad epitope coverage, by both CD4 and CD8 T cells. There is less restriction to S protein immunity than for Ig responses, though any correlation with disease outcome remains to be determined. Correlation of clinical outcomes with laboratory markers of cell-mediated immunity, not only with antibody response, may shed further light on how to optimize induction of protective immunity after both natural infection and vaccination. A preliminary report of just such an investigation was recently published [52] for subjects aged 18–55 years, up to 8 weeks after vaccination with a single dose of ChAdOx1 nCoV-19. CD4 T cell responses were characterized by interferon-γ and tumor necrosis factor-α cytokine secretion, with predominantly IgG1 and IgG3 antibodies. Some CD8$^+$ T cells were also induced of monofunctional, polyfunctional and cytotoxic phenotypes, with, to date, little documented clinical significance. A more exhaustive study of CD8 T cell immunity following natural infection was also reported recently [53]. A highly heterogeneous response was seen across numerous CD8+ epitopes and across multiple (6) HLAs, with up to 52 unique epitopes recorded, against both structural and non-structural targets in the SARS-CoV-2 proteome, though again any correlation with the outcome has yet to be made [53].

Some attempt to gain more insight into the mechanism(s) of T cell resistance comes from animal studies by Zhuang and co-workers [54]. Their data indicate that the type I interferon pathway was critical for generating optimal antiviral T cell responses after SARS-CoV-2 infection of mice, and that T cell vaccination alone could even provide partial protection from severe disease in infected animals.

2. How Does the Clinical Efficacy of SARS-CoV-2 Vaccines Align with Induction of Immunity?

2.1. Innate Immunity

In the introduction [2–12] mention was made of the potential, largely unexplored, role of innate immunity in SARS-CoV-2 infection. Innate immunity is triggered by a family of so-called pattern recognition receptors, and is known to induce interferons and multiple cytokines, activating cells of both the myeloid and lymphoid differentiation pathway for protection against pathogens [2]. Live-attenuated vaccines for tuberculosis, measles, and polio have all been shown to "train" the innate immune system, through histone

J. Pers. Med. **2021**, *11*, 1253

modifications and epigenetic reprogramming of monocytes to develop an inflammatory phenotype, thus enhancing broad resistance to other infectious diseases, of which SARS-CoV-2 infection may be an example [55,56].

A recent study comparing innate immune response to Influenza and SARS-CoV-2 in nasal washes from infected adults suggested an important difference in innate immunity following SARS-CoV-2 infection [57], with decreased IFN-associated transcripts in neutrophils, macrophages and epithelial cells compared with influenza-infected individuals, and decreased epithelial cell-cell interactions. GWAS studies have also implied an important link between the IFN pathway and disease severity [58]. In an important new publication, Inanova et al. [59] compared various immune parameters in subjects post natural infection or SARS-CoV-2 vaccination (SARS-CoV-2 BNT162b2 mRNA). Both infection and vaccination induced innate and adaptive immune responses, but only in SARS-CoV-2 infected patients, and not vaccinated individuals, was this characterized by augmented interferon responses. This was in turn correlated with the upregulation of cytotoxic genes in the peripheral T cells and innate-like lymphocytes in the same cohort. In addition, as assessed by B and T cell receptor repertoires, in SARS-CoV-2 infected patients most clonal B and T cells in infected patients were effector cells, while in vaccinated subjects the expanded cells were primarily circulating memory cells. Further complicating attempts to understand immune protection following deliberate vaccination are data that we have summarized elsewhere suggesting natural herd immunity was already developing on population scales across Europe before the vaccine rollout had really begun [60]. A recent publication suggests another promising approach to elevate broad spectrum intra-nasal anti-viral Innate Immunity in the upper respiratory tract, using local delivery of an engineered defective viral genome which ultimately leads to enhanced both local and distal type I interferon responses [61].

2.2. B Cell Immunity following Vaccination

Studies in a naturally infected cohort of individuals who had recovered from mild SARS-CoV-2 infection showed evidence for SARS-CoV-2 specific IgG, neutralizing antibodies, and memory B and memory T cells persisting beyond months [62]. Memory T cells secreted cytokines and expanded upon antigen re-encounter, and memory B cells expressed receptors capable of neutralizing virus when expressed as monoclonal antibodies. Similarly, Dan et al. reported memory cell survival beyond 8 months in both B and T cells following infection [63], though it seemed B cell memory responses were more persistent than T cell immunity, although the clinical significance of this was not addressed. This observation on long-term persistence of neutralizing IgG following natural infection is consistent with studies from a German cohort assessed up to 9 months post-infection [64] and other studies showing persistent viral neutralizing antibody correlated with outcome [65], and even that viral rebound after early clearance is associated with lower induction and lower levels of RBD-specific IgA and IgG antibodies [66].

How does the development of a protective Ig response compare after natural infection versus vaccination? In particular, what implications are there for vaccine induced immunity to infection, given the (relatively) rapid antigenic drift in SARS-CoV-2 reported over the last 8 months [67]. Mutations on the S protein, in particular, can, in theory, affect binding to either (or both) of the cell receptor ACEII or antibody binding. A shared mutation that increases binding to ACEII, and transmissibility is present in the variants B.1.1.7, (UK) P.1, (Brazil); and B.1.351, (South Africa). The B.1.351 and P.1 variants also display another mutation which decreases binding of neutralizing antibodies, leading to (partial) immune escape and favoring reinfections [67]. The contribution of a background of increased immunity (in the "at risk" population) to the emergence of new mutations remains to be explored. A recent analysis of publicly available genomic sequence and epidemiological data during the 2nd Wave in Victoria, Australia discusses the likelihood of rapid amplification of SARS-CoV-2 in the face of a failed innate immune response (as in the elderly co-morbid patients). Thus these publicly available data already suggest

J. Pers. Med. **2021**, *11*, 1253

that capricious expansion of a common genomic sequence is favored with limited further putative deaminase-mediated mutation at APOBEC and ADAR-deaminase motifs (C-sites, A-sites) in the SARS-CoV-2 genomes isolated from such patients [68].

Analysis of antibody and memory B cell responses of a cohort of 20 volunteers given either of two mRNA vaccines against SARS-CoV-2 showed the plasma neutralizing activity and relative numbers of RBD-specific memory B cells was similar in vaccinated and naturally infected cohorts. However, activity against SARS-CoV-2 variants was reduced significantly [69]. A similar reduction, albeit small, in neutralizing activity against the B.1.1.7 SARS-CoV-2 and in binding to the RBD motif was reported by Collier et al. [70] after vaccination with a mRNA-based vaccine, with more substantial loss of neutralizing activity following introduction of a second variant in the B.1.1.7 background, which they hypothesize may represent a threat to the efficacy of this vaccine. Similar concerns are raised by reports from other groups [71,72]. ACEII binding and neutralizing Ab, isolated following natural infection with a number of different SARS-CoV-2 variants, also highlighted preservation of RBD binding to some more conserved sites.

A more comprehensive summary using 506,768 SARS-CoV-2 genome isolates, including mutations of the S-RBD from patients, was reported to explore the efficacy of immunity to the growing list of SARS-CoV-2 variants, also concluded that most variants were associated with increased binding to ACEII, and thus likely greater infectiousness. Many new RBD mutants were characterized which could affect neutralizing Ig binding to the RBD, including mutations now described in the California variant B.1.427, and the Mexico variant B.1.1.222, which markedly enhances the infectivity of the latter. The authors conclude that "the genetic evolution of SARS-CoV-2 on the RBD, which may be regulated by host gene editing, viral proofreading, random genetic drift, and natural selection, (can) give rise to more infectious variants that will potentially compromise existing vaccines and antibody therapies" [73,74]. A similar concern was raised by Venkatakrishnan et al. [75]. Despite this gloomy forecast, however, there is clear evidence that the current vaccines in use have led to a clinically significant protective response to infection in those at risk [76,77], as was emphasized in a recent report exploring hospitalization post-vaccination [78].

2.3. T Cell Immunity following Vaccination

As mentioned previously, it seems self-evident that a systematic analysis of T cell epitopes recognized by subjects following natural infection, correlated with disease outcome, is essential to guide interpretation of monitoring patient responses, and to develop vaccines that might prove efficacious in protection. A USA government-led clinical trial [79] was designed with just this in mind in 2020 (now in data analysis phase, but yet to report). Blood samples from SARS-CoV-2 infected patients who have recovered from the infection were screened using a genome-wide, high-throughput screening technology [80], with the hope that identification of T cell receptors and immunogenic viral epitopes on SARS-CoV-2 which may contribute to development of long-lasting protection against SARS- CoV-2 will be achieved. Preliminary reports from other groups, using a more restricted research design, already hold out hope that these studies will have some utility. Thus a longitudinal analysis (up to 6 months post-infection) revealed decreasing S and nucleocapsid-specific antibody responses while in contrast functional T cell responses remained persisted and even increased, over the same period, with many dominant T cell epitopes identified [81]. A more recent genome-wide screen approach was used to explore CD8 immunity in convalescent SARS-CoV-2 individuals [82]. From a pool of ~3140 MHC Class I-binding peptides covering the complete SARS-CoV-2 genome over 120 immunogenic peptides were identified, with a subset of these found to represent immunodominant SARS-CoV-2 T cell epitopes. A pre-existing T cell recognition signature was seen in naïve individuals, possibly reflecting exposure to previous coronavirus infections. More importantly, a robust T cell activation profile could be characterized in previously infected patients, which was most marked in those with severe disease, and there was a minimal response seen in those with mild disease or in naïve (uninfected) individuals [82].

J. Pers. Med. **2021**, *11*, 1253

Further studies have attempted to explore the nature of recognition of viral variants in vaccinated/infected versus naïve subjects, in order to compare the data with that observed from comparison of Ig responses in similar groups (see above). Subjects receiving either Pfizer-BioNTech (BNT162b2) or Moderna (mRNA-1273) mRNA-based SARS-CoV-2 vaccine were characterized, and found to show broad T cell responses to the SARS-CoV-2-S protein, with only 4/23 targeted peptides potentially affected by mutations in the UK (B.1.1.7) and South African (B.1.351) variants. CD4+ T cells from vaccine recipients recognized the 2 variant spike proteins as effectively as they recognized the ancestral virus S-protein from the ancestral virus, in contrast to antibody data discussed above. Interestingly, a 3-fold increase in the CD4+ T cell responses to influenza S-peptides was seen after vaccination, implying a cross-protection (following SARS-CoV-2 vaccination) against some endemic coronaviruses [83]. Others have also reported that SARS-CoV-2-specific T cells from vaccinated individuals recognize variant SARS- CoV-2 isolates and that that vaccinated convalescents have more persistent nasopharynx-homing SARS- CoV-2- specific T cells compared to infection-naïve counterparts [84]. However, mention should be made of a conflicting report by Gallagher et al. [85] which used standard functional assays to assess T-cell immunity to SARS- CoV-2 in uninfected, convalescent, and vaccinated individuals. While vaccinated individuals showed stronger T-cell responses to the wild-type spike and nucleocapsid proteins, compared with convalescent patients, quite diminished T-cell responses to spike variants (B.1.1.7, B.1.351, and B.1.1.248) were observed in vaccinated but otherwise healthy donors, in parallel to the Ig data discussed before. Other than differences in the assays used, acknowledging again an absence of any correlation with clinical utility, there is no obvious explanation for the discrepancies with the studies reported in [85] vs. [81–84].

The importance of understanding T cell immunity to SARS-CoV-2 is confirmed by a recent report investigating the logistics of using in vitro expanded SARS-CoV-2 immune T cells in adoptive immunotherapy in immunocompromised subjects [86]. This group expanded SARS- CoV-2 specific T cells from convalescent donors using GMP facilities and combinations of membrane, spike, and nucleocapsid peptides. All induced IFN-γ production, in 27 (59%), 12 (26%), and 10 (22%) respectively in convalescent donors, and in 2 of 15 unexposed controls. Polyfunctional CD4-restricted T-cell epitopes were identified within a conserved region of membrane protein, which induced polyfunctional T-cell responses. The authors suggest these may have utility in the development of both effective vaccine and T-cell therapies for use in immunocompromised patients with blood disorders or following bone marrow transplantation. An exhaustive review of current candidate vaccines in phase 3 trial has recently been published [87].

3. Unexpected Adverse Effects of SARS-CoV-2 Vaccination

It seems apropos to conclude the present discussion with some thoughts on adverse effects noted from SARS-CoV-2 vaccination. Heralding the rapid and novel introduction of mRNA vaccines into the clinical armamentarium, a new formulation of synthetic mRNA strands encoding the SARS-CoV-2-S glycoprotein, packaged in lipid nanoparticles to deliver mRNA to cells, Verbeke et al. suggest we stand on the threshold of a "new dawn" in vaccinology [88]. However, as they acknowledge, there are still huge gaps in our understanding. Already data from the two widely used mRNA vaccines BNT162b2 and mRNA-1273, suggest that the nucleoside-modified mRNA approach allows for delivery of higher maximal tolerable doses and might thus in part explain why these, rather than the adenovirus encoded S-protein in a more conventional vaccine, allows for more rapid generation of antibody responses [88]. It remains unexplained why the two similar (nucleoside-modified) mRNA vaccines elicited quite different S-specific CD8+ T cell responses. There are a number of plausible hypotheses, including, but not limited to, possible differences in innate responses to the two candidates; and the mRNA sequence design (e.g., UTR inclusion, codon optimizations) which might have contributed to the potency and reactogenicity (minor adverse effects) of the vaccines. It is beyond doubt, that more in-depth knowledge on the in vivo delivery efficiency and the particular innate immune

J. Pers. Med. **2021**, 11, 1253

effects of the different mRNA vaccines will contribute to the design of even safer and more effective mRNA vaccines in the future.

The need to address these issues is highlighted by the recent CDC briefing, held with the plan to alleviate many concerns within the public over what may be (in the longer-scheme of things) minor issues [89]. As a brief summary they emphasize:

A. Although still not fully understood, even the most effective of vaccines does not prevent illness 100% of the time-vaccine breakthrough occurs, though generally with less disease severity.

B. Since it takes some 10–14 days post-vaccination to develop immunity, if an individual was infected shortly before/after vaccination, it is predicted they may still become infected. In addition (see above) infection may occur with a variant for which the current vaccines are not providing effective immunization for.

C. While to date no unusual patterns have been detected in the data of people infected post-vaccination, CDC has an ongoing goal to identify any unusual patterns, such as trends in age or sex, the vaccines involved, underlying health conditions, and whether particular SARS-CoV-2 variants are causing sickness.

D. There is abundant data now to suggest that vaccines help protect people who are vaccinated from getting COVID-19 or from getting severely ill from SARS-CoV-2. Nevertheless, because people can still get sick and possibly spread the virus to others after being fully vaccinated, the current recommendation remains that people continue to take simple public health measures to protect themselves and others-see also [90]. Indeed, the efficacy of vaccination for protection against documented infection re-mains a controversial issue [91].

Others have focused attention on clearly documented adverse effects from SARS-CoV-2 vaccines already in use. First and foremost, amongst these is vaccine-induced immune thrombotic thrombocytopenia (VITT) in the aftermath of vaccination with the adenoviral vector SARS-CoV-2 vaccine ChAdOx1 nCoV-19 [92]. Rare patients (less than 1 in 100,000) develop thrombosis and thrombocytopenia 5–24 days after vaccination, often with thromboses at unusual sites (cerebral venous sinus; portal, hepatic and splanchnic veins), test strongly positive in PF4/polyanion enzyme immunoassays (EIAs), and show serum-induced platelet activation which is maximal in the presence of PF4. It is not clear what components of the vaccine are responsible for the enhanced response to an unrelated host protein (PF4), and why it occurs only after exposure to the adenovirus vector. It may be that PF4 is a bystander component within an immune complex that activates platelets. Thiele et al. assessed the frequency of anti-PF4/polyanion antibodies in healthy vaccinees and assessed whether PF4/polyanion EIA-positive sera exhibited platelet-activating properties after vaccination with ~140 each of ChAdOx1 nCoV-19 or BNT162b2 (BioNTech/Pfizer) vaccines [93]. Although 19 of 281 participants tested positive for anti-PF4/polyanion antibodies post-vaccination (All: 6.8% [95%CI, 4.4–10.3]; BNT162b2: 5.6% [95%CI, 2.9–10.7]; ChAdOx1 nCoV-19: 8.0% [95%CI, 4.5–13.7%]), none of the PF4/polyanion EIA-positive samples induced platelet activation in the presence of PF4. They concluded that positive PF4/polyanion EIAs could occur after SARS-CoV-2 vaccination with both mRNA- and adenoviral vector-based vaccines, but the majority of these antibodies likely had minor (if any) clinical relevance. The pathogenic platelet-activating antibodies causing VITT did not occur commonly after vaccination.

Additional groups have focused on the theoretical risk associated with the current vaccines, arguing that their "rush into service" has ignored potential concerns with their use, particularly the concern regarding induction of autoimmune reactivity [94]. As an example, the failure of SARS vaccines in animal trials involved pathogenesis consistent with an immunological priming that could involve autoimmunity in lung tissues due to previous exposure to the SARS spike protein [95]. A comparison of immunogenic epitopes in SARS-CoV-2-S proteins, and other SARS-CoV-2 proteins with human protein to search for homologous matching. The author concluded that only one immunogenic epitope in SARS-CoV-2 had no homology to human proteins, and that many of the overlaps with

J. Pers. Med. **2021**, *11*, 1253

human proteins could theoretically help explain some of the symptoms associated with the pathogenesis of SARS-CoV-2. In a similar vein, Lu et al. asked whether the rapid move to market the current SARS-CoV-2 vaccines might leave us at risk of causing neurologic disorders like those previously recognized, including vaccine-related demyelinating diseases, fever-induced seizure, and other deficits [96]. Others have focused on the issue of myocarditis following SARS-CoV-2 infection and/or vaccination [97], and other more subtle autoimmune type responses following SARS-CoV-2 infection [98]. It is self-evident, by comparison with past experience, that only time will tell how significant a problem this represents.

4. Concluding Remarks

In conclusion, we recall that pandemics of the type we have experienced over the past 18 months are far from new. Similar pandemics have punctuated human history over many millennia, often contributing to episodes of severe attenuation of populations, and in some instances leading even to the collapse of empires. In the past, however, the societal role for coping with such pandemics has been limited-confined in the main to alleviating suffering that resulted from the disease, and perhaps enabling the segregation of infective victims wherever possible. There was obviously no possibility at this stage of any globally coordinated response, nor of any large-scale intervention, to minimize transmission and thus accelerate the end of a pandemic. The advantage we possess now is scientific knowledge of the type we have discussed in this paper. If such knowledge is utilized honestly and dispassionately, a new utopia beckons; otherwise, we may be no better off now than in earlier epochs, and by some reckoning perhaps even worse.

All pandemics are of course self-limiting, eventually ending through the development of herd immunity to the infective agent. The global response to the current pandemic, involving severe and often punitive limitations of individual freedom is clearly unprecedented in history. The justification for such draconian measures is based on the assertion that scientific advances have made available a shortcut to the natural process of immunity that would greatly reduce the total number of infections, and the number of deaths. We show in this review that some aspects of the scientific arguments being currently deployed are either deficient or seriously flawed.

5. Summary

There is hope that we are now approaching an entrenchment phase in our response to the SARS-CoV-2 pandemic, with more widespread uptake of vaccines, protection of vulnerable population cohorts (especially the elderly), and adherence to better public health measures continuing to improve the overall outlook. At all levels, politically, sociologically, ethically, scientifically and medically, there have been instances of major mismanagement and misunderstanding, coupled with gross errors of judgement, which have clearly cost lives. As reviewed above, it can be argued that we still have failed to recognize the importance of implementation of basic science knowledge, both new research and understanding old observations, which even now would likely improve the future course of the disease. We need to remain vigilant in the face of having implemented so many previously untried and untested therapies for the appearance of new signs and symptoms in treated patients which are early indications of adverse events, for which VITT may be merely the tip of a large iceberg. As the philosopher, George Santayana once said "Those who cannot remember the past are condemned to repeat it". We need to make sure that the valuable lessons learned, at all levels, over the last 18 months are not forgotten.

Author Contributions: All authors contributed to the preparation of the manuscript, and have approved the final article submission. All authors have read and agreed to the published version of the manuscript.

Funding: This research did not receive any specific grant from funding agencies in the public, commercial, or not-for-profit sectors.

J. Pers. Med. **2021**, *11*, 1253

Acknowledgments: The authors thank Andrew Hapel and Pat Carnegie for many helpful discussions.

Conflicts of Interest: The authors declare no conflict of interest.

References

1. Gorczynski, R.M. Personalizing Vaccination for Infectious Disease in the 21st Century. *J. Vaccines Vaccin.* **2020**, *S5*, 5.
2. Netea, M.G. Training innate immunity: The changing concept of immunological memory in innate host defence. *Eur. J. Clin. Investig.* **2013**, *43*, 881–884. [CrossRef] [PubMed]
3. Samuel, C.E. Adenosine deaminases acting on RNA (ADARs) are both antiviral and proviral. *Virology* **2011**, *411*, 180–193. [CrossRef] [PubMed]
4. Vartanian, J.-P.; Henry, M.; Marchio, A.; Suspène, R.; Aynaud, M.-M.; Guétard, D.; Cervantes-Gonzalez, M.; Battiston, C.; Mazzaferro, V.M.; Pineau, P.; et al. Massive APOBEC3 Editing of Hepatitis B Viral DNA in Cirrhosis. *PLoS Pathog.* **2010**, *6*, e1000928. [CrossRef]
5. Lindley, R.A. A Review of the mutational role of deaminases and the generation of a cognate molecular model to explain cancer mutation spectra. *Med. Res. Arch.* **2020**, *8*, 8. [CrossRef]
6. Arts, R.J.W.; Moorlag, S.J.C.F.M.; Novakovic, B.; Li, Y.; Wang, S.Y.; Oosting, M.; Kumar, V.; Xavier, R.J.; Wijmenga, C.; Joosten, L.A.B.; et al. BCG vaccination protects against experimental vi-ral infection in humans through the induction of cytokines associated with trained immunity. *Cell Host Microbe* **2018**, *23*, 89–100. [CrossRef]
7. Guo, J.U.; Su, Y.; Zhong, C.; Ming, G.-L.; Song, H. Hydroxylation of 5-Methylcytosine by TET1 Promotes Active DNA Demethyla-tion in the Adult Brain. *Cell* **2011**, *145*, 423–434. [CrossRef]
8. Scourzic, L.; Mouly, E.; Bernard, O.A. TET proteins and the control of cytosine demethylation in cancer. *Genome Med.* **2015**, *7*, 9. [CrossRef]
9. Rieckmann, A.; Villumsen, M.; Sørup, S.; Haugaard, L.K.; Ravn, H.; Roth, A.; Baker, J.L.; Benn, C.S.; Aaby, P. Vaccinations against smallpox and tuberculosis are associated with better long-term survival: A Danish case-cohort study 1971–2010. *Int. J. Epidemiol.* **2016**, *46*, 695–705. [CrossRef]
10. Covián, C.; Fernández-Fierro, A.; Retamal-Díaz, A.; Díaz, F.E.; Vasquez, A.; Lay, M.K.; Riedel, C.; Gonzalez, P.A.; Bueno, S.M.; Kalergis, A.M. BCG-Induced Cross-Protection and Development of Trained Immunity: Implication for Vaccine Design. *Front. Immunol.* **2019**, *10*, 2806. [CrossRef]
11. Bacillus Calmette-guérin Vaccination to Prevent Infections of the Elderly (ACTIVATE). Available online: https://clinicaltrials.gov/ct2/show/NCT03296423 (accessed on 16 October 2021).
12. BCG Vaccine for Health Care Workers as Defense Against COVID 19 (BADAS). Available online: https://clinicaltrials.gov/ct2/show/NCT04348370 (accessed on 16 October 2021).
13. Acharya, D.; Liu, G.-Q.; Gack, M.U. Dysregulation of type I interferon responses in SARS-CoV-2. *Nat. Rev. Immunol.* **2020**, *20*, 397–398. [CrossRef] [PubMed]
14. Blanco-Melo, D.; Nilsson-Payant, B.E.; Liu, W.-C.; Uhl, S.; Hoagland, D.; Møller, R.; Jordan, T.X.; Oishi, K.; Panis, M.; Sachs, D.; et al. Imbalanced Host Response to SARS-CoV-2 Drives Development of COVID-19. *Cell* **2020**, *181*, 1036–1045.e9. [CrossRef]
15. Hadjadj, J.; Yatim, N.; Barnabei, L.; Corneau, A.; Boussier, J.; Smith, N.; Péré, H.; Charbit, B.; Bondet, V.; Chenevier-Gobeaux, C.; et al. Impaired type I interferon activity and exacerbated inflammatory responses in severe Covid-19 patients. *Science* **2020**, *369*, 718–724. [CrossRef]
16. Netea, M.G.; Giamarellos-Bourboulis, E.J.; Domınguez-Andrés, J.; Curtis, N.; van Crevel, R.; van de Veerdonk, F.L.; Bonten, M. Trained Immunity: A tool for reducing susceptibility to and the severity of SARS-CoV-2 infection. *Cell* **2020**, *181*, 969–977. [CrossRef]
17. Zhang, Q.; Bastard, P.; Liu, Z.; Le Pen, J.; Moncada-Velez, M.; Chen, J.; Ogishi, M.; Sabli, I.K.D.; Hodeib, S.; Korol, C.; et al. Inborn errors of type I IFN immunity in patients with life-threatening SARS-CoV-2. *Science* **2020**, *370*. [CrossRef]
18. Moderbacher, C.R.; Ramirez, S.I.; Dan, J.M.; Dan, J.M.; Grifoni, A.; Hastie, K.M.; Weiskopf, D.; Belanger, S.; Abbott, R.K.; Kim, C.; et al. Antigen-Specific Adaptive Immunity to SARS-CoV-2 in Acute COVID-19 and Asso-ciations with Age and Disease Severity. *Cell* **2020**, *183*, 996–1012. [CrossRef] [PubMed]
19. Sette, A.; Crotty, S. Adaptive immunity to SARS-CoV-2. *Cell* **2012**, *184*, 1–20.
20. Lucas, C.; Wong, P.; Klein, J.; Castro, T.B.R.; Silva, J.; Sundaram, M.; Ellingson, M.K.; Mao, T.; Oh, J.E.; Israelow, B.; et al. Longitudinal analyses reveal immunological misfiring in severe SARS-CoV-2. *Nature* **2020**, *584*, 463–469. [CrossRef]
21. Hansen, C.H.; Michlmayr, D.; Gubbels, S.M.; Mølbak, K.; Ethelberg, S. Assessment of protection against reinfection with SARS-CoV-2 among 4 million PCR-tested individuals in Denmark in 2020: A population-level observational study. *Lancet* **2021**, *397*, 1204–1212. [CrossRef]
22. Steele, E.J.; Lindley, R.A. Analysis of APOBEC and ADAR deaminase-driven Riboswitch Haplotypes in SARS-CoV-2 RNA strain variants and the implications for vaccine design. *Res. Rep.* **2020**, *4*, e1–e146. Available online: https://companyofscientists.com/index.php/rr (accessed on 16 October 2021).
23. Tan, C.W.; Chia, W.N.; Qin, X.; Liu, P.; Chen, M.I.; Tiu, C.; Hu, Z.; Chen, V.C.W.; Young, B.E.; Sia, W.R.; et al. A SARS-CoV-2 surrogate virus neutralization test based on an-ti-body-mediated blockage of ACE2-spike protein-protein interaction. *Nat. Biotechnol.* **2020**, *38*, 1073–1078. [CrossRef]

J. Pers. Med. **2021**, *11*, 1253   13 of 16

24. Robbiani, D.F.; Gaebler, C.; Muecksch, F.; Lorenzi, J.C.C.; Wang, Z.; Cho, A.; Agudelo, M.; Barnes, C.O.; Gazumyan, A.; Finkin, S.; et al. Convergent antibody responses to SARS-CoV-2 in con-valescent individuals. *Nature* **2020**, *584*, 437–442. [CrossRef]
25. Arashkia, A.; Jalilvand, S.; Mohajel, N.; Afchangi, A.; Azadmanesh, K.; Salehi-Vaziri, M.; Fazlalipour, M.; Pouriayevali, M.H.; Jalali, T.; Nasab, S.D.M.; et al. Severe acute respiratory syndrome-coronavirus-2 spike (S) protein based vaccine candidates: State of the art and future prospects. *Rev. Med. Virol.* **2020**, *31*, e2183. [CrossRef]
26. Criscuolo, E.; Diotti, R.A.; Strollo, M.; Rolla, S.; Ambrosi, A.; Locatelli, M.; Burioni, R.; Mancini, N.; Clementi, M.; Clementi, N. Weak correlation between antibody titers and neu-tralizing activity in sera from SARS-CoV-2 infected subjects. *J. Med. Virol.* **2021**, *93*, 2160–2167. [CrossRef] [PubMed]
27. Wilson, P.; Stamper, C.; Dugan, H.; Li, L.; Asby, N.; Halfmann, P.; Zheng, N.-Y.; Huang, M.; Stovicek, O.; Wang, J.; et al. Distinct B cell subsets give rise to antigen-specific antibody responses against SARS-CoV-2. *Res. Sq.* **2020**. preprint. [CrossRef]
28. Rathe, J.A.; Hemann, E.A.; Eggenberger, J.; Li, Z.; Knoll, M.L.; Stokes, C.; Hsiang, T.-Y.; Netland, J.; Takehara, K.K.; Pepper, M.; et al. SARS-CoV-2 Serologic Assays in Control and Un-known Populations Demonstrate the Necessity of Virus Neutralization Testing. *J. Infect. Dis.* **2021**, *223*, 1120–1131. [CrossRef] [PubMed]
29. Niu, L.; Wittrock, K.N.; Clabaugh, G.C.; Srivastava, V.; Cho, M.W. A Structural Landscape of Neutralizing Antibodies Against SARS-CoV-2 Receptor Binding Domain. *Front. Immunol.* **2021**, *12*, 647934. [CrossRef]
30. Fu, D.; Zhang, G.; Wang, Y.; Zhang, Z.; Hu, H.; Shen, S.; Wu, J.; Li, B.; Li, X.; Fang, Y.; et al. Structural basis for SARS-CoV-2 neutralizing antibodies with novel binding epitopes. *PLoS Biol.* **2021**, *19*, e3001209. [CrossRef] [PubMed]
31. Rogers, T.F.; Zhao, F.; Huang, D.; Beutler, N.; Burns, A.; He, W.T.; Limbo, O.; Smith, C.; Song, G.; Woehl, J.; et al. Isolation of potent SARS-CoV-2 neutralizing antibodies and pro-tection from disease in a small animal model. *Science* **2020**, *369*, 956–963. [CrossRef]
32. Liu, R.; Americo, J.L.; Cotter, C.A.; Earl, P.L.; Erez, N.; Peng, C.; Moss, B. One or two injections of MVA-vectored vaccine shields hACE2 transgenic mice from SARS-CoV-2 upper and lower respiratory tract infection. *Proc. Natl. Acad. Sci. USA* **2021**, *118*, e2026785118. [CrossRef] [PubMed]
33. Weisberg, S.P.; Connors, T.; Zhu, Y.; Baldwin, M.; Lin, W.H.; Wontakal, S.; Szabo, P.A.; Wells, S.B.; Dogra, P.; Gray, J.I.; et al. Antibody responses to SARS-CoV2 are distinct in chil-dren with MIS-C compared to adults with SARS-CoV-2. Version 1. *medRxiv* **2020**, 20151068. [CrossRef]
34. Wilkie, B.N. Respiratory tract immune response to microbial pathogens. *J. Am. Vet. Med. Assoc.* **1982**, *181*, 1074–1079. [PubMed]
35. Schiavone, M.; Gasperetti, A.; Mitacchione, G.; Viecca, M.; Forleo, G.B. Response to: COVID-19 re-infection. Vaccinated individuals as a potential source of transmission. *Eur. J. Clin. Investig.* **2021**, *51*, e13544. [CrossRef]
36. Bleier, B.S.; Ramanathan, M.; Lane, A.P. COVID-19 Vaccines May Not Prevent Nasal SARS-CoV-2 Infection and Asymptomatic Transmission. *Otolaryngol. Head Neck Surg.* **2021**, *164*, 305–307. [CrossRef] [PubMed]
37. Matsuda, K.; Migueles, S.A.; Huang, J.; Bolkhovitinov, L.; Stuccio, S.; Griesman, T.; Pullano, A.A.; Kang, B.H.; Ishida, E.; Zimmerman, M.; et al. A replication-competent adenovirus-vectored influenza vaccine induces durable systemic and mucosal immunity. *J. Clin. Investig.* **2021**, *131*. [CrossRef]
38. Fröberg, J.; Diavatopoulos, D.A. Mucosal immunity to severe acute respiratory syndrome coronavirus 2 infection. *Curr. Opin. Infect. Dis.* **2021**, *34*, 181–186. [CrossRef]
39. CDC Update: Science Brief: Background Rationale and Evidence for Public Health Recommendations for Fully Vaccinated Peo-ple Centers for Disease Control and Prevention, SARS-CoV-2 2021. Updated 2 April 2021. Available online: https://www.cdc.gov/coronavirus/2019-ncov/science/science-briefs/fully-vaccinatedpeople.html (accessed on 16 October 2021).
40. Smith, N.; Goncalves, P.; Charbit, B.; Grzelak, L.; Beretta, M.; Planchais, C.; Bruel, T.; Rouilly, V.; Bondet, V.; Hadjadj, J.; et al. Distinct systemic and mucosal immune responses during acute SARS-CoV-2 infection. *Nat. Immunol.* **2021**, *22*, 1428–1439. [CrossRef]
41. Lopez, J.; Mommert, M.; Mouton, W.; Pizzorno, A.; Brengel-Pesce, K.; Mezidi, M.; Villard, M.; Lina, B.; Richard, J.-C.; Fassier, J.-B.; et al. Early nasal type I IFN immunity against SARS-CoV-2 is compromised in patients with autoantibodies against type I IFNs. *J. Exp. Med.* **2021**, *218*. [CrossRef]
42. Cheemarla, N.R.; Watkins, T.A.; Mihaylova, V.T.; Wang, B.; Zhao, D.; Wang, G.; Landry, M.L.; Foxman, E.F. Dynamic innate immune response determines susceptibility to SARS-CoV-2 infection and early replication kinetics. *J. Exp. Med.* **2021**, *218*, e20211211. [CrossRef]
43. Sterlin, D.; Mathian, A.; Miyara, M.; Mohr, A.; Anna, F.; Claër, L.; Quentric, P.; Fadlallah, J.; Devilliers, H.; Ghillani, P.; et al. IgA dominates the early neutralizing antibody response to SARS-CoV-2. *Sci. Transl. Med.* **2021**, *13*. [CrossRef] [PubMed]
44. Butler, S.E.; Crowley, A.R.; Natarajan, H.; Xu, S.; Weiner, J.A.; Bobak, C.A.; Mattox, D.E.; Lee, J.; Wieland-Alter, W.; Connor, R.I.; et al. Distinct Features and Functions of Systemic and Mucosal Humoral Immunity Among SARS-CoV-2 Convalescent Individuals. *Front. Immunol.* **2021**, *11*, 618685. [CrossRef] [PubMed]
45. Ketas, T.J.; Chaturbhuj, D.; Cruz-Portillo, V.M.; Francomano, E.; Golden, E.; Chandrasekhar, S.; Debnath, G.; Diaz-Tapia, R.; Yasmeen, A.; Leconet, W.; et al. Antibody responses to SARS-CoV-2 mRNA vaccines are detectable in saliva. *bioRxiv* **2021**, *11*, 434841. [CrossRef] [PubMed]
46. Hassan, A.O.; Kafai, N.M.; Dmitriev, I.P.; Fox, J.M.; Smith, B.K.; Harvey, I.B.; Chen, R.E.; Winkler, E.S.; Wessel, A.W.; Case, J.B.; et al. A Single-Dose Intranasal ChAd Vaccine Protects Upper and Lower Respiratory Tracts against SARS-CoV-2. *Cell* **2020**, *183*, 169–184. [CrossRef] [PubMed]

J. Pers. Med. **2021**, *11*, 1253

47. Sui, Y.; Li, J.; Zhang, R.; Prabhu, S.K.; Andersen, H.; Venzon, D.; Cook, A.; Brown, R.; Teow, E.; Velasco, J.; et al. Protection against SARS-CoV-2 infection by a mucosal vaccine in rhesus macaques. *JCI Insight* **2021**, *6*. [CrossRef]
48. Pierce, C.A.; Sy, S.; Galen, B.; Goldstein, D.Y.; Orner, E.; Keller, M.J.; Herold, K.C.; Herold, B.C. Natural mucosal barriers and COVID-19 in children. *JCI Insight* **2021**, *6*. [CrossRef]
49. Quinti, I.; Mortari, E.P.; Salinas, A.F.; Milito, C.; Carsetti, R. IgA Antibodies and IgA Deficiency in SARS-CoV-2 Infection. *Front. Cell. Infect. Microbiol.* **2021**, *11*, 655896. [CrossRef]
50. Çölkesen, F.; Kandemir, B.; Arslan, Ş.; Çölkesen, F.; Yıldız, E.; Korkmaz, C.; Vatansev, H.; Evcen, R.; Aykan, F.S.; Kılınç, M.; et al. Relationship between selective IgA deficiency and COVID-19 prognosis. *Jpn. J. Infect. Dis.* **2021**. [CrossRef]
51. Hellerstein, M. What are the roles of antibodies versus a durable, high quality T-cell response in protective immunity against SARS-CoV-2? *Vaccine X* **2020**, *6*, 100076. [CrossRef]
52. Ewer, K.J.; Barrett, J.R.; Belij-Rammerstorfer, S.; Sharpe, H.; Makinson, R.; Morter, R.; Morter, R.; Flaxman, A.; Wright, D.; Bellamy, D.; et al. T cell and antibody responses induced by a single dose of ChAdOx1 nCoV-19 (AZD1222) vaccine in a phase 1/2 clinical trial. *Nat. Med.* **2021**, *27*, 270–278. [CrossRef]
53. Kared, H.; Redd, A.D.; Bloch, E.M.; Bonny, T.S.; Sumatoh, H.R.; Kairi, F.; Carbajo, D.; Abel, B.; Newell, E.W.; Bettinotti, M.P.; et al. SARS-CoV-2–specific CD8+ T cell responses in convalescent COVID-19 individuals. *J. Clin. Investig.* **2021**, *131*. [CrossRef]
54. Zhuang, Z.; Lai, X.; Sun, J.; Chen, Z.; Zhang, Z.; Dai, J.; Liu, D.; Li, Y.; Li, F.; Wang, Y.; et al. Mapping and role of T cell response in SARS-CoV-2–infected mice. *J. Exp. Med.* **2021**, *218*. [CrossRef]
55. Chumakov, K.; Avidan, M.S.; Benn, C.S.; Bertozzi, S.M.; Blatt, L.; Chang, A.Y.; Jamison, D.T.; Khader, S.A.; Kottilil, S.; Netea, M.G.; et al. Old vaccines for new infections: Exploiting innate immunity to control COVID-19 and prevent future pandemics. *Proc. Natl. Acad. Sci. USA* **2021**, *118*. [CrossRef]
56. Parmar, K.; Siddiqui, A.; Nugent, K. Bacillus Calmette-Guerin Vaccine and Nonspecific Immunity. *Am. J. Med. Sci.* **2021**, *361*, 683–689. [CrossRef]
57. Gao, K.M.; Derr, A.G.; Guo, Z.; Nundel, K.; Marshak-Rothstein, A.; Finberg, R.W.; Wang, J.P. Human nasal wash RNA-seq reveals distinct cell-specific innate immune responses between influenza and SARS-CoV-2. *JCI Insight* **2021**. [CrossRef] [PubMed]
58. Zhu, H.; Zheng, F.; Li, L.; Jin, Y.; Luo, Y.; Li, Z.; Zeng, J.; Tang, L.; Li, Z.; Xia, N.; et al. A Chinese host genetic study discovered IFNs and causality of laboratory traits on COVID-19 severity. *iScience* **2021**, *24*. [CrossRef]
59. Ivanova, E.N.; Devlin, J.C.; Buus, T.B.; Koide, A.; Cornelius, A.; Samanovic, M.I.; Herrera, A.; Mimitou, E.P.; Zhang, C.; Desvignes, L.; et al. Discrete immune response signature to SARS-CoV-2 mRNA vaccination versus infection. *medRxiv* **2021**, 255677. [CrossRef]
60. Steele, E.J.; Gorczynski, R.M.; Lindley, R.A.; Tokoro, G.; Wallis, D.H.; Temple, R.; Wickramasinghe, N.C. An End of the COVID-19 Pan-demic in Sight? *Infect. Dis Ther.* **2021**, *2*, 1–5.
61. Xiao, Y.; Lidsky, P.V.; Shirogane, Y.; Aviner, R.; Wu, C.-T.; Li, W.; Li, W.; Zheng, W.; Talbot, D.; Catching, A.; et al. A defective viral genome strategy elicits broad protective immunity against respiratory viruses. *Cell* **2021**. [CrossRef]
62. Rodda, L.B.; Netland, J.; Shehata, L.; Pruner, K.B.; Morawski, P.A.; Thouvenel, C.D.; Takehara, K.K.; Eggenberger, J.; Hemann, E.A.; Waterman, H.R.; et al. Functional SARS-CoV-2-Specific Immune Memory Persists after Mild SARS-CoV-2. *Cell* **2021**, *184*, 169–183. [CrossRef] [PubMed]
63. Dan, J.M.; Mateus, J.; Kato, Y.; Hastie, K.M.; Yu, E.D.; Faliti, C.E.; Grifoni, A.; Ramirez, S.I.; Haupt, S.; Frazier, A.; et al. Immunological memory to SARS-CoV-2 assessed for up to 8 months after infection. *Science* **2021**, *371*, eabf4063. [CrossRef]
64. Rockstroh, A.; Wolf, J.; Fertey, J.; Kalbitz, S.; Schroth, S.; Lübbert, C.; Ulbert, S.; Borte, S. Correlation of humoral immune responses to different SARS-CoV-2 antigens with virus neutralizing antibodies and symptomatic severity in a German SARS-CoV-2 cohort. *Emerg Microbes Infect.* **2021**, *10*, 774–781. [CrossRef] [PubMed]
65. Dispinseri, S.; Secchi, M.; Pirillo, M.F.; Tolazzi, M.; Borghi, M.; Brigatti, C.; De Angelis, M.L.; Baratella, M.; Bazzigaluppi, E.; Venturi, G.; et al. Neutralizing antibody responses to SARS-CoV-2 in symptomatic COVID-19 is persistent and critical for survival. *Nat. Commun.* **2021**, *12*, 2670. [CrossRef]
66. Hu, F.; Chen, F.; Ou, Z.; Fan, Q.; Tan, X.; Wang, Y.; Pan, Y.; Ke, B.; Li, L.; Guan, Y.; et al. A compromised specific humoral immune response against the SARS-CoV-2 receptor-binding domain is related to viral persistence and periodic shedding in the gastrointestinal tract. *Cell Mol. Im-Munol.* **2020**, *17*, 1119–1125. [CrossRef] [PubMed]
67. Boehm, E.; Kronig, I.; Neher, R.A.; Eckerle, I.; Vetter, P.; Kaiser, L. Novel SARS-CoV-2 variants: The pandemics within the pandemic. *Clin. Microbiol. Infect.* **2021**, *27*, 1109–1117. [CrossRef] [PubMed]
68. Lindley, R.A.; Steele, E.J. Analysis of SARS-CoV-2 haplotypes and genomic sequences during 2020 in Victoria, Australia, in the context of putative deficits in innate immune deaminase anti-viral responses. *Scand. J. Immunol.* **2021**, *94*, e13100. [CrossRef]
69. Wang, Z.; Schmidt, F.; Weisblum, Y.; Muecksch, F.; Barnes, C.O.; Finkin, S.; Schaefer-Babajew, D.; Cipolla, M.; Gaebler, C.; Lieberman, J.A.; et al. mRNA vaccine-elicited antibodies to SARS-CoV-2 and circulating variants. *Nature* **2021**, *592*, 616–622. [CrossRef]
70. Collier, D.A.; De Marco, A.; Ferreira, I.A.T.M.; Meng, B.; Datir, R.P.; Walls, A.C.; Kemp, S.A.; Bassi, J.; Pinto, D.; Silacci-Fregni, C.; et al. Sensitivity of SARS-CoV-2 B.1.1.7 to mRNA vac-cine-elicited antibodies. *Nature* **2021**, *593*, 136–141. [CrossRef]
71. Yuan, M.; Huang, D.; Lee, C.-C.D.; Wu, N.C.; Jackson, A.M.; Zhu, X.; Liu, H.; Peng, L.; van Gils, M.J.; Sanders, R.W.; et al. Structural and functional ramifications of antigenic drift in recent SARS-CoV-2 variants. *Science* **2021**, *373*, 818–823. [CrossRef]

J. Pers. Med. **2021**, *11*, 1253

72. Chen, X.; Chen, Z.; Azman, A.S.; Sun, R.; Lu, W.; Zheng, N.; Zhou, J.; Wu, Q.; Deng, X.; Zhao, Z.; et al. Comprehensive mapping of neutralizing antibodies against SARS-CoV-2 variants induced by natural infection or vaccination. *medRxiv* **2021**, *5*, 21256506. [CrossRef]

73. Wang, R.; Chen, J.; Gao, K.; Wei, G.-W. Vaccine-escape and fast-growing mutations in the United Kingdom, the United States, Singapore, Spain, India, and other COVID-19-devastated countries. *Genomics* **2021**, *113*, 2158–2170. [CrossRef]

74. Chakraborty, C.; Bhattacharya, M.; Sharma, A.R. Present variants of concern and variants of interest of severe acute respiratory syndrome coronavirus 2: Their significant mutations in S-glycoprotein, infectivity, re-infectivity, immune escape and vaccines activity. *Rev. Med. Virol.* **2021**, e2270. [CrossRef]

75. Venkatakrishnan, A.J.; Anand, P.; Lenehan, P.; Ghosh, P.; Suratekar, R.; Siroha, A.; O'Horo, J.C.; Yao, J.D.; Pritt, B.S.; Norgan, A.; et al. Antigenic minimalism of SARS-CoV-2 is linked to surges in COVID-19 community transmission and vaccine breakthrough infections. *medRxiv* **2021**, 21257668. [CrossRef]

76. Bailly, B.; Guilpain, L.; Bouiller, K.; Chirouze, C.; N'Debi, M.; Soulier, A.; Demontant, V.; Pawlotsky, J.-M.; Rodriguez, C.; Fourati, S. BNT162b2 Messenger RNA Vaccination Did Not Prevent an Outbreak of Severe Acute Respiratory Syndrome Coronavirus 2 Variant 501Y.V2 in an Elderly Nursing Home but Reduced Transmission and Disease Severity. *Clin. Infect. Dis.* **2021**. [CrossRef] [PubMed]

77. Bernal, J.L.; Andrews, N.; Gower, C.; Robertson, C.; Stowe, J.; Tessier, E.; Simmons, R.; Cottrell, S.; Roberts, R.; O'Doherty, M.; et al. Effectiveness of the Pfizer-BioNTech and Oxford-AstraZeneca vaccines on covid-19 related symptoms, hospital admissions, and mortality in older adults in England: Test negative case-control study. *BMJ* **2021**, *373*. [CrossRef]

78. Moline, H.L.; Whitaker, M.; Deng, L.; Rhodes, J.C.; Milucky, J.; Pham, H.; Patel, K.; Anglin, O.; Reingold, A.; Chai, S.J.; et al. Effectiveness of COVID-19 Vaccines in Preventing Hospitalization Among Adults Aged ≥65 Years—COVID-NET, 13 States, February–April 2021. *Morb. Mortal. Wkly. Rep.* **2021**, *70*, 1088–1093. [CrossRef]

79. Blood Collection Study From COVID-19 Convalescents Previously Hospitalized to Identify Immunogenic Viral Epitope. Available online: https://www.clinicaltrials.gov/ct2/show/NCT04397900 (accessed on 16 October 2021).

80. Kula, T.; Dezfulian, M.H.; Wang, C.I.; Abdelfattah, N.S.; Hartman, Z.C.; Wucherpfennig, K.W.; Lyerly, H.; Elledge, S.J. T-Scan: A Genome-wide Method for the Systematic Discovery of T Cell Epitopes. *Cell* **2019**, *178*, 1016–1028.e13. [CrossRef]

81. Bilich, T.; Nelde, A.; Heitmann, J.S.; Maringer, Y.; Roerden, M.; Bauer, J.; Rieth, J.; Wacker, M.; Peter, A.; Hörber, S.; et al. T cell and antibody kinetics delineate SARS-CoV-2 peptides mediating long-term immune responses in COVID-19 convalescent individuals. *Sci. Transl. Med.* **2021**, *13*. [CrossRef]

82. Saini, S.K.; Hersby, D.S.; Tamhane, T.; Povlsen, H.R.; Hernandez, S.P.A.; Nielsen, M.; Gang, A.O.; Hadrup, S.R. SARS-CoV-2 genome-wide T cell epitope mapping reveals immunodominance and substantial CD8 + T cell activation in COVID-19 patients. *Sci. Immunol.* **2021**, *6*, 7550. [CrossRef]

83. Woldemeskel, B.A.; Garliss, C.C.; Blankson, J.N. SARS-CoV-2 mRNA vaccines induce broad CD4+ T cell responses that recognize SARS-CoV-2 variants and HCoV-NL63. *J. Clin. Investig.* **2021**, *17*, e149335. [CrossRef]

84. Neidleman, J.; Luo, X.; McGregor, M.; Xie, G.; Murray, V.; Greene, W.C.; Lee, S.A.; Roan, N.R. mRNA vaccine-induced SARS-CoV-2-specific T cells rec-ognize B.1.1.7 and B.1.351 variants but differ in longevity and homing properties depending on prior infection status. *bioRxiv* **2021**, 443888. [CrossRef]

85. Gallagher, K.M.E.; Leick, M.B.; Larson, R.C.; Berger, T.R.; Katsis, K.; Yam, J.Y.; Grauwet, K.; MGH COVID-19 Collection & Processing Team; Maus, M.V. SARS-CoV-2 T-cell immunity to variants of concern following vaccination. *bioRxiv* **2021**, 442455. [CrossRef]

86. Keller, M.D.; Harris, K.M.; Jensen-Wachspress, M.A.; Kankate, V.V.; Lang, H.; Lazarski, C.A.; Durkee-Shock, J.; Lee, P.-H.; Chaudhry, K.; Webber, K.; et al. SARS-CoV-2-specific T cells are rapidly expanded for therapeutic use and target conserved regions of the membrane protein. *Blood* **2020**, *136*, 2905–2917. [CrossRef] [PubMed]

87. Kyriakidis, N.C.; López-Cortés, A.; González, E.V.; Grimaldos, A.B.; Prado, E.O. SARS-CoV-2 vaccines strategies: A comprehensive review of phase 3 candidates. *NPJ Vaccines* **2021**, *6*, 1–17. [CrossRef] [PubMed]

88. Verbeke, R.; Lentacker, I.; De Smedt, S.C.; Dewitte, H. The dawn of mRNA vaccines: The SARS-CoV-2 case. *J. Control. Release* **2021**, *333*, 511–520. [CrossRef] [PubMed]

89. The Possibility of COVID-19 after Vaccination: Breakthrough Infections. Available online: https://www.cdc.gov/coronavirus/2019-ncov/vaccines/effectiveness/why-measure-effectiveness/breakthrough-cases.html (accessed on 16 October 2021).

90. Keehner, J.; Horton, L.E.; Binkin, N.J.; Laurent, L.C.; Pride, D.; Longhurst, C.A.; Abeles, S.R.; Torriani, F.J. Resurgence of SARS-CoV-2 Infection in a Highly Vaccinated Health System Workforce. *N. Engl. J. Med.* **2021**, *385*, 1330–1332. [CrossRef] [PubMed]

91. Subramanian, S.V.; Kumar, A. Increases in COVID-19 are unrelated to levels of vaccination across 68 countries and 2947 counties in the United States. *Eur. J. Epidemiol.* **2021**. [CrossRef]

92. Cines, D.B.; Bussel, J.B. SARS-CoV-2 Vaccine–Induced Immune Thrombotic Thrombocytopenia. *N. Engl. J. Med.* **2021**, *384*, 2254–2256. [CrossRef]

93. Thiele, T.; Ulm, L.; Holtfreter, S.; Schönborn, L.; Kuhn, S.O.; Scheer, C.; Warkentin, T.E.; Bröker, B.M.; Becker, K.; Aurich, K.; et al. Frequency of positive anti-PF4/polyanion antibody tests after COVID-19 vaccination with ChAdOx1 nCoV-19 and BNT162b2. *Blood* **2021**, *138*, 299–303. [CrossRef]

J. Pers. Med. **2021**, *11*, 1253

94. Lyons-Weiler, J. Pathogenic priming likely contributes to serious and critical illness and mortality in COVID-19 via autoimmunity. *J. Transl. Autoimmun.* **2020**, *3*, 100051. [CrossRef]

95. Tseng, C.-T.; Sbrana, E.; Iwata-Yoshikawa, N.; Newman, P.C.; Garron, T.; Atmar, R.L.; Peters, C.J.; Couch, R.B. Correction: Immunization with SARS Coronavirus Vaccines Leads to Pulmonary Immunopathology on Challenge with the SARS Virus. *PLoS ONE* **2012**, *7*. [CrossRef]

96. Lu, L.; Xiong, W.; Mu, J.; Zhang, Q.; Zhang, H.; Zou, L.; Li, W.; He, L.; Sander, J.W.; Zhou, D. The potential neurological effect of the COVID-19 vaccines: A review. *Acta Neurol. Scand.* **2021**, *144*, 3–12. [CrossRef] [PubMed]

97. Bozkurt, B.; Kamat, I.; Hotez, P.J. Myocarditis With COVID-19 mRNA Vaccines. *Circulation* **2021**, *144*, 471–484. [CrossRef] [PubMed]

98. Dotan, A.; Muller, S.; Kanduc, D.; David, P.; Halpert, G.; Shoenfeld, Y. The SARS-CoV-2 as an instrumental trigger of autoimmunity. *Autoimmun. Rev.* **2021**, *20*, 102792. [CrossRef] [PubMed]

SECTION 7

The End of the Pandemic and Emergence and Spread of Omicron

Review Article

Exploding Five COVID-19 Myths on its Origin, Global Spread and Immunity

Edward J. Steele[1,2,3]*, Reginald M. Gorczynski[4], Herbert Rebhan[1], GensukeTokoro[5], Daryl H. Wallis[5], Robert Temple[6] and N. Chandra Wickramasinghe [3,5,7,8]

[1]C.Y.O' Connor ERADE Village Foundation, Piara Waters, Perth, WA, Australia

[2]Melville Analytics Pty Ltd, Melbourne, VIC, Australia

[3]Centre for Astrobiology, University of Ruhuna, Matara, Sri Lanka

[4]University Toronto Health Network, Toronto General Hospital, University of Toronto, Toronto, ON, Canada

[5]Institute for the Study of Panspermia and Astroeconomics, Gifu, Japan

[6]The History of Chinese Science and Culture Foundation, Conway Hall, London, United Kingdom 9University of Buckingham, Buckingham, UK

[7]National Institute of Fundamental Studies, Kandy, Sri Lanka

[8]University of Buckingham, Buckingham, UK

*Corresponding author: Edward J. Steele, C.Y.O' Connor ERADE Village Foundation, Piara Waters, Perth, WA, Australia; E-mail: e.j.steele@bigpond.com

Received: September 23, 2020; Accepted: October 04, 2020; Published: October 12, 2020

Abstract

By critically analysing and exploding the key foundation myths that have arisen around the origin, mode of spread and immunity on COVID-19 we lay out the evidence and critical arguments supporting an immediate end to all COVID-19 justified lockdowns. These emergency laws, invoked by many previously free and democratic societies, involve social distancing, obligatory wearing of masks, limited crowd sizes and gatherings (funerals, weddings, religious gatherings, sporting fixtures etc), the closures of schools and many small and large businesses not deemed necessary to containing the virus, border closures, and thus free travel movements, domestic and international. The basic premise in all these dictums is that the primary mechanism of spread of COVID-19 is assumed via person-to-person contacts only. We show this premise to be false. Our recommendations are anchored in the key relevant evidence and observations of the past two years gathered by us and published in a series of papers through 2020 and 2021. Our analysis documents the plausible putative first cause to the arrival of COVID-19 from space in a carbonaceous meteorite bolide in the stratosphere over China on October 11 2019; and then its blanket China-wide viral-laden meteorite dust contamination through November-December 2019 followed by further global dispersal of these viral-laden meteorite dust clouds by prevailing stratospheric and tropospheric wind systems, including human passaged virus aerosol-plumes adding to lower level (tropospheric) viral laden clouds. We explain why all lockdowns of any type cannot possibly work in principle against viral dispersal and transportation of this type – emergence of new clusters of disease, with poor evidence of connectivity through contact, clearly does not support person-to-person infections as the primary cause of spread. The initiation of mass infective events ("Mystery Cases") in each regional and localised COVID-19 epidemic is caused by unsuspecting victims most likely catching the virus by rubbing up against a virus contaminated environment. We also deal with the efficacy of current vaccination roll outs on population-wide scales. It is most unfortunate that currently available mRNA expression vector vaccines, delivered by the intramuscular route ("Jab in the Arm"), may not only be dangerous in inducing many putative adverse reactions as their human safety is untested, they also cannot protect in principle against common cold and other respiratory pathogen infections like COVID-19 that arrive via the oral-nasal route. That evidence is discussed along with our recommendations for mankind's preparedness for future suddenly emerging pandemics of this type.

Introduction

We have published recent papers that review the evidence that the prevailing global wind systems are the primary distributors of COVID-19 viral-rich clouds [1-3] and a detailed summary of the analysis of a clear set of mystery outbreaks in Victoria, Australia May-June 2021 [4] which constitute unequivocal evidence of a non-person-to-person introduction of the virus. These airborne viral in-falls from the troposphere have resulted in significant region-wide environmental viral contaminations, both small and large scale across the globe, of meteorite-derived viral-laden dust clouds. These include sudden strikes of COVID-19 outbreaks on crew and passengers on ships at sea [5,6] islands such as Sri Lanka that had avoided the epidemics until Oct 6 2020 [7] and the remote Chilean O'Higgins Army Outpost in Antarctica where most of the personnel were struck down suddenly and simultaneously with COVID-19 in late Dec 2020 [3].

While some infections can theoretically be caught by victims from breathing in viral-laden dust particles in the air, the case Incidence maps which show the stability of an infected zone outbreak in carefully analysed specified regions (as an example, selected parts of the State of Victoria in Australia and State New South Wales, covering pre-Winter and Winter months May-Sept both 2020 and 2021) suggest

DOI: https://doi.org/10.31038/IDT.2021223

https://researchopenworld.com/exploding-five-covid-19-myths-on-its-origin-global-spread-and-immunity/

Infect Dis Ther, Volume 2(2): 1–15, 2020

Edward J. Steele (2021) Exploding Five COVID-19 Myths on its Origin, Global Spread and Immunity

alternate explanations. We surmise that most infections are caught by unsuspecting victims from contact with a virus-contaminated environment (e.g. contaminated fingers or contaminated face masks themselves) with subsequent transfer to portals of entry via oral-nasal passages, initiating an infection in the lining of the respiratory tract. Case Incidence maps for Victoria, Australia and the prevailing weather directions of rain visiting Victoria from Southern Ocean are shown in Figure 1a and 1b.

The viral-laden dust clouds would need to be brought down to ground by local precipitation (rain). This likely occurred through most of 2020 across the globe given the localised stability of regional outbreaks (USA, Europe, Pakistan, Japan, South Korea, South Africa and the Indian subcontinent), particularly through April-May 2020 on the 40° N Latitude band prior to the strike on New York City. Early outbreaks in South Korea and Japan were also centred on this latitude line [1]. On either side of this line, during this 2020 time

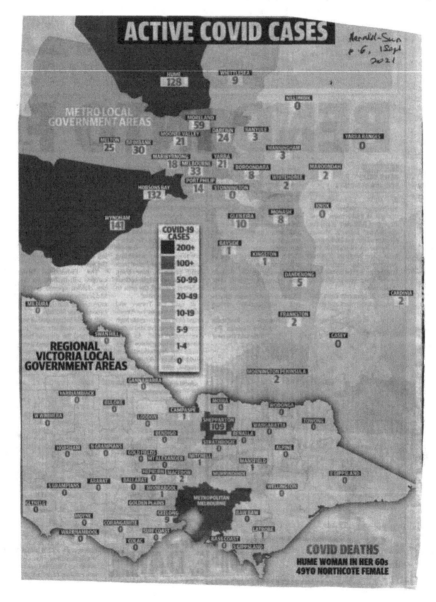

Figure 1a: Map of COVID-19 outbreaks (40-50% Mystery cases) in Victoria Winter 2021. Note the whole town of Shepparton 190 km north of Melbourne was a cluster of numerous and sudden mystery outbreaks (unlinked genomically in sequence to Melbourne 'Delta' outbreaks according to newspaper reports) as Melbourne was sealed off by a 'ring of steel' hard lock down with night time curfews, no movement in or out of Melbourne, no travel through country regions, and the border with New South Wales was sealed by police, army and surveillance drones.

Edward J. Steele (2021) Exploding Five COVID-19 Myths on its Origin, Global Spread and Immunity

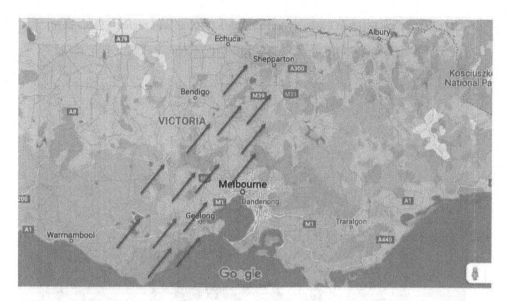

The pre-winter and winter weather with cold rain always visits Victoria from South West to North Direction creating a WEST->EAST weather gradient across the state - the COVID-19 infections occurred in same gradient in May-Sept 2020 and May – Sept in 2021. The East of the state has been essentially virus free in both winter seasons.

Figure 1b: Infection arc of Figure 1a showing very similar to prevailing Winter weather into Victoria from the Southern Ocean. Notice that the East of the State (Figure 1a) is basically virus free. The same pattern was observed in 2020 (see Appendix A).

interval, there were many countries which represented infection "null zones", which soon became engaged north and south of the 40° N line (France, United Kingdom, most countries in Europe and Russia and Scandinavian countries). Subsequently we have suggested that the putative meteorite viral-laden dust clouds then washed down and entered the Southern Hemisphere over the Atlantic Ocean [2]. The viral clouds were then brought to Australia in 2020 along the 40° S latitude Line, via the W->E Roaring Forties prevailing winds to Victoria and to a far lesser extent into NSW, Australia (May-Sept 2020, and then again in 2021, including the significant out breaks in French Polynesia 2020-21 as well as small outbreaks in New Zealand [3]. In Australia in both winters Western Australia (Perth), South Australia (Adelaide), Tasmania (Hobart, Launceston), and Queensland (Brisbane) were all null zones, only suffering transient outbreaks via infected international passengers entering by jet planes. It is very important to understand such null zones, as they confirm the annual regularity of the prevailing wind and weather systems – the COVID-19 strikes in Australasia were clearly governed by these predictable weather systems.

Later in the year 2020, and into 2021, the main spreads and regional in-falls could well have been of human passaged COVID-19 rich viral dust clouds generated by the significant tropospheric plumes of viral aerosols above United Kingdom, India, South Africa, Brazil and other countries through the later months 2020 and through 2021 [4]. Other genomic and epidemiological evidence to be referred to

here is an analysis of >12,000 full length COVID-19 genomes and associated epidemiology data publicly available from the 2nd Wave COVID-19 epidemic in Victoria, Australia June-Sept 2020 [8]. This analysis builds on the COVID-19 full length genome analysis in clear hotspot epidemics in [9]. Here we expose to critical scrutiny the unscientific myths in wide mainstream media circulation (and also actively promoted by the same media particularly the global News Ltd media) which has driven the global response of all governments and their health authorities.

What Actually Happened in China Late 2019 and Early 2020?

Before exposing the key circulating myths we must have a clear-eyed view of what *actually* transpired in China late 2019 through January 2020, and into the explosive exponential rise in COVID-19 case numbers per day in January 2020 [9]. The earliest confirmed cases in retrospect emerged from late October-early November [10]. The widely discussed data is based on the Wuhan epidemic in Hubei province central China but it is clear from *all the data* collected at the time from across China that a series of China-wide explosive epidemics *occurred simultaneously* (Figure 2). Any explanation has to manage this clear fact - tens to hundreds of millions of Chinese were exposed and succumbed to COVID-19 infections over a short time period, too fast for any type of person-to-person (P-to-P) spread as is commonly assumed by mainstream epidemiological theory and bat-

Edward J. Steele (2021) Exploding Five COVID-19 Myths on its Origin, Global Spread and Immunity

The COVID-19 Case Incident Pattern Central China (Wuhan and regions) Feb 7 2020

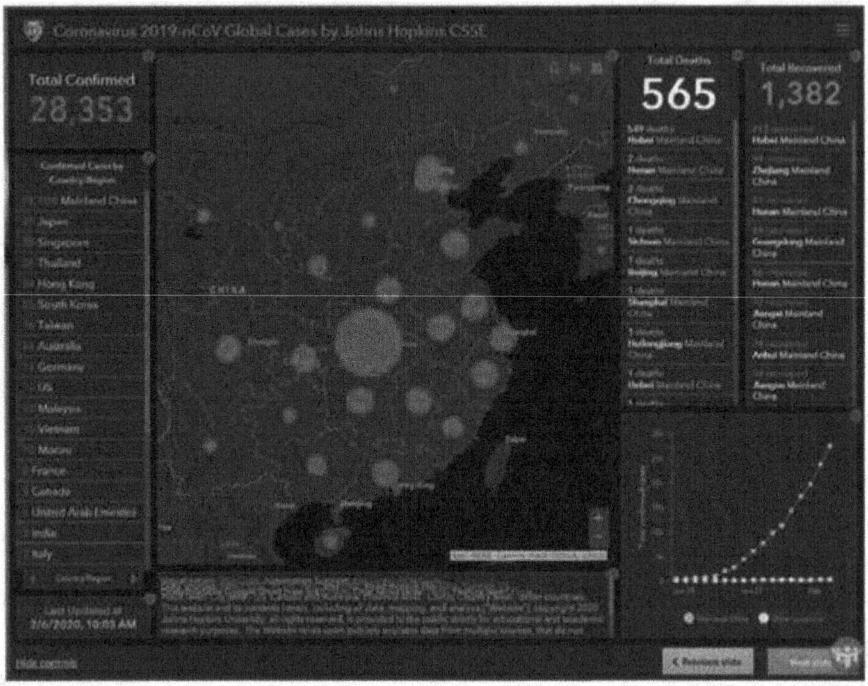

Fig. 7 Case density map—China itself. Johns Hopkins University as February 7, 2020. Johns Hopkins University's Centre for Systems Science and Engineering.

Figure 2: This is Figure 7 discussed in depth in Ref [11], Steele EJ, Gorczynski RM, Lindley RA, Tokoro G, et al. (2020) **Origin of new emergent Coronavirus and Candida fungal diseases-Terrestrial or Cosm**ic? *Advances in Genetics* 106, 75-100 https://doi.org/10.1016/bs.adgen.2020.04.002

human and most Lab leak conspiracy theories.

Current Myth#1

The COVID-19 pandemic began with a sudden explosive animal - to - human jump on China-wide scale of the earlier SARS-CoV-1 now in a bat or pangolin reservoir in South East Asia.

Both we and mainstream viral molecular evolutionists (e.g. Professor Andrew Rambaut, University Edinburgh; Professor Ed Holmes, University of Sydney) agree such a jump is statistically impossible on the basis of all existing SARS-CoV-2 "like" sequences isolated from putative bat, pangolin or cat reservoirs. We discuss these data and calculate the odds of a "jump" giving a COVID-19 sequence match [6]. For the closest known bat sequence, 96.2% similar to COVID-19 across the full length 29903 nucleotide (nt) positions of the Wuhan or Hu-1 reference sequence, the probability of getting a match of a correct nucleotide substitution at approx. 1100 positions is of the order one successful trial in 10^{684} random trial jumps. If we are generous and assume there is a sequence of 99% similarity to COVID-19 lurking in some unknown bat or pangolin animal reservoir it is 10^{184}. If the reader has difficulty grasping the essence of such astronomical numbers a good comparator number is 10^{84}, the

number of Hydrogen nuclei in the known Big Bang Universe (H atoms quantitatively dominate the known Universe). So getting a successful jump outstrips, by many orders of magnitude, the molecular and statistical resources of the known universe. *To re-state the obvious conclusion: this infection did not come from an infected bat via wet market contact* (supported also by all the early reports that exclude such 'origin' sources on other grounds [11-13].

Current Myth#2

The COVID-19 pandemic began with a sudden explosive release of a genetically engineered virus just like COVID-19 (the full length 29903 nt Hu-1 sequence) from the Wuhan Institute of Virology. This has been actively and strongly pushed by Professor Nikolai Petrovsky (Flinders University), Sharri Markson the lead investigative journalist in News Ltd in Australia, other writers in The Australian newspaper, many Fox News Channel (News Ltd) talking Heads eg Tucker Carlson Tonight and others on FNC) and many writers in The Wall street Journal (News Ltd) and The London Times (News Ltd, including Professor Luc Montagnier [14]). It is a fair assessment that the News Ltd media in particular has actively pushed this Cold War Conspiracy. Theory propaganda globally on a massive scale. Ex-president Trump also argued the

Edward J. Steele (2021) Exploding Five COVID-19 Myths on its Origin, Global Spread and Immunity

same case with his 'China Virus' accusations in 2020, despite having been told this story was most likely false "in a big power telephone communication" on Feb 6 2020 with President Xi - see Appendix B, pages xviii-xix Bob Woodward's book *Rage*: "It goes through the air," Trump said. "That's always tougher than the touch. You don't have to touch things. Right? But the air, you just breathe the air and that's how it's passed. And so that's a very tricky one. That's a very delicate one."

Notice that none of the material put out by those advocating a human-engineered cause (Petrovsky, Markson, Carlson, Montagnier et al) ever attempts to grapple with a wealth of precise facts that need to be considered (see Figure 2). Our own explanation of a natural cosmic cause is plausible in terms both of timing and location, given the Oct 11 2019 meteorite strike over Nth East China, [15,16], and all existing historical and recent knowledge on life bearing carbonaceous meteorites arriving in the stratosphere prior to COVID-19 [17-19]. Our analysis comes to grips with this explosive first strike (Figure 2) of putatively tens of millions of mystery infections imposed across a vast area of China (Dec 20219-Jan 2020) and the subsequent sequelae of epidemics (and genetics of the virus) on the ground in the first few months after Oct 11 2019, first in China, then elsewhere in South East Asia, Western Pacific, then Iran, Italy, Spain and New York City [1,6,9]. Of course, following a mystery infection (falling from the sky) there would then be person to person (P-to-P) spread to close contacts and to close uninfected family members (the genetic data from the Wuhan sequences suggest 1 or at most two P-to-P transfers, [9]). This we do not deny. Such a human passaged transmission would have begun immediately in China, resulting eventually in a rising aerosol plume of human passaged COVID-19 virions being lofted into the troposphere above China. The infective strikes on the cruise ships in the South China Sea and Sea of Japan (*Diamond Princess, Westerdam*), the *USS Theodore Roosevelt* aircraft carrier (May 2020, north Pacific Ocean) and the sudden strike in late February 2020 on the other side of the Pacific Ocean on the *Grand Princess* cruise ship, support lower level West -to-East global transport of the Wuhan human passaged viral plume cloud across the Pacific in this time interval [3]. This is consistent with the available genetic evidence viz. unmutated and lightly mutated Hu-1 sequences (L or in Pango, B) among infected passengers/crew on that ship [9].

The meteorite viral-laden dust cloud arising from a cometary strike over Jilin, North East China on the 40° N line on the night Oct 11 2019 was, we believe, the likely first deposit of viral-laden dust into the stratosphere above China - and its East to West stratospheric jet stream transport ensured global spread - coincident with a first ground strike by the direct faster fall of a fragment of the viral-laden meteorite cloud to ground blanketing China through November and December 2019, although still centred on Wuhan. The estimate of the earliest cases in November fit this explanation [10]. This explanation is consistent with all known facts about the early months as the pandemic ignited in China. It is far more plausible and parsimonious than the animal jump or Lab leak theories, and does not require multiple additional, and implausible assumptions (further discussed below and Appendix C). The cause of the many genuine 'mystery cases' observed in Victoria (and NSW) in Australia in 2020 [8], and 2021 needs to be interpreted in the same way, but on a far smaller scale of infection numbers [4].

The stability of the infection arc over two winters in Victoria (Figure 1 and Appendix B for 2020) implies prevailing weather patterns. The null zones of Perth (Western Australia), Adelaide (South Australia), Hobart & Launceston (Tasmania), Brisbane (Queensland), despite all the political finger pointing in Australia, are most simply explained as arguing that all those other Australian states were lucky- they were not in the "teeth" of prevailing weather winds and in consequence they have avoided the political, social and economic mayhem which has followed the "conventional dogma explanations".

Implausibility of Lab Leak Theories

We next turn attention to confront in detail and properly assess the "Lab Leak Conspiracy" theories that are gaining widespread apparent momentum and respectability in the public mind. As stated above these models require multiple additional, and in our view implausible, assumptions, which are discussed in depth in a series of numbered points (below and Appendix C). In exploring in detail the implications of the 'Predictions' of this theory, as we would for any scientific theory, which must be tested also for coherence and robustness, and here to, by necessity, we will limit the number of tacit and overt assumptions (and Appendix C). The advantage of the latest claims is we can examine the predictions. The claim now is that an engineered COVID-19 virus culture at very high titre and thus dose was somehow deposited in the stratosphere and thus entered into the global weather system over China. In our view this is a concocted and politically convenient cold war conspiracy fantasy (Sharri Markson Wed 15 Sept 2021 p.1 *The Australian* newspaper "Revealed: US failed to act on Covid-19 intelligence, says Wei Jingsheng", the latter is a Chinese defector to the USA).

In exploring the implications and predictions of this assertion for coherence and scientific plausibility, readers must also stay aware of the scientific plausibility of the argument, critique any data put forward to support it, and ask themselves whether it even "makes sense" to imply a 'human purpose' and 'motivation' for a first strike stratospheric cause which fits the observed and sudden China-wide infection data (*vide supra*). We have already made clear that in our view all the available scientific data is consistent with the pandemic being a natural phenomenon - like that which occurred 100 years ago in an era before viruses were not fully characterised and a time when DNA/RNA genetic manipulation biotechnology did not exist. As we shall show the assumptions needed to defend a conspiracy alternative are *ad hoc*, without independent evidence, and so also are the number of additional concepts needed to reconcile with the available epidemiologic and genetic data

Points to Consider as Arguments in Favour of a "Lab Leak Conspiracy"

1. A balloon launch or drone plane flight released a viral 'bomb' in the stratosphere over China. There is no reported evidence, from China, US or European satellites of a balloon launch, drone flight, or spy-plane which could be responsible, in Oct-Dec 2019. No coherent argument (political) has been suggested for who might have been responsible for such a strike, and why.

2. If it was from outside China, one would expect the Chinese military to have neutralised it quickly and for there to have been political repercussions-it is hard not to expect repercussions detected by the rest of the world if a launch occurred from within China itself. The viral vector vehicle is postulated to harbour a pure culture of COVID-19 virions with an exact genomic sequence to the Hu-1 (Wuhan) reference sequence, and would need to be in the stratosphere on the 40° N line above China in the period Oct-Dec 2019 to fit the known subsequent global spread and time lines. Simultaneous infection of multiple Chinese cities, with the biggest dose over Hubei/Wuhan, has also to be explained-does this imply multiple deliberate releases?

3. How and where was the exact COVID-19 29,903 nt sequence made? Was it at the Wuhan Institute of Virology, or the National Institutes of Health (NIH), Bethesda Maryland, where Dr. Fauci's group are based, and are known collaborators with the Wuhan laboratory (according to Tucker Carlson and many other news outlets). Furthermore, if the infection source was a product of a bioweapon development program, why was a common cold coronavirus chosen, which has such low mortality effects, causing death in <1% of the exposed population (with deficits in Type I and III Interferon responses [21-26]? One could claim that this was a "trial run", but that also brings up the question (if this really does represent a trial bioweapon) *how is it planned that the designers of this agent would be protected?*

This short summary shows that Sharri Markson, Luc Montagnier, Wei Jingsheng, Nikolai Petrovsky and all the other writers elsewhere and at News Ltd on the influential *The Australian* newspaper in particular (Nick Cater, Adam Creighton, Paul Monk) have not thought through the implications of these proposals. There must be, as was the case with the 9/11 strike on the World Trade Centre, a significant amount of discoverable 'human-factor' associated-evidence behind this stratospherically launched viral attack over China and thus the world in Oct-Dec 2019, if there is any credibility to this theory-none has been reported. Scientific analyses of data and observations and building of explanatory models works in a different way. Science sticks to known facts, plausible mechanisms, with an absolute minimum number of useful assumptions, to explain the observed facts in a coherent way. As soon as the tested theory starts to flounder without the introduction of an ongoing series of *ad hoc* assumptions, the theory is abandoned and new, testable, hypothesis considered. *Our published explanation has, to date, consistently explained the myriad of global data, without any need for further modification.*

• **Current Myth#3**

COVID-19 is a very severe respiratory disease resulting in death in many people.

All the current evidence strongly suggests that a very small immune defenceless group of patients lacking type I and type III interferon innate immunity responses are vulnerable and at high risk of death to COVID-19 infection [20-25]. In longitudinal studies these innate immune deficits are revealed, as expected, very early in infection in patients with a poor prognosis [24] (Figure 2c in that paper). Therapies to quell the respiratory crisis clearly need to be implemented very early in the infection in order to prevent life threatening pneumonia and other respiratory compromise. Included amongst such conventional therapies are pulse steroids (including prednisone; inhaled budesonide; dexamethasone) along with anti-viral agents (remdesivir) and other more novel immunobiologic interventions (monoclonal antibodies). Ivermectin therapy, although controversial, has also been suggested as a novel treatment [26]. What proportion of the population falls into the "immune defenceless elderly co-morbid group"? In surveying Cases and Deaths world-wide for some 18 months, and applying reasonable correction factors for the Numerator and Denominators in different countries and an assessment of the coverage and reliability of the tests and death outcomes in different countries and regions an estimate of 0.1% of all Covid-19 exposures appear to result in severe outcome, viz. death by COVID-19. A concrete example illustrates the calculation on data released on September 12 2021 at the NSW Dept Health Website, https://www.nsw.gov.au/covid-19/find-the-facts-about-covid-19#nsw-covid-19-datasets

For all COVID-19 Cases to date (for 2020 -21) there have been 41,999 confirmed cases of COVID-19 (severity has not been appended or made public here). There have been 14,701,732 PCR tests in a population of about 7 million over 2020 -21 to Sept 12 2021. The number of lives lost 2020-21 is 226. The great bulk of the deaths (as in Victoria in 2020 [9]) would occur in the ≥ 60 yr group (≥97%) or ≥ 70 yr group (≥94%). Clearly COVID-19 infection caused by *any variant* (raw meteorite dust or human passaged plume dust) causes high mortality in a *very small vulnerable subset of the elderly population*, as was evident in Wuhan in Jan 2020 and New York City (Mar-April 2020). What is this fraction? In NSW the Death rate is 0.54% on the above numbers, if you correct the Numerator (x2) and Denominator (divide by 2) for undetected cases and those dying with COVID-19 you arrive at a proportion close to the global estimate mentioned already of 0.1% deaths of all COVID-19 exposed cases in New South Wales in 2020-21. In the USA the correction to the Denominator is obligatory as in April-May 2020 the White House Chief Medical Advisor Dr Deborah Birx made it clear on several occasions in public that all deaths in COVID-19 positive patients would be scored as "COVID-19 deaths". This has catastrophic consequences for an accurate appraisal of all the data coming out of the USA- *the data, as presented, simply is not reliable*, and needs to be corrected the way it has been done above. Indeed, the same erroneous calculation has almost certainly been going on all over the world - and is clearly also evident in public information released by the Victorian and New South Wales Departments of Health, their Chief Health Officers and their Health Ministers. viz a sensational headline of young people dying of COVID-19, only to be revealed later or fine print of the same report that many of the patients had very severe comorbidities (a curated and backed up digital file of most newspaper reports of this type in Australia 2020-21 has been maintained by the authors and the assertions can be backed up by news reports).

We posit the inescapable conclusion that the COVID-19 pandemic *is a pandemic of a (slightly more severe?) common coronavirus*

Edward J. Steele (2021) Exploding Five COVID-19 Myths on its Origin, Global Spread and Immunity

(influenza-like) infection which >99% of people shrug off as they have throughout previous cold and flu outbreaks in past years. This has been dealt with in the past without widespread isolation, wearing of masks, and being locked at home with businesses and schools closed down. Indeed in past Influenza seasons the mortality rates in geriatric,

Table 1: INFLUENZA v COVID-19: By the numbers.

Australian Influenza Cases in 2019

NSW	112,841
Vic	66,015
Qld	66,407
WA	22,720
SA	22,754
ACT	3,952
TAS	2,937
NT	1,458

Source: National Notifiable Diseases Surveillance System, Oct 2019.

Australian COVID-19 Cases in 2020-21

NSW	20,466
Vic	21,618
Qld	1,972
WA	1,064
SA	870
ACT	300
TAS	235
NT	201

Source: covid19data.com.au, 25 Aug 2021.

Australian Influenza Deaths in 2019

NSW	334
Vic	138
Qld	264
WA	80
SA	119
ACT	10
TAS	0
NT	5

Source: NSW Health, Victorian Influenza Snapshot, Qld Health, SA Health, ACT Health NT Health.

Australian COVID-19 Deaths in 2020-21

NSW	129
Vic	820
Qld	7
WA	9
SA	4
ACT	3
TAS	13
NT	0

Source: covid19data.com.au, 25 Aug 2021.

aged care /nursing home facilities have often been higher during influenza epidemics (Table 1, summarised from Melbourne's *Herald-Sun* p.32 29 August 2021). A comparison with influenza in Australia 2019 prior to COVID-19 shows that the seasonal influenza outbreaks in that year took a greater toll in cases and similar numbers in deaths. The numbers are biased because of the situation in Victoria [8]. There was massive political incompetence and chaos in Victoria in 2020 (and into 2021) – a reflection of the poor government and health system incompetence. Also, all the aged carers (usually Asian women with families to feed on poor wages) worked across *multiple aged care and nursing homes a*nd were very efficient viral vectors- a veritable bonfire of the nursing and aged care homes, almost simultaneous ignitions on scale. It was mainly caused by the single clone the L241f.1vic haplotype identified which the health authorities tracked and released genomic sequences of – although they did not release the genomes of the approx. 40% of mystery genome sequences (>3500) where it is hard not to see those infections not playing a role in the aged care and nursing homes. This is covered in detail [8].

However, we have deduced, no real viral cloud in-fall occurred in the other Australian states. More than 95% of COVID-19 infections were in Victoria in 2020. The other states had mainly infected travellers from overseas or interstate from Victoria. Mystery infections in Victoria in 2020 were about 40% of all cases (often publicly confirmed as unlinked by genomic sequencing to known nursing home clusters) - these 3500-4000 genomes have yet to be released into the public scientific domain by the Peter Doherty Institute despite repeated requests in writing by the authors. Very few deaths this year so far in both Victoria and NSW, and mystery cases when reported are running at least at 50% of all PCR positive cases. All the details are not being released by the health authorities. It is conceivable that in 2021 lessons have indeed been learnt and aged care facilities may well be applying immediate therapies to the infected elderly to quell the respiratory crisis (and prevented employees working across multiple facilities). The infection flare-ups discussed below (Figure 3) appear now in large migrant 3-generation families under one roof in West-North suburbs of Melbourne (but same infection arc as 2020), and South-West arc of infections in Sydney, NSW.

So COVID-19 is potentially dangerous for those with *severe innate immune deficit in type I and III interferon responses [8]* and references above. The target vulnerable group that requires special immediate therapeutic care are our elderly citizens in geriatric, aged care and nursing homes – as has always been the case in past cold and flu seasons in Australia. Indeed, in the early phases of this pandemic, the *global* argument for any restrictions ("lockdowns") was to give time for health care systems everywhere to "get their ducks in order" so they were not overwhelmed and could be better prepared to deal with infections in those most at risk-that valid argument was rapidly forgotten, and people seemed to accept the early response strategy as a valid long-term one, without ever questioning why this viral infection should merit such long-term draconian responses. It is apparent with COVID-19 that elderly grandparents that still live with a wider three-generation family under one household roof are now especially vulnerable - as is typically the case for many recently arrived migrant families in the communities of western Sydney and western /northern

Edward J. Steele (2021) Exploding Five COVID-19 Myths on its Origin, Global Spread and Immunity

COVID-19 Cases per Day during Epidemics VIC and NSW June-Sept 2021
Spikes and Flares in case per Day indicated by red arrow

Victoria (Mainly West to North Melbourne)

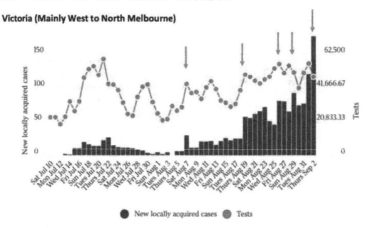

Source: Victoria Department of Health

NSW (mainly West to South West Sydney)

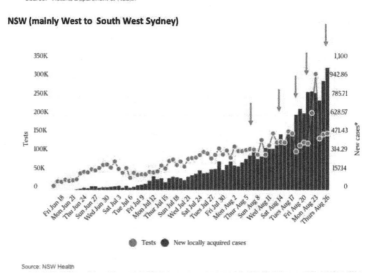

Source: NSW Health

Figure 3: Cases per day plots in Victoria and NSW May-August 2021.

Melbourne in Australia, in particular.

Current Myths#4

Nature of "Virulence' with COVID-19? "Highly virulent rampaging and transmissible variants" (UK Mutant, South African mutant, Indian Delta etc).

Virulence is a term now widely and loosely used in the media and by political leaders and Chief Health Officers, without any good consensus as to its biologic meaning. In the current "Delta" outbreaks in Victoria and NSW the public is told that "Delta" seems to be "speeding through the community" indeed so fast it out runs the contact tracing teams, and it must therefore represent a highly virulent

and transmissible variant, and thus a forebearer of a dangerous disease. When the sudden outbreaks in Shepparton, 190 km north of Melbourne began to appear from August 21 2021, one might have hoped for a pause for critical thinking by Victorian Premier Daniel Andrews and Chief Health Officer Brett Sutton. A "ring of steel" had been erected around Melbourne (from Aug 11) and hard stage 4 lock downs (and night curfews) had begun much earlier. This meant that no one from Melbourne could have travelled to/from Shepparton- and given the northern border with NSW was sealed (by police, army and drones) no one from the highly infected northern state of NSW could have come to Shepparton. We argue that only one infection route could and should have been considered....... "It must have come via

Edward J. Steele (2021) Exploding Five COVID-19 Myths on its Origin, Global Spread and Immunity

an airborne route". There is no public evidence that this explanation has been considered. At the time of preparing this paper, Sept 12-13 2021, the hard Stage 4 lockdown is still in place, cases per day are going up, 50-60% of all cases are genuine "mystery cases", mandatory masks required inside and outside, QR tracking everywhere, hysterical headlines every day "to get tested" then "get jabbed". Full night curfews are still in place. Only AFL Footballers (and NRL Footballers) seem to be able to move around. Many businesses have literally gone broke and many families will never recover. The number of bordered up businesses in the neighbourhood of EJS (Prahran, Toorak, Armadale, and South Yarra) is staggering. Long term social and health damage has been caused in Victoria, we are now in our 8th month of hard Stage 4 lock down.

However, we must be very clear, these lockdowns have had *zero impact* on the spread or apparent 'virulence' of the virus and course of the epidemics. The lockdown during the 2nd wave in Victoria in 2020 also had no effect, leaving us with the following conclusion [3]: "With respect to the symmetrical nature of the bell-shaped curves (Figure 4 below) describing the distributions of cases per day seen in such well documented epidemics such as the Victorian 2nd Wave an important deduction can be drawn about the impact of extreme 'lockdown' social distancing measures aimed at reducing viral reproduction rate Ro to less than 1. We have statistically analysed the Gaussian features of the Victorian 2nd Wave (which peaked on August 1-2, 2020). The best Gaussian fit with R^2 gives 0.8999 which implies an almost perfect statistical fit to a symmetrical bell-shaped curve. Such a result would be consistent with the epidemic curve being overwhelmingly dominated by the growth and decay of a localised atmospheric in-fall event. The hard Stage 4 lockdown in Victoria came into effect on August 2, 2020. Given this perfect symmetry we conclude that the hard lock down measures had little impact, if any, on the course of the 2nd Wave COVID-19 epidemic in Victoria, Australia. This conclusion is consistent with the independent analyses of the impact of extreme lockdown measures on the course of the COVID-19 lockdowns introduced in a number of States in the USA during 2020 [27]."

Further Comment on COVID-19 Virulence

In our view the high virulence of a variant is an illusion caused by occurrence of multiple simultaneous 'mystery cases' occurring over a defined short time periods- a month or two via airborne region wide viral contamination. The impression of speed of transmission is created as unsuspecting victims catch CVOVID-19 via touching their contaminated environment. What then is the nature of this suddenly emergent pandemic? Since COVID-19 first emerged in China in Dec 2019- Jan 2020 we have been trying to quell and eliminate a variant annual respiratory viral infection (similar to a common cold) – most (>99.9%) of all infected people handle the virus by Innate Immunity and Adaptive Immune Responses in the cells and tissues lining the mouth, nose, respiratory tract and lung- there is a vulnerable group about 0.1% of all infected people. *The best response* would have been to provide therapies and pro-active care of all *Immune Defenceless Elderly Co-Morbid citizens* through the respiratory crisis: Vulnerable age group for death by COVID-19 is ≥ 70 yrs and median is somewhere around 80-90 yr. COVID-19 is therefore basically a common seasonal

respiratory virus, but if there is an Innate Immune Deficit that would result in uncontrolled replication and potential pneumonia [8].

Another Media Claim: Rampaging Virulent Variants?

Answer: No it just appears that way.

According to the main stream media and political leaders the human passaged COVID-19 variants currently engaging Australia and Northern Hemisphere infected zones (2021) such as the UK Mutant (alpha'), Indian Plume Mutants ('Delta', Kappa') are apparently highly rampaging and virulent transmissible variants. This is not true. They have been spread and globally transported as viral-dust clouds first by prevailing tropospheric winds from the plumes of human passaged viral aerosols that arose in the original host country, and were then brought to ground by precipitation (rain) in defined regions. Figure 1 is illustrative: In Australia the prevailing weather systems have struck repeatedly in Victoria (South West-West- North arc of Melbourne into Northern regions (Shepparton, and maybe also further north east to ACT). The East of the State of Victoria has been virus free, 2020, 2021; in Sydney, NSW a similar defined arc Bondi-South West-West Sydney suburbs in 2021. Thus a viral-laden contaminated environment causing large numbers of effectively (in time) simultaneous "mystery cases "of community transmissions i.e. the variant(s) only appear as "Rampaging Virulent variants".

However, they are dangerous in geriatric, aged care/nursing homes and in large three generation migrant families viz. closed clusters of Immune Defenceless elderly Co-morbid communities, where massive viral amplifications to trillions of virions contaminating all peoples and fomite surfaces in immediate environment. Thus carers, medical staff, family members and close associate *who then all develop a flu-like illness* (due to sheer viral dose loads at infection) are at risk of infection and likely to become PCR Positive. These are the ramping flare-ups in PCR Positive numbers per Day often seen in the published Cases Per Day Plots in both Victoria and NSW in 2021 (Figure 4) - and in the Victorian 2nd wave in 2020 (Figure 2). These striking features are NOT being discussed or mentioned in the mainstream media or press conferences. Such patients will be High PCR cycle number positives (i.e. very low numbers of virus or viral fragments in oral-nasal swab); and the primary infected amplifying elderly patients are expected to be very low PCR cycle number positive cases.

The other evidence against is that the " UK Mutant" entered Australia by jet plane in Jan-Feb 2021 at multiple portals of entry (Perth, Adelaide, Brisbane, Melbourne etc) and also dispersed contacts to regional cities in Australia, with large numbers (hundreds) of putative contacts- hotel cleaners, drivers, departure and arrival lounges, trains, buses, kiosk workers at food counters, taxis etc: The UK mutant DID NOT spread person-to-person in Australia (but may well have amplified in communities of Immune Defenceless Elderly co-morbids if such an entry had happened, but it did not. So again the group that should be monitored and cared for are our elderly citizens. As we have discussed [8] these negative transmission data led the Australian epidemiologist at The Australian National University, Professor Peter Collignon, to release his considered opinion to *The Australian* newspaper [28]: "...*In retrospect, the Melbourne lockdown*

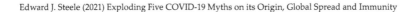

Edward J. Steele (2021) Exploding Five COVID-19 Myths on its Origin, Global Spread and Immunity

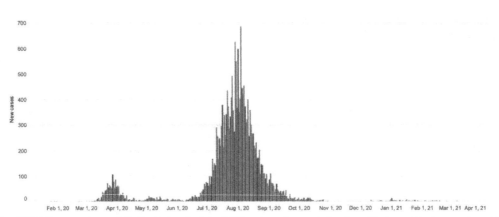

Figure 4: New SARS-CoV-2 cases per day recorded in Victoria, Australia, during 2020. These data can be accessed at https://www.dhhs.vic.gov.au/victorian-coronavirus-covid-19-data

was unnecessary... From my perspective, if you've got very little community transmission, I'm not sure that a short lockdown achieves much extra, if you've got good contact tracing and good testing," he said. ... "If I look at the lockdowns done in Adelaide, Brisbane, Perth, and now Melbourne, it didn't turn up one more case than contact tracing did. ... "The UK strain has not spread uncontrollably and wildly." Further research is required to understand why the putative highly virulent "UK Mutant" did not spread when introduced via multiple entry points into Australia in the first few months of 2021.

Current Myths#5

Efficacy of current Jab in the Arm vaccines?

We have discussed [8, 29] why all "Jab in the Arm" vaccines, whilst stimulating systemic immunity in the blood stream (IgG and IgM complement fixing and other classes of serum antibodies and later potentially enduring cytotoxic T lymphocyte adaptive immunity) may not be the best antigen-delivery route for activating enduring mucosal immunity (non-complement fixing yet very avid neutralising secretory IgA including mucosal adaptive T cell responses). This can be expected based simply on current textbook knowledge and past experimental experiences. This explains why many examples are now emerging of a failure of twice vaccinated individuals to be protected against catching COVID-19 e.g. many high profile politicians, sportsmen, whole US baseball teams travelling on the road, and of course the current wide-spread infections in the State of Israel despite most of the population being double vaccinated. Further, the phenomenon of antibody dependent enhancement (ADE) means that such individuals are at additional risk to formation of complement fixing antigen-antibody complexes in lung capillary airways if they become subsequently COVID-19 infected compounding the severity of the pathogenic cytokine storms [30]. This unintended adverse consequence has been discussed at length by Professor Dolores Cahill in a recent May 21 2021 interview [31]. Indeed apart from all the other deep and genuine concerns widely held by scientists and in the community about the safety and adverse affects of these novel engineered mRNA expression vector vaccines [31], it is clear also to us, that the vaccine roll out has played *little if any role* at all in the clear decline of the severity

of the pandemic in Northern Hemisphere infected zones [32]. Thus in exemplar countries, with a substantial vaccine roll out at time of writing, Sweden, Denmark, Netherlands, United Kingdom, France, Germany, Italy, and Israel it is clear the decline in respiratory disease severity as assessed by the metric "% COVIDI-19 associated Death" was well advanced and effectively over *before* the vaccine roll out began (Figure 5 for Denmark).

In the case of Denmark there is clear supportive independent evidence that natural herd immunity induced by prior oral-nasal infections throughout 2020 prior to the vaccine roll out was the clear cause of the type of decline in COVID case severity curve typical of many countries in Figure 5. Thus, to directly quote from [8]: "Natural infections with SARS-CoV-2 (in recovered patients) would therefore be expected to induce protective dimeric sIgA mucosal immunity. Certainly the recent longitudinal population scale study in Denmark implies that prior infection with SARS-CoV-2 affords upwards of 80% protection in the population under 65yr against reinfection between the first and second major surges of SARS-CoV-2 in Denmark in 2020; with the protective rate in the re-infected elderly vulnerable group a half lower again at 47% [33]. These are encouraging findings suggesting, at the time of writing, that natural 'herd immunity' could be well underway in Denmark and similar Northern hemisphere infected zones in 2020 and into likely surges and waves of SARS-

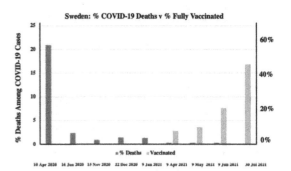

Figure 5: Percent Deaths Among COVID-19 cases versus the timing of the Vaccination roll out (% population vaccinated) in Denmark.

Edward J. Steele (2021) Exploding Five COVID-19 Myths on its Origin, Global Spread and Immunity

CoV-2 in 2021." There is also reason to believe, given the failure of a typical 'virulent' mutant (UK Mutant) to spread widely and quickly by P-to-P spread in Australia that the human passaged variants are attenuating- typical during decline phases of all epidemics as the host v parasite interaction tempers the replicative efficacy of the pathogen.

Our Recommendations

Given that all the fundamental assumptions of all governments and all their chief health advisors and epidemiologists have been wrong about every aspect of the COVID-19 pandemic - from its origin, its global mode of spread and the best way to medically treat and induce vaccine-immunity against oral-nasal acquired cold and flu infection, we recommend the following:

1. All lockdown measures to stop P-to-P be immediately lifted viz. social distancing, mask wearing, curfews, crowd controls, border closures, restrictions on business operations, school closures, church closures, sporting club closures, fitness centre closures etc.

2. Abolish vaccination rollouts and stop vaccine mandates and passports: All government (and main stream media) propaganda about vaccines protecting individuals needs to cease; all vaccine mandates of all types cease (for work, business trading, travel domestic and international) be lifted.

3. All State and International borders be immediately opened.

4. Immediate financial compensation scheme by the Federal Government to help all Australian citizens affected by any of these clearly erroneous and wrong emergency power laws especially small business owners.

5. An apology is in order for wrongful actions that have caused harm. From: Governments and their Chief Health Officers and associated organisations that implemented all lockdown and vaccine procedures. In Australia, The Therapeutic Goods Administration (TGA) includes major scientific organisations that actually gave a scientific blessing to the Federal and State Governments justifying their actions (The Peter Doherty Institute, The Australian Academy of Science) all need to apologise.

As we have suggested on numerous occasions the world needs to accept that suddenly emerging diseases from space have been a regular feature of our history and the evolution of life on Earth. Thus, the need for early warning surveillance, via orbiting satellite platforms and sampling the meteorite and cosmic dust on the external surface of the International Space Station. This would seem a logical step now for mankind to take as a unified collective. Since many suddenly emergent pandemic diseases are often cold or flu viruses that target the respiratory tract it would be sensible to design all such future vaccines to mimic the natural infection portal of entry via nose and mouth. Vaccines designed to be delivered via the oral-nasal route would certainly induce acquired mucosal secretory IgA immunity which is the most likely population-wide identifiable immune factors responsible the currently observed population-scale 'Herd Immunity' [32,33].

References

1. Wickramasinghe NC, Steele EJ, Gorczynski RM, Temple R, Tokoro G, et al. (2020) Predicting the Future Trajectory of COVID-19. *Virology: Current Research* 4: 1. https://www.hilarispublisher.com/open-access/predicting-the-future-trajectory-of-covid19-44601.html

2. Wickramasinghe NC, Wallis MK, Coulson SG, Kondakov A, Steele EJ, et al. (2020) Intercontinental Spread of COVID-19 on Global Wind Systems. *Virology: Current Research* 4: 1. https://www.hilarispublisher.com/open-access/intercontinental-spread-of-covid19-on-global-wind-systems-45198.html

3. Steele EJ, Gorczynski RM, Lindley RA, Tokoro G, Wallis DH, et al. (2021) Cometary Origin of COVID-19 (2021) *Infect Dis Ther* 2: 1-4. https://researchopenworld.com/cometary-origin-of-covid-19/

4. Steele EJ, Gorczynski RM, Carnegie P, Tokoro G, Wallis DH, et al. (2021) COVID-19 Sudden Outbreak of Mystery Case Transmissions in Victoria, Australia, May-June 2021: Strong Evidence of Tropospheric Transport of Human Passaged Infective Virions from the Indian Epidemic. *Infect Dis Ther* 2: 1-28. https://researchopenworld.com/covid-19-sudden-outbreak-of-mystery-case-transmissions-in-victoria-australia-may-june-2021-strong-evidence-of-tropospheric-transport-of-human-passaged-infective-virions-from-the-indian-epidemic/

5. Howard GA, Wickramasinghe NC, Rebhan H, Steele EJ, Gorczynski RM, et al. (2020) Mid-Ocean Outbreaks of COVID-19 with Tell-Tale Signs of Aerial Incidence *Virology: Current Research* 4: 2. https://www.hilarispublisher.com/open-access/midocean-outbreaks-of-covid19-with-telltale-signs-of-aerial-incidence.pdf

6. Steele EJ, Gorczynski RM, Rebhan H, Carnegie P, Temple R, et al. (2020) Implications of haplotype switching for the origin and global spread of COVID-19. *Virology: Current Research* 4: 2. https://www.hilarispublisher.com/open-access/implications-of-haplotype-switching-for-the-origin-and-global-spread-of-covid19.pdf

7. Wickramasinghe NC, Steele EJ, Nimalasuriya A, Gorczynki RM, Tokoro G, et al. (2020) Seasonality of Respiratory Viruses Including SARS-CoV-2. *Virology: Current Research* 4: 2. https://www.hilarispublisher.com/open-access/seasonality-of-respiratory-viruses-including-sarscov2-51923.html

8. Lindley RA, Steele EJ (2021) Analysis of SARS-CoV-2 haplotypes and genomic sequences during 2020 in Victoria, Australia, in the context of putative deficits in innate immune deaminase anti-viral responses. *Scand J Immunol.* 00:e13100 https://doi.org/10.1111/sji.13100

9. Steele EJ, Lindley RA (2020) Analysis of APOBEC and ADAR deaminase-driven Riboswitch Haplotypes in COVID-19 RNA strain variants and the implications for vaccine design. *Research Reports.* doi:10.9777/rr.2020.10001 https://companyofscientists.com/index.php/rr.

10. Pekar J, Worobey M, Moshiri N, Scheffler K, Wertheim JO (2021) Timing the SARS-CoV-2 index case in Hubei province. *Science* 372: 412-417. [crossref]

11. Steele EJ, Gorczynski RM, Lindley RA, Tokoro G, Temple R, et al. (2020) Origin of new emergent Coronavirus and Candida fungal diseases-Terrestrial or Cosmic? *Advances in Genetics* 106: 75-100. https://doi.org/10.1016/bs.adgen.2020.04.002

12. Huang C, Wang Y, Li X, Ren L, Zhao J, et al. (2020) Clinical Features of Patients Infected with 2019 Novel Coronavirus in Wuhan. *Lancet* 395: 497-506. [crossref]

13. Cohen, J (2020) Wuhan seafood market may not be source of novel virus spreading globally. *Science* https://www.sciencemag.org/news/2020/01/wuhan-seafood-market-may-not-be-source-novel-virus-spreading-globally

14. Luc Montagnier Gilmore Health https://www.gilmorehealth.com/chinese-coronavirus-is-a-man-made-virus-according-to-luc-montagnier-the-man-who-discovered-hiv/

15. Wickramasinghe NC, Steele EJ, Gorczynski RM, Temple R, Tokoro G, et al. (2020) Comments on the Origin and Spread of the 2019 Coronavirus. *Virology: Current Research* 4: 1. https://www.hilarispublisher.com/open-access/comments-on-the-origin-and-spread-of-the-2019-coronavirus-33365.html

16. Wickramasinghe NC, Steele EJ, Gorczynski RM, Temple R, Tokoro G, et al. (2020) Growing Evidence against Global Infection-Driven by Person-to-Person Transfer of COVID-19. *Virology Current Research* 4: 1. https://www.hilarispublisher.com/open-access/growing-evidence-against-global-infectiondriven-by-persontoperson-transfer-of-covid19.pdf

17. Hoyle F, Wickramasinghe NC (1979) Diseases from Space JM Dent & Son London

18. Steele EJ, Al Mufti S, Augustyn KA, Chandrajith R, Coghlan JP, et al (2018) Causes of Cambrian Explosion-Terrestrial or Cosmic? *Prog. Biophys Mol Biol* 136: 3-23. [crossref] https://doi.org/10.1016/j.pbiomolbio.2018.03.004

Edward J. Steele (2021) Exploding Five COVID-19 Myths on its Origin, Global Spread and Immunity

19. Steele EJ, Gorczyski RM, Lindley RA, Liu Y, Temple R, et al (2019) Lamarck and Panspermia-On the efficient spread of living systems throughout the cosmos. *Prog Biophys. Mol. Biol.* 149: 10-32. [crossref] https://doi.org/10.1016/j.pbiomolbio.2019.08.010

20. Acharya D, Liu G, Gack MU (2020) Dysregulation of type I interferon responses in COVID-19 *Nat. Rev. Immunol* 20: 397–98. [crossref]

21. Blanco-Melo D, Nilsson-Payant BE, Liu WC, Uhl S, Hoagland D, et al. (2020) Imbalanced Host Response to SARS-CoV-2 Drives Development of COVID-19. *Cell* 181: 1036-1045. [crossref]

22. Hadjadj J, Yatim N, Barnabei L, Corneau A, Boussier J, et al. (2020) Impaired type I interferon activity and exacerbated inflammatory responses in severe Covid-19 patients. *Science* 369: 718-724. [crossref]

23. Sette A, Crotty S (2021) Adaptive immunity to SARS-CoV-2 and COVID-19. *Cell* 184: 861-880. [crossref]

24. Lucas C, Wong P, Klein J, Castro TBR, Silva J, et al. (2020) Longitudinal analyses reveal immunological misfiring in severe COVID-19. *Nature* 584: 463-469. [crossref]

25. Zhang Q, Bastard P, Liu Z, Le Pen J, Moncada-Velez M, et al. (2020) Inborn errors of type I IFN immunity in patients with life-threatening COVID-19. *Science* 370: eabd4570. [crossref]

26. Bryant A, Lawrie TA, Dowswell T, Fordham EJ, Mitchell S, et al. (2021) Ivermectin for Prevention and Treatment of COVID-19 Infection: A Systematic Review, Meta-analysis, and Trial Sequential Analysis to Inform Clinical Guidelines. *American Journal of Therapeutics* 28: e434–e460. [crossref]

27. Luskin DL (2020) The failed experiment of COVID-19 lockdowns. *The Wall Street Journal.* https://www.wsj.com/articles/the-failed-experiment-of-covid-lockdowns-11599000890

28. Baxendale R, Robinson N (2021) Spread of UK coronavirus variant limited to close contacts. *The Australian.*

29. Gorczynski RM, Lindley RA, Steele EJ, Wickramasinghe NC. 2021 Nature of acquired immune responses, epitope specificity and resultant protection from SARS-CoV-2. Under submission

30. Lee WS, Wheatley AK, Kent SJ, DeKosky BJ (2020) Antibody-dependent enhancement and SARS-CoV-2 vaccines and therapies. *Nat. Microbiol* 5: 1185-1191. https://www.nature.com/articles/s41564-020-00789-5

31. Professor Dolores Cahill in a recent May 21 2021 interview on *Asia Pacific Today*: https://rumble.com/vjhasl-professor-dolores-cahill-says-the-mrna-vaccines-cause-injury-and-death..html

32. Steele EJ, Gorczynski RM, Lindley RA, Tokoro G, Wallis DH, et al. (2021) An End of the COVID-19 Pandemic in Sight? *Infectious Diseases and Therapeutics* 2: 1-5. https://researchopenworld.com/an-end-of-the-covid-19-pandemic-in-sight/

33. Hansen CH, Michlmayr D, Gubbels SM, Mølbak K, Ethelberg S (2021) Assessment of protection against reinfection with SARS-CoV-2 among 4 million PCR-tested individuals in Denmark in 2020: a population-level observational study. *The Lancet* 397: 1204-1212.

Citation:

Steele EJ, Gorczynski RM, Rebhan H, Tokoro G, Wallis DH, et al. (2021) Exploding Five COVID-19 Myths on its Origin, Global Spread and Immunity. *Infect Dis Ther* Volume 2(2): 1-15.

Edward J. Steele (2021) Exploding Five COVID-19 Myths on its Origin, Global Spread and Immunity

Appendix-A

Melbourne's *Herald Sun* Sat 1 Aug 2020

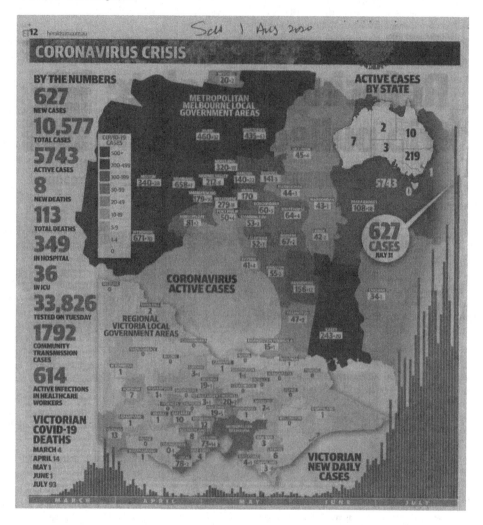

Appendix-B

Bob Woodward's 2020 book *RAGE* (From Robert Temple)

Please note Trump was repeating what Xi Jinping had told him: the virus goes through the air ... you just breathe the air and that's how it's passed. You don't have to touch things. The conversation between Xi Jinping and Donald Trump was on February 6, 2020. Trump passed Xi's comments on to Woodward on February 8. The passage occurs in the Prologue to Bob Woodward's 2020 book " RAGE". The passage occurs in the Prologue to the book, and here it is: "Trump called me at home about 9:00 p.m. on Friday, February 7, 2020. Since he had been acquitted in the Senate impeachment trial two days earlier, I expected he would be in a good mood. "Now we've

got a little bit of an interesting setback with the virus going in China," he said. He had spoken with President Xi Jinping of China the night before. 'Setback?' I was surprised the virus was on his mind, rather than his acquittal. There were only 12 confirmed cases in the United States. The first reported coronavirus death in the United States was three weeks away. The news had been all impeachment all the time. The Chinese were very focused on the virus, Trump said. "I think that goes away in two months with the heat," Trump said. 'You know as it gets hotter that tends to kill the virus. You know, you hope." He added, "We had a great talk for a long time. But we have a good relationship. I think we like each other a lot."

I reminded the president that in earlier interviews for this book he had told me he had harshly confronted President Xi about the Made in

Edward J. Steele (2021) Exploding Five COVID-19 Myths on its Origin, Global Spread and Immunity

China 2025 plan to overtake the United States and become the world's leading producer in high-tech manufacturing in 10 industries from driverless cars to biomedicine. "That's very insulting to me," Trump had told Xi. The president had also said with fierce pride that he was "breaking China's ass on trade" and caused China's annual growth rate to go negative. "Oh yeah, we've had some arguments," Trump acknowledged. So what had President Xi said yesterday? "Oh, we were talking mostly about the virus," Trump said. Why? I wondered. "Mostly?" "And I think he's going to have it in good shape," Trump said, "but you know, it's a very tricky situation." What made it "tricky"? "It goes through the air," Trump said. "That's always tougher than the touch. You don't have to touch things. Right? But the air, you just breathe the air and that's how it's passed. And so that's a very tricky one. That's a very delicate one. It's also more deadly than even your strenuous flus." "Deadly" was a very strong word. Something was obviously going on here that I was not focused on. (Pages xviii-xix of Woodward's book)

Appendix-C (This expanded 16 point version prepared by Edward J Steele, Herbert Rebhan)

Implausibility of Lab Leak Theories - Sixteen Points to Consider

1. A balloon launch or drone plane flight release of a viral 'bomb' in the stratosphere over China. The first question is where is the evidence of a balloon launch or drone flight Oct-Dec 2019 and where did it take place? What type of balloon and carriage or drone? How did it go undetected in China? Or undetected by US and European spy satellites?

2. If it was from a country foreign to China, the Chinese military would have neutralised it perhaps quickly? So was the launch itself then in China? if not China, somewhere else, such as strategic competitor South Korea? Japan? Taiwan?, USA/Guam,? Or from an aircraft carrier or ship in the Pacific Ocean? The viral vector vehicle would be releasing a pure culture of COVID-19 virions with an exact genomic sequence to the Hu-1 (Wuhan) reference sequence. It would need to be in the stratosphere on the $40°$ N line presumably above China in the period Oct-Dec 2019 (to fit global spread observations and known time lines)? Why at that point in history? But the release was big enough to blanket all of China on a wide scale, at about the same time?– but the biggest dose was over Hubei/Wuhan.

3. The other variant explanation is it was released from a high flying aircraft (spy plane?). Again, which country did it? and why was it not detected by satellite surveillance systems? If it came from outside China, surely it would have been detected and neutralised given China's high technology and space infrastructure?

4. Then we will want to know how and where was the exact COVID-19 29,903 nt sequence made? Wuhan Institute of Virology? Or was it at the National Institutes of Health (NIH), Bethesda Maryland- the latter is in the mix since Dr. Anthony Fauci's group were collaborators with the Wuhan laboratory (according to Tucker Carlson and many other news outlets).

5. So, finding the evidence for that balloon, drone or plane launch is important to satisfy the predictions listed. And at that time period?

What type of balloon/plane/drone and who made it? The evidence must be recorded in the computers of satellite surveillance platforms, or other intelligence listening/observing channels - as there are now many 'spies in the skies'.

6. The issue of where the plane/balloon/drone was launched from is important. Was it from: China?, Taiwan? Guam? South Korea? Japan? Alaska? Russian Siberia? What was the make of the launch vehicles and who made them? China? USA? Taiwan? Japan? North Korea?. Etc etc.) – again there must be satellite surveillance evidence of where the balloon or plane or drone departed from. It must exist somewhere. So, this is an important part of the predictions of the Lab Leak theory to explore further.

7. But before we go further, take notice the escalating set of *ad hoc* assumptions that already need to be tested. We are putting ourselves in the position of the Sci Fi fantasist: there must be other possibilities not thought of - because that is the nature of fantasy as opposed to science. One will never pin it down rationally. It has a fantastic life all of its own.

8. But if a product of a bioweapon development program why now with this garden variety common cold coronavirus? And why one that seriously causes bad respiratory outcomes (death) in only about 0.1% of the exposed population (with deficits in Type I and III Interferon responses [20-25]. Maybe the common cold is a test run? But by Who, and Why? Yes why design it this way? Why not kill all competitor enemies, particularly those of military age? Why not use a known virus of superior lethality and proven effectiveness, such as the Spanish Flu variant sequence (that is known and is located at least at NIH, and maybe in laboratories elsewhere- but anyone could synthesise it from public sequence information) - **and how was it planned that the designers of this agent would be protected?**

9. Notice again the multiplication of implausible assumptions- **this is a clear signature of a non-scientific fantasy**. Indeed we need the assistance of a real Sci Fi fantasist here – someone like Arthur C. Clark to give it authenticity.

10. The "human purpose and motivation factors" (Cold War Conspiracy) are necessary and must be plausible in this story- because that is the whole point of the story.

11. But there may be other non-State bad actors- like ISIS or Al Quaeda. After 9/11 the United States eventually found all the evidence, some quickly, then launched the missions to bomb their bases in Afghanistan and kill Osama Bin Laden, and then strike Iraq as Saddam Hussein threatened nuclear attacks on Israel and neighbours so he had to go as well. This short summary shows that Sharri Markson, Luc Montagnier, Wei Jingsheng, Nikolai Petrovsky and all the other writers elsewhere and at News Ltd on the influential *The Australian* newspaper in particular (Nick Cater, Adam Creighton, Paul Monk) have not thought through the fantastic implications of their proposals and conclusions. There must be, as was the case with the 9/11 strike on the World Trade Centre, a significant amount of discoverable 'human-factor' associated-evidence behind this stratospherically launched viral attack over China and thus the world in Oct-Dec 2019 that supports their theory.

Edward J. Steele (2021) Exploding Five COVID-19 Myths on its Origin, Global Spread and Immunity

12. So this human motivated attack was first made on China i.e. ALL of China Dec 2019-Jan 2020- but central China in the biggest viral dose- and there are many How? and Why? questions generating the predictions we list.

13. Because the first big explosive outbreaks are centered on the Chinese industrial heartland, is that the reason a foreign state would target China? But why do that as many countries trade and depend on Chinese products? And if not foreign inspired why would China do that to potentially destroy its extraordinary industrial hinterland?

14. So it goes full circle – it would have to be a strategic competitor like Taiwan or USA?

15. But then why arrange matters with the first strike, and knowledge of stratospheric jet streams, so the viral bombing run continued to first Tehran, then Lombardy/Italy, then Spain, …why those countries first, and why their elderly co-morbid citizens?

16. And then on to the "Mother of all Targets"…New York City!? Why in that order? And again why these targets first? There was also some viral dusting of South Korea and Japan early in Feb 2020- Why so?

All these questions are not trivial. But then you also have to pause to ask yourself this- where does all this fantastic mental effort end? The answer is, that with fantasy stories, **there is no end to creative SciFi imagination.** Scientific analyses of data and observations and then predictions are very different. Science sticks to known facts, plausible mechanisms, with a bare minimum number of useful assumptions, to explain the widest possible domain of observed facts in a coherent way - without multiplying the number of *ad hoc* assumptions. This is why our published explanation is preferred over all Lab Leak theories involving human intention.

Review Article

Overview SARS-CoV-2 Pandemic as January-February 2022: Likely Cometary Origin, Global Spread, Prospects for Future Vaccine Efficacy

Edward J. Steele[1,2*], Reginald M. Gorczynski[3], Robyn A. Lindley[1,4,5], Patrick R. Carnegie[6], Herbert Rebhran[7], Shirwan Al-Mufti[8], Daryl H Wallis[9], Gensuke Tokoro[9], Robert Temple[10], Ananda Nimalasuriya[11], George A Howard[12], Mark A. Gillman[13], Milton Wainwright[2,8], Stephen Coulson[9], Predrag Slijepcevic[14], Max K. Wallis[9], Alexander Kondakov[15] and N. Chandra Wickramasinghe[2,8,9,16]

[1]Melville Analytics Pty Ltd, Melbourne, VIC, Australia

[2]Centre for Astrobiology, University of Ruhuna, Matara, Sri Lanka

[3]University Toronto Health Network, Toronto General Hospital, University of Toronto, Toronto, ON, Canada

[4]GMDxgen Pty Ltd, Melbourne, Victoria, Australia

[5]Department of Clinical Pathology, The Victorian Comprehensive Cancer Centre, Faculty of Medicine, Dentistry & Health Sciences, University of Melbourne, Melbourne, Victoria, Australia

[6]School of Biological Sciences and Biotechnology, Murdoch University, WA, Australia

[7]C.Y.O' Connor ERADE Village Foundation, Piara Waters, Perth, WA, Australia

[8]Buckingham Centre for Astrobiology, University of Buckingham, MK18 1EG, UK

[9]Institute for the Study of Panspermia and Astroeconomics, Gifu, Japan

[10]History of Chinese Science and Culture Foundation, Conway Hall, London, UK

[11]Kaiser Permanente Riverside Medical, 10800 Magnolia Ave # 1, Riverside, CA 92505, USA

[12]Restoration Systems, LLC, Raleigh, NC, USA

[13]South African Brain Research Institute, 6 Campbell Street, Waverly, Johannesburg, South Africa

[14]School of Health Sciences, Brunel University, London, UK

[15]193/Sinyavinskaya str 16/11, Moscow, Russia

[16]National Institute of Fundamental Studies, Kandy, Sri Lanka

Corresponding author: Edward J. Steele, Melville Analytics Pty Ltd Melbourne, VIC, Australia; **E-mail:** e.j.steele@bigpond.com

Received: February 25, 2022; **Accepted:** March 03, 2022; **Published:** March 10, 2022

Abstract

As the SARS-CoV-2 pandemic is nearing its eventual end we focus on what we believe are two key omissions from the mainstream scientific literature and which have significant implications for how mankind manages the next global pandemic. We therefore review data, observations, analyses and conclusions from our series of papers published through 2020 and 2021 on its likely cometary origin and global spread. We also revisit our long held understanding of the superior effectiveness of intra-nasal vaccines against respiratory tract pathogens that involve induction of dimeric secretory IgA antibodies. While these two oversights seem disparate, together they provide us with new insights into our collective awareness of how we might view and address the next global pandemic. We begin with our hypothesis of the likely cometary origin of the SARS-CoV-2 virus via a bolide strike in the stratosphere on the night of October 11 2019 on the 40° N line over Jilin in NE China. Further global spread most likely occurred via prevailing wind systems transporting both the pristine cometary virus followed by continuing strikes from the same primary source as well as prior human-passaged virus transmitted by person to person spread and through contaminated dust in global wind systems. We also include a discussion of our prior work on data relating to vaccine protective efficacy. Finally we review the totality of evidence concerning the likely origin and global spread of the predominant variants of the virus 'Omicron' (+Delta mix?) from early to mid-December 2021 and extending into the first week January 2022. We describe the striking data showing the large numbers of infectious cases per day and outline the scale of what appears to be a global pandemic phenomenon, the causes of which are unclear and not completely understood. Firstly, these essentially *simultaneous* and sudden global-wide epidemic COVID-19 out breaks, appear to be *largely correlated with events external to the Earth, probably causing globally correlated precipitation events*. They appear related broadly to "Space Weather" events that render the Earth vulnerable to cosmic pandemic pathogen attack particularly during times of the minima of the Sunspot Solar Cycle which we are now currently passing through. Secondly, we argue that these sudden global-wide epidemic outbreaks of COVID-19 are specifically largely influenced by global wind transport and deposition mechanisms, the physics of which we need to further explore and comprehend. We conclude on an optimistic note for mankind. Given our prior knowledge of the effectiveness against respiratory tract pathogens of mucosal immunity involving induction of dimeric secretory IgA antibodies, we consider that the recently published intra-nasal vaccine data from laboratories based at the University of California, San Francisco and, independently at Yale University. These latter studies hold out great promise for the future development of both *pan-specific and specific* immunity against future pandemics caused by suddenly emergent respiratory pathogens, whether viral, bacterial or fungal.

Keywords: Global spread COVID-19, Origin COVID-19, Panspermia, Space weather, Vaccines respiratory pathogens

DOI: 10.31038/IDT.2022311

https://researchopenworld.com/overview-sars-cov-2-pandemic-as-january-february-2022-likely-cometary-origin-global-spread-prospects-for-future-vaccine-efficacy/

Infect Dis Ther, Volume 3(1): 1–16, 2022

Edward J. Steele (2022) Overview SARS-CoV-2 Pandemic as January-February 2022: Likely Cometary Origin, Global Spread, Prospects for Future Vaccine Efficacy

Introduction

The authors encompass a multi-disciplinary team across the scientific disciplines of Biology, Medicine and Physics in the broadest meaning of those categories of scientific understanding. We follow in the footsteps of the prior foundation studies published in many key historical works on Astronomy, Astrophysics and Astrobiology incorporating references to many peer reviewed papers (many in the journal *Nature*) by Fred Hoyle and N. Chandra Wickramasinghe [1-8]. Many authors on the current list of co-authors have made significant contributions to recent publications on diverse related matters, with some of these presciently dating just prior to the emergence of the COVID-19 pandemic [9-13]. This previous experience has heightened our analytical ability to scientifically track and plausibly explain the cometary origin and global spread of COVID-19. A number of reviews of the relevant datasets and conclusions therefore have already been published through 2020 and 2021 [14-16], including a compendium of chapters on 'Cosmic Genetic Evolution' all of which places the COVID-19 pandemic in its appropriate cosmic perspective [17]. Thus, a number of papers published by us since February 14 2020 review the data supporting our first claims of COVID-19's putative meteorite origins over China, following a cometary bolide strike on the 40° N Latitude line over Jilin, NE China on the night of October 11, 2019 [18]. We note here that the causative virus-carrying bolide may not have arrived at the top of the Earth's atmosphere as a cohesive body, but as an aggregation of dust particles, with individual radii of the order of micrometres. It is well known that of the order of 100 tonnes of such material are incident on the upper atmosphere daily. Approximately two thirds of micron sized micrometeorites can plausibly be assumed to be of cometary origin. Modelling of their dynamics in the atmosphere shows that a significant fraction of these particles reach the surface of the Earth without experiencing destructive heating [19].

Our subsequent publications in the early weeks of the pandemic focused on the relative lack of evidence for person-to person transmission as the primary infection mechanism for COVID-19 [20]. Indeed, detailed analyses of the active region-wide epidemic episodes around the globe during 2020 and 2021 occurred initially (late 2019 to March through April 2020) mainly on the 30-50° N latitude band with limited outbreaks taking place outside this band [21]. We developed explanations of the unfolding data relating to the pandemic as it engulfed the world from the later months of 2019. In our modelling we took full account of genetic, immunologic and epidemiologic evidence, as well as the role of geophysical and atmospheric processes including a possible continuation of a space input of the virus.

In summary, our main analyses were as follows:

a. The genetic analysis of the SARS-CoV-2 viral genomes and the deaminase-mediated haplotype variation and adaptation strategy of the coronavirus as it navigated infections in different susceptible/vulnerable human hosts and genetic backgrounds first in China then Spain, France and New York with eventual infection documented in Australia from January through to September 2020 [15,18,20-23].

b. The immunologic analysis of the host-parasite relationship and vaccine efficacy of systemic versus mucosal-local antigen routes of immunization [22-24].

c. The epidemiologic analyses of both the temporal order of epidemics and their global location, including the role of prevailing winds systems, remote outpost strikes (O'Higgins Chilean Army outpost in Antarctica), sudden island strikes and strikes on ships at sea [15,16,25,26].

d. The geophysics and atmospheric physics of the major convection cells plus jet streams sweeping up and depositing virus-bearing dust, including human-passaged aerosol transferring them in the northern hemisphere with limited connection to the south [21,27-29]. Global connectivity is effective on the 10-day time-scale. The evidence of long-distance tropospheric transportation in the Northern Hemisphere is provided by the COVID-19 genomic sequence data from the *Grand Princess* cruise ship off San Francisco (engaged late February 2020) which displayed the exact same largely unmutated genomic sequence (Hu-1) as determined in China during December 2019 and January 2020 [16,22].

e. The role of human-passaged (and created) regional variants lofted or plumed attached to microdust particles into the troposphere and the global wind systems, in likely attenuated form [16,28,29] see also reference in these papers to the independent assessment of the role of global wind transportation systems in past influenza pandemics in [30] Hammond et al. 1989. Thus these authors noted the large-scale eddy circulation as causing occasional lofting and patchy deposition of virus carriers. It saw survival of the influenza virus in the air and solar radiation as important, though did not know of survival against UV in clumps, or embedded in micro-dust particles.

All of our prior analyses and conclusions and its relation to the wider scientific literature on SARS-CoV-2/COVID-19 can be found in our past publications, which can be accessed at https://www.academia.edu/50814212/ Papers and Summary Interviews on Origin and Global Spread of COVID 19 Wickramasinghe and colleagues. The URL links to all relevant video interviews involving N. Chandra Wickramasinghe and Edward J Steele can be found in this list and at *The Cosmic Tusk* website of George A. Howard. https://cosmictusk.com

We have also considered and refuted the main popular explanations that were spreading uncritically abroad in both the scientific and popular media, concerning the protective efficacy of all systemic-delivered vaccines and the putative origins of COVID-19, the latter as either a jump from a latent SARS-CoV-1 animal reservoir (bat, pangolin, cat) or as a human-engineered COVID-19 genome. In the latter case this infection, identical in genomic sequence to the original Hu-1 reference (isolated in China in December 2019, NC_045512.2), was postulated to have been released from a Chinese laboratory (Wuhan Institute of Virology) either accidently or deliberately. We show both these origin explanations are scientifically implausible or impossible on genetic grounds [15,29]. Indeed, the Wuhan Lab Leak and related narratives are clearly implausible and simply do not explain *what was actually observed* in the first month or two of the pandemic.

Edward J. Steele (2022) Overview SARS-CoV-2 Pandemic as January-February 2022: Likely Cometary Origin, Global Spread, Prospects for Future Vaccine Efficacy

Against this backdrop, we have analysed a putative "Space Weather" and "solar-wind pulse" like event [10,11] which, although poorly understood at the present time, may well account for the manner in which the pandemic signature became evident globally. At the time of writing this review the pandemic appears to have waned in severity via the natural processes of natural Herd Immunity, attenuation of the human-passaged variants and viral decay in the environment [31,32]. From the Cases per Day Curves (Figures 1-8) we think these observations have been the major new phenomenon of the pandemic that has become manifest in the data from the middle of December 2021.

Omicron/Delta Outbreaks though December 2021 and January 2022 in Global Synchrony

Cases-per-day plots for selected locations (captured as screen shots on January 3 2022) are shown in Figures 1-5 to illustrate the extreme synchronous or simultaneous eruptions of COVID-19 epidemics (Omicron/Delta mix?) in the Northern Hemisphere regions Figures 1-3 (United Kingdom, Denmark, France, Italy, Ontario, Quebec, New York, Florida, Hawaii, Aruba), and in the Southern Hemisphere, Figures 4 and 5, embracing populated regions in South America, Africa and Australia (Buenos Aires, Angola, Kenya, Mozambique, and in Australia : South Australia, Victoria, New South Wales and Queensland). In Table 1 we list all regions of the world that display *conformal* exponentially rising cases per day curves over the *same* time interval as illustrated by the selected examples in Figures 1-5. Countries or regions with low or equivocal rises in case numbers are listed in Table 2. In some regions there was a clear peak of the presumed Omicron outbreak beginning about a week or two earlier with case numbers per day coming down in

those regions (Table 3). However, many countries are 'null zones' with respect to this time period experiencing no rising epidemic profile (Table 4).

The reader can scrutinise the data at the URL site for '*Coronavirus disease statistics*' shown in the legend to the figures. The predominant pandemic 'strain' evident in most regions of the world prior to these extraordinary explosive and temporally coordinated epidemic outbreaks was the 'Delta' strain (and related Indian-plumed strains) from the massive Indian epidemic of April-May 2021, which we hypothesized was released as a very large aerosol of many millions of trillions of virions into the troposphere for redistribution to globally distant regions via prevailing W-E, E-W and N-S wind systems [28]. The Omicron variant was found first in Botswana on November 2, 2021 and was widely assumed to have emerged first in South Africa. We discuss speculative causes of the emergence of the Omicron variant and the probable region of its origin in Section 3.

What plausible explanations can be provided for the data in Figures 1-5 and Table 1-4, and in particular the essentially simultaneous eruptions of region-specific epidemics of COVID-19 in so many different regions across the world? This is not a question that can be easily resolved. The strong indications are of a globally correlated phenomenon that we do not fully understand. One explanation could be connected to space weather events associated with the deep Sun-Spot minimum between Solar Cycles 24 and 25 [10,11]. Unseasonal weather that has been reported both in the Northern and Southern hemispheres (e.g.UK and Australia) during this time period may give a hint in this direction. The sheer numbers and global coverage of infection essentially eliminates Person-to-Person spread as the sole or main causative explanation.

Table 1: Countries and Regions all showing clear Synchronous Epidemics as shown in Figures 1-5 as captured January 3 2022 (use URL Figures 1-5)

Albania, Angola, Argentina (Buenos Aires City and Region in main), **Aruba, Australia** (SA, Vic, NSW, Tas, Qld but not WA, NT, the latter could be airplane visitors), **Barbados, Belize, Bermuda, Bolivia, Botswana, British Virgin Islands, Burundi, Canada** (Alberta, British Columbia, Manitoba, New Brunswick, Newfoundland and Labrador, Northwest Territories, Nova Scotia, Ontario, Prince Edward Island, Quebec, Saskatchewan), **Cape Verde, Cayman Islands, Comoros, Cote d'Ivoire, Croatia, Curacao, Cyprus, Denmark, Dominion Republic, Ecuador, Ethiopia, Faroe Islands, Fiji, Finland, France, Gabon, Ghana, Gibraltar, Greece, Guinea, Guyana, Iceland, Ireland, Israel, Italy, Jamaica, Kenya, Kuwait, Lebanon, Luxemburg, Madagascar, Malawi, Mali, Malta, Mauritania, Mexico, Montenegro, Mozambique, Netherlands, Panama, Peru, Portugal, Qatar, Reunion, Rwanda, Saint Barthelemy, Saint kitts and Nevis, San Marino, Sierra Leone, Sint Maarten, South Sudan** (coming down rapidly), **Spain, Sweden, Switzerland, Togo, Uganda, United Kingdom** (England, Northern Ireland, Scotland, Wales), **United States** (Alabama, Arkansas, California, Colorado, Connecticut, Delaware, Florida, Georgia, Hawaii, Illinois, Louisiana, Massachusetts, Mississippi, Nevada, New Jersey, New York, North Carolina, Ohio, Oregon, Pennsylvania, Puerto Rico, Rhode Island, South Carolina, Tennessee, Texas, US Virgin Islands, Virginia, Washington, Washington D.C.), **Zambia.**

Table 2: Countries and Regions showing only a Low or Equivocal Synchronous Epidemics as shown in Figures 1-5 as captured January 3 2022 (use URL Figures 1-5)

Andorra, Algeria, Austria, Bahrain, Belgium, Bulgaria, Burkina Faso, Caribbean Netherland, Canada (Nunavut), **Chad, Columbia, Estonia, Greenland, Grenada, Hong Long, Latvia, Liberia, Mauritius, Mayotte, Monaco, Morocco, Niger, Saint Lucia, Saint Martin, Sao Tome and Principe, Saudi Arabia, Serbia, Senegal, Seychelles, Suriname, The Bahamas** (Visitors from infected zones?), **Turkey, Turks and Caicos Islands, United States** (Indiana, Kansas, Kentucky, Michigan, Minnesota, Nebraska, New Hampshire, North Dakota, Northern Mariana Islands, Oklahoma, Utah, Vermont, West Virginia, Wisconsin), **Uruguay.**

Table 3: Countries and Regions all showing an explosive epidemic beginning a week or two earlier relative to those shown in Figures 1-5 as captured January 3 2022 (use URL Figures 1-5)

Namibia, Nigeria, Norway, South Africa, South Korea, Trinidad and Tobago, Zimbabwe

Table 4: Countries and Regions all showing no explosive epidemic or obvious begining a week or two earlier as Figures 1-5 as captured January 3 2022 (use URL Figures 1-5)

Afghanistan ,Anguilla, Antigua and Barbuda, Armenia, Azerbaijan, Bangladesh, Belarus, Benin, Bhutan, Bosnia and Herzegovina, Brazil, Brunei, Cambodia, Cameroon, Central Africa Republic, Chile, China , Dominica, Egypt, El Salvador, Equatorial Guinea, Eswatini, Falkland Islands, French Guinea, French Polynesia, Guadeloupe, Guatemala, Guernsey, Guinea-Bissau, Haiti, Honduras, India, Indonesia, Iran, Iraq, Isle of Man, Japan, Jersey, Jordan, Kazakhstan, Kosovo, Kyrgyzstan, Laos, Lesotho, Libya, Liechtenstein, Lithuania, Macao, Malaysia, Maldives, Martinique, Moldova, Mongolia, Montserrat, Myanmar, Nepal, New Caledonia, New Zealand, Nicaragua, North Macedonia, Oman, Pakistan, Palestine, Philippines, Poland, Republic of Congo, Romania, Russia, Saint Pierre and Miquelon, Saint Vincent and the Grenadines, Singapore, Slovakia, Somalia, Slovenia, Sri Lanka, Sudan, Syria, Taiwan, Tajikistan, Tanzania , Thailand, The Gambia, Timor-Leste, Tunisia, Ukraine, United States (American Samoa, Guam, Iowa-maybe a little earlier?), **Uzbekistan, Venezuela, Vatican City, Vietnam, Yemen.**

Edward J. Steele (2022) Overview SARS-CoV-2 Pandemic as January-February 2022: Likely Cometary Origin, Global Spread, Prospects for Future Vaccine Efficacy

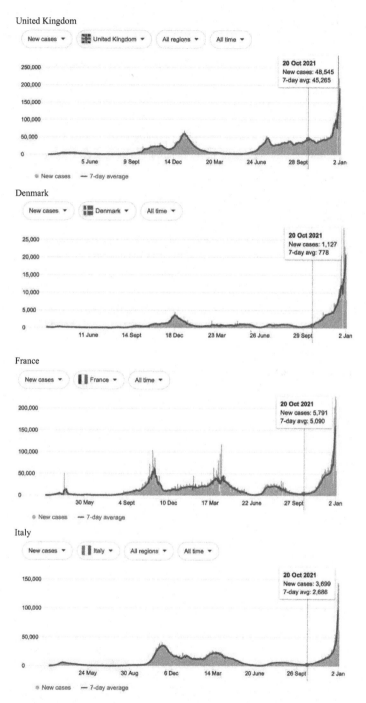

Figure 1: COVID-19 Case Rises in Selected Global Locations- Europe: United Kingdom, Denmark, France, Italy. Exponential rises in new COVID-19 cases per day as captured January 3 2022 from the Google searched site: "Coronavirus disease statistics". The URL opens at the Australia dashboard but all countries and regions can be searched via the Cases and Deaths search Menus for that region. Click or copy and paste URL into your browser : https://www.google.com.au/search?hl=en&ei=vWxyX7ipM4-m9QP18If4CQ&q=Coronavirus+disease+statistics&oq=Coronavirus+disease+statistics&gs_lcp=CgZwc3ktYWIQAzICCAAyAggAOgQIABBHOgcIABCxAxBDOgQIABBDULZUWPh1YJF7aABwAXgAgAH2AYgBvA6SAQYwLjEwLjGYAQCgAQMgAQdnd3Mtd2l6yAEGwAEB&sclient=psy-ab&ved=0ahUKEwj4-47e-4zsAhUPU30KHXX4AZ8Q4dUDCAw&uact=5

Edward J. Steele (2022) Overview SARS-CoV-2 Pandemic as January-February 2022: Likely Cometary Origin, Global Spread, Prospects for Future Vaccine Efficacy

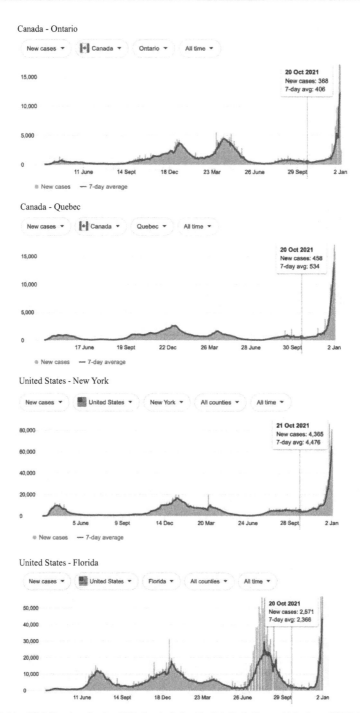

Figure 2: COVID-19 Case Rises in Selected Global Locations- Canada and USA: Ontario, Quebec, New York, Florida. Exponential rises in new COVID-19 cases per day as captured January 3 2022 from the Google searched site: "Coronavirus disease statistics". The URL opens at the Australia dashboard but all countries and regions can be searched via the Cases and Deaths search Menus for that region. Click or copy and paste URL into your browser : https://www.google.com.au/search?hl=en&ei=vWxyX7ipM4-m9QP18If4CQ&q=Coronavirus+disease+statistics&oq= Coronavirus+disease+statistics&gs_lcp=CgZwc3ktYWIQAzICCAAyAggAOgQIABBHOgcIABCxAxBDOgQIABBDULZUWPh1YJF7aABwAXgAgAH2AYgBvA6SAQYwLjEwLjGYAQCgAQ GqAQdnd3Mtd2l6yAEGwAEB&sclient=psy-ab&ved=0ahUKEwj4-47e-4zsAhUPU30KHXX4AZ8Q4dUDCAw&uact=5

Edward J. Steele (2022) Overview SARS-CoV-2 Pandemic as January-February 2022: Likely Cometary Origin, Global Spread, Prospects for Future Vaccine Efficacy

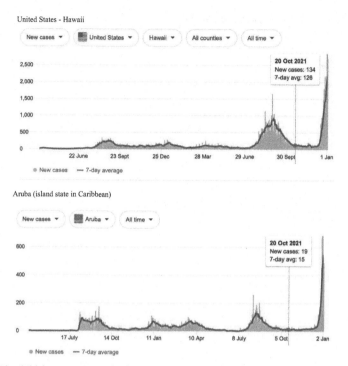

United States - Hawaii

Aruba (island state in Caribbean)

Figure 3: COVID-19 Case Rises in Selected Global Locations- Hawaii and Aruba . Exponential rises in new COVID-19 cases per day as captured January 3 2022 from the Google searched site : "Coronavirus disease statistics". The URL opens at the Australia dashboard but all countries and regions can be searched via the Cases and Deaths search Menus for that region. Click or copy and paste URL into your browser : https://www.google.com.au/search?hl=en&ei=vWxyX7ipM4-m9QP18If4CQ&q=Coronavirus+disease+statistics&oq=Coronavirus+disease+statistics&gs_lcp=CgZwc3ktYWIQAzICCAAyAggAOgQIABBHOgcIABCxAxBDOgQIABBDULZUWPh1YJF7aABwAXgAgAgAH2AYgBvA6SAQYwLjEwLjGYAQCgAQGqAQdnd3Mtd2l6yAEGwAEB&sclient=psy-ab&ved=0ahUKEwj4-47e-4zsAhUPU30KHXX4AZ8Q4dUDCAw&uact=5

A more plausible scientific explanation lies in massive region-wide in falls from the sky (the troposphere) of prior human-passaged then aerosol-plumed COVID-19 virions lofted into the troposphere and introduced into prevailing wind systems. Given current Omicron case densities, we tentatively assume a northern European origin followed by transport of viral aerosol-clouds across the Atlantic from an origin in the UK/North Europe (?), into the Pacific and Atlantic prevailing winds onto to Africa and thence to Australia.

We are still left with the conundrum of why now, and why at the same time all over the globe? The data in Figures 1-5 are but a small subset of the large number of global-wide regions in the Northern Hemisphere, Equatorial Regions, Island States, and Southern Hemisphere *all struck like this at the same time* (Tables 1 and 2). In addition, over this time period, many Atlantic cruise ships with double vaccinated and pre-screened passengers also became suddenly engaged with COVID-19 (assumed Omicron see [33,34]) including a fully vaccinated US Navy ship [35]. There was also the well-documented sudden outbreak from December 14 involving large numbers of fully vaccinated personnel at a remote Belgian Research Station in Antarctica thousands of miles from civilization [36]. This is indeed strikingly reminiscent of similar strikes on ships at sea and remote locations during the early phases of the pandemic in 2020 [15,16,25], including the sudden strike on the island of Sri Lanka Oct 4-5 2020 [26], and more recently on Taiwan presumed to have occurred as a result of Indian-plumed Delta virus

which struck suddenly for first time from 14 May 2021 [28]. All indications are of a globally-correlated environmental trigger that we cannot fully understand at the present time.

One possible explanation is that globally dispersed viral aerosol-clouds (Omicron/Delta variant mix?) were released and lofted following human passage, and were widely distributed in the troposphere remaining viable although not immediately falling to Earth or ocean over many different regions of the world. A putative global trigger in mid-December 2021 might be postulated that brought such viral particles to earth virtually simultaneously around the world. This may have been ultimately facilitated by, but not been dependent upon, rain/precipitation [28,29]. The resulting virus-contaminated environments would then ignite outbreaks of mystery unlinked Omicron/Delta cases on a large scale giving the appearance of superfast infective spreading in a given populated contaminated region as we have previously discussed in detail for the outbreaks of mystery infections in Victoria, Australia [28,29]. This is a plausible explanation for the synchronous sudden rises of COVID-19 globally. The fact there are many "null" zones (Table 4) and 'low' or equivocal regions (Table 2) adds to the patchy cloud-like nature of the viral distribution in the troposphere prior to and coinciding with the solar cycle minimum. That is, it arises as deposition from the convection-driven upper troposphere which is patchy over a range of distance scales.

Edward J. Steele (2022) Overview SARS-CoV-2 Pandemic as January-February 2022: Likely Cometary Origin, Global Spread, Prospects for Future Vaccine Efficacy

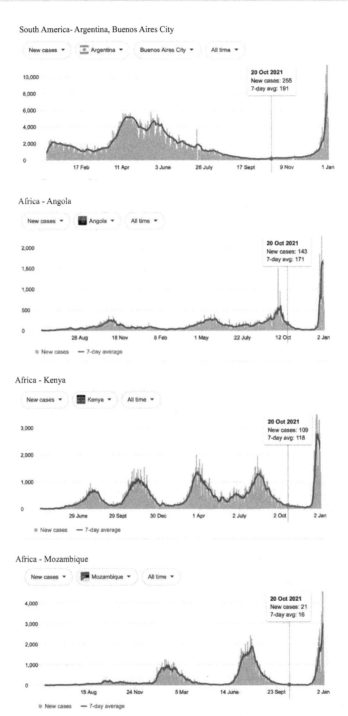

Figure 4: COVID-19 Case Rises in Selected Global Locations- South America and Africa: Buenos Aires, Angola, Kenya, Mozambique. Exponential rises in new COVID-19 cases per day as captured January 3 2022 from the Google searched site: "Coronavirus disease statistics". The URL opens at the Australia dashboard but all countries and regions can be searched via the Cases and Deaths search Menus for that region. Click or copy and paste URL into your browser : https://www.google.com.au/search?hl=en&ei=vWxyX7ipM4-m9QP18If4CQ&q=Coronavirus+dise ase+statistics&oq=Coronavirus+disease+statistics&gs_lcp=CgZwc3ktYWIQAzICCAAyAggAOgQIABBHOgcIABCxAxBDOgQIABBDULZUWPh1YJF7aABwAXgAgAH2AYgBvA6SAQYwL jEwLjGYAQCgAQGqAQdnd3Mtd2l6yAEGwAEB&sclient=psy-ab&ved=0ahUKEwj4-47e-4zsAhUPU30KHXX4AZ8Q4dUDCAw&uact=5

Edward J. Steele (2022) Overview SARS-CoV-2 Pandemic as January-February 2022: Likely Cometary Origin, Global Spread, Prospects for Future Vaccine Efficacy

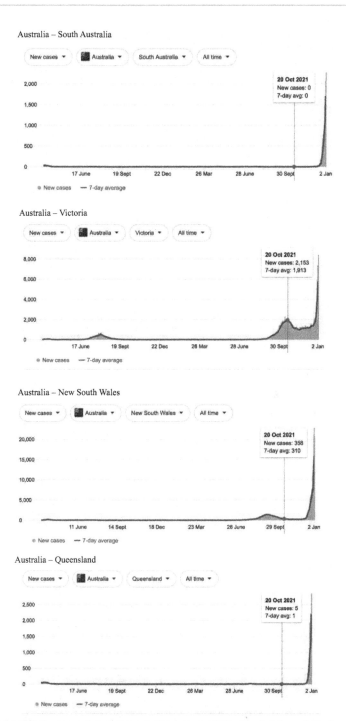

Figure 5: COVID-19 Case Rises in Selected Global Locations- Australia: South Australia, Victoria, New South Wales, Queensland . Exponential rises in new COVID-19 cases per day as captured January 3 2022 from the Google searched site: "Coronavirus disease statistics". The URL opens at the Australia dashboard but all countries and regions can be searched via the Cases and Deaths search Menus for that region. Click or copy and paste URL into your browser : https://www.google.com.au/search?hl=en&ei=vWxyX7ipM4-m9QP18If4CQ&q=Coronavirus+disease+statistic s&oq=Coronavirus+disease+statistics&gs_lcp=CgZwc3ktYWIQAzICCAAyAggAOgQIABBHOgcIABCxAxBDOgQIABBDULZUWPh1YJF7aABwAXgAgAH2AYgBvA6SAQYwLjEwLjGYAQ CgAQGqAQdnd3Mtd2l6yAEGwAEB&sclient=psy-ab&ved=0ahUKEwj4-47e-4zsAhUPU30KHXX4AZ8Q4dUDCAw&uact=5

Edward J. Steele (2022) Overview SARS-CoV-2 Pandemic as January-February 2022: Likely Cometary Origin, Global Spread, Prospects for Future Vaccine Efficacy

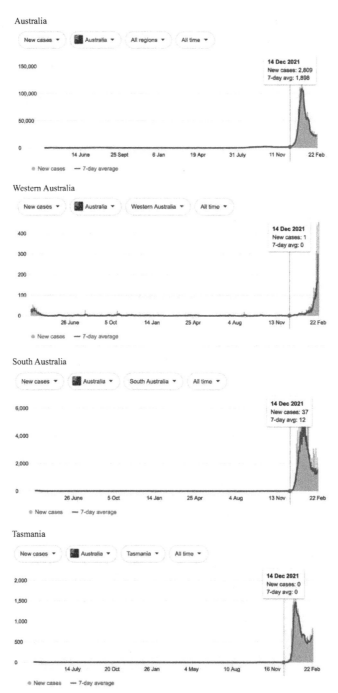

Figure 6: COVID-19 Case Rises in the whole Australia, and Western Australia, South Australia, Tasmania (similar right hand side shoulders observed for Northern Territory, Australian Capital Territory). Exponential rises in new COVID-19 cases per day as captured February 24 2022 from the Google searched site : "Coronavirus disease statistics". The URL opens at the Australia dashboard but all countries and regions can be searched via the Cases and Deaths search Menus for that region. Click or copy and paste URL into your browser : https://www.google.com.au/search?hl=en&ei=vWxyX7ipM4-m9QP18If4CQ&q=Coronavirus+disease+statistics&oq=Coronavirus+disease+statistics&gs_lcp=CgZwc3ktYWIQAzICCAAyAggAOgQIABBHOgcIABCxA xBDOgQIABBDDULZUWPh1YJF7aABwAXgAgAH2AYgBvA6SAQYwLjEwLjGYAQCgAQGqAQdnd3Mtd2l6yAEGwAEB&sclient=psy-ab&ved=0ahUKEwj4-47e-4zsAhUPU30KHXX4AZ8 Q4dUDCAw&uact=5

Edward J. Steele (2022) Overview SARS-CoV-2 Pandemic as January-February 2022: Likely Cometary Origin, Global Spread, Prospects for Future Vaccine Efficacy

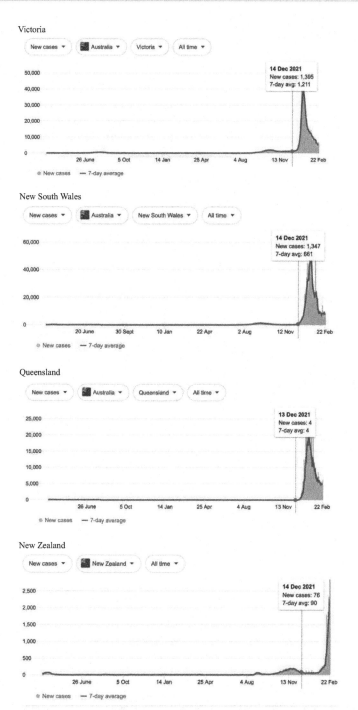

Figure 7: COVID-19 Case Rises in Victoria, New South Wales, Queensland and New Zealand (similar rising 'hockey stick' cases per day graph seen for French Polynesia, and Chile). Exponential rises in new COVID-19 cases per day as captured February 24 2022 from the Google searched site: "Coronavirus disease statistics". The URL opens at the Australia dashboard but all countries and regions can be searched via the Cases and Deaths search Menus for that region. Click or copy and paste URL into your browser: https://www.google.com.au/search?hl=en&ei=vWxyX7ipM4-m9 QP18If4CQ&q=Coronavirus+disease+statistics&oq=Coronavirus+disease+statistics&gs_lcp=CgZwc3ktYWIQAzICCAAyAggAOgQIABBHOgcIABCxAxBDOgQIABBDULZUWPh1YJF7aA BwAXgAgAH2AYgBvA6SAQYwLjEwLjGYAQCgAQGqAQdnd3Mtd2l6yAEGwAEB&sclient=psy-ab&ved=0ahUKEwj4-47e-4zsAhUPU30KHXX4AZ8Q4dUDCAw&uact=5

Edward J. Steele (2022) Overview SARS-CoV-2 Pandemic as January-February 2022: Likely Cometary Origin, Global Spread, Prospects for Future Vaccine Efficacy

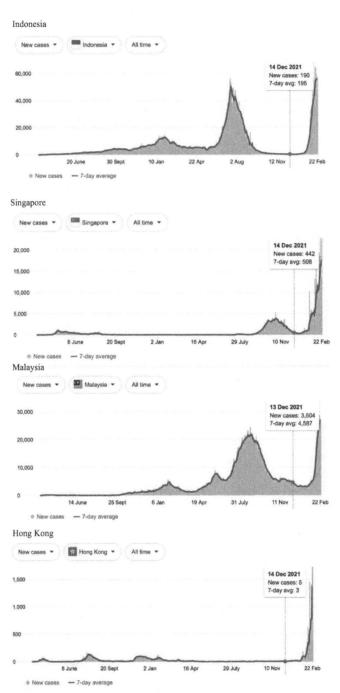

Figure 8: COVID-19 Case Rises in Indonesia, Singapore, Malaysia, Hong Kong (similar rising 'hockey stick' cases per day graph seen for Bhutan, Brunei, Thailand, Vietnam, Cambodia, Myanmar, South Korea, Mongolia possible shoulder in Japan). Exponential rises in new COVID-19 cases per day as captured February 24 2022 from the Google searched site: "Coronavirus disease statistics". The URL opens at the Australia dashboard but all countries and regions can be searched via the Cases and Deaths search Menus for that region. Click or copy and paste URL into your browser : https://www.google.com.au/search?hl=en&ei=vWxyX7ipM4-m9QP18If4CQ&q=Coronavirus+disease+statistics&oq=Coronavirus+disease+statistics&gs_lcp=CgZw c3ktYWIQAzICCAAyAggAOgQIABBHOgcIABCxAxBDOgQIABBDULZUWPh1YJF7aABwAXgAgAH2AYgBvA6SAQYwLjEwLjGYYAQCgAQGgAQGqAQdnd3Mtd2l6yAEGwAEB&sclient=psy-ab&ved=0ahUKEwj4-47e-4zsAhUPU30KHXX4AZ8Q4dUDCAw&uact=5

Edward J. Steele (2022) Overview SARS-CoV-2 Pandemic as January-February 2022: Likely Cometary Origin, Global Spread, Prospects for Future Vaccine Efficacy

Another possibility, given the global nature of the present observations, and thus which cannot be ignored as a causative factor, is the known vulnerability of the Earth to pandemics during the minima of the sunspot Solar Cycle [10,11]. Thus it could be an ill-defined and poorly understood physical event broadly classed as a "Space Weather" event associated with the sunspot cycle minimum, particularly now between cycles 24 and 25, where we may be most vulnerable to "pathogen attack" from the outside the Earth: viz.

"..the Earth's magnetosphere, and the interplanetary magnetic field in its vicinity, are modulated by the solar wind that in turn controls the flow of charged particles onto the Earth [4]. During times of sunspot minima, particularly deep sunspot minima, a general weakening of magnetic field occurs which would be accompanied by an increase in the flux of cosmic rays (GCR's) and also of electrically charged interstellar and interplanetary dust particles"... bringing charged particles (virus-laden dust particles) to earth. Wickramasinghe et al. 2019 [11].

Getting back to the original events in late 2019 we can advance another specific scenario on what *actually happened* across China which was initiated in the stratosphere over N-E China in late December 2019, and then in early January 2020 after the initial input of cometary virus-carrying dust. The virus became strongly amplified in humans across China until lock-down measures came into full force. Despite efforts to wash down the streets, the virus's long lifetime and persistence in viable condition on dust particles enabled it to spread widely in the environment. When appropriate wind conditions arrived, the virus-carrying dust was readily swept up in tropospheric winds into the East-Asian subtropical jet stream, carrying it across the Pacific to southern USA and Western Europe. Precipitation into local wind systems thus caused infection on a state-wide and country-wide scale. In 2021 similar wind-borne viral-laden dust spread over the entire sub-continent of India causing sudden eruptions of COVID-19 infections (via PANGO variants Alpha, Kappa, and Delta at least). These country-wide sudden eruptions have been noted before although they have not been fully understood [14,16,28,29].

Finally, we should consider another putative "pulse-like" causative factor that contributed to the synchronous nature of the sudden outbreaks of Omicron/Delta infections around the world. This phenomenon was not previously explored except in the broadest of terms in our earlier publications [12,13]. It is most probably related to the fact that most viruses in their cell-to-cell infection cycle are transported as enveloped *clusters* of mature virions [37]. This may be important if an influence associated with "Space Weather" external to the Earth somehow triggered the liberation of smaller clusters of virions associated with tropospheric dust clouds over any given region. A dust particle of 2-3 microns could theoretically envelope 40-60 COVID-19 virions. If these were suddenly liberated to fall to ground as smaller clusters (doubletons or triplets) that would result in a ten-fold sudden increase in putative infective virion clusters floating down to contaminate a terrestrial environment. The nature of this virion liberation "trigger" is unknown (temp/pressure/radiation?) so this is still a highly speculative scenario that we present for further exploration.

However, we can now add further observations, as the manuscript was being prepared for final submission. This is again consistent with a series of "pulse-like" infection events enveloping a large fraction of the globe at the *same* time (prior 24-48 h). (This has been noted as January 14 2022 from the "*Coronavirus disease statistics*" database.) The following countries appear to have been all engaged in an exponential sharp rise in COVID-19 new cases per day, a synchronous effect that was not evident in the earlier survey of January 3 2022. These countries are: Brazil, Bosnia Herzegovina, Costa Rica, Cuba, Djibouti, Egypt, French Guiana, Guatemala, Guinea-Bissau, Haiti, Hungary, Liechtenstein, Lithuania, Martinique, Maldives, Montserrat, Morocco, Monaco, North Macedonia, Norway, Pakistan, Poland, Slovenia, India, Nepal, Bhutan, Kyrgyzstan, Philippines, Japan, Romania, Sao Tome and Principe, Taiwan, Thailand, Trinidad and Tobago, Tunisia, Turks and Caicos Islands, Ukraine, Mongolia, and Venezuela. All these regions could be part of the same mid-December 2021 tropospheric in-fall process just described but show an apparent delay due to data reporting and database updating.

In addition, we surveyed plots of new cases per day from the same database as captured 24 February 2022. We detected a clear further set of global-wide synchronous eruptions of COVID-19 epidemics - presumed Omicron/Delta (mix) - in Oceania Figures 6 and 7 (all Australian states and territories, New Zealand, and French Polynesia, extending to Chile) and many countries throughout South East Asia and North East Asia (Figure 8). These synchronous eruptions we speculate have occurred by simultaneous tropospheric viral-cloud in-falls contaminating the environment of populated regions occurring most likely in early February 2022. All populated regions of Australia appear to have been struck like Western Australia (Figure 6) at the same time. WA stands out with a clear "hockey stick" infection curve as it came off a very low base. This is consistent with the evident shoulders and blips on the right hand sides of the curves for NSW, VIC, TAS, and QLD. A plausible explanation is this extended shoulder is due to this second synchronous in-fall but masked by the already high Cases per Day in these other Australian states. In a related survey of the database (captured 18-19 February 2022) we detected another set of synchronous epidemic eruptions beginning about January 10 2022 and peaking late January early February 2022, these include : Algeria, Armenia, Azerbaijan, Bangladesh, Czechia, Faroe Islands, Georgia, Iran, Iraq, Jordan, Kazakhstan, Kosovo, Latvia, Libya, Moldova, Nepal, New Caledonia, Oman, Palestine, Paraguay, Russia, Slovakia, Taiwan, Yemen.

Therefore since mid-December 2021 two further separate global-wide synchronous epidemic eruptions can be detected, from about Jan 10, then from early February 2022. We highlight in particular Western Australia in Figure 6 as that vast Australian region had never before experienced a genuine tropospheric COVID-19 epidemic strike until just recently (Figure 6) - yet that state of Australia was lock-downed repeatedly and isolated from the rest of Australia and the wider world by stringent enforced border and travel restrictions. In addition, mask mandates and social distancing regulations (crowd sizes sports events, movie theaters, churches and so on) were enforced outside homes and work places, including mandatory vaccinations for most WA workers during 2020 and 2021 despite very few if any COVID-19 cases being

Edward J. Steele (2022) Overview SARS-CoV-2 Pandemic as January-February 2022: Likely Cometary Origin, Global Spread, Prospects for Future Vaccine Efficacy

recorded in the state (mainly in travelers coming by road and airplane from other infected zones in Australia and from overseas who were immediately isolated and quarantined). The recent large Omicron/Delta (mix?) strike completely surprised the WA Department of Health and Medical authorities as they could not explain any of the suddenly emergent infection events recorded across the state by conventional person-to-person transmissions. The apparent 'super spreading' was particularly strange given the population was largely fully vaccinated.

Given these striking globally-coordinated cases per day events detected by data monitoring just COVID-19, we cannot rule out additional surprises. We speculate that other unknown dust-associated pathogens (viral, bacterial, eukaryotic *spp*) in the troposphere have also been brought to Earth by the same general Space Weather/Solar-pulse processes during the current Sun Spot minimum between solar cycles 24 and 25. We have laid out here a range of explanations, some over-lapping, because we are dealing with a "globally correlated phenomenon that we do not fully understand." We have done so to ensure that as many plausible alternatives are available for further discussion and consideration in order that we may ultimately understand what happened.

Speculations How Omicron may have Arisen and Where?

All news reports in Australia, USA, South America, Africa and European countries, that are all engaged in the synchronous exponential eruptions, focus on Omicron as the main variant which is rapidly replacing Delta. From all available reports and early clinical experience, the respiratory disease severity of Omicron is less than Delta. This is consistent with death rate data (confirmed at URL links in Figures 1-5) that are consistently very low, and is approaching or remains below other estimates of death rates attributed to COVID-19 (whether Original Hu-1, Alpha, Delta and now Omicron). In approximately 0.1% of all COVID-19 exposed cases [29] death is the serious outcome mainly in the 'Immune Defenseless Elderly Co-Morbid' patient group. Highly vulnerable patients require administration of prompt respiratory therapies to navigate their respiratory crises that follow from the infection. Such patients often display clear deficits in innate immunity, often feeding into deficits in adaptive immunity and so are particularly at risk [38-44]. Other clinical studies [45] also show that patients in this subgroup specifically display deficits in Type I and type III interferon (IFN) inducible antiviral immunity and thus appear 'immune defenceless' to coronavirus respiratory tract infections and so are at a very high risk for severe outcomes including death.

How could a human-passaged variant like Omicron arise? Omicron is clearly a derivative of "Delta" a PANGO lineage name of the L241f haplotype of the Steele-Lindley replicative-haplotype scheme (Steele and Lindley 2020) with many changes in the mRNA encoding the spike protein suggestive of mutation accrual via human passage (person to person spread, P-to-P). The analysis of how a single putative cloned variant we named "L241f.1vic" spread through aged care and nursing facilities in Melbourne, Australia beginning from about 10 May 2020 through June 2020 then erupting on scale in such facilities through July and August 2020 is very informative

[23]. From the full-length genomic analysis of many thousands of publicly available SARS-Cov-2 genomes (>12,000 made available by the Victorian Dept of Health through The Peter Doherty Institute) we showed previously that there were two types of clearly identifiable patients. The first displayed *unmutated* versions of the virus over the entire 29903 nt genomic length. These types were particularly evident in the last two weeks of June 2020 through most of July 2020. It appeared very much like the virus was being amplified on scale in hosts that were *unable to mutate* the RNA virus genomes at APOBEC (cytosine to uracil) and ADAR (adenosine to inosine) deamination sites [22,23]. The second group of patients, clustering in a late August time window, displayed mutated versions of the virus, again largely at APOBEC and ADAR cytosine and adenosine deamination motifs. It was concluded thus [23] to quote conclusion directly:

The data reported herein are thus consistent with the following P-to-P infection model which is also the operational hypothesis under test: clusters of immune defenceless elderly co-morbid citizens in many aged care and nursing facilities were all systematically struck with devastating force (high infection rates and death rates), with a single unmutated (or lightly mutated) SARS-CoV-2 haplotype variant (L241f.1vic). Through late June, July, August and September in 2020, this putatively cloned variant must have been spread unimpeded by carriers who were asymptomatic or lightly symptomatic infected health- care professionals and carers working across multiple age care institutions [30-33]. The large-scale amplifications of the L241.1vic variant—instanced by the size of the multiple 'New case' spikes (shown in Figure 1), particularly through July 2020—could have produced many trillions of L241f.1vic virions in each location thus contaminating numerous surfaces (fomites, personal effects of all types) and could have contaminated or infected human carriers in each institution. This then fuelled the further putative quantitative dominant rapid spread of this apparently capricious L241f.1vic variant into the local community and particularly to other aged care facilities leading to further putative viral amplifications in elderly co-morbid subjects. If anything, the Victorian experience underlines why elderly co-morbid citizens require very special care, protection and therapies during cold and flu seasons [31,32].

It was then speculated that the putative highly contagious, yet clearly attenuated, "UK Mutant" (Alpha) that emerged in September in 2020 in parts of southern England was generated the same way. We also think Omicron arose by similar cycles of deaminase-mediated mutagenesis in healthy almost asymptomatic carriers, then became amplified (cloned unmutated) in Immune Defenseless Elderly Co-morbids – then after one or two more cycles via healthy intermediate 'vectors', infecting new cohorts of Immune Defenseless Elderly Co-Morbids where it was amplified and cloned. A plumed aerosol of literally millions on trillions of Omicron virions into the immediate troposphere and prevailing wind transportation could have easily distributed Omicron in the prevailing wind systems (e.g. from Northern Europe to South Africa where first detected). This model of alternating cycles of deaminase-mutagenesis and cloning amplification could have created a plume in a real high-density hotspot. Was it around or near UK where most Omicron have been recorded initially? At the present time we acknowledge these are speculations, but given the existence of detailed genomic records from

Edward J. Steele (2022) Overview SARS-CoV-2 Pandemic as January-February 2022: Likely Cometary Origin, Global Spread, Prospects for Future Vaccine Efficacy

the millions of genomes now sequenced and in computer databases, these speculations can, and will be tested in the fullness of time.

Future Vaccine Developments for Next Pandemic of Cold or Flu Respiratory Tract Pathogens?

There are many public health lessons to be learnt from the COVID-19 pandemic. Near-Earth balloon launches, stratospheric airplane and orbiting platform sampling of incoming meteorite dust have all been stressed as important early warning strategies on many previous occasions in other places (discussed recently in [9,16,29,46]. However a pandemic public health management strategy employing a *more effective vaccination method* needs urgent consideration. The aim should be quite different from the current very simplistic strategy of intramuscular "jab-in-the arm" vaccination (irrespective whether traditional antigens are used or the poorly safety tested mRNA expression vector vaccines). Public health vaccination which mimics natural 'Herd' immunity" is the desired outcome, whether to coronaviruses, influenza viruses and many other respiratory tract pathogens including bacterial *ssp.* that cause respiratory pneumonias and severe bronchitis.

Here we review how to optimize intranasal defective /attenuated live virus vaccination for all likely future types of pandemic respiratory viruses and finally discuss promising newly published experimental data which offers some hope for the future. We and many others have discussed the failure of the current jab in the arm intramuscular mRNA vaccines to protect against COVID-19 – yet they have been mandated by many governments and public health bureaucracies [24,29,47]. Further, the mRNA vaccines which also have high adverse effect rates are ineffective on first immunological principles because of the *wrong route of delivery*. The current 'jab-in-the-arm' route of immunization cannot possibly protect against COVID-19 infection gaining entry to and growing in mucosal cells of the respiratory tract. For that the mucosal secretory IgA antibody system needs *local* activation [23,24,29]. In a rush to bring COVID-19 vaccines to market, it seems that science and medicine neglected a large body of work already available on the nature of immunity and host resistance to respiratory viral infections, and how best to mimic this by vaccination, and instead became seduced by advances in 21st century molecular engineering principles into production of a vaccine whose utility and clinical efficacy even now remains unknown- more troubling is that any serious long-term sequalae are entirely unexplored. This is discussed graphically and underlined in recent interviews as well in https://youtu.be/Ijc4mjiIquk and in the *Asia Pacific TV* interview with Mike Ryan https://rumble.com/vmrmmq-the-origins-of-covid-19-and-why-the-vaccines-dont-work.html

Based on a wealth of scientific/immunologic data gleaned over decades, as well as experience in vaccination against respiratory viral disease, it is self-evident that protective vaccination needs to be via the oral-nasal route to activate the mucosal immune response, which is responsible for Natural Immunity and "Herd Immunity" in the population. The natural decline in the incidence of severe COVID-19 outcomes (COVID-19 associated death) was *well underway before the vaccine roll out* in European and USA Infection zones through 2020 and early 2021 [32]. This is brought about most effectively by effective

'Herd Immunity' which has been documented in a large longitudinal and population base study, conducted in Denmark through 2020 [31].

We have previously discussed the two most important forms of immunity to be activated in the mucosal cells and associated lymphoid cells of the respiratory lining. The first of these is Innate Immunity- a general elevation of these activities would strengthen the "Anti-Viral Wall" in all nasal cells and mucosal lining cells. This barrier is defective in 'Immune Defenseless Elderly Co-Morbids' which are the primary vulnerable group in the COVID-19 pandemic. Note that this group equates to < 1% of all infected patients see Netea et al. [41] and discussed elsewhere in detail [23] based on data from many clinical studies throughout 2020 [38-45]. In our analysis of the data >99% of the population handles COVID-19 effectively via natural immune mechanisms- to these patients it is just a "Common Cold". Both Innate Immune Interferon Type I and III anti-viral barriers in all cells would be activated, and then adaptive acquired mucosal immunity.

Secondly, Adaptive Acquired Mucosal Immunity requires, as we discuss, the induction of dimeric secretory IgA antibodies – these antibodies are demonstrably highly avid (strong binding and thus neutralizing of toxins, viruses and adhesins preventing cell adherence and cell entry) that do not activate the Complement cascade thus do not add to "inflammatory cytokine storms." Indeed, secretory IgA is expected to competitively block antigen binding and thus nullify the antibody-dependent enhancement (ADE) by the blood borne IgG and IgM complement fixing antibodies particularly in advanced COVID-19 infections of the elderly vulnerable group [23,24]. This sequelae of ADE pathology in vaccinated individuals who then go on to catch COVID-19 for first time is discussed more fully elsewhere [29].

To ensure that intranasal vaccination is effective it is desirable that activation of the innate immune response via the Toll receptors in addition to induction of secretory IgA against the virus. An agonist, INNA-51 of the Toll-2 receptor, was patented in 2018 (WO2018176099, Treatment of respiratory infection with a TLR2 agonist). It is currently being used in a Phase 2 trial of intranasal vaccination to prevent COVID-19 with the AstraZeneca antigen [48]. A better antigen could be an inactivated virus such as Sinovac as many more epitopes would be delivered than with AstraZeneca's viral vector containing just the SARS-CoV-2 spike protein.

Two recent papers describing experiments in mice (a small mammal with an immune system similar to, but not identical to, humans in principle) involving intra-nasal vaccine development and assessment of efficacy in protection from disease, have now been published in December 2021. Xaio and associates [49] created a defective or harmless coronavirus that cannot replicate properly, and delivered it via the intra-nasal route so as to induce both Innate Immunity (to *any other* viral challenge oro-nasal) and Adaptive Immunity (that is antigen specific secretory IgA). In the other study Oh and associates [50] set up intranasal priming with influenza infection or with adjuvanted recombinant neuraminidase flu vaccine. This induced local lung-resident B cell populations that secrete protective mucosal antiviral secretory IgA. In these complimentary studies, using these different intra-nasal, mucosal lining activation strategies the workers induced both elevated *pan-specific* Innate

Edward J. Steele (2022) Overview SARS-CoV-2 Pandemic as January-February 2022: Likely Cometary Origin, Global Spread, Prospects for Future Vaccine Efficacy

Immunity as recommended by Netea and associates [41] protecting against many other unrelated respiratory track pathogens, but also the necessary dimeric secretory IgA *adaptive specific immunity* akin to more tradition vaccination strategies. Recent published work adds to this conclusion [51].

We would argue that studies such as these offer the hope that can now look forward to the production of easily delivered, safe and effective vaccines against many epidemic respiratory viruses, irrespective of variant or viral type, so we will be well armed in advance of the next pandemic of respiratory tract infections. This would represent a real scientific advance and a saving grace for humanity.

Acknowledgements

We thank Max Rocca, Heath Goddard, and Dayal T. Wickramasinghe for discussions and Brig Klyce also for bringing our attention to Afkhami et al 2022 [51].

Conflicts of Interest

None of the co-author team has a conflict of interest apart from understanding the scientific reasons for the origin, global spread and efficacy of human immunity to SARS-CoV-2.

Multi-author Contributions

Conceptualisation EJS, NCW, RGG, GAH: *Draft writing*: EJS, NCW, RMG *Reading the primary clean draft*: All co-authors. *Active Contributions to primary draft via edits and additions*: RAL, PRC, MW, SC, MKW Integration of all minor changes: EJS, NCW, RMG.

Multi-author Expertise

The areas of expertise of the multi-author team are:

Edward J. Steele: Biomedical science, Immunology, Ancestral Haplotypes, Mutagenesis, Biotechnology, Evolution, Panspermia, Cosmic Biology.

Reginald M. Gorczynski: Biomedical science, Medicine, Immunology, Evolution, Panspermia, Cosmic Biology.

Robyn A. Lindley: Biomedical science, Immunology, Biotechnology, Mutagenesis, Evolution, Panspermia, Cosmic Biology.

Patrick R. Carnegie: Biomedical science, Immunology, Biotechnology.

Herbert Rebhran: Biomedical science, Ancestral Haplotypes, Veterinary Surgeon, Cosmic Biology)

Shirwan Al-Mufti: Astronomy, Astrobiology, Astrophysics, Evolution, Panspermia, Cosmic Biology.

Daryl H. Wallis: Astronomy, Astrobiology, Scanning Electron microscopy, Meteorite Analysis, Evolution, Panspermia, Cosmic Biology.

Gensuke Tokoro: Biotechnology, Vaccines, Astroeconomics, Panspermia, Cosmic Biology.

Robert Temple: Evolution, History & Philosophy Science, Panspermia, Cosmic Biology.

Ananda Nimalasuriya: Medicine, Panspermia, Cosmic Biology.

George A Howard: Deep Earth Evolution, Archaeology, Ice Ages, Environment Restoration, Panspermia, Cosmic Biology.

Mark A. Gillman: Biomedical science, Neuropharmacology – Pain & Pleasure, Evolution, Panspermia, Cosmic Biology.

Milton Wainwright: Biomedical science, Microbiology, Balloon Loft Stratosphere Sampling, Evolution, Panspermia, Cosmic Biology.

Stephen Coulson: Astrobiology, Mathematics, Astrophysics, Panspermia, Cosmic Biology.

Predrag Slijepcevic: Biomedical science, Microbiology, Evolution, Panspermia, Cosmic Biology.

Max K. Wallis: Astrobiology, Geophysics, Space Science, Mathematics, Astrophysics, Panspermia, Cosmic Biology.

Alexander Kondakov: Astrobiology, Panspermia, Cosmic Biology.

N. Chandra Wickramasinghe: Astronomy, Astrobiology, Biomedical science, Mathematics, Astrophysics, Evolution, Panspermia, Cosmic Biology.

References

1. Hoyle F, Wickramasinghe NC (1978) *Life Cloud*. J.M. Dent Ltd, London.

2. Hoyle F, Wickramasinghe NC (1979) *Diseases from Space*. J.M. Dent Ltd, London.

3. Hoyle F, Wickramasinghe NC (1981) *Evolution from Space*. J.M. Dent Ltd, London.

4. Hoyle F, Wickramasinghe NC (1985) *Living Comets*. Univ. College, Cardiff Press, Cardiff.

5. Hoyle F, Wickramasinghe NC (1991) *The Theory of Cosmic Grains*. Kluwer, Dordrecht.

6. Hoyle F, Wickramasinghe NC (1993) *Our Place in the Cosmos: the Unfinished Revolution*. J.M. Dent Ltd, London.

7. Hoyle F, Wickramasinghe NC (1999) *Astronomical Origins of Life: Steps towards Panspermia*. Reprints from Astrophys. Space Sci 268: 1-3. Kluwer Academic Publishers, Dordrecht, The Netherlands.

8. Wickramasinghe C (2020) *Diseases from Outer Space: Our Cosmic Destiny*. 2nd Edition of Diseases from Space, World Scientific Publishing Company, Singapore.

9. Wainwright M, Rose CE, Baker AJ, Wickramasinghe NC, Omairi T (2015) Biological Entities Isolated from Two Stratosphere Launches-Continued Evidence for a Space Origin. *J. Astrobiol Outreach* 3:2. https://www.walshmedicalmedia.com/archive/jao-volume-3-issue-2-year-2015.html

10. Wickramasinghe NC, Steele EJ, Wainwright M, Tokoro G, Fernando M, et al. (2017) Sunspot Cycle Minima and Pandemics: The Case for Vigilance? *J Astrobiol Outreach* 5:2. https://www.walshmedicalmedia.com/open-access/sunspot-cycle-minima-and-pandemics-the-case-for-vigilance-2332-2519-1000159.pdf

11. Wickramasinghe NC, Wickramsainghe DT, Senanayake S, Qu J, Tokoro G, et al. (2019) Space Weather and Pandemic Warnings? *Curr. Sci* 117: 1554. http://www.lifefromspace.com/resources/CurrentScience2020.pdf

12. Steele EJ, Al-Mufti S, Augustyn KA, Chandrajith R, Coghlan JP, et al. (2018) Causes of Cambrian Explosion-Terrestrial or Cosmic? *Prog. Biophys Mol Biol* 136: 3-23. [crossref]

13. Steele EJ, Gorczyski RM, Lindley RA, Liu Y, Temple R, et al. (2019) Lamarck and Panspermia-On the efficient spread of living systems throughout the cosmos. *Prog Biophys. Mol. Biol* 149: 10-32. [crossref]

14. Steele EJ, Gorczynski RM, Lindley RA, Tokoro G, Temple R, et al. (2020) Origin of new emergent Coronavirus and Candida fungal diseases- Terrestrial or Cosmic? *Adv. Genetics* 106: 75-100. [crossref]

15. Steele EJ, Gorczynski RM, Rebhan H, Carnegie P, Temple R, et al. (2020) Implications of haplotype switching for the origin and global spread of COVID-19. *Virology: Current Research* 4: 2020. DOI: 10.37421/Virol Curr Res.2020.4.115

Edward J. Steele (2022) Overview SARS-CoV-2 Pandemic as January-February 2022: Likely Cometary Origin, Global Spread, Prospects for Future Vaccine Efficacy

16. Steele EJ, Gorczynski RM, Lindley RA, Tokoro G, Wallis DH, et al. (2021) Cometary Origin of COVID-19 *Infect Dis Ther* 2: 1-4. https://researchopenworld.com/cometary-origin-of-covid-19/ DOI: 10.31038/IDT.2021212

17. Steele EJ, Wickramasinghe NC (2020) (Eds). Cosmic Genetic Evolution Academic Press-Elsevier: Advances in Genetics. Volume 106, Serial Editor Dhavendra Kumar, London and San Diego. https://www.elsevier.com/books/cosmic-genetic-evolution/steele/978-0-12-821518-0

18. Wickramasinghe NC, Steele EJ, Gorczynski RM, Temple R, Tokoro G, et al. (2020) Comments on the Origin and Spread of the 2019 Coronavirus. *Virology: Current Research* 4: 1. DOI: 10.37421/vcrh.2020.4.109

19. Coulson SG, Wickramasinghe NC. (2003) Frictional and radiation heating of micron-sized meteoroids in the Earth's upper atmosphere. *Mon. Not. Roy. Astron. Soc* 343: 1123-1130.

20. Wickramasinghe NC, Steele EJ, Gorczynski RM, Temple R, Tokoro G, et al. (2020) Growing Evidence against Global Infection-Driven b Person-to-Person Transfer of COVID-19. *Virology Current Research* 4:1. DOI: 10.37421/vcrh.2020.4.110

21. Wickramasinghe NC, Steele EJ, Gorczynski RM, Temple R, Tokoro G, et al. (2020) Predicting the Future Trajectory of COVID. *Virology Current Research* 4:1. DOI: 10.37421/vcrh.2020.4.111

22. Steele EJ, Lindley RA (2020) Analysis of APOBEC and ADAR deaminase-driven Riboswitch Haplotypes in COVID-19 RNA strain variants and the implications for vaccine design. *Research Reports* https://www.companyofscientists.com/index.php/rr

23. Lindley RA, Steele EJ (2021) Analysis of SARS-CoV-2 haplotypes and genomic sequences during 2020 in Victoria, Australia, in the context of putative deficits in innate immune deaminase anti-viral responses. *Scand J Immunol.* https://doi.org/10.1111/sji.13100

24. Gorczynski RM, Lindley RA, Steele EJ, Wickramasinghe NC (2021) Nature of Acquired Immune Responses, Epitope Specificity and Resultant Protection from SARS-CoV-2. *J. Pers. Med* 11: 1253. https://doi.org/10.3390/jpm11121253

25. Howard GA, Wickramasinghe NC, Rebhan H, Steele EJ, Gorczynski RM, et al (2020) Mid-Ocean Outbreaks of COVID-19 with Tell-Tale Signs of Aerial Incidence. *Virology Current Research* 4:1. DOI: 10.37421/vcrh.2020.4.114

26. Wickramasinghe NC, Steele EJ, Nimalasuriya A, Gorczynski RM, Tokoro G, et al. (2020) Seasonality of Respiratory Viruses Including SARS-CoV-2. *Virology Current Research* 4:2. DOI: 10.37421/vcrh.2020.4.117

27. Wickramasinghe NC, Wallis MK, Coulson SG, Kondakov A, Steele EJ, et al. (2020) Intercontinental Spread of COVID-19 on Global Wind Systems. *Virology Current Research* 4:1. DOI: 10.37421/vcrh.2020.4.113

28. Steele EJ, Gorczynski RM, Carnegie P, Tokoro G, Wallis DH, et al (2021) COVID-19 Sudden Outbreak of Mystery Case Transmissions in Victoria, Australia, May-June 2021: Strong Evidence of Tropospheric Transport of Human Passaged Infective Virions from the Indian Epidemic. *Infect Dis Ther* 2: 1-28. DOI: 10.31038/IDT.2021214

29. Steele EJ, Gorczynski RM, Rebhan H, Tokoro G, Wallis DH, et al. (2021) Exploding Five COVID-19 Myths On the Origin, Global Spread and Immunity. *Infect Dis Ther* 2: 1-15. DOI: https://doi.org/10.31038/IDT.2021223

30. Hammond GW, Raddatz RL, Gelskey DE (1989) Impact of atmospheric dispersion and transport of viral aerosols on the epidemiology of Influenza. *Reviews of Infectious Disease* 11: 494-497. [crossref]

31. Hansen CH, Michlmayr D, Gubbels SM, Mølbak K, Ethelberg S (2021) Assessment of protection against reinfection with SARS-CoV-2 among 4 million PCR-tested individuals in Denmark in 2020: A population-level observational study. *The Lancet* 397: 1204-1212. DOI: https://doi.org/10.1016/S0140-6736(21)00575-4

32. Steele EJ, Gorczynski RM, Lindley RA, Tokoro G, Wallis DH, et al. (2021) An End of the COVID-19 Pandemic in Sight? *Infect Dis Ther* 2: 1-5. DOI: 10.31038/IDT.2021222

33. Lee H. (2021) CDC Investigates 86 Cruise Ships With COVID-19 Outbreaks Dec 28 2021. https://www.theepochtimes.com/cdc-investigates-86-cruise-ships-with-covid-19-outbreaks_4181845.html

34. Khalip A, Pereira M (2021) COVID outbreak ends cruise for thousands on German ship in Lisbon https://www.reuters.com/world/europe/covid-outbreak-ends-cruise-thousands-german-ship-lisbon-2022-01-02/

35. AP|Washington 2021 (Dec 25) US Navy pauses warship deployment to South America amid Covid-19 outbreak. https://www.business-standard.com/article/international/us-navy-pauses-warship-deployment-to-south-america-amid-covid-19-outbreak-121122500109_1.html

36. BBC News Coronavirus Pandemic: Antarctic Outpost hit by Covid-19 outbreak. https://www.bbc.com/news/world-europe-59848160

37. Combe M, Garijo R, Geller R, Cuevas JM, Sanjaun R (2015) Single-cell analysis of RNA virus infection identifies multiple genetically diverse viral genomes within single infectious units. *Cell Host Microbe* 18: 424-432. [crossref]

38. Achary D, Liu G-Q, Gack MU (2020) Dysregulation of type I interferon responses in COVID-19. *Nat. Rev Immunol* 20: 397- 398. [crossref]

39. Blanco-Melo D, Nilsson-Payant BE, Liu W-C, Uhl S, Hoagland D, et al. (2020) Imbalanced Host Response to SARS-CoV-2 Drives Development of COVID-19. *Cell* 181: 1036-1045. [crossref]

40. Hadjadj J, Yatim N, Barnabei L, Corneau A, Boussier J, et al. (2020) Impaired type I interferon activity and exacerbated inflammatory responses in severe Covid-19 patients. *Science* 369: 718-724. DOI: 10.1126/science.abc6027

41. Netea MG, Giamarellos-Bourboulis EJ, Domınguez-Andre's J, Curtis N, Reinoutvan C, et al. (2020) Trained Immunity: A tool for reducing susceptibility to and the severity of SARS-CoV-2 infection. *Cell* 181: 969-977. [crossref]

42. Zhang Q, Bastard P, Liu Z, Le Pen J, Moncada-Velez M, et al. (2020) Inborn errors of type I IFN immunity in patients with life-threatening COVID-19. *Science* 370: eabd4570. [crossref]

43. Moderbacher CR, Ramirez SI, Dan JM, Grifron A, Hastie KM, et al. (2020) Antigen-specific adaptive immunity to SARS-CoV-2 in acute COVID-19 and associations with age and disease severity. *Cell* 183: 996-1012. [crossref]

44. Sette A, Crotty S (2021) Adaptive immunity to SARS-CoV-2 and COVID-19. *Cell* 184: 861-880. [crossref]

45. Lucas C, Wong P, Klein J, Castro TBR, Silva J, et al. (2020) Longitudinal analyses reveal immunological misfiring in severe COVID-19. *Nature* 584: 463-469. [crossref]

46. Qu J, Wickramasinghe NC (2020) The world should establish an early warning system for new viral infectious diseases by space-weather monitoring. *MedComm* 1: 423 -426. [crossref]

47. Subramanian SV, Kumar A. (2021) Increases in COVID-19 are unrelated to levels of vaccination across 68 countries and 2947 counties in the United States. *Eur J Epidemiol* 36: 1237-1240. https://doi.org/10.1007/s10654-021-00808-7

48. Deliyannis G, Wong CY, McQuilten HA, Bachem A, Clarke M, et al. (2021) TLR2-mediated activation of innate responses in the upper airways confers antiviral protection of the lungs. *JCI Insight* 6: e140267. [crossref]

49. Xiao Y, Lidsky PV, Shirogane Y, Aviner R, Wu CT, et al. (2021) A defective viral genome strategy elicits broad protective immunity against respiratory viruses. *Cell* 184: 6037-6051. [crossref]

50. Oh JE, Song E, Moriyama M, Wong P, Zhang S, et al (2021) Intranasal priming induces local lung-resident B cell populations that secrete protective mucosal antiviral IgA. *Science Immunology* 6: eabj5129. [crossref]

51. Afkhami S, D'Agostino MR, Zhang A, Stacey HD, Marzok A, et al. (2022) Respiratory mucosal delivery of next-generation COVID-19 vaccine provides robust protection against both ancestral and variant strains of SARS-CoV-2. *Cell* 185: 896–915. [crossref]

Citation:

Steele EJ, Gorczynski RM, Lindley RA, Carnegie PR, Rebhran H, et al. (2022) Overview SARS-CoV-2 Pandemic as January-February 2022: Likely Cometary Origin, Global Spread, Prospects for Future Vaccine Efficacy. *Infect Dis Ther* Volume 3(1): 1-16.

SECTION 8

Coronavirus Evolutionary Footprint on Human Genome

Review Article

Open Access

Footprints of Past Pandemics in the Human Genome

N Chandra Wickramasinghe[1,2,3,4*], Edward J. Steele[2,5,6], Daryl H. Wallis[3], Milton Wainwright[3], Gensuke Tokoro[4], Herbert Rebhan[5], Reginald M Gorczynski[7] and Robert Temple[8]

[1]Buckingham Centre for Astrobiology, University of Buckingham, MK18 1EG England, UK

[2]Centre for Astrobiology, University of Ruhuna, Matara, Sri Lanka

[3]National Institute of Fundamental Studies, Kandy, Sri Lanka

[4]Institute for the Study of Panspermia and Astroeconomics, Gifu, Japan

[5]C Y O'Connor, ERADE Village Foundation, Piara Waters, Perth 6112 WA, Australia

[6]Melville Analytics Pty Ltd, Melbourne, VIC, Australia

[7]University Toronto Health Network, Toronto General Hospital, University of Toronto, Toronto, ON, Canada

[8]The History of Chinese Science and Culture Foundation, Conway Hall, London, United Kingdom

Abstract

Viral pandemics over centuries and millennia have left indelible signatures on our genomes. Deciphering these signatures could give us profoundly important information on our evolutionary history that appears to have been directed by the arrival of new viruses from the deep cosmos. A recent study that shows a residual signature of SARS-CoV-2 (in the form of multiple generational expression of host-specific SARS-CoV targeting viral interacting proteins known as VIPs) in the genomes of a South Asian population suggests that a major COVID-19 type infectious episode may have occurred about 25,000 years ago. The need to monitor the stratosphere for the arrival of new pathogenic viruses, or even the return of old viruses such as Small Pox, is stressed.

Keywords: SARS-CoV-2 • Footprints • Pandemic infectious episodes • Evolutionary history

Introduction

In this article we discuss the growing evidence to support the view that at least some of the viruses that cause diseases in plants and animals including humans are of extra-terrestrial cosmic origin. This was raised first specifically for the fully-sequenced human genome by Wickramasinghe [1], and expanded to review evidence for the range of integrated full-length viral genomes and their fragments, of DNA and RNA viruses, both retro-viral and non-retroviral, by Wickramasinghe and Steele [2]. This is but one part of the body of evidence that is pointing towards an extra-terrestrial origin of life on our planet, in contradiction to the conventional view that life originated de novo on the Earth from a primordial soup of organics. This alternative viewpoint argues that life is unequivocally a cosmic phenomenon, and one that takes root on every habitable planetary abode throughout the cosmos.

Nearly four decades ago Hoyle and Wickramasinghe, from their studies of interstellar and cometary dust, arrived at the startling conclusion that a large proportion of cosmic dust is comprised of bacteria and viruses, a fraction of which must exist in viable form Hoyle and Wickramasinghe It was argued that the origin of life on habitable planets like Earth inevitably involved the arrival of microorganisms in viable form, thereby circumventing the concept of small-scale planet-bound abiogenesis, an issue which is fraught with both inconsistencies and extreme statistical improbabilities [3,4]. As a consequence of these ideas, it was further proposed that the occurrence of pandemic diseases of viral origin in plants and animals is an anticipated corollary that in turn would have a crucial impact on the evolution of life. Indeed, the several stages of human evolution must have been profoundly affected by these myriad viral genetic integration signatures. They are the most striking feature of the human genomic DNA sequence structure-"the forest rather than the trees against which protein-coding genes are conventionally embedded."

In the book "Living Comets" published in 1985 Hoyle and Wickramasinghe wrote [5]. Thus:

"An illusion was put about widely a few years ago that it would be impossible for viruses from space to mount pathogenic attacks on terrestrial plants and animals with the specificity that is actually observed, for example with measles being a specifically human disease. But this was merely an expression of opinion. Worse, it was untrue. Human viruses attack tissue-cell cultures of other primates, and most human viruses can be cultured even in chick embryo, a taxonomic class apart from humans.

The specificity does not come therefore from individual cells or from the viruses themselves, but from our immune systems. This should really be no surprise because our immune systems can be specific even to the extent of rejecting tissue from close relatives of our own species.

It appears very likely that our very genetic make-up has an origin external to Earth. As well as causing pathogenic attacks, viruses can simply add themselves to our chromosomes, placidly multiplying only as our cells divide. In this way we derive new genes as a matter of fact, not conjecture. Since it needs only an elementary mathematical calculation to show that genes are so astonishingly complex that they could never be produced by random internal shuffling of bases on our DNA, it is then but a short step to the realisation that all of our genes are of external origin, added by viruses [1-4]. Complete immunity to viral invasion can therefore be seen to be impossibility for an evolving biological system."

Corresponding Author: N Chandra Wickramasinghe, Buckingham Centre for Astrobiology, University of Buckingham, MK18 1EG England, UK, E-mail: ncwick@gmail.com

Received: June 30, 2020; **Accepted:** July 14, 2021; **Published:** July 21, 2021

https://www.hilarispublisher.com/open-access/footprints-of-past-pandemics-in-the-human-genome.pdf
https://www.hilarispublisher.com/archive/vcrh-volume-5-issue-4-year-2021.html

Wickramasinghe NC, et al.   Virol Curr Res, Volume 5: 4, 2021

The Role of Viruses-Evidence from DNA

After the human genome was fully sequenced in 2001 our cosmic ancestry was laid bare and many of the predictions of the cosmic theory of the 1980s were verified. The discovery that only 25,000 genes exist to code for all our proteins left the origin and the role of the vast majority of our seemingly redundant DNA unexplained. There seems now little doubt that much of this genetic inheritance is comprised of DNA whose origin is viral in nature. This DNA shows up as LINEs (Long Interspersed Nuclear Elements) (21%), and SINEs (Short Interspersed Nuclear Elements) (13%). The LINES are directly functionally related to retroviruses as reverse transcriptase encoding elements which assist the integration and retro-transposition of other shorter SINE elements (e.g. Alu elements). The HERVs (Human Endogenous Retroviruses) and LTRs (Long Terminal Repeats) comprise about 9% of the human genome (see Ref.6 Appendix B). These are all relics of viruses that have infected our ancestral lineage over the past millions of years and have left their footprint in our DNA. During the past 4.2 billion years of terrestrial evolution of life on this planet viruses have played a key role. When a virus invades and productively infects a cell it multiplies with the "assistance" of the invaded cell. In other instances viruses can instead insert genetic (viral) elements which can alter the previous cell program without causing any overt deleterious changes to the cell. Such program insertions by viruses may have been responsible for many stages of evolution over millennia for the vast ensemble of life forms (species) both on Earth and elsewhere in the cosmos.

In general, it will not happen that a virus on entering a cell will have precisely the right elements for insertion of genetic material into the life-form in question at its current stage of evolution. During evolution there will thus necessarily have been a multitude of "abortive trials", likely with massive viral replication and cell death, before a successful program insertion is accomplished and evolutionary advances occur. It is our hypothesis that a cosmic imperative is for viruses to act as a driver of evolution, in which viruses seek cells, not vice versa.

Viral sequences added through the mechanism of pandemic disease could provide evolutionary potential that leads to new genotypes and new species at one end of the scale, and to new traits and the capacity to express our genes in novel ways at the other. It is becoming clear that our entire existence on this planet is contingent on the continuing ingress of cosmic viruses, which we had hitherto thought were merely the vehicles for death and disease. Their positive role in evolution that was predicted in the 1980's may only just be beginning to be seen. Major evolutionary steps in the development of complex life forms leading to Homo sapiens are thus all externally derived, and evolution is essentially driven from the universe outside. If this is so the overall impression will be of a pre-programming in the higher levels of development of intelligence that is manifest in biology.

Evidence from Geology

The facts relating to the evolution of life on the Earth progressing through a long series of punctuated steps have been available for several decades [7]. Long periods of slow and tedious evolutionary progress are frequently interrupted by sudden bursts of evolution and innovative speciation, with or without accompanying episodes of extinctions, which we can often attribute either to comet collisions or climatic catastrophes of one form or another [8]. It is this process of speciation that Hoyle and Wickramasinghe already discussed in the 1980's and attributed to viral additions [9] (Figure 1).

A recent observation in the field of geology that is inconsistent with the standard theory that life emerged in a primordial soup on the Earth is the discovery that the very first evidence of microbial life on Earth was found locked away within crystals of zirconium in rocks that formed 4.1-4.2 billion years ago now exposed in the Jack Hills outcrop in Western Australia [10]. This discovery lies to rest the possibility of the origin of life in a primordial soup brewing on Earth at a time when the planet was being relentlessly bombarded by comets and meteorites. The evidence is in favour of the alternative viewpoint that the first life on Earth in the form of bacteria came from impacting comets.

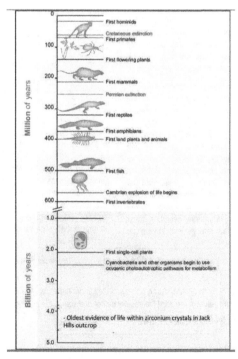

Figure 1. Evolution of plants and animals, from the time of the first introduction of life 4.2 billion years ago.

Wickramasinghe NC, et al.   Virol Curr Res, Volume 5: 4, 2021

The delivery of micro biota from comets to the Earth would of course have continued from that early moment 4.2 billion years ago to the present time, bringing the set of microbial genes from a vast cosmic ensemble that directed the evolution of life on our planet in the manner first proposed by Hoyle and Wickramasinghe in 1981 [9] and all the relevant supportive evidence recently reviewed by Steele et al. [4,6] The existence of virus-related DNA in vast quantity in our genomes testifies to the operation of such a process taking place over billions of years of evolutionary history [1,2].

Deep History of Ancestral Pandemics

DNA sequence studies over the past decades have clearly shown that the evolution from early primates leading up to Homo sapiens was marked by a long series of viral pandemics, each of which could well have represented a "brush with extinction", but the evolving line survived through eventually to reach us today. The branching points in the evolutionary lineage are marked by the discovery of HERVS and ERVS as shown schematically in Figure 2.

Viral inserts via direct viral-encoded reverse transcription as for the retroviruses is clear. In the case of non-retroviral RNA infections this would require host cellular-derived reverse transcription, such as for the single-stranded coronaviruses like COVID-19. Such inserts appear involved at the branching points in the evolutionary tree depicted in Figure 2 are arguably also implicated in a long sequence of pandemics of disease. In each postulated pandemic of disease [11]. In each postulated pandemic of viral disease over the past 45 million years a surviving cohort of our ancestral line would have directly acquired the retroviral genes indicated (Figure 2).

A recent study of the genomes of an East-Asian population group has shown evidence of multiple generational human gene signatures of strong positive genetic adaptations which occurred in these populations, in multiple genes that interact with coronaviruses, including SARS-CoV-2. These signatures of viral-interacting proteins show up as a strong peak after retracing mutational steps generation-by-generation through 900 generations in the past [11]. This evidence is reproduced from Souilmi et al [11]. below indicating a major Covid-19 type pandemic some 25,000 years ago (Figure 3).

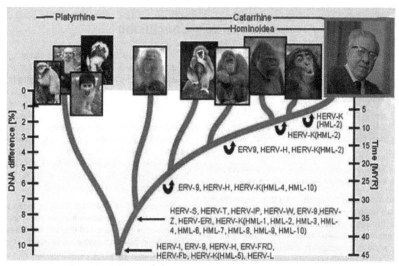

Figure 2. Schematic evolution of the hominid line leading up to Homo sapiens.

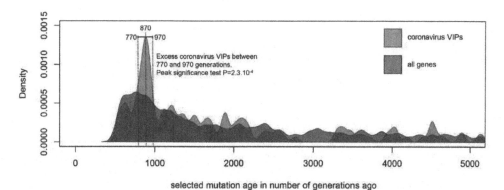

Figure 3. Evidence of COVID-19 pandemic 870 generations ago in the form of multiple generational expressions through the genome of SARS-CoV specific proteins known as VIPs. From Figure 2 in Souilimi et al [11].

Wickramasinghe NC, et al.   Virol Curr Res, Volume 5: 4, 2021

Reports of the sudden spread of plagues and pestilences have punctuated human history throughout the centuries [12]. The various epidemics, scattered through time and across the world are sometimes in a few instances recognisable as similar to modern diseases, a striking example being smallpox. Skin lesions strongly suggestive of smallpox have been found in the Egyptian mummy of Ramses V (1145 BCE). Furthermore, clinical descriptions consistent with smallpox are described in medical writings both from ancient India and China at around the same time. The absence of any comparable descriptions of pandemics in classical Greece and throughout early Christendom in Europe suggests an absence of the disease from human populations for over 1500 years, until it reappeared in China possibly in the 5th century of the Common Era. Thereafter it remains endemic in the world's human population until its final deliberate eradication in the 20th century. A major puzzle for understanding the re-emergence of smallpox after an absence for 1600 years is the lack of an animal reservoir into which the virus might have receded, humans being the only known host of the Variola major virus. An alternative viewpoint considers the data to make a prima facie case for a comet with period 1600 years-if the last episode of infection is assumed to have happened in 500 AD in China (vide supra), a return of the same comet is alarmingly imminent.

The identifiable recurrence of smallpox (Variola major) through history is an exception. More often, from written descriptions alone, ancient epidemics bear little or no resemblance to either modern disease or to one another. However, they all share the common property of afflicting entire population centres, countries or even widely separated parts of the Earth in a matter of days or weeks.

The Greek Historian Thucydides said of one such isolated event, the plague of Athens of 429 BC [12,13], thus:

"It is said to have begun in that part of Ethiopia above Egypt. On the city of Athens it fell suddenly and first attacked the men in Piraeus; so that it was even reported by them that the Peloponnesians had thrown poison into the cisterns."

Thucydides writes further that many families were simultaneously struck by a disease with a combination of symptoms hitherto unknown.

The prevailing orthodoxy that viruses responsible for all major pandemics have their origin in animal reservoirs (birds, pig, bats) is a conjecture with no substantial evidential backing. The fact that both influenza viruses and corona viruses both represent broad viral families with counterparts in animals does not imply a plausible mechanism of transfer. Indeed, it has been argued that for the COVID-19 virus to be transferred from a bat, via a pangolin to a human requires random mutations that would far exceed the available probability space in the whole universe [14].

The orthodox narrative asserts that pandemics of viral or bacterial origin throughout human history were all initiated with the advent of farming and animal husbandry, thus allowing zoonotic viruses from wild and domestic animals systematically to access and infect humans. As we have already mentioned the cross-over from zoonotic variants to humans in the case of the COVID-19 pandemic involved an insurmountable probability barrier, and similar impediments may apply to other instances throughout history. In addition, the claim that the 2012 MERS-CoV outbreak was caused by viral jumps to humans in the Middle East via infected camels is not supported by existing evidence [15]. Indeed the evidence of a COVID-19 pandemic in a South Asian group of humans 25,000 years ago [11] already highlights the inconsistency in this idea. At this late stage of the Iron Age human populations were still thinly scattered across the globe and agriculture had barely been discovered.

The recent discovery by Zhang et al. in 2021 [16] is very significant in regard to COVID-19 genomic sequences eventually appearing as significant germline signatures in the human genome. These authors have shown that the fragments of the COVID-19 genome, particularly the highly expressed coding region for the nuclear capsid protein (NC) at the 3' end of the genome, are directly fused to multiple different protein-coding gene segments at many exon sites across the entire human genome. This provides molecular underpinning for the findings of Souilmi, et al. [11]. About two thirds of all integrated sequences appear to have been mediated at endonuclease site motifs that allow target site reverse transcription (RT) by the RT enzyme encoded by LINE1 elements. We can only speculate that the other 33% of integrants have been target site reverse transcribed and integrated by the other known dominant cellular reverse transcriptase, the DNA repair enzyme DNA Polymerase-η (eta) [17,18] and assisted by recently discovered RT activity also in the DNA repair enzyme DNA Polymerase-θ (theta) [19]. At this stage all reported integrations have been into the nuclear DNA of somatic cells, and germline integrants have not been searched for, but given the sheer number of humans of all races infected with COVID-19, running into the many tens of millions, we should anticipate that significant germline human genomic sequences of COVID-19 and its many protein coding segments (fused in many cases to different human genetic coding exons) may appear in human genomes of future generations-these in turn may be associated with inborn genetic errors as mankind's legacy of the 2020-2021 COVID-19 pandemic.

Conclusion

As discussed by Hoyle and Wickramasinghe in many places the Earth interacts with the debris streams of comets that carry bacteria and viruses; and such comets have periods ranging from a few years to tens of thousands of years. In one particular instance, Comet Encke with a period of 3.3 years, a case was made to argue for a close correspondence with the appearances of this comet and cycles of Whooping cough from 1940 until routine vaccinations essentially eliminated the disease in 1980 [13]. As for longer period comets, the best known is Comet Hyakutake which reached its last perihelion in 1996 and which has an orbital period of 70,000 years. The putative comet responsible for the COVID-19 virus would be estimated to have a period of between 20,000 and 25,000 years, and a smallpox virus bearing comet a period of 1600 years.

Bacteria and other biological entities down to viral sizes have been isolated from the stratosphere over several years and the only reasonable explanation in our view is that they are of extra-terrestrial origin. From the stratospheric sampling carried out by Harris et al and others [20-23] we have estimated that some 10^8 bacteria and 10^{10} viruses per square metre arrive from space at the Earth's surface every day. Very recently the startling report of bacterial DNA discovered by PCR techniques on the outside of the International Space Station (ISS) orbiting at 400 km above the Earth has been reported [24], but has largely gone unnoticed.

In an unrelated project carried out by a team of international scientists the total flux of bacteria and viruses falling through the atmosphere on the tops of the Sierra Nevada Mountains has recently examined by Reche et al. [25]. The average downward flux of viruses from this height, presumably mainly lofted from the ground, was discovered to be 800 million per square metre per day close to the estimate that we made earlier from stratospheric sampling. If both the space-incident microorganisms and terrestrial microbes are mingled into this latter estimate their genetic differences could turn out to be difficult to detect. Efforts to separate these components are clearly of paramount importance, and after our current experience of COVID-19 this should be considered an international scientific priority [26]. The evidence that comets continue to bring bacteria and viruses including COVID-19 [26] to the Earth, and routinely thus contribute to the microbiomes of all life forms, aiding evolution in the long term, and sometimes cause pandemics, is still regretfully being ignored by mainstream science.

Wickramasinghe NC, et al.

Virol Curr Res, Volume 5: 4, 2021

References

1. Wickramasinghe, N Chandra. "DNA Sequencing and Predictions of the Cosmic Theory of Life." *Astrophys Space Sci* 343(2012):1-5.

2. Wickramasinghe, N Chandra, and Edward J Steele. "Dangers of Adhering to an Obsolete Paradigm: Could Zika Virus Lead to a Reversal of Human Evolution." *J Astrobiol Outreach* 4(2016):2332-2519.

3. Hoyle, Fred, and N Chandra Wickramasinghe. "Astronomical Origins of Life." *Kluwer Academic Press* (2000).

4. Steele, Edward J, Reginald M Gorczynski, Robyn A Lindley and Yongsheng Liu, et al. "Lamarck and Panspermia-On the Efficient Spread of Living Systems Throughout the Cosmos." *Prog Biophys Mol Biol* 149(2019):10-32.

5. Hoyle, Fred, and N Chandra Wickramasinghe. "Living Comets" University College, Cardiff Press. *Cardiff* (1985).

6. Steele, Edward J, Shirwan Al-Mufti, Kenneth A Augustyn and Rohana Chandrajith, et al. "Cause of Cambrian explosion-terrestrial or cosmic?." *Prog Biophys Mol Bio* 136(2018):3-23.

7. Gould, Stephen Jay, and Niles Eldredge. "Punctuated Equilibria: The Tempo and Mode of Evolution Reconsidered." *Paleobiology* 3(1977):115-151.

8. Hoyle, Fred, and N Chandra Wickramasinghe. "Comets, Ice Ages, and Ecological Catastrophes." *Astrophys Space Sci* 53(1978):523-526.

9. Hoyle, Fred, N Chandra Wickramasinghe. "Evolution from Space". *J M Dent Ltd London* (1981)

10. Bell, Elizabeth A, Patrick Boehnke, Mark Harrison, and Wendy L Mao. "Potentially Biogenic Carbon Preserved in a 4.1 Billion-Year-Old Zircon." *Proc Natl Acad Sci* 112(2015):14518-14521.

11. Souilmi, Yassine, Elise Lauterbur, Ray Tobler and Christian D. Huber et al. "An Ancient Viral Epidemic Involving Host Coronavirus Interacting Genes More Than 20,000 Years Ago in East Asia." *Curr Biol* 9822(2021):15-16.

12. Hoyle, Fred, and N Chandra Wickramasinghe. "Diseases from Space." *J M Dent Ltd* (1979).

13. Hoyle, Fred, and Wickramasinghe N Chandra. "Our Place in the Cosmos: the Unfinished Revolution." *J M Dent* (1993).

14. Steele, Edward J, Reginald M Gorczynski, Herbert Rebhan and Patrick Carnegie, et al. "Implications of Haplotype Switching for the Origin and Global Spread of COVID-19." *Virol Curr Res* 4(2020):1-4.

15. Killerby, Marie E, Holly M Biggs, Claire M Midgley and Susan I Gerber, et al. "Middle East Respiratory Syndrome Coronavirus Transmission." *Emerg Infect Dis* 26(2020): 191-198.

16. Zhang, Liguo, Alexsia Richards M, Inmaculada Barrasa and Stephen H Hughes, et al. "Reverse-Transcribed SARS-CoV-2 RNA can Integrate into the Genome of Cultured Human Cells and can be Expressed in Patient-Derived Tissues." *Proc Natl Acad Sci* 118(2021):22-23.

17. Franklin, Andrew, Peter J Milburn, Robert V Blanden, and Edward J Steele. "Human DNA Polymerase-η, an A-T Mutator in Somatic Hypermutation of Rearranged Immunoglobulin Genes, is a Reverse Transcriptase." *Immunol Cell Biol* 82(2004):219-225.

18. Franklin, Andrew, Edward J Steele, and Robyn A Lindley. "A Proposed Reverse Transcription Mechanism for (CAG) N and Similar Expandable Repeats that Cause Neurological and Other Diseases." *Heliyon* 6(2020):e03258.

19. Chandramouly, Gurushankar, Jiemin Zhao, Shane McDevitt and Timur Rusanov, et al. "Polθ Reverse Transcribes RNA and Promotes RNA-Templated DNA Repair." *Sci Adv* 7(2021):1771-1773.

20. Harris, Melanie J, Nalin Chandra Wickramasinghe, David Lloyd and JV Narlikar, et al. "Detection of Living Cells in Stratospheric Samples." *Int Curr Opt Photonics* 4495(2002):192-198.

21. Wainwright, Milton, N Chandra Wickramasinghe, JV Narlikar, and P Rajaratnam. "Microorganisms Cultured from Stratospheric Air Samples Obtained at 41 KM." *FEMS Microbiology Letters* 218(2003):161-165.

22. Wainwright, Milton, N Chandra Wickramasinghe, M Harris, and T Omairi. "Confirmation of the Presence of Viable But Non-Culturable Bacteria in the Stratosphere." *Int J Astrobiology* (2004)3:13-15.

23. Wainwright, Milton, N Chandra Wickramasinghe and Tokoro Gensuke. "Neopanspermia-Evidence that Life Continuously Arrives at the Earth from Space." *Advances in Astrophysics* (2021):6-18.

24. Grebennikova, Tatiana V, AV Syroeshkin, EV Shubralova and OV Eliseeva, et al. "The DNA of Bacteria of the World Ocean and the Earth in Cosmic Dust at the International Space Station." *Sci World J* 32(2018):1-5.

25. Reche, Isabel, Gaetano D Orta, Natalie Mladenov and Danielle M. Winget et al. "Deposition Rates of Viruses and Bacteria above the Atmospheric Boundary Layer." *ISME J* 12(2018):1154-1162.

26. Edward J, Steele, Reginald M Gorczynski, Robyn A Lindley and Gensuke Tokoro, et al. "Cometary Origin COVID-19." *Infect Dis & Therapeutics* 2(2021):1-4.

How to cite this article: Wickramasinghe, N Chandra, Gensuke Tokoro, Daryl H. Wallis and Milton Wainwright et al. "Footprints of Past Pandemics in the Human Genome." *Virol Curr Res* (2021) 5: 134.

SECTION 9

Public Health Lessons

What Public Health Lessons have we Learnt to Handle the Next Inevitable Pandemic?

Steele EJ, Wickramasinghe NC, Gorczynski RM

The social, financial and economic destruction caused by the COVID-19 pandemic has been immense. By general consensus at the time of writing, in all main stream scientific and popular press media, the over reaction by public health and government authorities has been the main problem (Chapters 14, 15, 18 and 19 — ineffective lockdowns, curfews, social distancing and isolation/quarantine laws, mandatory mask rules, forced mandated vaccinations for entry or to retain employment).

These public health and epidemiological failures have now become overt and apparent all over the world. Pandemic control responses have been out of proportion to the known risk presented by COVID-19. It was evident within the first months of 2020 that "Immune Defenceless Elderly Co-morbid" patients were at most risk of death *by* COVID-19 (median age ≥ 84 yr) — and this group conservatively constituents 0.1% of all COVID-19 exposed cases (Fauci *et al.* 2020, Chapters 13, 17 and 18). Thus 99.9% of the human population was not at risk of dying by COVID-19 at any time during the pandemic. It can now be seen clearly as a common cold or mild flu. Such infections, of course, are serious in inducing respiratory pneumonias (as in all past cold and flu seasons) in our vulnerable elderly citizens in geriatric wards and nursing homes. This group actually needed *early therapies* aimed at quelling the respiratory crisis: targeting both the virus and/or the inflammatory cytokine storm-induced bronchitis (e.g. antibodies; non-specific anti-viral agents such as ivermectin, Bryant *et al.* 2021, Kory *et al.* 2021; anti-inflammatories and antibiotics for secondary bacterial pneumonias).

To be blunt, all public health and political authorities have been trying to quell and eliminate the spread of a relatively harmless common cold virus — largely detected by the highly sensitive PCR — and more recently rapid antigen tests (RAT) — and *not by diagnosis of cold or flu symptoms*. Most positive detections, perhaps >90%, have been in asymptomatic individuals or those who have recovered. All this has contributed to the hysterical response from about March 2020 and led to *many mistakes*, including a false belief that an intra-muscular "jab in the arm" vaccine — of a novel genetically engineered "spike" protein mRNA expression vector preparation — would be a clear saviour of mankind and end the pandemic. There is no evidence it has had any effect on the natural decline of the pandemic (Chapters 16–18). For the Spanish Flu, in 1918–1919, where diagnosis was based on symptoms, the pandemic was essentially over in two years. It is conceivable that the current faulty pandemic control and mitigation public health policies, based on PCR/RAT diagnosis tests, could easily extend the COVID-19 pandemic into a 3rd or 4th year on present observations of public health decisions in many countries and states.

It can still be argued that an inadequately researched program was launched by governments and pharmaceutical companies led in the USA by "Operation Warped

Speed". This was launched on the trusting citizens of the world. The vaccines were not adequately safety tested, without any real testing for protective efficacy, and we now know from many, many government public health authorities e.g. data releases in United Kingdom, Israel, they are both unable to protect individuals from catching COVID-19 (Subramanian and Kumar 2021) and have what would previously have been an unacceptably high adverse event rate (post vaccine injury, early death) which under normal circumstances would lead to them being withdrawn from the market as a "protective or therapeutic medicine".

So the handling of the COVID-19 pandemic has been a massive public health failure. As we discuss further (Chapter 19), as well as adequate safety testing, the oral-nasal route of immune stimulation now needs to be rigorously applied in all future vaccine development for respiratory tract pathogens (the most common causative agents of human pandemics over the past 100 years, since the Spanish Flu of 1918–1919). Current indications in Melbourne, Australia (Minear 2022) is for the "jab in the arm" Covid-19 booster and flu shots to be rolled out for all elderly in geriatric and nursing facilities in the southern winter months (June–Sept) — so, at present, it appears that current vaccine mistakes are likely to be repeated.

Near-Earth early warning surveillance and upper atmosphere sampling will help planning on what type(s) of pathogens are lurking in the stratospheric viral/pathogen dust clouds. As we have discussed in several places in this book satellite robotic platforms could be put in position, including regular sampling and testing of the external surface of the International Space Station (Chapters 2 and 3). These efforts could be complimented by lower-level balloon loft sampling as well as, stratospheric sampling via aircraft collections.

COVID-19 is a common cold pandemic, molecularly tracked to a degree never before seen in history. We have an opportunity to learn from the past 2–3 year experience and to get many things right for the next pandemic.. Many of the causative pathogens in the recent past (100 years) have been cold or flu-like respiratory tract diseases — thus stimulating oro-nasal mucosal secretory IgA immunity coupled to obligatory safety testing is crucial. On first strike with a meteorite-associated respiratory virus the exact identity may take time to develop specific vaccines for safe oro-nasal stimulation. But in the intervening period we have already "on the shelf" defective/attenuated coronaviruses and influenza virus preparations, likely to be safe, that could be used first (Xiao *et al.* 2021, Oh *et al.* 2021). Such locally-applied vaccines of defective related or unrelated viruses will initially stimulate heightened non-specific mucosal Innate Immunity (Netea *et al.* 2020). This could buy time while the specific pandemic variant is being cloned and cultured for specific acquired adaptive vaccine development. So these completely safe "defective" prior variants could be used *in lieu*.

Lock downs, curfews, crowd size limits, contact tracing and social distancing mitigation do not work when the *primary arrival of all epidemic outbreaks* is from the sky or troposphere. Unsuspecting individuals catch such infections from their contaminated environment. That is the key to understanding apparent "super spreader" events viz. ignition of multiple mystery infections at once. So "contagious virulence" will be more apparent than real. However the full extent of person to person (P-to-P) transmission would need to be established as early as possible, with the full knowledge that contaminated environment (fomites) ignites the primary infections.

Masks in theory might provide some protection and disruption if P-to-P aerosol is the primary spread mode. However, masks would have greatest protective effect if worn at in-fall. However, such events cannot usually be predicted in advance in a sudden emergent epidemic. Thus, attention reverts again to the contaminated environment as the primary source reservoir of the pathogens. With masks worn at actual in-fall itself the main danger could well be contaminated fingers by touching the outside of the mask then touching one's nose and mouth.

So, the main public health lesson from COVID-19 is for the proper in advance, therapeutic care and attention to our elderly, particularly in closed geriatric facilities and nursing homes. Active intra-muscular vaccinations in such a group may have marginal utility and could be positively dangerous given the known frail and aberrant systemic immunity in aged individuals.

REFERENCES

Bryant AB, Lawrie TA, Dowswell T, Fordham EJ, Mitchell S, Hill SR, Tham TC (2021) Ivermectin for Prevention and Treatment of COVID-19 Infection: A Systematic Review, Meta-analysis, and Trial Sequential Analysis to Inform Clinical Guidelines. *Amer. J. Therapeutics* **28**, e434–e460.

Fauci AS, Lane HC, Redfield RR (2020) Covid-19 — Navigating the Uncharted. *N. Engl. J. Med.* **382**, 1268–1269.

Kory P, Medurim GU, Varon J, Iglesias J, Marik PE (2021) Review of the Emerging Evidence Demonstrating the Efficacy of Ivermectin in the Prophylaxis and Treatment of COVID-19 *Amer. J. Therapeutics* **28**, e299–e318.

Minear T (2020) Double up for Winter — Elderly could Receive Covid and Flu Jabs. *The Herald Sun* (Melbourne) p. 11 Mon Feb 28 2022.

Netea MG, Giamarellos-Bourboulis EJ, Domınguez-Andre's J, Curtis N, Reinoutvan C, *et al.* (2020) Trained Immunity: A Tool for Reducing Susceptibility to and the Severity of SARS-CoV-2 infection. *Cell* **181**, 969–977.

Subramanian SV, Kumar A (2021) Increases in COVID-19 are Unrelated to Levels of Vaccination across 68 Countries and 2947 Counties in the United States. *Eur. J. Epidemiol.* **36**, 1237–1240.

Xiao Y, Lidsky PV, Shirogane Y, Aviner R, Wu C-T, Li W, *et al.* (2021) A Defective Viral Genome Strategy Elicits Broad Protective Immunity against Respiratory Viruses. *Cell* **184**, 6037–6051.

Oh JE, Song E, Moriyama M, Wong P, Zhang S, Jiang R, *et al.* (2021) Intranasal Priming induces Local Lung-resident B Cell Populations that Secrete Protective Mucosal Antiviral IgA. *Science Immunology* **6**, Issue 66 • DOI:10.1126/sciimmunol.abj5129.

Following the Science for COVID-19: Societal Constraints and Limitations

Dear Editor

We the undersigned wholeheartedly endorse the views expressed in your recent editorial relating to the COVID-19 pandemic (1). There are many examples from the history of medicine that support the assertion that when good science is suppressed patients die. When Ignaz Semmelweis' advocacy of handwashing to prevent deaths from infections in maternity wards was roundly ridiculed, the fatalities continued unabated. For new and unsolved problems in science a blind adherence to orthodoxy could literally prove fatal — the solution of such problems always lying in the morass of heterodoxy. Determining the form which this heterodoxy might take is always the challenge.

The difficulty of "following the science" in the case of the ongoing COVID-19 pandemic is that in many aspects the discussion of the science itself has often been ill-defined and moreover betrays a lack of understanding of all aspects of the problem. The first uncertainty relates to the origin of the virus itself. The hypothesis of a corona virus passing from bats via an intermediate animal to humans is widely accepted though by no means proven nor, as we have argued in detail, scientifically plausible from haplotype analyses of COVID-19 genomes and related isolates (2,3).

In a series of articles, we have developed the unorthodox proposal that the Covid-19 virus, like many other pandemic viruses, may have an extraterrestrial origin and was initially dispersed in the high atmosphere from a disintegrating cometary bolide (3–10). The first major infall of the virus from this primary source in the Hubei province of China would have inevitably led to a massive amplification of the virus in humans, a fraction of which would have been lofted back to the upper atmosphere to be carried in global wind systems across the world. Furthermore, we have shown that this novel hypothesis actually explains much of the evolving science on COVID-19 which we have seen over the past twelve months (5,9,10). Although initially the idea that this virus originated extraterrestially seems outrageous, as Sherlock Holmes might have said: "Once you have eliminated the impossible, then whatever remains, however improbable, must be the truth."

In our model of the pandemic we argue that trillions of virions entered the Earth's upper atmosphere sometime in the latter part of 2019. Virus-laden dust clouds were thereafter able to break through to ground level locations, and spread of the pandemic around the world subsequently occurred through a combination of such infall, viruses transported in global wind systems, and eventually by person-to-person spread. This

https://www.bmj.com/content/371/bmj.m4425/rr-34

Rapid Response letter in the *British Medical Journal* to the Editorial by Kamran Abbasi (Executive Editor)

Covid-19: politicisation, "corruption," and suppression of science *BMJ* 2020; 371

DOI: https://doi.org/10.1136/bmj.m4425 (Published 13 November 2020) Cite this as: BMJ 2020;371:m4425

model accounts for a swathe of data that is otherwise difficult to explain — for example the sudden emergence of new foci of infection as recently happened in Sri Lanka where a cluster of thousand or more cases arose suddenly with no hard evidence of any identifiable "superspreader" (9,10). Similar mysterious outbreaks have occurred elsewhere around the world including on ships at sea — many of these were instances where entire cohorts of passengers and crew were repeatedly tested negative for COVID-19 prior to embarkation.

Other aspects of the current pandemic that are poorly understood include a lack of knowledge about the precise modes of person to person transmission. This in turn leads to uncertainties about the best strategies to be deployed for minimising transmission. There is also a need, in our view, to respond urgently to well-attested facts relating to differential morbidities in various cohorts of the population, for example the older age groups with comorbidities. We need more information on the nature of the protective immune response against COVID-19 and how this might vary in different cohorts.

Finally, we note that recent data showing a correlation of COVID-19 case rates with high levels of local atmospheric particulate pollution is worthy of adding to the "science" that the authorities might choose to follow. Micron-sized pollutant dust particles in the atmosphere could not only mop up infalling virions from the troposphere, but also accrete virions that are exhaled by victims, and such dust particles can be shown to take considerable lengths of time — many hours — to settle to ground level (11,12). A high level of smog and pollution is therefore to be regarded as a significant additional risk factor for COVID-19 in locations where the infections prevail-the high rates in the Lombardy district of Italy, and in heavily industrialized urban centres around the world are consistent with this notion. In view of the links to atmospheric pollution new ways of protection of the more vulnerable cohorts may need to be considered.

Sincerely

N.C. Wickramasinghe, MA, PhD, ScD, FRSA, FRAS, University of Buckingham, UK; National Institute of Fundamental Studies, Sri Lanka; Centre for Astrobiology, University of Ruhuna, Matara, Sri Lanka

R.M. Gorczynski, MD, PhD, Professor Emeritus, Depts Surgery & Immunology, University of Toronto, ON, Canada

Anthony Perera, MBChB, FRCS, Consultant Orthopaedic Surgeon, University Hospital of Wales, Cardiff

A. Nimalasuriya, MBBS, MD, Consultant Physician, Kaiser Permanente Riverside Medical, 10800 Magnolia Ave # 1, Riverside, CA 92505, USA

Patrick Carnegie, PhD, School of Biological Sciences and Biotechnology, Murdoch University, WA, Australia

Milton Wainwright, PhD, Institute for the Study of Panspermia and Astroeconomics, Gifu, Japan; Centre for Astrobiology, University of Ruhuna, Matara, Sri Lanka

Predrag Slijepcevic, PhD, Department of Life Sciences, College of Health, Medicine and Life Sciences, Brunel University, London, UK

Max K. Wallis, MA, PhD, FRAS, Institute for the Study of Panspermia and Astroeconomics, Gifu, Japan

Stephen G. Coulson, BSc, PhD, FRAS, Institute for the Study of Panspermia and Astroeconomics, Gifu, Japan

Daryl H. Wallis, BSc, PhD, FRAS, Institute for the Study of Panspermia and Astroeconomics, Gifu, Japan

Gensuke Tokoro, Director, Institute for the Study of Panspermia and Astroeconomics, Gifu, Japan Centre for Astrobiology, University of Ruhuna, Matara, Sri Lanka

Robert Temple, Director, History of Chinese Science and Culture Foundation, Conway Hall, London UK

Herbert Rebhan, CYO'Connor ERADE Village Foundation, 24 Genomics Rise, Piara Waters, 6112

Edward J. Steele, PhD, CYO'Connor ERADE Village Foundation, 24 Genomics Rise, Piara Waters, 6112; Melville Analytics Pty Ltd, Melbourne, Vic, Australia

REFERENCES

https://www.bmj.com/content/371/bmj.m4425?utm_source=etoc&utm_medium=ema...

Steele EJ, Lindley RA (2020) Analysis of APOBEC and ADAR Deaminase-driven Riboswitch Haplotypes in COVID-19 RNA Strain Variants and the Implications for Vaccine Design. Research Reports. doi: 10.9777/rr.2020.10001

Steele EJ, Gorczynski RM, Rebhan H, Carnegie P, Temple R, Tokoro G, *et al.* (2020) Implications of Haplotype Switching for the Origin and Global Spread of COVID-19. *Virol. Curr. Res.* Volume 4:2, 2020. DOI: 10.37421/Virol Curr Res.2020.4.115

Steele EJ, Gorczynski RM, Lindley RA, Tokoro G, *et al.* (2020) Origin of New Emergent Coronavirus and Candida Fungal Diseases — Terrestrial or Cosmic? — *Adv. Genetics* **106**, 75–100.

Hoyle F, Wickramasinghe NC (1979) Diseases from Space (J.M. Dent & Son Lond) (see also revised edition published by World Scientific Publishing Co.); Hoyle F, Wickramasinghe NC (1990) Influenza — Evidence Against Contagion. *Journal of the Royal Society of Medicine* **83**, 258–261.

Wickramasinghe C, Wainwright M, Narlikar JV (2003) SARS — A Clue to its Origins. *The Lancet* **361**, 1832.

Steele EJ, Al-Mufti S, Augustyn KK, Chandrajith R, Coghlan JP, Coulson SG, Ghosh S, Gillman M, *et al.* (2018) "Cause of Cambrian Explosion: Terrestrial or Cosmic?" *Prog. Biophys. Mol. Biol.* **136**, 3–23.

Steele EJ, Gorczynski RM, Lindley RA, Liu Y, Temple R, Tokoro G, Wickramasinghe DT, Wickramasinghe NC (2019) "Lamarck and Panspermia — On the Efficient Spread of Living Systems Throughout the Cosmos". *Prog. Biophys. Mol. Biol.* **149**, 10–32.

Wickramasinghe NC, Wallis MK, Coulson SJ, *et al.* (2020) Intercontinental Spread of COVID-19 on Global Wind Systems. *Virol. Curr. Res.* (4:2). Volume 4:1,2020.
DOI: 10.37421/Virol Curr Res.2020.4.113

Wickramasinghe NC, Steele EJ, Nimalasuriya A, *et al.* (2020) Seasonality of Respiratory Viruses Including SARS-CoV-2 Virol Curr Res Volume 4:2, 2020 DOI: 10.37421/VCRH.2020.4.117

Coccia, M (2020) Factors Determining the Diffusion of COVID-19 and Suggested Strategy to Prevent Future Accelerated Viral Infectivity Similar to COVID. *Sci. Total Environ.* **729**, 138474. https://doi.org/10.1016/j.scitotenv.2020.138474

Zhu Y, Xie J, Huang F, Cao L (2020) Association Between Short-term Exposure to Air Pollution and COVID-19 Infection: Evidence from China. *Sci. Total Environ.* **727**, 138704. DOI: 10.1016/j.scitotenv.2020.138704

Competing interests: No competing interests

Printed in the United States
by Baker & Taylor Publisher Services